IITK Directions

Volume 6

IITK Directions is an institutional series of the Indian Institute of Technology Kanpur. IITK Directions aims at presenting original contributions and reviews of important and cutting-edge topics by the faculty members and other stakeholders of IIT Kanpur in a consolidated manner. It is a platform that reflects upon the ongoing research and development activities, major achievements, and evolving trends. Each volume in the series focuses on a particular area of science and technology with chapters written by the faculty members, students and research staff. Each chapter is written in a journalistic tone for the peer group – readability and accessibility being important parameters. The volumes contain a survey of the subject as a whole and the extent of contributions recorded by the Institute faculty and students who participate so extensively in research.
The volumes in this series will be useful to researchers, practitioners, students, industry leaders, government officials and policy makers. Above all, the series serves as platform to publish the most cutting edge research summaries and evaluate the applications and impact of the research work undertaken at IIT Kanpur.

More information about this series at https://link.springer.com/bookseries/15345

Krishanu Biswas • Sri Sivakumar •
Nilesh Gurao
Editors

Electron Microscopy in Science and Engineering

Springer

Editors
Krishanu Biswas
Department of Materials Science and Engineering
Indian Institute of Technology Kanpur
Kanpur, India

Sri Sivakumar
Department of Chemical Engineering
Indian Institute of Technology Kanpur
Kanpur, India

Nilesh Gurao
Department of Materials Science and Engineering
Indian Institute of Technology Kanpur
Kanpur, India

ISSN 2509-6591 ISSN 2509-6605 (electronic)
IITK Directions
ISBN 978-981-16-5100-7 ISBN 978-981-16-5101-4 (eBook)
https://doi.org/10.1007/978-981-16-5101-4

This Springer imprint is published by the registered company Springer Nature Singapore Pte Ltd.
The registered company address is: 152 Beach Road, #21-01/04 Gateway East, Singapore 189721, Singapore

Series Editor's Preface

Several electron microscopes installed across various engineering and science departments at IIT Kanpur, India, have been used extensively to solve various problems catering to the need of both internal and external users. The current issue of Directions on Electron Microscopy (EM) is focused on the extensive use of scanning and transmission electron microscopy in multiple research frontiers including small-scale deformation studies, in situ testing, micro-composition analysis, advanced imaging, study of phase transformation behavior, morphological characterization of cells and viruses, electron-back-scatter diffraction, etc., that are currently being investigated at IIT Kanpur. The contents also provide a detailed and comprehensive view of the basic features and advanced capabilities of EM facilities to the scientific community.

I am thankful to the authors for their active participation in contributing the articles and to the editors for extensive review in raising the quality of the publication.

Based on the earlier experience, we expect this issue too to reach a wider community through the Springer platform.

A. R. Harish
Dean, Research and Development
Indian Institute of Technology Kanpur
Kanpur, India

Preface

Electron microscopy (EM) has become integral part of research and development of almost all the fields of science and engineering. 'Seeing is believing' is used as a common slogan for any experimental observation to justify the claims made, and hence, this is a common practice to make electron microscopes as 'part-and-parcel' of research activities. Electron microscopes vary a lot depending on the need and the observations we would like to make. The most common one is scanning electron microscope (SEM), whereas the sophisticated transmission electron microscope (TEM) and reflection electron microscope (REM) belong to a niche class of characterization tools. The first one uses a technique of raster scanning of high-energy electron beams to produce gamut of signals, utilized for imaging (standard and orientation imaging) and spectroscopy. On the other hand, TEM is an original type of microscope, allowing us to form images due to direct scattering of electron by means of passing through a high-voltage electron beam. Both imaging and spectroscopic analyses can routinely be performed in TEM with high resolution (sub nm level) and extremely high precision. The last type of EM, the REM, in general, uses the technique of detection of elastically scattered electron beam, reflected in any specimen. The commonly used methods involve reflection high-energy electron diffraction (RHEED) and reflection high-energy loss spectroscopy (RHELS), providing a host of information from the specimen under investigation.

In the last ten years, a substantial number of electron microscopy (EM) facilities have been set up in IIT Kanpur. A large number of scanning electron microscopes (SEMs) have been installed and utilized by researchers across various engineering (BSBE, CHE, CE, EE, ME, MSE) and science (CHM, ES, PHY) departments. Some of these microscopes are managed by individual departments, and some are housed in various central facilities (ACMS, AIC, Ion Beam Facility (IBF), Nanoscience and Soft Nanotechnology (Nano Center). The SEM facilities attached to the individual department are mainly utilized by the researchers from the respective departments. ACMS, IBF, Nano Center, being one of the major centers, housing large number of characterization facilities catering to the need of a large number of researchers from various departments, centers, and interdepartmental programs. In 2015, a new center, known as Advanced Imaging Center (AIC), has been established to house state-of-the-art facilities for high-resolution transmission electron microscopes. The TITAN® microscope has widely been utilized by institute communities for various research projects. This facility is capable of atomic resolution imaging, fast compositional analyses, and Lorenz microscopy for magnetic samples. In addition, there is a TEM (120 kV) for high-contrast cryomicroscopy with low beam dosage. Similarly, ACMS has augmented EM facilities recently with the addition of new SEMs and remote access to National Facility for Atom Probe Tomography (NFAPT) at IIT Madras. The ion beam facility has the dual-beam focused ion beam facility for wider use in the institute. IIT Kanpur is also going to establish a national facility of cryo-electron microscopy to cater to the need of burgeoning need of the researchers working at the interface of biological and other associated applied fields.

Therefore, these facilities have extensively been utilized by the large number of researchers, actively involving in the institute as well as other institutes from the region. It can be anticipated that the usage of EM facilities will see an exponential rise due to the increase of the research scholars and the need to perform high-quality research. Hence, it is pertinent to

provide a snapshot of these facilities with research performed utilizing these facilities, specifications, and capabilities of EM facilities available in various departments and central facilities. The special issue of direction will provide a detailed and comprehensive view of the basic features and advanced capabilities of the existing EM facilities to the scientific community within the institute as well as outside users. The present issue is intended to provide both 'breadth' and 'depth' of various EM facilities available in the institute.

We would like to thank all the contributing authors for their valuable contribution, patience, and meticulous corrections, the office of Dean (Research & Development), present (Prof. H. R. Harish), immediate past Dean (Prof. S. Ganesh) for providing all logistics and approval for the issue. It is also important to thank the Springer team, whose friendly reminders kept us engaged in the job of completion. We shall feel happy and elated if the community finds the content of the issue useful and worthy.

Kanpur, India

Krishanu Biswas
Sri Sivakumar
Nilesh Gurao

Contents

About the Editors

Dr. Krishanu Biswas Ranjit Singh Chair Professor at Department of Material Science and Engineering, Indian Institute of Technology (IIT) Kanpur has made significant contribution towards understanding of several important scientific and technological aspects of metallurgy and materials engineering. He obtained his Ph.D. from Indian Institute of Science (IISc) and B. Tech. from National Institute of Technology (NIT) Durgapur, India. His research interests ranges from complex concentrated alloys, high entropy materials, electron microscopy, novel processing of ceramic composites, development of alloy catalysis for energy and environment. He has received a number of awards, fellowships and professional reorganization. He has published over 190 papers in international repute peer reviewed journals, three patents, ten book chapters, two books and delivered 50 invited talks in different national and international conferences. He has completed several projects from Indian Space Research Organization (ISRO) and Indian National Science Academy (INSA) to bigger projects from Department of Science and Technology (DST), Department of Biotechnology (DBT), Board of Research on Nuclear Sciences (BRNS). He is a member of Indian National Young Academy of Sciences (INYAS) and Global Young Academy (GYA). He is also recipient of Young Faculty fellowship from IIT Kanpur.

Dr. Sri Sivakumar is currently working as professor in Department of Chemical Engineering, Indian Institute of Technology (IIT) Kanpur. He also serves as Associate Faculty in Materials Science Programme and Co-ordinator of Centre for Nanoscience and Advanced Imaging Centre. He obtained his B.Sc. (Tech) and M.Sc. (Tech) degree from University Institute of Chemical Technology (ICT), Mumbai in 1997 and 2001 respectively. He obtained his Ph.D. degree from University of Victoria in 2006. Dr. Sivakumar carried out his post-doctoral research at the University of Melbourne. Dr. Sivakumar's research focuses on development of functional nanomaterials for biological and environmental/catalytic applications. He has authored over 100 publications, four book chapters, 11 patents and edited one book. He has obtained thirteen grants worth of Rs. 13 crores from government agencies as well as from industry (Chevron, HPCL, Aarti Industries, and TCS). Furthermore, he has graduated 17 Ph.D. students and is currently supervising ten Ph.D. students. Professor Sivakumar works on synthesis of functional nanomaterials for catalysis and biomedical applications. His work on catalysis includes both chemical and electro catalysis.

Dr. Nilesh Gurao is currently an Associate Professor at the Department of Materials Science and Engineering at Indian Institute of Technology (IIT) Kanpur. He obtained his Ph.D. in Materials Engineering from Indian Institute of Science (IISc), Bengaluru, India in 2010 and Bachelors in Technology from Visvesvaraya National Institute of Technology, India in 2005 prior to attending the University of Saskatchewan, Saskatoon, Canada for a postdoctotoral position. He has established the Microstructure-Texture-Stress Laboratory at IIT Kanpur and has graduated five Ph.D. and 12 master's students till date. The research work from the group has resulted in multiple projects with different government and private funding agencies and high quality journal publications. Dr. Gurao is a recipient of the INSA Young Scientist award

from the Indian National Science Academy and the Young Metallurgist of the Year award from Ministry of Steel, Government of India. His current research interests include mechanical behavior of materials, crystallographic texture, crystal plasticity simulations and diffraction studies with special emphasis on in situ diffraction experiments across real and reciprocal space.

Small-Scale Deformation Experiments Inside an SEM

Sumit Basu

1 Introduction

The first prototype of the scanning electron microscope (SEM) was built in 1937 by Manfred von Ardenne in Germany. Commercialization of the SEM by the Cambridge Scientific Instrument Company began in 1965. Reports of in-situ deformation and fracture experiments on small-scale samples conducted inside the vacuum chamber of started appearing soon after, in mid-70s and 80s (Ujiiye et al. 1971; Dingley 1973; Stephens and Hoeppner 1988; Roberts and Lehtinen 1976; Nakagawa et al. 1980).

In-situ deformation experiments are now routinely performed, and all modern microscopes provide ports on the vacuum chamber that can be used to interface deformation stages with control instrumentation outside (see, Fig. 1). Deformation stages (which basically are miniature universal testing machines or UTMs), often with a facility to heat the sample during deformation, are also available. These miniature UTMs are customized to 'dovetail' snugly into the movable stage of microscopes of all major makes. A compression stage assembled from off-the-shelf components and instrumented at IIT Kanpur is shown in Fig. 2.

Small-scale deformation experiments offer a few very unique opportunities to the materials scientist. Micro-deformation mechanisms that operate during deformation and fracture of materials can often be clearly visualized on the surface of small samples. In-situ visualization of micro-mechanical events leading to plastic deformation and failure has been explored most widely for steel (Alaie et al. 2015; gang Liu et al. 2019; Prochazka et al. 2017; Li et al. 2019; Yang et al. 2015), titanium (Barkia et al. 2015; Jun et al. 2016; Jieping et al. 1989; Bao et al. 2010), and its alloys (Niwa and Ito 1987; Zhang et al. 2018; Li et al. 2014; Zhang et al. 2019), though other metals like aluminum alloys (Motsi et al. 2014), e.g., nickel (Perusin et al. 2004) and chromium (Fritz et al. 2017) have been studied as well. Often, imaging of the micro-deformation process is accompanied by simultaneous electron backscatter diffraction (EBSD)-based crystallographic characterization (Wu et al. 2016; Li et al. 2008; min Wang et al. 2005; Bruck et al. 1989).

For non-metals too, several innovative experiments have been reported. Investigation of brittle fracture in thermal barrier coatings (Wu et al. 2008; Arai et al. 2010), cell wall plasticity in open cell forms (Zhou et al. 2004), cell deformation in wood (Adusumalli et al. 2010), and breakage mechanisms in micron-sized silica, alumina, and titania particles (Romeis et al. 2015; Sarobol et al. 2016; Herre et al. 2017) are examples where insights into the micro-deformation processes leading to fracture could not have been obtained without resorting to small-scale in-situ experiments. A slideshow accompanying this article showcases some in-situ deformation experiments that have been conducted at IIT Kanpur.

Is it possible to perform more quantitative experiments in-situ? For instance, can we accurately determine the uniaxial stress–strain response or the fracture toughness of a micron-sized sample while observing the micro-mechanisms driving its deformation? Such experiments are especially useful when we need to quantify structure property relationships in hazaradous materials like irradiated steel (Bruck et al. 1989), which can be handled only in very small quantities.

Electronic Supplementary Material
The online version of this chapter (https://doi.org/10.1007/978-981-16-5101-4_1) contains supplementary material, which is available to authorized users.

S. Basu (✉)
Department of Mechanical Engineering, Indian Institute of Technology Kanpur, Kanpur, Uttar Pradesh 208016, India
e-mail: sbasu@iitk.ac.in

K. Biswas et al. (eds.), *Electron Microscopy in Science and Engineering*, IITK Directions 6,
https://doi.org/10.1007/978-981-16-5101-4_1

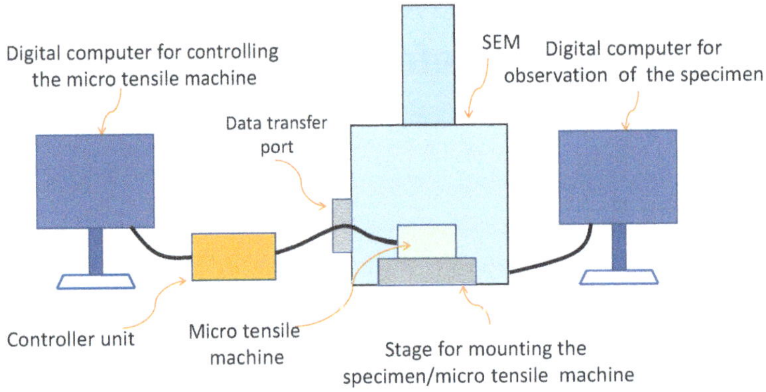

Fig. 1 Schematic of an in-situ micro-deformation set up. The deformation stage is placed inside the vacuum chamber of the SEM. It communicates with the control hardware placed outside through connectors on a port on the chamber

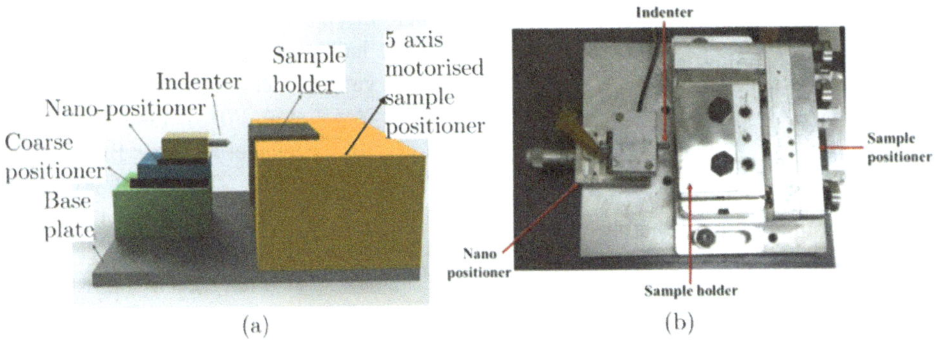

Fig. 2 Block diagram of a micro-compression device assembled at IIT Kanpur is shown in (**a**). Top view of the actual device is shown in (**b**). This device is designed to fit into the stage of a Zeiss Sigma VM FESEM

2 In-Situ Digital Image Correlation

2.1 A Brief Introduction to DIC

A miniature stage like the one shown in Fig. 2 is equipped with a load cell and a linear actuator, both of which communicate with softwares outside the vacuum chamber (see Fig. 1). The load applied to the specimen is directly obtained from the load cell. However, the position of the actuator gives the displacement imparted to the gripped end of the specimen. This can be converted into an average strain over the entire specimen. In case of non-homogeneous deformation, the average strain is not a reliable measure. If accurate and localized strain measurement is required (as would be the case when deformation is large and localized, e.g., at shear bands), more sophisticated techniques will be required. How can we measure the strain accurately over a surface while it is being simultaneously deformed and exposed to an electron beam inside the vacuum chamber? As far as conducting quantitative in-situ experiments is concerned, this is a difficult hurdle.

Fortunately, in recent years, an elegant solution has emerged in the form of two-dimensional digital image correlation (DIC), which is a full-field technique for measuring displacements and strains over a specified domain on the surface of the sample (Chu et al. 1985; Bruck et al. 1989; Sutton et al. 2007, 2009). A brief description of the method is given here. Several detailed reviews of the theoretical underpinnings and implementation of the method are available (Sutton et al. 2009; Pan et al. 2009; Hild and Roux 2006).

First, a random speckle pattern is generated all over a domain on the flat surface of the deforming body (lying, say, on the $x-y$ plane), over which displacements $u(x, y)$, $v(x, y)$ are to be determined. In two-dimensional DIC, it is assumed that out of plane displacements are absent. The speckle pattern can be generated by spraying black and white paint on the surface. Alternatively, the natural texture of the surface can be used. In any case, the domain over which displacements and its gradients are measured must have a random gray-scale intensity distribution. For ex-situ DIC, the surface of the specimen is imaged with a digital camera while it is deforming. An image of the deformed domain is compared with the initial reference domain to find the displacement and strain fields.

If a point (x, y) in the reference image maps to a point (x^*, y^*) in the deformed, it is assumed that the intensity $f(x, y)$ in the reference image is equal to $f^*(x^*, y^*)$ in the

deformed. Note that both f and f^* are functions that take only integer values between 0 and 255, corresponding to the gray-scale levels.

Consider the domain shown on the left of Fig. 3 which deforms as shown on the right. A sub-domain of $m \times n$ pixels shown by the red rectangle in the left figure deforms to the red quadrilateral in the right one. Provided the sub-domain is small, the displacement of an arbitrary point Q (to Q') inside it can be related to that of its center P (to P'). If the coordinates of P are (x_0, y_0) and that of Q are $(x_0 + \Delta x, y_0 + \Delta y)$, the deformed position of Q' can be written as

$$x_{Q'} = x_Q + u_0 + \partial u \partial x|_P \Delta x + \partial u \partial y|_P \Delta y,$$
$$y_{Q'} = y_Q + v_0 + \partial v \partial x|_P \Delta x + \partial v \partial y|_P \Delta y.$$

Here, (u_0, v_0) are displacements of the center of the sub-domain and $x_Q = x_0 + \Delta x, y_Q = y_0 + \Delta y$.

In the above, the quantities $u_0, v_0, \partial u \partial x, \partial u \partial y, \partial v \partial x, \partial v \partial y$ are unknown for a given sub-domain. They are obtained using the assumption that, for the best choice of these six quantities, the correlation between the intensities of the $m \times n$ pixels in the red rectangle and the red quadrilateral will be the highest among all possible red quadrilaterals that can be placed in the image of the deformed domain. In other words, a measure of the correlation

$$C = \sum_{m \times n} [f(x, y) - f^*(x^*, y^*)] \sum_{m \times n} f^2(x, y), \tag{1}$$

attains a maximum when we hit upon the correct set of the six quantities. The search is carried out in a systematic manner using standard algorithms that are described in, e.g., Bruck et al. (1989).

2.2 Issues Associated with In-Situ DIC

The above procedure works well for macroscopic samples ex-situ. For experiments conducted inside the vacuum chamber of an SEM, several additional issues need to be addressed. Many of these are related to the manner in which an image is produced in the SEM. A labeled schematic showing the major components of a typical field emission scanning electron microscope (FESEM) is presented in Fig. 4a.

The electron beam emerging from the field emitter follows the central axis and passes sequentially through micron-sized apertures and is focused by the electro-magnetic fields of the lens system. Finally, the scan coils that are part of the objective lens displace the beam through computer control so that it is focused to a sequence of points on the area of interest (see, Fig. 4b). The gray-scale value of a pixel on each digital image is a measure of the interaction of the electron beam with a corresponding point on the sample as recorded by a electron detector (e.g., an Everhart–Thornley detector for secondary electrons emanated from the surface on interaction with the incoming beam). The image produced by the raster scanning action of the beam is different from the 'true image' produced in a light microscope.

In an SEM micrograph, all pixels are not imaged at the same time. This is unlike an 'true image' taken under normal light. Assume that the scanning of the area on the sample involves W locations along a line, repeated for H lines (see, Fig. 4b). It is mapped onto a gray-scale image, where $\zeta : (\boldsymbol{m}, \boldsymbol{n})$ denotes a pixel position. In a stack of N images taken in succession, if the time at which scanning for image

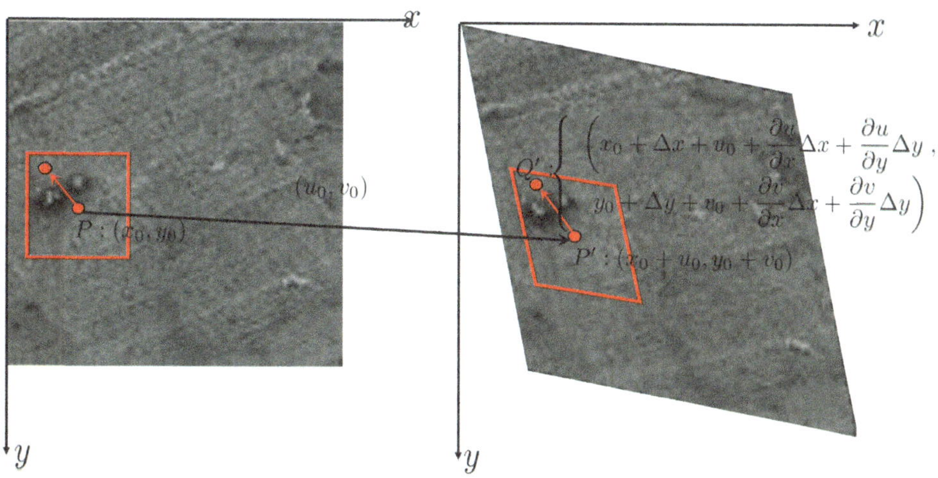

Fig. 3 The complete initial domain over which displacement field is computed by DIC is shown in the left. This domain deforms in the manner shown on the right. The point $P : (x_0, y_0)$ lies at the center of the red rectangular sub-domain, which deforms to the red quadrilateral. Deformed positions of neighboring points P and Q in the initial sub-domain are denoted by P' and Q'. The displacement components of point P are given by $u_0(x, y)$ and $v_0(x, y)$

i was started is t_i, the time at which the pixel at ζ is scanned, will be given by:

$$t(\zeta) = t_i + (m - 1)t_l + (n - 1)t_d, \quad (2)$$

where t_d is the time spent by the beam on each location (marked by a solid circle in Fig. 4b) on the sample, t_d is the time required to reposition the beam from the end of a line to the beginning of the next. The time required to scan a line $t_l = Wt_d + t_p$.

The major artifacts in an SEM image and their underlying reasons are well established (Jin and Li 2015; Snella 2010; Kammers and Daly 2013; Maraghechi et al. 2018, 2019). These can be divided into time independent and dependent ones.

The most important time-independent artifact is spatial distortion. As explained in Maraghechi et al. (2018), spatial distortion is probably caused by the slight non-uniformity of the electromagnetic field created by the objective lens. Images with lower magnification exhibit higher spatial distortion because the beam in these cases, needs to deviate significantly from the central axis. In doing so, it is affected by the non-uniform fields that exist near the outer periphery of the objective lens (Kammers and Daly 2013).

Drift distortions on the other hand are time-dependent artifacts that are present at all magnifications. These distortions occur due to relative motion between the beam and the surface of the specimen. Among other reasons, they are caused by interaction of the beam with a sample surface that has acquired charges or is undergoing thermal deformation. The extent of drift distortion can change nonlinearly with time and its temporal variation is often dependent on the conditions in which the test is performed.

An example of drift distortion is shown in Fig. 5. Exactly the same region in a stationary sample is scanned at two different points of time. The results are shown in Fig. 5a, b. The rectangular box in Fig. 5a, b is centered at the same pixel location. A close look at the feature inside the box shows that it has shifted a bit in the later image. The extent of the shift can be quantified by performing a DIC using the first image as the reference and the second as the deformed (see, Fig. 6a, b). This reveals that the second image has shifted due to drift by $\sim 15 - 20$ pixels in both the x and y directions.

Some of the artifacts can be reduced by adjusting the SEM parameters. Faster scanning (to reduce the difference between t_i and $t(\zeta)$), higher beam voltage leading to smaller spot sizes, and software-based averaging techniques may help in alleviating some of the distortions. However, it should be noted that many of these adjustments add noise to the SEM image. In fact, filtering noise from the images obtained is an essential first step in applying DIC to them. Correlations tend to be erratic if this is not done properly.

Lastly, the issue of creating a proper speckle pattern on a sample has to be kept in mind while performing in-situ deformation experiments that rely on DIC. The natural texture was used in all cases reported here. But this may not be always possible. We have attempted to create nanospeckle patterns by 'sprinkling' nanoparticles on the surface of interest. Fluorescent nanoparticles have been used to map nanoscale displacement fields around silica micro-particles (embedded in an elastomer matrix deformed in tension) through DIC (Berfield et al. 2006).

3 Toward Effective Distortion Correction Techniques

Methods for correcting for both drift and spatial distortions have been proposed by Sutton et al. (2007, 2009). More recently, a unified framework for digital correlation incorporating corrections for distortions has been proposed (Maraghechi et al. 2018). We have implemented the methods due to Sutton et al. (2007, 2009) where images need to be post-processed before regular DIC techniques are applied. Post-processing includes initial de-noising and correcting for spatial and drift distortions.

The effects of all the artifacts are described through a set of virtual examples. In Fig. 7a, a 600×500 pixel-sized virtual sample with an equilateral triangular cut-out at the center is prepared using MATLAB. Random noise is added to the non-white pixels to incorporate an essential feature of a real SEM micrograph. Imagine that we are scanning a 319×287 pixel-sized sub-domain (i.e., $H = 287$ and $W = 319$) around the triangular cut-out in this sample. The total scanning time is $T = H(Wt_d + t_p)$

Imagine that the sample deforms in simple shear at a slow rate $\dot{\gamma}$, such that $1/\dot{\gamma} \gg T$. In this case, the equilateral triangle distorts marginally during the scan as shown in Fig. 7b. However, if $1/\dot{\gamma} \simeq T$, the distortion becomes significant as shown in Fig. 7c. This distortion is simply due to the fact that all pixels in the sub-domain are not scanned simultaneously. Spatial distortion, added to this, causes significantly blurring of the edges of the triangle (see, Fig. 7d). Finally, we have added a fictitious downward displacement due to drift distortion that is simply a linear function of time (and, unrealistically, not a function of position). This causes further distortion of the triangular feature. Performing correlation between Fig. 7e and the corresponding sub-domain of (a) will not reveal that the underlying mechanical deformation being imparted is just a simple shear.

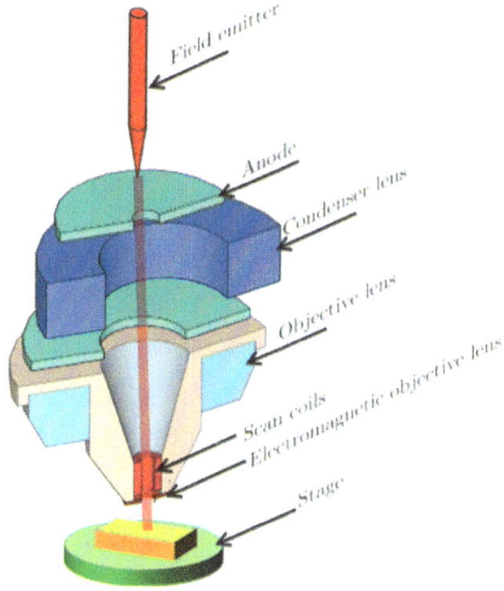

(a)

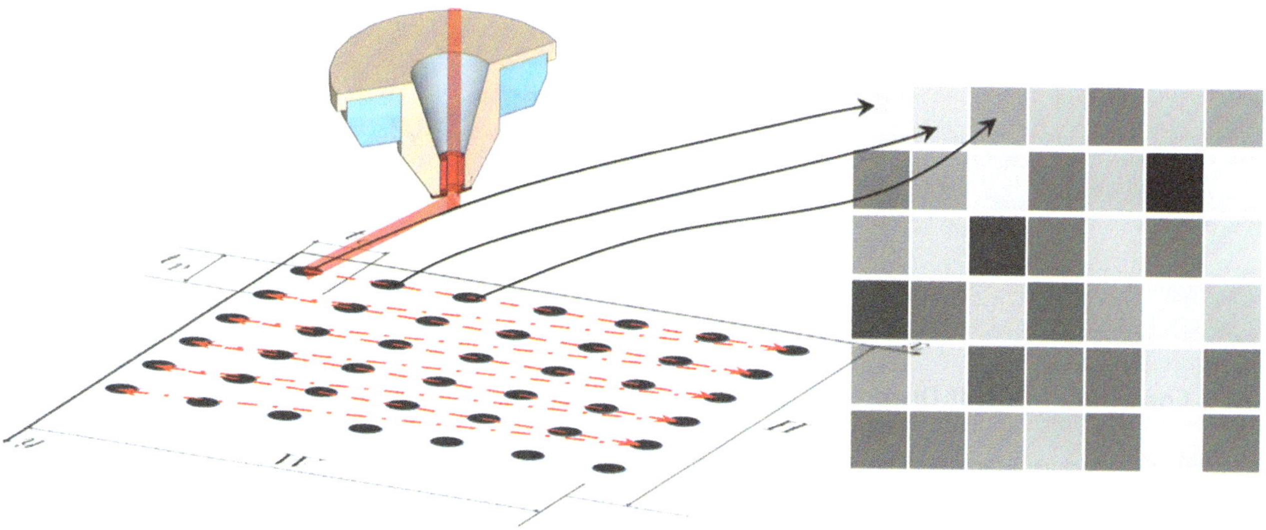

(b)

Fig. 4 Major components in the beam column of a FESEM are shown in (**a**). The process by which a digital image is produced from a raster scan of the sample surface with the electron beam is shown in (**b**)

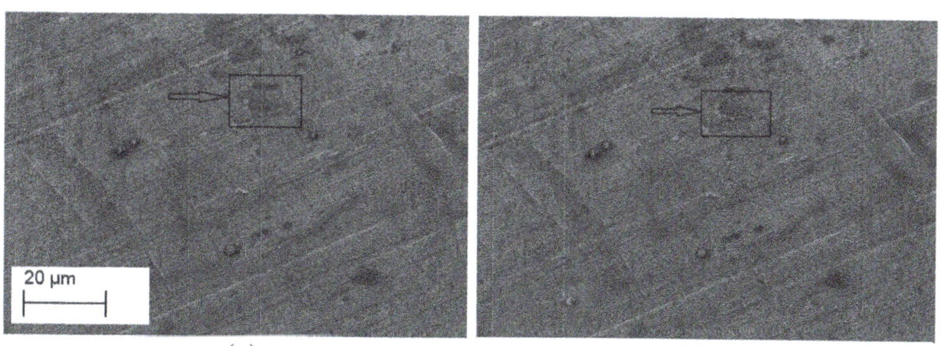

(a) (b)

Fig. 5 FESEM images of exactly the same region in a sample taken a few seconds apart. The black rectangle is used to mark the same sub-region in both the images. Drift of the feature inside the rectangle has caused it to shift slightly. The natural texture in the images is used to compute the full-field displacements over the region. The u component is shown in (**c**) while V is in (**d**)

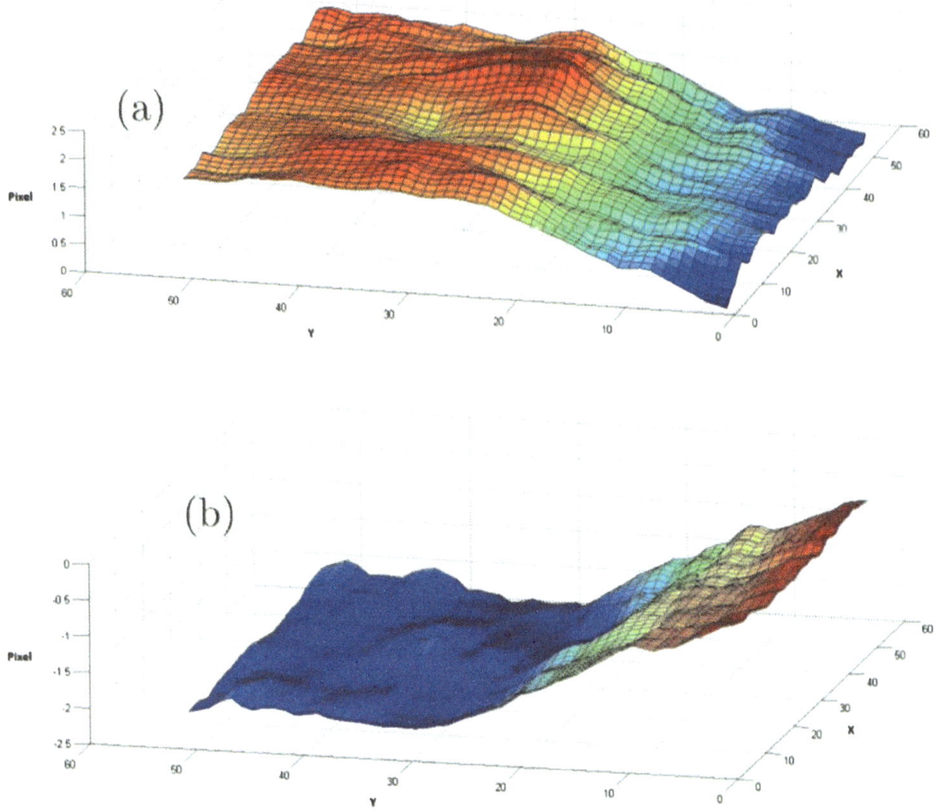

Fig. 6 Natural texture in the images in Fig. 5 are used to compute the displacements over the entire region. The u component over this region is shown in (**a**) and the v in (**d**). The x and y axes are divided into 50 equally spaced points each

3.1 Correcting for Drift Distortion

Consider Fig. 8, where the deformation event of Fig. 3 is shown again. A point P at $\boldsymbol{X}$ in the reference image suffers a deformation to map onto a point Q at $\zeta = \boldsymbol{X} + \boldsymbol{u}$ in the deformed. However, apart from the mechanical deformation, it suffers a further drift displacement $\boldsymbol{d}$, which is a function of the time $t(\zeta)$ at which the location ζ is scanned. The challenge is to recover the actual location ζ, reached by deformation, from $\boldsymbol{x} = \boldsymbol{X} + \boldsymbol{u} + \boldsymbol{d}(\boldsymbol{t}(\zeta))$. To achieve this, some information about the variation of $\boldsymbol{d}$ at the location ζ with time is required.

To acquire information on $\boldsymbol{d}(\boldsymbol{t}(\zeta))$, a calibration procedure needs to be performed (Sutton et al. 2007) just before conducting the actual deformation experiments. The idea is illustrated in Fig. 9. A total of nine image pairs are taken. A pair i (where $i = 1, 3, 5 \ldots 9$) is captured in quick succession without moving the sample. In between pairs, a purely x or purely y translation is imparted. The total translation in either direction is approximately about 25 % of the total field of view.

Between the image pairs i and $i + 1$ ($i = 1, 3, 5 \ldots 9$), only drift distortion exists. Suppose that a point $\boldsymbol{x}_i$ in image i maps to a point $\boldsymbol{x}_{i+1}$ in image $i + 1$. If we perform a DIC between images i and $i + 1$, we will obtain the displacement at $\boldsymbol{x}$ as

$$\boldsymbol{u}(\boldsymbol{x}) = \boldsymbol{x}_{i+1}(\boldsymbol{t}(\boldsymbol{x}_{i+1})) - \boldsymbol{x}_i(\boldsymbol{t}(\boldsymbol{x}_i)), \tag{3}$$

where $t(\boldsymbol{x}_{i+1})$ and $t(\boldsymbol{x}_i)$ are the times at which the points are scanned.

Now, for both images i and $i + 1$, the position in the calibration stage is the same, ζ_i. Thus $\boldsymbol{x}_i = \zeta_i + \boldsymbol{d}(\boldsymbol{x})(\boldsymbol{t}(\boldsymbol{x}_i))$ and $\boldsymbol{x}_{i+1} = \zeta_i + \boldsymbol{d}(\boldsymbol{x})(\boldsymbol{t}(\boldsymbol{x}_{i+1}))$. Since the sample is stationary, and no spatial distortion is present $\boldsymbol{u}(\boldsymbol{x})$ computed through DIC equals the change in drift $\Delta\boldsymbol{d}(\boldsymbol{x}_i) = \boldsymbol{d}(\boldsymbol{x})(\boldsymbol{t}(\boldsymbol{x}_{i+1})) - \boldsymbol{d}(\boldsymbol{x})(\boldsymbol{t}(\boldsymbol{x}_i))$ at $\boldsymbol{x}_i$ between images i and $i + 1$. The drift velocity at $\boldsymbol{x}_i$ can then be calculated as

$$\boldsymbol{v}(\boldsymbol{x}_i) \simeq \frac{\Delta\boldsymbol{d}(\boldsymbol{x}_i)}{\boldsymbol{t}(\boldsymbol{x}_{i+1}) - \boldsymbol{t}(\boldsymbol{x}_i)}. \tag{4}$$

This is taken to be the drift velocity at time $\boldsymbol{t}(\boldsymbol{x}_{i+1}) + \boldsymbol{t}(\boldsymbol{x}_i)/2$.

From the definition of t,

$$t(\boldsymbol{x}_i) = t_i + (\zeta_x + \boldsymbol{d}_x(\boldsymbol{x}_i) - 1)\boldsymbol{t}_d + (\zeta_y + \boldsymbol{d}_y(\boldsymbol{x}_i) - 1)\boldsymbol{t}_p, \tag{5}$$

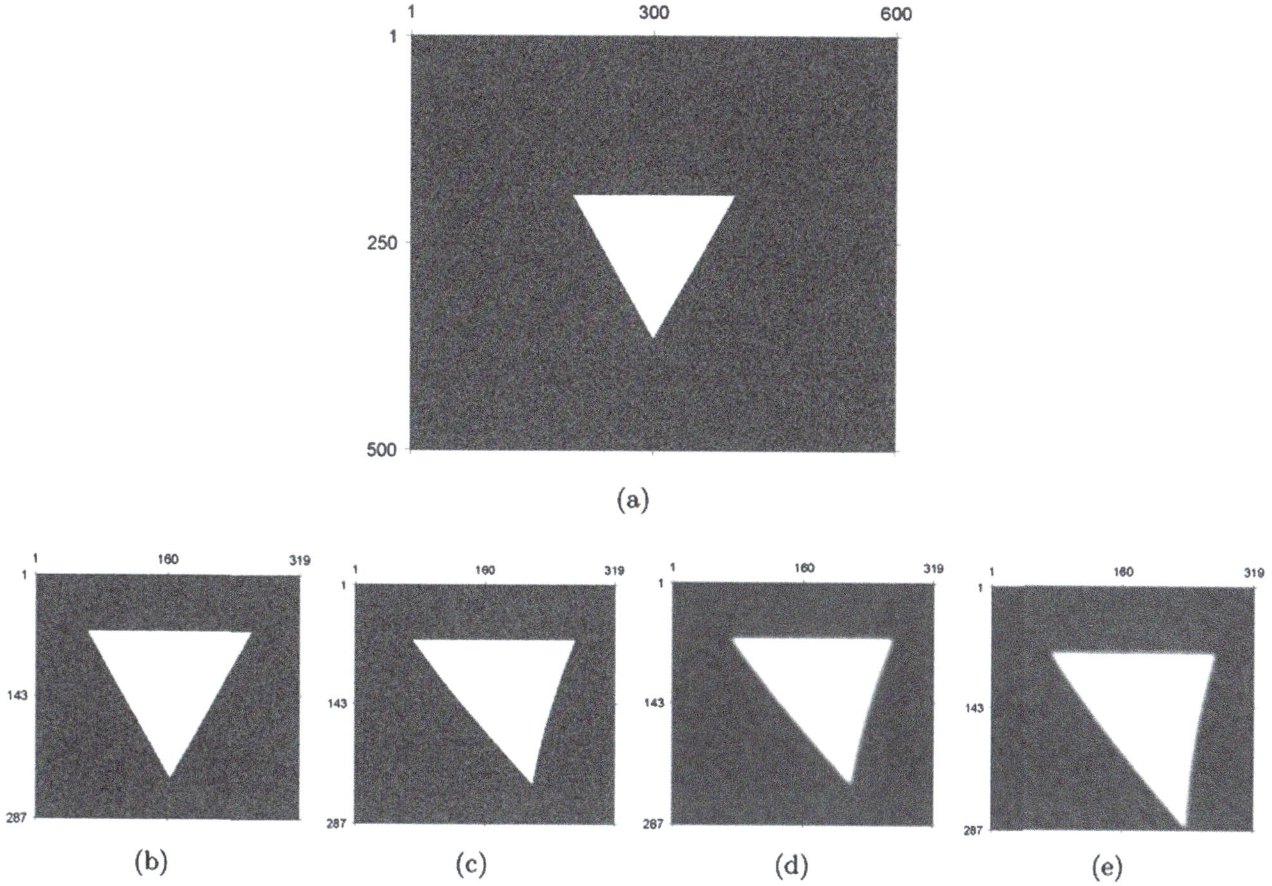

Fig. 7 **a** A 600 × 500 pixel-sized virtual domain with a cut-out in the form of an equilateral triangle is created in MATLAB. Random noise has been added to the intensities of the dark part. A 319 × 287 pixel-sized sub-domain around the triangle is scanned. The deformed configurations when the sub-domain is deformed under simple shear with very slow and very fast shear rates are shown in (**b**) and (**c**), respectively. For fast deformation, the effect of spatial distortion is shown in (**d**). Additionally, the effect of an unrealistic drift distortion linear in time and independent of position is shown in (**e**)

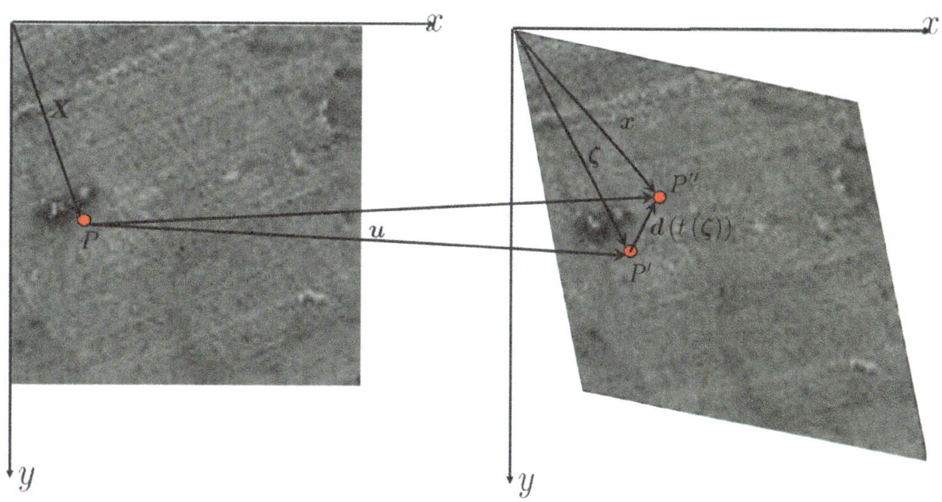

Fig. 8 The point P in the reference image is mapped to P' by mechanical deformation. But distortion causes a further drift $\boldsymbol{d}$ that makes the point appear at P''

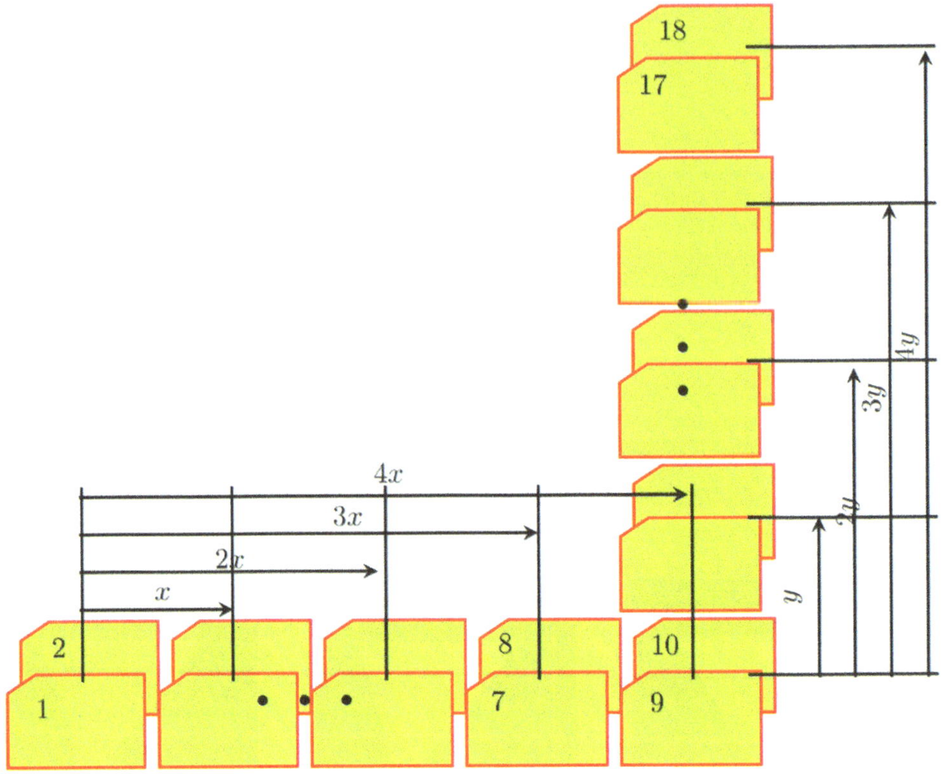

Fig. 9 In the calibration phase, nine pairs of images are taken. For each pair, the stage is translated by first by an amount x and then by y. For a pair, two images are captured in quick succession

and

$$t(\boldsymbol{x}_{i+1}) = \boldsymbol{t}_{i+1} + (\zeta_x + \boldsymbol{d}_x(\boldsymbol{x}_{i+1}) - \boldsymbol{1})\boldsymbol{t}_d + (\zeta_y + \boldsymbol{d}_y(\boldsymbol{x}_{i+1}) - \boldsymbol{1})\boldsymbol{t}_p, \quad (6)$$

so that,

$$\boldsymbol{t}(\boldsymbol{x}_{i+1}) - \boldsymbol{t}(\boldsymbol{x}_i) = \boldsymbol{T} + \boldsymbol{\Delta t}_i + \boldsymbol{\Delta d}_x(\boldsymbol{x}_i)\boldsymbol{t}_d + \boldsymbol{\Delta d}_y(\boldsymbol{x}_i)\boldsymbol{t}_p, \quad (7)$$

where,

$$\Delta d_x(\boldsymbol{x}_i) = (\boldsymbol{d}_x(\boldsymbol{x}_{i+1}) - \boldsymbol{d}_x(\boldsymbol{x}_i)), \boldsymbol{\Delta d}_y(\boldsymbol{x}_i) = (\boldsymbol{d}_y(\boldsymbol{x}_{i+1}) - \boldsymbol{d}_y(\boldsymbol{x}_i)). \quad (8)$$

Finally, the difference between the start times for images i and $i+1$ is $t_{i+1} - t_i = T + \Delta t_i$, where Δt_i is the interval between the end of scanning of i and beginning of $i+1$.

A set of nine pairs of images used for calibration are shown in Fig. 9. Pairs 1–5 are obtained by translating the stage in the x direction while 5–9 are in the y direction. The x and y components of the drift velocity $\boldsymbol{v}$, u_{dr} and v_{dr} are plotted against time in Fig. 10 for a generic point on the odd-numbered images. Cubic splines are fitted to the data for u_{dr} and v_{dr}. This exercise has to be repeated for every pixel in the odd-numbered images. For any pixel location $\boldsymbol{x}$ in an image i $(i = 1, 3, 5 \ldots 9)$, the drift corrected position is obtained as

$$\zeta = \boldsymbol{x}(\boldsymbol{t}(\boldsymbol{x})) - \int_0^{\boldsymbol{t}(\boldsymbol{x})} \boldsymbol{v}dt. \quad (9)$$

3.2 Correcting for Spatial Distortion

After the odd-numbered images are corrected for drift, they can be used to correct for spatial distortion. The rigid body displacement of an image i from the first image is known to be ζ_i. Now, a DIC between the first image and drift corrected image i will yield a displacement $\boldsymbol{u}_i(\boldsymbol{x}_i)$. The spatial distortion is extracted as $\boldsymbol{s}(\boldsymbol{x}_i) = \boldsymbol{u}_i(\boldsymbol{x}_i) - \zeta_i$ for all $\boldsymbol{x}_i$ and i. The spatial distortion is independent of time and remains nominally constant over the duration of an experiment.

The load displacement response of a rather slow miniature dog-bone specimen under uniaxial tension in the x direction is shown in Fig. 11. The u displacements obtained from 12 images taken at monotonically increasing loads are corrected for both drift and spatial distortions.

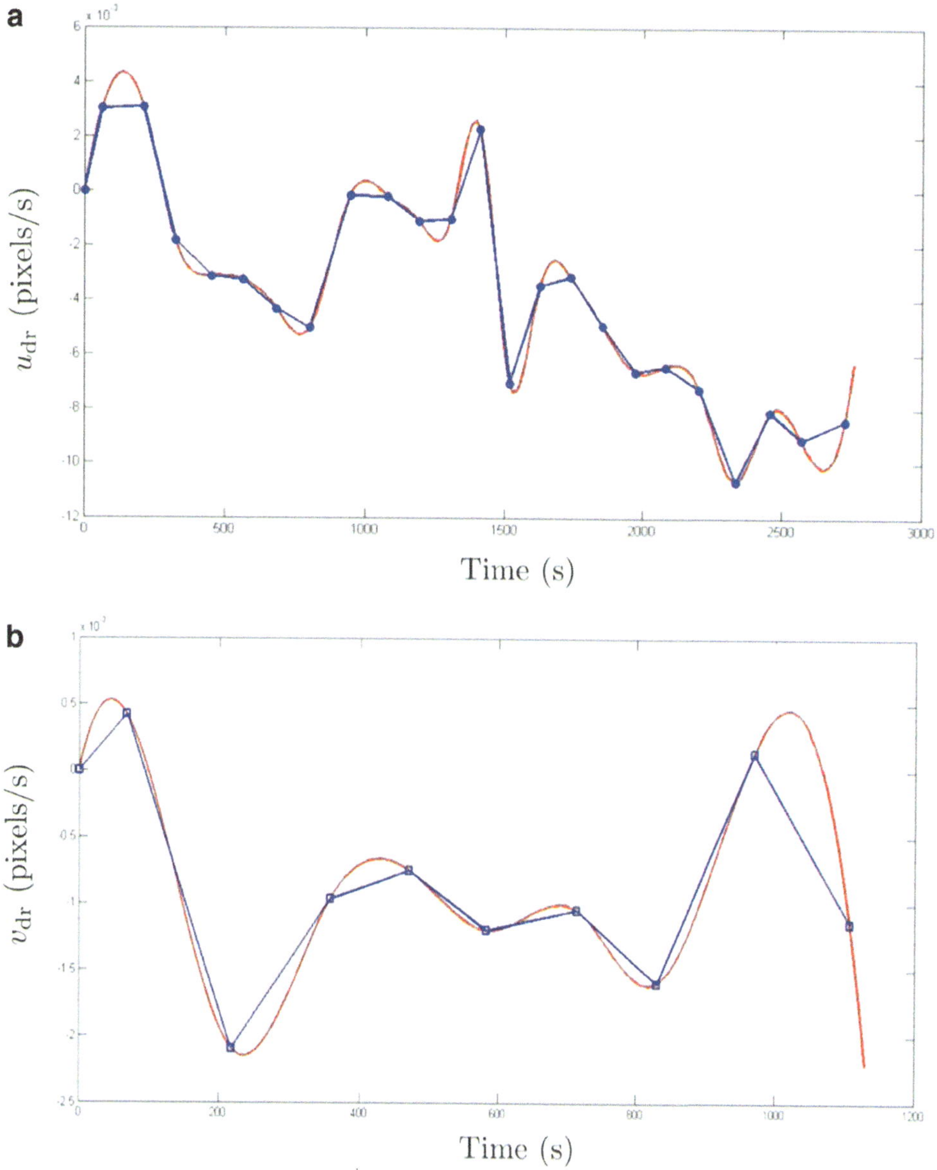

Fig. 10 Drift velocity components, **a** u_{dr} in the x direction and **b** v_{dr} in the y direction are obtained from the calibration phase of the in-situ experiment as functions of time. Cubic splines are fitted to the data in order to have a smooth functional form that can be readily used for drift correction in the actual testing phase

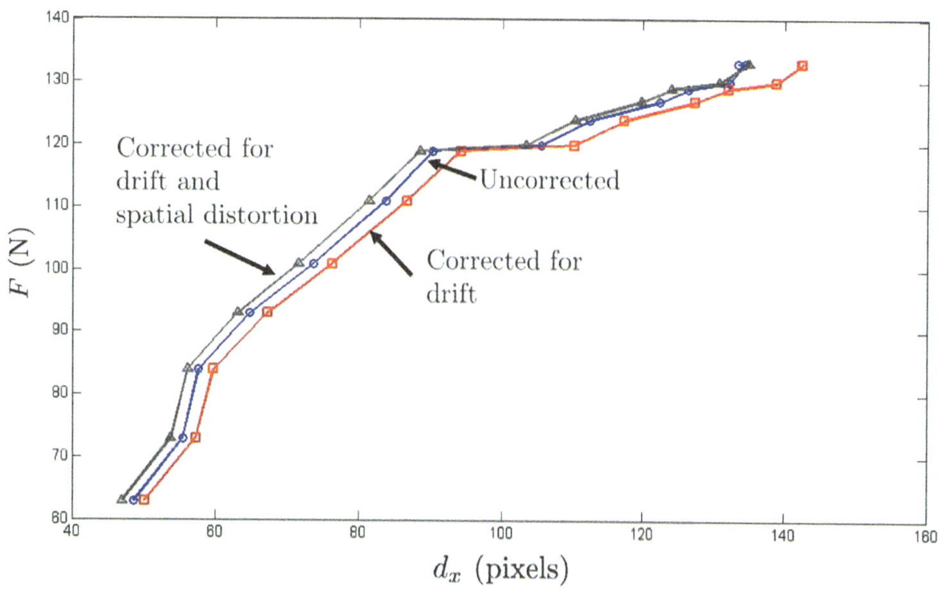

Fig. 11 Load displacement responses of a miniature dog-bone specimen deformed in uniaxial tension in-situ. The uncorrected response and those after correction for only drift and both drift and spatial distortions are shown

4 Conclusions

Conducting quantitative in-situ deformation experiments inside the vacuum chamber of a scanning electron microscope is useful under many circumstances. However, owing to the nature of image generation in an SEM, quantitative measurements of full-field displacements and strains pose unique challenges. We have shown that the raster scanning process by which the electron beam generates a digital image leads to artifacts that can potentially derail attempts to apply digital image correlation-based techniques to compute displacements. In this article, we have discussed recently proposed methods for correcting drift and spatial distortions in SEM images. These two imaging artifacts seem to have the largest effects on the displacements on the surface of a specimen. We are in the process of conducting many small-scale experiments where algorithms for correction discussed in this article are applied to several different materials under a range of two-dimensional deformation protocols. Development of a software package that seamlessly integrates deformation measurement through DIC following corrections for drift and spatial distortions is also underway.

Acknowledgements The algorithms for DIC and correction of imaging artifacts have been implemented in MATLAB at IIT Kanpur by Suhas Vilas Powar in the period 2014–2015. Micro-compression stages for conducting in-situ tests were assembled and instrumented by Rachit Nayak also in 2015. A miniature tensile stage was procured as part of a project funded by the Department of Science and Technology, Govt. of India, titled 'Modeling Of Interface Deformation And Failure Through A Combination Of Finite Element Analysis And Digital Image Correlation,' in 2009, in collaboration with Prof. P. Venkitanarayanan. Various test results mentioned as part of this article are taken from the works of Dr T Guruprasad, Dr Chatanya K Desai, S Arun Kumar, Moonish Mustafa, and Ankur Patel.

References

Adusumalli R-B, Raghavan R, Ghisleni R, Zimmermann T, Michler J (2010) Deformation and failure mechanism of secondary cell wall in spruce late wood. Appl Phys A: Mater Sci Process 100(2):447–52

Alaie A, Kadkhodapour J, Ziaei Rad S, Asadi Asadabad M, Schmauder S (2015) Formation and coalescence of strain localized regions in ferrite phase of dp600 steels under uniaxial tensile deformation. Mater Sci Eng : A (Structural Materials: Properties, Microstructure and Processing) 623: 133 – 44

Arai M, Wu X, Fujimoto K (2010) Inelastic deformation of freestanding plasma-sprayed thermal barrier coatings. J Solid Mech Mater Engi 4(2):2212–234

Bao Lei, Lecomte J-S, Schuman C, Philippe M-J, Zhao X, Esling C (2010) Study of plastic deformation in hexagonal metals by interrupted in-situ ebsd measurement. Adv Eng Mater 12(10):1053–1059

Barkia B, Doquet V, Heripre E, Guillot I (2015) Characterization and analysis of deformation heterogeneities in commercial purity titanium. Mater Characterization 108:94–101

fritz2017 fritz2017 Fritz R, Wimler D, Leitner A, Maier-Kiener V, Kiener D (2017) Dominating deformation mechanisms in ultrafine-grained chromium across length scales and temperatures. Acta Mater 140:176–187

Gussev MN, Leonard KJ (2019) In situ sem-ebsd analysis of plastic deformation mechanisms in neutron-irradiated austenitic steel. J Nuclear Mater 517:45–56

Bruck HA, McNeill SR, Sutton M, Peters WHIII (1989) Digital image correlation using newton-raphson method of partial differential correction. Experimental Mech 29:261–267

Chu TP, Ranson WF, Sutton M (1985) Applications of digital-image-correlation techniques to experimental mechanics. Experimental Mech 25:232–244

Dingley DJ (1973) In situ studies of deformations of metals in an s.e.m, pp 112–117

Liu X, Wang C, Gui J, Xiao Q, Guo B (2019) Effect of mns inclusions on deformation behavior of matrix based on in-situ experiment. Mater Sci Engi: A (Structural Materials: Properties, Microstructure and Processing) 746: 239–247

Herre P, Romeis S, Makovi M, Przybilla T, Paul J, Schwenger J, Torun B, Grundmeier G, Spiecker E, Peukert W (2017) Deformation behavior of nanocrystalline titania particles accessed by complementary in situ electron microscopy techniques. J Am Ceramic Soc 100(12):5709–22

Hild F, Roux S (2006) Digital image correlation: from displacement measurement to identification of elastic properties: a review. Strain 42:69–80

Zhang J, Gu H, Zhou H, Zhang S, Laird C (1989) Tensile deformation and fracture in high purity titanium: in situ observation by scanning electron microscopy. Mater Scie Eng A (Structural Materials: Properties, Microstructure and Processing) A114: 89–96

Jin P, Li X (2015) Correction of image and drift distortion in a scanning electron microscopy. J Microscopy 260:268–280

Jun T-S, Sernicola G, Dunne FPE, Britton TB (2016) Local deformation mechanisms of two-phase ti alloy. Mater Sci Eng: A (Structural Materials: Properties, Microstructure and Processing) 649: 39–47

Kammers AD, Daly S (2013) Digital image correlation under scanning electron. Experimental Mech 53:1743–1761

Li H, Boehlert CJ, Bieler TR, Crimp MA (2014) Analysis of the deformation behavior in tension and tension-creep of ti-3al-2.5v (wt pct) at 296 k and 728 k (23 c and 455 c) using insitu sem experiments. Metall Mater Trans A 45(13): 6053–6066

Li J, Mishara RK, Kubic R (2008) In-situ ebsd analysis on the microstructures during deformation. J Chinese Electron Microscopy Soc 27(6):439–442

Li S, Wang Y, Wang X (2019) In situ observation of the deformation and fracture behaviors of long-term thermally aged cast duplex stainless steels. Metals 9(2): 258 (9 pp)

Maraghechi S, Hoefnagels JPM, Peerlings RHJ, Geers MGD (2018) Correction of scan line shift artifacts in scanning electron microscopy: an extended digital image correlation framework. Ultramicroscopy 187:144–163

Maraghechi S, Hoefnagels JPM, Peerlings RHJ, Rokos O, Geers MGD (2019) Correction of scanning electron microscope imaging artifacts in a novel digital image correlation framework. Experimental Mech 59:489–516

Wang M, Lu W, Zhang D, Qin J, Fan T, Ji B, Zhu F, Ji S (2005) An ebsd and tem study on the microstructural evolution of in situ synthesized (tib + tic)/ti matrix composites during superplastic deformation. Mater Trans 46(8):1833–1838

Motsi GT, Olubambi PA, Sono TJ, Shoke L (2014) In situ electron microscopy studies on the tensile deformation mechanisms in aluminium 5083 alloy. Adv Mater Res 1019:103–11

Nakagawa K, Maeda K, Takeuchi S (1980) Plastic deformation of cdte single crystals. i. microscopic observations. J Phys Soc Jpn 49(5): 1909–1915

Niwa N, Ito K (1987) In-situ sem observation of deformation process in uniaxial tension of ti-13-11 alloy. Annual Report of the Engineering Research Institute, Faculty of Engineering, University of Tokyo 46:207–12

Pan B, Qian K, Xie H, Asundi A (2009) Two dimensional digital image correlation for in-plane displacement and strain measurement: a review. Measurement Sci Technol 20:062001

Perusin S, Viguier B, Salabura JC, Oquab D, Andrieu E (2004) Behaviour of the oxide scale during sem in situ plastic deformation of pure nickel foil. Mater Sci Eng A. Properties, Microstructure and Processing, Structural Materials

Prochazka J, Kuerova L, Bystriansky M (2017) Evaluation of in-situ deformation experiments of trip steel, vol 179, pages 012059 (7 pp)

Roberts W, Lehtinen B (1976) An in situ sem study of void development around inclusions in steel during plastic deformation. Acta Metallurgica 24(8):745–58

Romeis S, Paul J, Herre P, Hanisch M, Klupp Taylor RN, Schmidt J, Peukert W (2015) In situ deformation and breakage of silica particles inside a sem. Proc Eng 102:201–210

Sarobol P, Chandross M, Carroll JD, Mook WM, Bufford DC, Boyce BL, Hattar K, Kotula PG, Hall AC (2016) Room temperature deformation mechanisms of alumina particles observed from in situ micro-compression and atomistic simulations. J Thermal Spray Technol 25(1–2):82–93

Snella MT (2010) Drift correction for scanning electron microscopy. Master's thesis, Massachusetts Institute of Technology

Stephens RR, Hoeppner DW (1988) New apparatus for studying fatigue deformation at high magnifications. Rev Sci Instruments 59(8):1412–19

Sutton M, Li N, Garcia D, Cornille N, Orteu JJ, McNeill SR, Schreier HW, Li X, Reynolds AP (2007) Scanning electron microscopy for quantitative small and large deformation measurements part ii: experimental validation for magnifications from 200 to 10,000. Experimental Mech 47:789–804

Sutton M, Li N, Joy DC, Reynolds AP, Li X (2007) Scanning electron microscopy for quantitative small and large deformation measurements part i: Sem imaging at magnifications from 200 to 10,000. Experimental Mech 47:775–787

Sutton MA, Orteu JJ, Hubert S (2009) Image correlation for shape. Motion and deformation measurements, Springer, US

Ujiiye N, Kimoto S, Kawasaki Y (1971) Observation of deformation and fracture in metals-a dynamic application of sem, pp 97–104

Wu XH, Arai M, Fujimoto K, Sun Q (2008) Inelastic deformation of free-standing plasma-sprayed thermal barrier coatings, vol 7375, p 73755M (6 pp)

Wu Z, Sandlobes S, Wu L, Hu W, Gottstein G, Korte-Kerzel S (2016) Mechanical behaviour of zn-al-cu-mg alloys: Deformation mechanisms of as-cast microstructures. Mater Sci Eng: A (Structural Materials: Properties, Microstructure and Processing) 651: 675–687

Fuqiang Yang, Renbo Song, Yaping Li, Ting Sun, Kaikun Wang (2015) Tensile deformation of low density duplex fe-mn-al-c steel. Mater Desi 76:32–9

Song Zhang, Yilong Liang, Qifan Xia, Meigui Ou (2019) Study on tensile deformation behavior of tc21 titanium alloy. J Mater Eng Performance 28(3):1581–90

Xuehua Zhang, Shuangyin Zhang, Qinyang Zhao, Yongqing Zhao, Rong Li, Weidong Zeng (2018) In-situ observations of the tensile deformation and fracture behavior of a fine-grained titanium alloy sheet. J Alloys Compounds 740:660–8

In-Situ Micromechanical Testing in Scanning Electron Microscopy

R. Sarvesha and Sudhanshu S. Singh

1 Introduction

In-situ electron microscopy is a fast-growing and leading field in the materials research. It is an indispensable tool in understanding the material behavior in real-time. Additionally, the rapid miniaturization of the components for technological devices, that approaches micron and nanoscale dimensions, requires accurate size-specific properties (Gianolaet 2011) as it has been shown that the properties at a small length scale can be significantly different from the bulk counterpart (Dimiduk et al. 2005; Uchic et al. 2004; Volkert et al. 2008). Besides, in the multi-phase materials, the properties measured at a small length scale can be used as input to carry out microstructure-based modeling, which further assists in understanding the bulk deformation behavior (Guo et al. 2014).

To understand the material behavior in real-time, and at small length scales, a number of improvements in the microscopy techniques have been made over the years. Several two-dimensional (2D) microscopy techniques [e.g., optical, Raman, scanning electron microscopy (SEM), electron backscattered diffraction (EBSD), electron channeling contrast imaging (ECCI)] and three-dimensional (3D) techniques [e.g., transmission electron microscopy (TEM), X-ray tomography, neutron imagining, atom probe tomography (APT), focused ion beam (FIB) tomography] cover a range of length scales (Singh et al. 2014a,2015,2017; Gianolaet 2011; Volkert et al. 2008; Guo et al. 2014; Legros et al. 2010). Among these, the electron microscopy technique is well suited to elucidate the microstructural changes, with time, for micron- and submicron-sized specimens.

In-situ electron microscopy can be used to understand different phenomena depending upon the attachments equipped in SEM. For instance, a customized or commercial mechanical testing jig assists in unraveling the complex deformation mechanisms (Singh et al. 2014a). Further, EBSD and digital image correlation (DIC) techniques can assist in understanding the strain partitioning between different phases or grains in the materials. Novel microscopy techniques, such as electron channeling contrast imaging (ECCI) (Slama et al. 2019), can further assist in the quantification of the deformation systems generated under the application of load. FIB machining and deposition enable the sample preparation, which aids in evaluating the site-specific properties at small length scales using specialized attachments, such as nanoindentation system in a SEM (Sarvesha et al. 2020; Guo et al. 2014; Singh et al. 2014b). In recent years, irradiation properties of the nuclear materials have been studied by irradiating different ions, such as Fe+ , W+, He+, on the microscale test structures in assistance with FIB (Armstrong et al. 2015). Furthermore, a couple of *in-situ* SEM studies have also been carried out to evaluate the corrosion properties in environmental SEM (Proff et al. 2010), where a special *in-situ* jig was used to simulate the corrosion environment (Kim et al. 2020).

A powerful way of capturing real-time deformation microstructure is acoustic emission (AE) along with the conventional *in-situ* measurements. The AE method is based on sound emitted due to the activation of deformation mechanisms or fracture during deformation and thus provides highly time-resolved information (Wisner et al. 2015).

Figure 1 summarizes the various *in-situ* tests performed in SEM. *In-situ* tests in combination with SE/BSE imaging and EBSD in SEM are the most attractive methods used to understand the deformation behavior. This article discusses a few case studies showing the use of *in-situ* electron microscopy in evaluating the deformation behavior of metallic systems (Sn whisker, 7075 aluminum alloys, and AZ80 magnesium alloy).

R. Sarvesha · S. S. Singh (✉)
Department of Materials Science and Engineering, IIT Kanpur, Kanpur, India
e-mail: sudhanss@iitk.ac.in

K. Biswas et al. (eds.), *Electron Microscopy in Science and Engineering*, IITK Directions 6,
https://doi.org/10.1007/978-981-16-5101-4_2

2 Case Studies

2.1 Case Study I: *In-Situ* Tensile Behavior of Sn Whiskers

Environment-friendly Pb-free solders are predominantly based on Sn-rich alloys, where whiskers are known to grow on the Sn plates (Mathew et al. 2009). An understanding of the mechanical response of Sn whisker is vital for the soldering community. Whiskers are single crystals and contain minimal defects, which assists in the free flow of electron, thus making them an excellent conductor. The phenomenon of Sn whisker formation has been studied for decades (Galyon 2005); however, only a few studies have been performed to evaluate the mechanical properties of Sn whiskers (Dunn 1987; Powell and Skove 2004). This is due to adversity involved in handling whiskers. This case study deals with the *in-situ* evaluation of tensile properties of Sn whisker using a micro–electro–mechanical system (MEMS) tensile stage in assistance with a focused ion beam (FIB) (Singh et al. 2014a).

Sn whiskers on a Sn plate, having a very high aspect ratio, are shown in Fig. 2a. The steps of *in-situ* sample preparation using FIB are shown in Fig. 2. Manipulator needle was brought close to the base of the Sn whisker (Fig. 2b) and carefully welded using Pt (Fig. 2c). Sn whisker was then cut using Ga ions, as shown in Fig. 2d. The whisker was then brought to the MEMS device and welded in the trenches using Pt, as shown in Fig. 2e–g. In the end, the needle was released by cutting the whisker using Ga ions (Fig. 2h).

The MEMS device is shown in Fig. 3a (details of construction of the MEMS stage are reported elsewhere (Han and Saif 2006; Han et al. 2007)), and welded whisker on it is shown in Fig. 3b. A quasistatic loading was applied during the tensile test until fracture. The fractured Sn whisker is shown in Fig. 3c. The magnified image of the whisker shows that its surface is irregular. Therefore, to evaluate the stress, the surface area was calculated using image processing software (ImageJ), as shown in Fig. 3d. Two successful tests were performed, and in both the case linear stress–strain behavior was observed for the Sn whisker (Fig. 3e). The values of Young's modulus of both the whiskers were measured to be 42 and 45 GPa, which are close to the theoretical value of the modulus for pure Sn. The fracture strength and strain to failure for the two tests were 720 MPa, 880 MPa, and 2%, 3%, respectively. The observed high fracture strength and limited ductility may be attributed to a lack of defects in the single crystal Sn whiskers.

Limited *ex-situ* experiments have been performed to evaluate the mechanical properties of Sn whiskers (Dunn 1987; Powell and Skove 2004). Powell and Skove (2004) observed the linear load–displacement behavior. However, the properties of the whiskers were not reported. Dunn (1987) obtained Young's modulus using the cantilever method. However, a large variability (8–85 GPa) was observed. One of the crucial shortcomings in Dunn's study was the measurement of the cross-sectional area in which the whisker was assumed to have a circular cross section. However, it should be noted that in the bending theory, Young's modulus varies with the fourth power of the radius, and thus, a small change in the radius would result in a significant deviation in the measurement of modulus. In comparison with the *ex-situ* testing, which had inherent limitations in handling the whiskers, the *in-situ* tensile testing in SEM assisted in evaluating the reliable mechanical properties of the Sn whisker.

2.2 Case Study II: Evaluation of Mechanical Properties of the Constituent Particles in Al 7075 by Micro-pillar Compression

Aluminum alloys are predominantly used as structural materials due to their high strength-to-weight ratio (Bucci et al. 2000; Starke and Staley 2011). These alloys contain second-phase particles (Fe-containing: Al_7Cu_2Fe and Si-containing: Mg_2Si), also called as constituent particles, which form during casting and do not dissolve in the

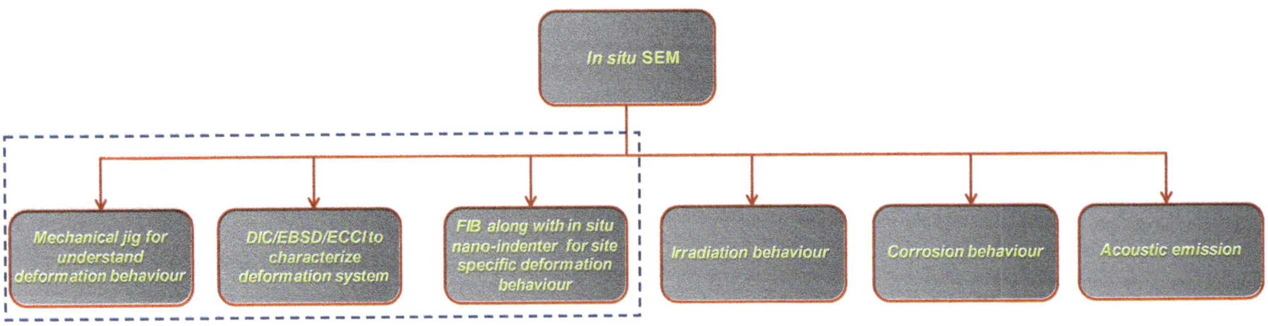

Fig. 1 Summary of the *in-situ* test performed in a scanning electron microscope

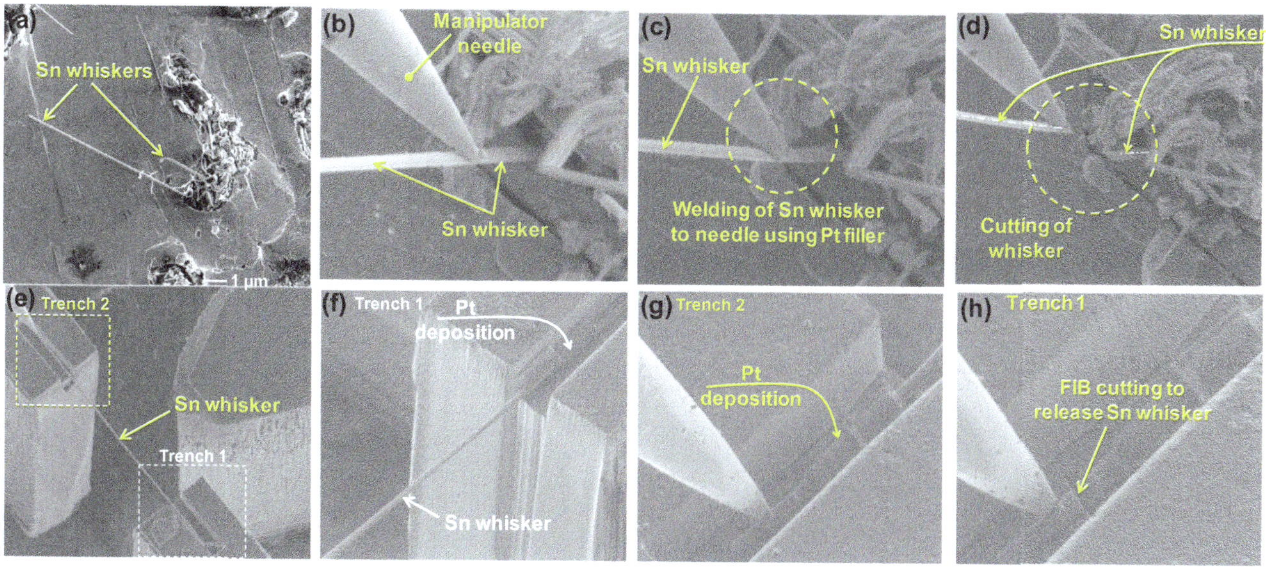

Fig. 2 **a** SEM image of Sn whiskers. Steps of whisker lift off and placement in MEMS inside FIB/SEM, **b** manipulator needle in contact with whisker, **c** welding of whisker using Pt filler, **d** FIB cutting of the whisker, **e–g** placement and welding of whisker in the trenches, and **h** FIB cutting to release the needle (Singh et al. 2014a)

subsequent thermomechanical treatment of the alloy (Payne et al. 2010; Xue et al. 2007). These particles have been observed to affect the overall deformation behavior of the alloy as they are the source for crack nucleation and propagation during static or dynamic loading (Pearson 1975; Weiland et al. 2009; Maire et al. 2011; Lugo et al. 2011). Hence, the overall mechanical response of the Al7075 alloy depends on the characteristic of constituent particles. This present case study deals with the evaluations of the stress–strain behavior of the constituent particles under uniaxial compression of micro-pillars (Singh et al. 2015).

The SEM micrograph (Fig. 4a) shows two types of constituent particles (one black and another white). The corresponding EDS analysis (Fig. 4b) indicates that the bright particle is Fe-bearing inclusions and the dark particle is Si-bearing inclusion. The approximate atomic ratio of Al, Cu, and Fe in Fe-bearing inclusion is 7:2:1, indicating them to be Al_7Cu_2Fe. Similarly, for Si-bearing inclusion, the atomic ratio of Mg and Si is 2:1, indicating them to be Mg_2Si. The micro-pillar fabrication sequence for Mg_2Si using dual-beam focused ion beam (FIB) is shown in Fig. 4c–f. The same procedure was followed for Al_7Cu_2Fe and Al7075 matrix. Initially, a circular trench of ~25 μm diameter was milled out (shown in Fig. 4c), which provides clearance for the flat punch during compression. A course pillar with ~7 μm was made at the inclusion center (refer to Fig. 4d). Further, the pillar diameter was reduced to ~3.5 μm (Fig. 4e), and milling was continued until an aspect ratio of 2.7–3.4 was maintained. During the final process, a low current was utilized, so the taper is less than 3° (shown in Fig. 4f).

The SEM micrographs before loading and after fracture of the pillars are shown in Fig. 5a1, b1, c1 and a2, b2, c2, respectively. The stress–strain behavior of the constituent particles and the matrix of the repeat test is shown in Fig. 5d. Linear stress–strain behavior is observed till fracture for the Al_7Cu_2Fe particles. The fracture stress is ~2.5 ± 0.2 GPa, and strain is approximately 2%. SEM micrograph of the fractured pillar (Fig. 5a2) indicates catastrophic failure. In the case of the Mg_2Si particle, the stress value increased linearly with strain in the initial region, followed by strain bursts. The significant strain hardening is due to the dislocation activity, which is also visible in the SEM micrograph (steps indicated by the arrow in Fig. 5b2). The compressive yield strength of Mg_2Si was calculated to be ~1.8 ± 0.1 GPa. The Al7075 matrix has similar stress–strain behavior as Mg_2Si with a lower yield strength of ~0.5 ± 0.1 GPa. The strength values are in-line with the hardness value obtained by nanoindentation (Kim et al. 2020), i.e., the highest hardness for Al_7Cu_2Fe particle followed by Mg_2Si particle and Al7075 matrix.

Previously, studies have been conducted on the evaluation of mechanical properties of Al_7Cu_2Fe and Mg_2Si by fabricating bulk samples through the powder metallurgy route. While both Al_7Cu_2Fe and Mg_2Si were found to be brittle (Laplanche et al. 2014; Wang et al. 2007; Muñoz--Palos et al. 1996; Takeuchi et al. 1996), limited plasticity for Mg_2Si was observed in this study. This difference in behavior could be attributed to the difference in microstructure like grain size, defect concentration, and type (such as residual porosity), etc. It has been recently shown in several micro-pillar compression studies that a brittle

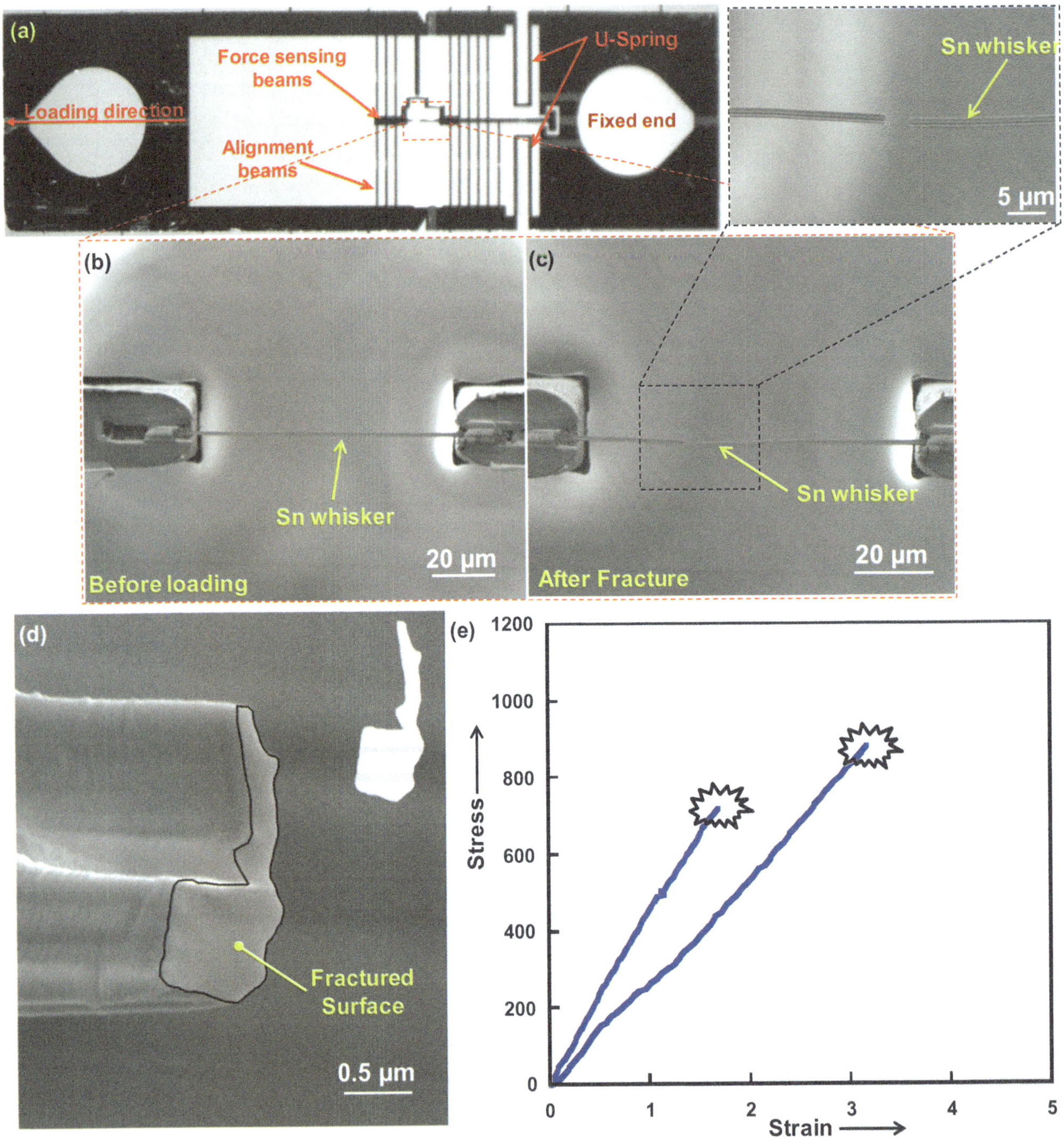

Fig. 3 **a** Optical micrograph of MEMS stage for tensile testing of whisker, **b** zoomed image of Sn whisker before loading, **c** fracture Sn whisker, **d** SE micrograph of fractured surface and inset is a binary image of the fractured surface, **e** nominal stress–strain in the behavior of Sn whisker (Singh et al. 2014a)

material (in bulk) can show plastic deformation at a small length scale (Östlundet 2009; Michler et al. 2007; Korte and Clegg 2011; Östlund 2011). Hence, reducing the size of the sample suppresses cracking, resulting in plastic deformation when the test sample is made significantly small (Östlundet 2009). Oswald (2003) evaluated the hardness and Young's modulus using nanoindentation and predicated stress–strain behavior. Even though the highest strength and modulus was reported for Al_7Cu_2Fe, a similar yield strength was predicated for Al-matrix and Mg_2Si due to their similar hardness

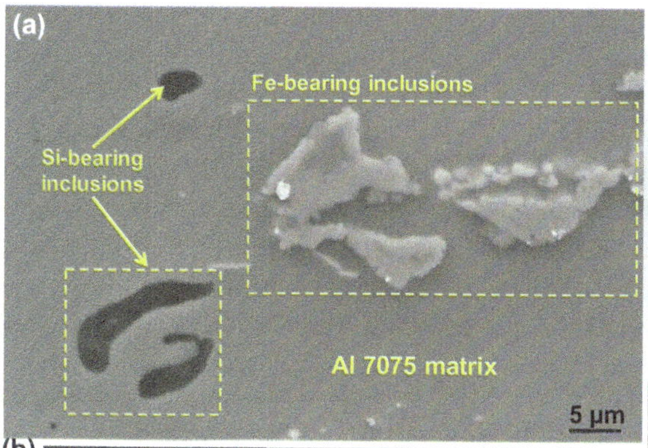

(b)

Fe-bearing Inclusions		Si-bearing Inclusions		Al 7075 matrix	
Elements	At%	Elements	At%	Elements	At%
Al	72.1 ± 0.9	Mg	58.2 ± 6.1	Al	93.6 ± 0.3
Cu	19.2 ± 0.9	Si	28.7 ± 2.1	Zn	2.6 ± 0.03
Fe	8.7 ± 0.6	O	8 ± 3.2	Mg	3.1 ± 0.3
		Al	5.1 ± 3.4	Cu	0.5 ± 0.04

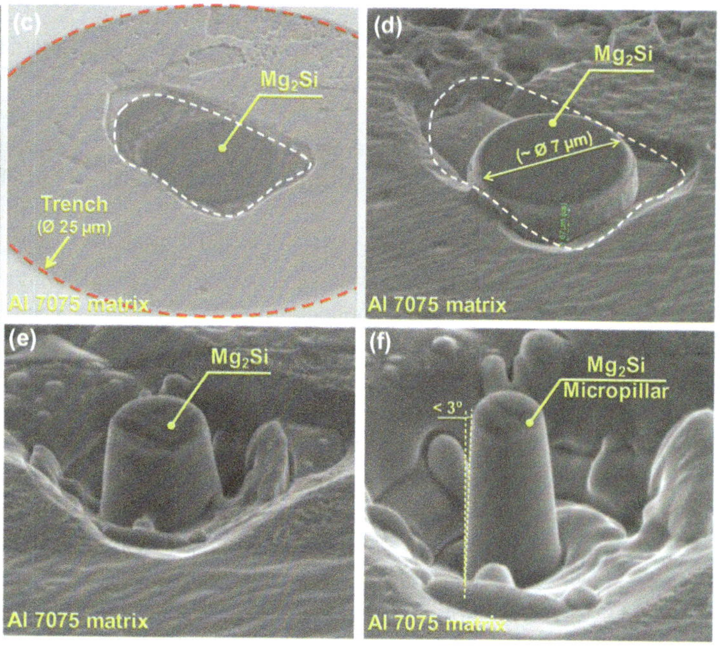

Fig. 4 **a** SEM image showing Fe- and Si-bearing inclusions in Al7075, **b** EDS analysis of the second-phase particles, and **c–f** micro-pillar fabrication using dual-beam FIB

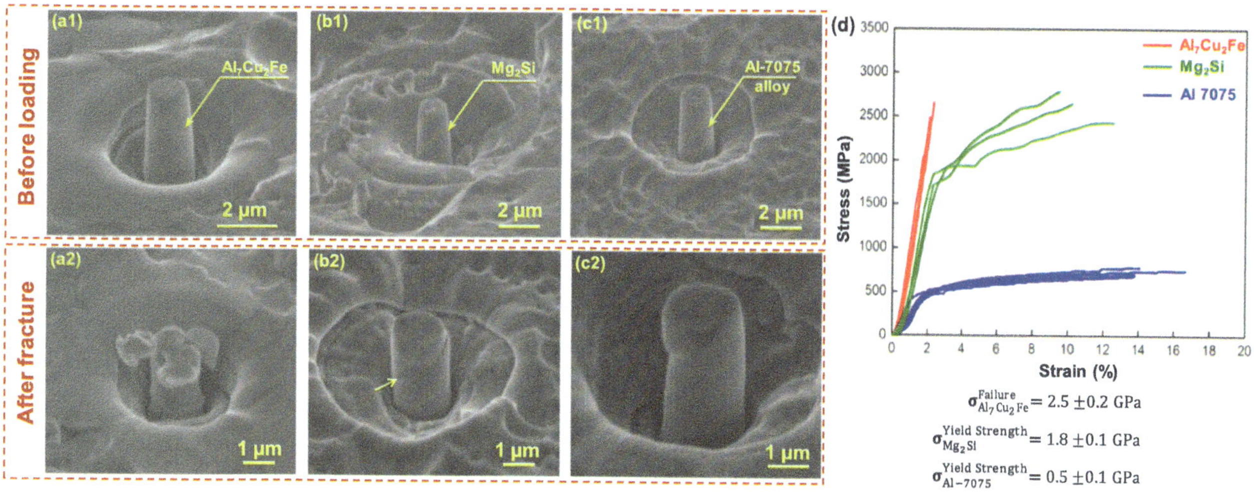

Fig. 5 **a1**, **b1**, **c1** and **a2**, **b2**, **c2** show Al_7Cu_2Fe, Mg_2Si, Al7075 micro-pillars before loading and after fracture, respectively, and (d) stress–strain behavior of the second-phase particles and the matrix (Singh et al. 2015)

values. However, the present study shows that Mg_2Si exhibits higher yield strength as compared to the matrix, which corroborates with the hardness values reported in other studies (Singh et al. 2014c).

In summary, the mechanical properties of the constituent particles were evaluated by micro-pillar compression testing, the knowledge of which will allow a better understanding of the bulk deformation behavior of Al7075 alloys.

2.3 Case Study III: Role of Second-Phase Particles on the Deformation Behavior of AZ80 Magnesium Alloys

The role of second-phase particles on the deformation behavior of AZ80 alloy has been divided into two separate studies. One study (Sarvesha et al. 2021) deals with understanding the role of these particles on the fracture process of

the alloy using *in-situ* tensile testing, and another study (Sarvesha et al. 2020) is on the measurement of mechanical properties of the particles using micro-pillar compression.

2.3.1 Effect of Second-Phase Particle on Crack Propagation in Magnesium alloy via *in-situ* Tensile Testing

Magnesium and its alloys exhibit the highest strength to-weight ratio, which assists in a weight reduction, thus have potential in the automobile, aerospace, and electronics industries (Kulekci 2008; Blawert et al. 2004). Mg-Al-Zn alloys, designated as AZ series alloys, which are a prominent class of magnesium alloys, contain Mg-Al precipitate and Al-Mn inclusions, (Zindal et al. 2018,2017). These second-phase particles have been found to affect the mechanical properties of magnesium alloys significantly (Lugo et al. 2011; Yakubtsov et al. 2008).

A typical as-cast optical micrograph (OM) of Mg-9.3Al-0.45Zn-0.15Mn is shown in Fig. 6a, which shows two types of micron-sized second-phase particles. The corresponding backscattered electron (BSE) image (Fig. 6b) shows gray and white particles due to difference in composition. The energy dispersive spectroscopy (EDS) map (Fig. 6c) shows that the gray particle is enriched with Mg and Al with Zn segregation. In contrast, the white particle is enriched with Mn and Al with the segregation of Fe and Si. Furthermore, the optical microscopic image (dark field mode) shows that Mg-Al precipitate has porosities, which is called a discontinuous eutectic precipitate. In addition, additional dark regions (indicated by arrows in Fig. 6a) correspond to continuous precipitates, which are formed adjacent to eutectic precipitate (refer SE micrograph in Fig. 6b). Electron backscatter diffraction (EBSD) maps suggest that the micron-sized Mg-Al precipitate corresponds to $Mg_{17}Al_{12}$ (space group $I\bar{4}3m$), which are polycrystalline and forms along the grain boundaries of the α-Mg matrix, whereas the Al-Mn inclusion corresponds to Al_8Mn_5 particle (space group R3m) and has a rhombohedral crystal structure.

Gatan *in-situ* tensile testing stage, along with the sample dimension, are shown in Fig. 7a, b, respectively. The sequence of secondary electrons (SE) micrographs at different strain (ε) levels (refer Fig. 7c) shows that crack propagation occurred predominantly through $Mg_{17}Al_{12}$ precipitates. The visible crack appeared at strain (ε) 0.0376. To further ascertain the strain at which the crack initiates in $Mg_{17}Al_{12}$, in-situ testing was performed with a focus on a single $Mg_{17}Al_{12}$ particle, as shown in Fig. 8a. It can be observed that at $\varepsilon = 0.017$, the crack initiates in the second-phase particle, which is in the linear portion of the stress–strain curve (shown in inset). With an increase in strain, more cracks appear perpendicular to the loading direction, as indicated by arrows in Fig. 8a.

Further, to understand the strain partitioning between the matrix and the precipitate, *in-situ* tensile testing, assisted with EBSD, was performed. A 70° pre-tilt in-situ stage (shown in Fig. 7a) was employed for EBSD scanning. The secondary electron (SE) micrographs (at 70° tilt) along with the EBSD maps, before loading and after fracture, are shown in Fig. 8b, c, respectively. Kernel average misorientation (KAM) maps in Fig. 8b, c are generated from EBSD scanning. KAM calculates the average misorientation between each pixel and its nearest neighbors and indicates strain in different phases during external loading. KAM map in Fig. 8b shows no strain in the matrix as well as in the particle before loading. However, after fracture, the strain is predominately distributed in the matrix, as the matrix shows higher KAM values (Fig. 8c). The KAM value of the precipitate is approximately zero, indicating the $Mg_{17}Al_{12}$ fractured in a brittle manner.

Previously, Yakubtsov et al. (2008) observed an increase in the ductility of AZ80 (Mg-8.2Al-0.51Zn) alloy with a decrease in the volume fraction of $Mg_{17}Al_{12}$precipitate. Lü et al. (2000) observed the crack formation near $Mg_{17}Al_{12}$ precipitate during tensile deformation, and it was postulated that the crack initiated at the interface between $Mg/Mg_{17}Al_{12}$. In the present study, it is evident from *in-situ* tensile testing, fracture initiates at $Mg_{17}Al_{12}$ at low strain and propagates through the $Mg_{17}Al_{12}$ phase.

2.3.2 Mechanical Property Evaluation of Second-Phase Particle in Magnesium Alloy by Micro-pillar Compression

It is clear from the previous study (Sect. 2.3.1) that the second-phase particles significantly affect the deformation characteristics of magnesium alloys. Therefore, it is essential to understand the mechanical properties of the individual particle. However, due to the small size of these particles, their mechanical properties cannot be evaluated by conventional techniques. Thus, this study deals with the evaluation of mechanical properties (stress–strain behavior) of these second-phase particles using *in-situ* micro-pillar compression (Sarvesha et al. 2020).

The micro-pillar fabrication process has already been discussed in Case II. The undeformed and deformed pillars of the matrix and second-phase particles are shown in Fig. 9, and the stress–strain behavior is shown in Fig. 10a. During compression, slip bands form on the α-Mg matrix surface (shown in Fig. 8a1 inset), which manifests as strain bursts in stress–strain curves (Fig. 10a)—a general characteristic of ductile metals/alloy (Schneider et al. 2013). In contrast, the stress–strain behavior of $Mg_{17}Al_{12}$ showed linear behavior until a massive strain burst (Fig. 10a). The corresponding SE micrograph shows a noticeable change in the shape of the $Mg_{17}Al_{12}$ pillar (Fig. 9b2), which could be due to strong

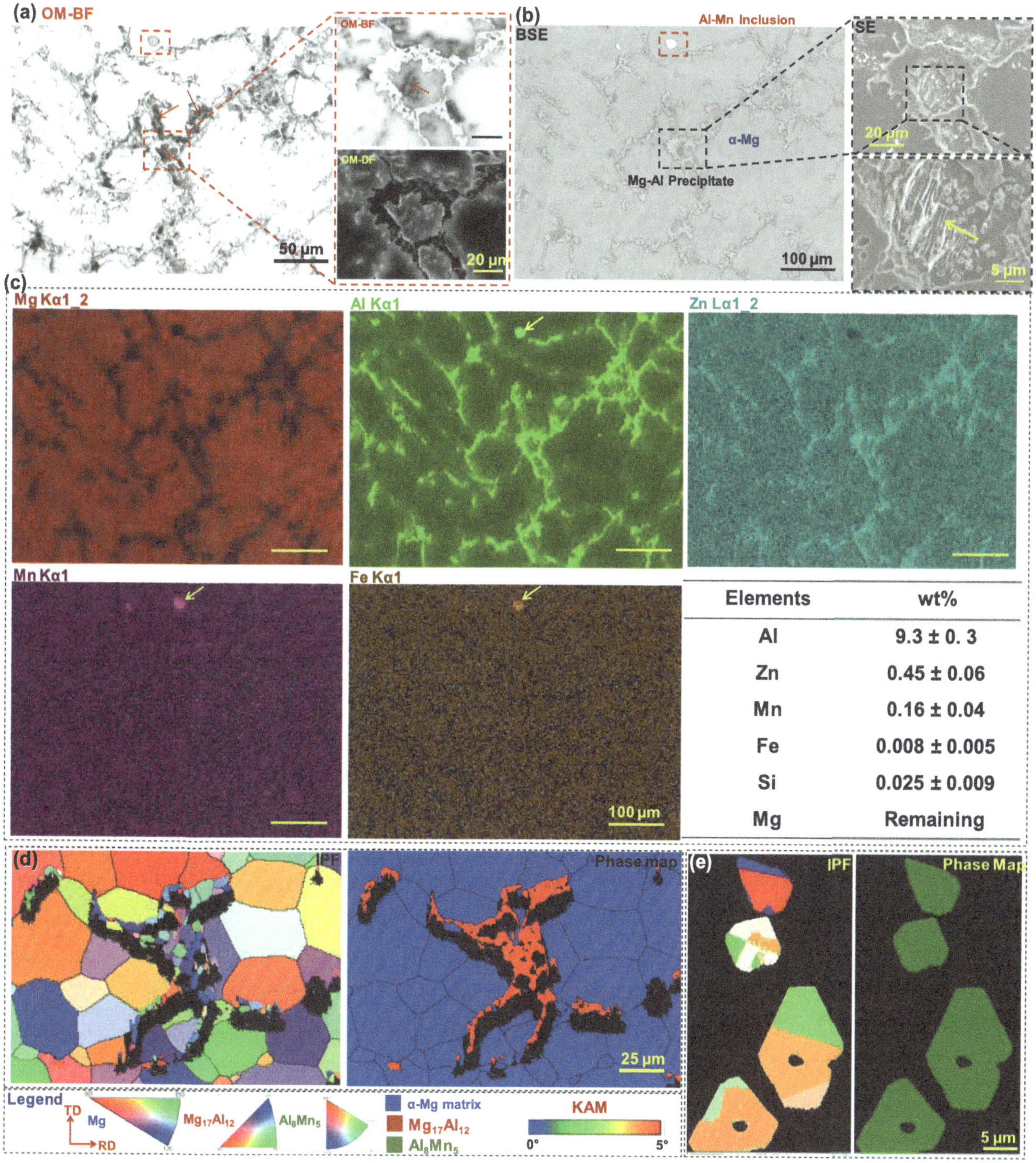

Fig. 6 **a** Optical micrograph (OM)-bright filed (BF) image, **b** SE micrograph, **c** EDS map of Mg, Al, Zn, Mn and Fe. **d**, **e** EBSD maps of $Mg_{17}Al_{12}$/α-Mg matrix and Al_8Mn_5 particle, respectively

strain localization without dislocation movement (Song et al. 2018). Further, it is evident from the stress–strain behavior of Al_8Mn_5 (Fig. 10a) particle that it exhibits the highest strength and ductility. SEM micrograph of the deformed Al_8Mn_5 pillar (Fig. 9c2) shows slip lines, which manifest as load drops in stress–strain curves (Fig. 10a). Al_8Mn_5 particle exhibits the highest yield strength of ~3084 ± 630 MPa, followed by $Mg_{17}Al_{12}$ with ~814 ± 141 MPa, and α-Mg matrix with ~134 ± 22 MPa.

The site-specific transmission electron microscopy (TEM) of Al_8Mn_5 deformed micro-pillar shows the dislocation structure (shown by the arrow in Fig. 10b). It can be

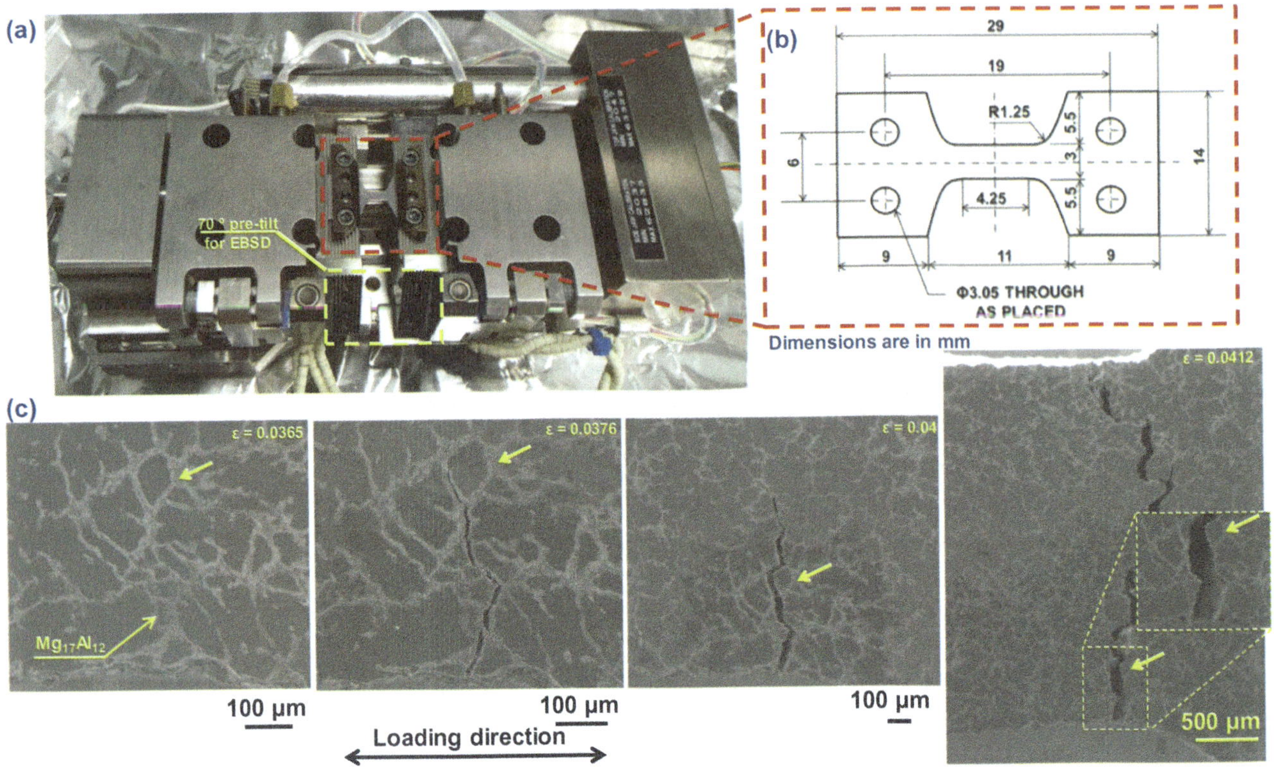

Fig. 7 **a** In-situ tensile testing stage, **b** sample dimension, **c** SEM images showing crack propagation through $Mg_{17}Al_{12}$ precipitates (arrow indicate reference region) in an as-cast sample

noticed that one type of dislocation structure is queued on the slip plane. The selective area diffraction pattern (SADP) along the [100] zone axis is shown in Fig. 10c. The angle between $(01\bar{1})$ and (021) is around 88.7°, which corresponds to the rhombohedral crystal structure (Zeng et al. 2018).

Additionally, to verify the deformation behavior of each phase, qualitative analysis was also performed using nanoindentation. The indentation was performed at 60 mN load for the Al_8Mn_5 particle and 35 mN load for the $Mg_{17}Al_{12}$ particle and the matrix. SEM micrographs, atomic force microscopy (AFM) images, and corresponding line profiles of the indents made on the Al_8Mn_5 particle, the $Mg_{17}Al_{12}$ particle, and the matrix are shown in Fig. 10d–f, respectively. The line profiles along the corner (*C*) to edge (*E*) were used to observe the pile-up and sink-in phenomenon. Line profiles for the Al_8Mn_5 particle clearly show pile-up along all the edges, whereas the $Mg_{17}Al_{12}$ particle does not show pile-up or sink-in along the edges. The α-Mg matrix shows both pile-up and sink-in (indicated in AFM in Fig. 10f). In addition, both pile-up and sink-in were visible along the same edge of the indent (shown in SE micrograph in Fig. 10f). It is already known that the plastically deformable materials show pile-up characteristics (Fischer-Cripps 2004). The observed pile-up's in the case of Al_8Mn_5 particle corroborate with the observation made previously, i.e., the Al_8Mn_5 particles exhibit ductility. In contrast, the absence of pile-up and sink-in in the case of $Mg_{17}Al_{12}$ particles indicates the absence of plastic deformation, which is also evident from micro-pillar compression (Fig. 9).

A couple of studies are available for the bulk deformation of $Mg_{17}Al_{12}$ (Ragani et al. 2011; Fukuchi and Watanabe 1980). However, no study has been carried out to evaluate the stress–strain behavior of Al_8Mn_5 particles. Ragani et al. (2011) fabricated bulk $Mg_{17}Al_{12}$ through levitation casting and measured the room temperature compressive fracture strength and strain to be ~325 MPa and ~2%, respectively. Fukuchi and Watanabe (1980) evaluated the bulk properties of $Mg_{17}Al_{12}$ at elevated temperature (between 360 and 435 °C), where particles were found to exhibit ductility. However, it should be noted that both the studies were carried out in the bulk form, which can show different properties than that at a small length scale. In fact, it has been shown that the mechanical response at large and small length scales might be different (Singh et al. 2015; Michler et al. 2007; Korte and Clegg 2011). In the present case, interestingly, the $Mg_{17}Al_{12}$ particle exhibits distinct behavior at room temperature, i.e., sudden failure after a significant strain burst, unlike the brittle nature reported in the bulk samples (Ragani et al. 2011).

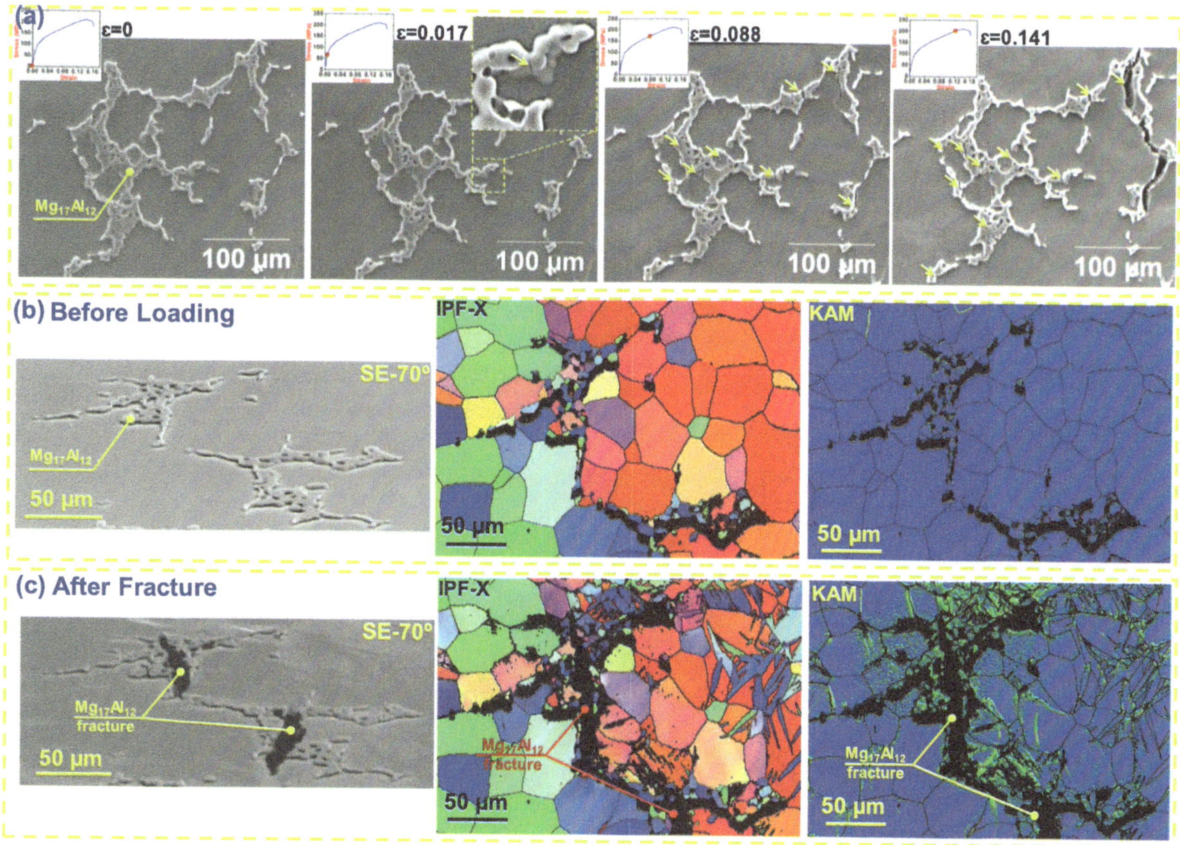

Fig. 8 **a** SEM micrographs of in-situ tensile testing of $Mg_{17}Al_{12}$ at different strain levels along with the stress–strain diagram. SE micrograph and corresponding area IPF-X and KAM map **b** before loading and **c** after fracture. (Loading is along *X* direction). (For legends, refer Fig. 6)

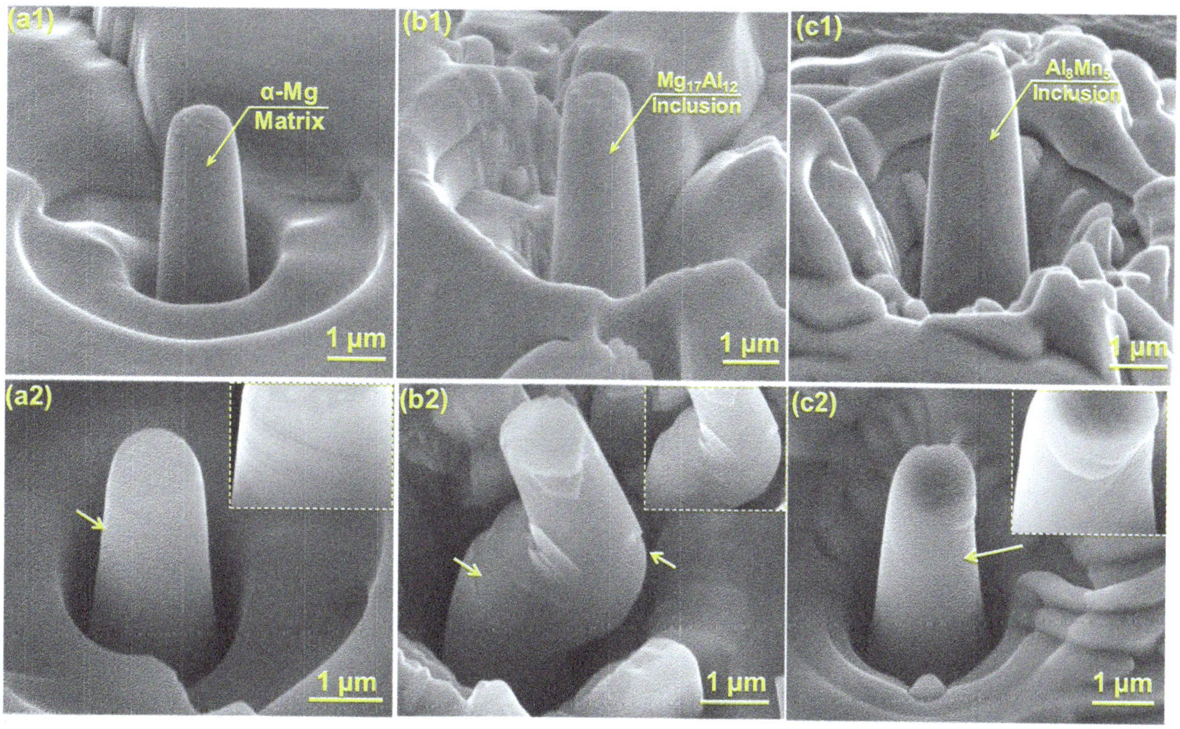

Fig. 9 **a1**, **b1**, **c1** and **a2**, **b2**, **c2** before and after deformation of α-Mg matrix, $Mg_{17}Al_{12}$, and Al_8Mn_5 micro-pillar, respectively (Sarvesha et al. 2020)

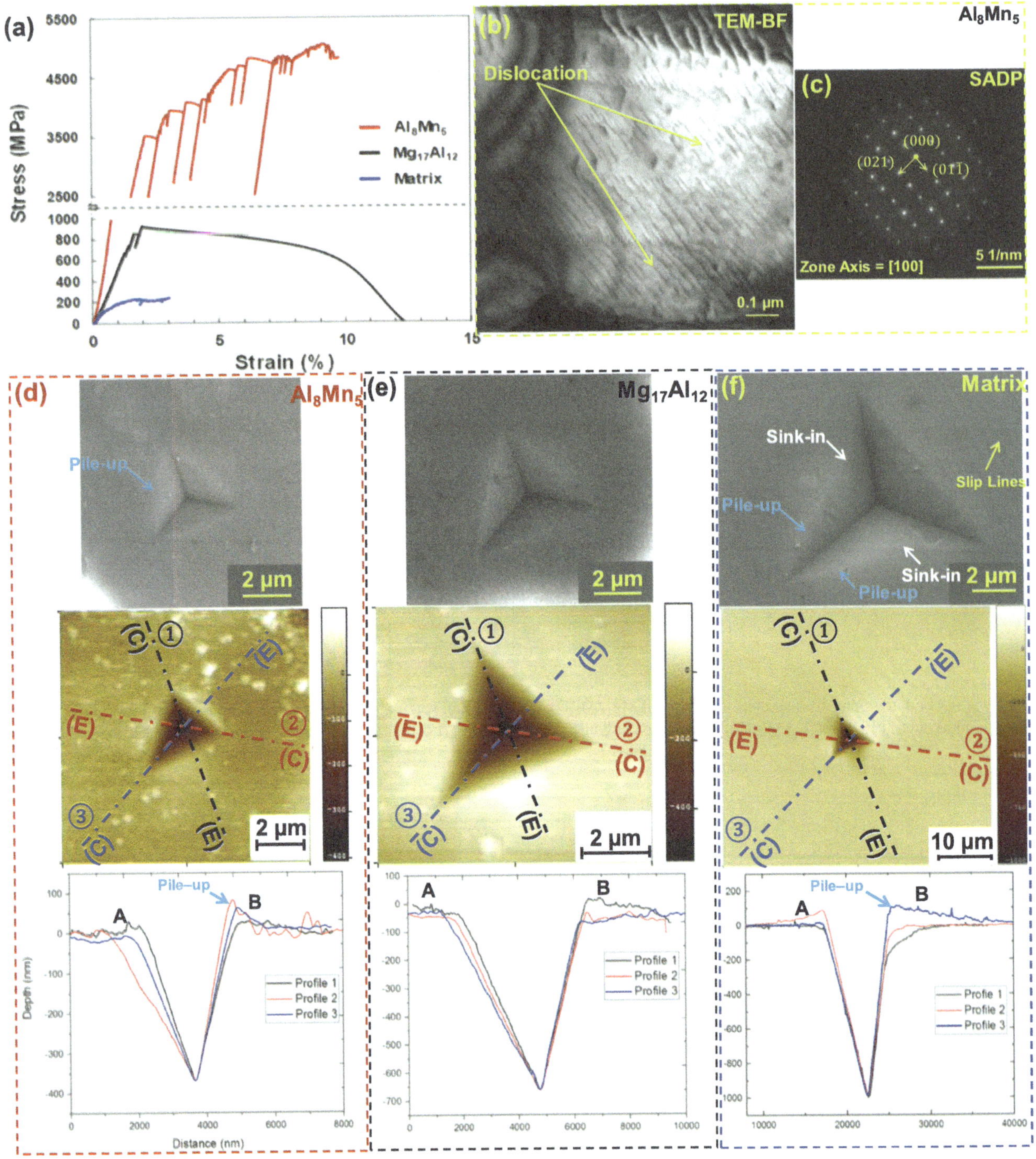

Fig. 10 **a** Stress–strain behavior of the matrix and particles, **b** TEM-BF, and **c** SADP of deformed Al_8Mn_5 pillar. **d–f** are the SE micrographs, AFM images, and line profile of the indents made using nanoindentation on Al_8Mn_5, $Mg_{17}Al_{12}$, and α-Mg matrix, respectively (Sarvesha et al. 2020)

3 Summary

The mechanical properties of materials change significantly with a reduction in size. Due to the inherent problems associated the conventional mechanical testing in understanding the deformation behavior of materials at a small length scale, *in-situ* electron microscopy has gained interest in recent years. The advancement in instrumentation in the electron microscopes, such as FIB and nanoindentation in SEM, has made it possible to understand the deformation behavior in real time. Also, techniques such as EBSD/ECCI/DIC assist in the quantification of the deformation characteristics of the materials. The present article shows the importance of electron microscopy in understanding the deformation behavior of metallic systems by using three case studies.

Acknowledgements SSS would like to thank Prof. Nikhilesh Chawla at Arizona State University for his valuable suggestions on case studies I and II. Authors also acknowledge the support of ACMS facility, IIT Kanpur, and Prof. Jayant Jain, IIT Delhi, for case study III.

References

Fischer-Cripps AC (2004) Nanoindentation, 2nd ed. Springer, New York

Armstrong DEJ, Hardie CD, Gibson JSKL, Bushby AJ, Edmondson PD, Roberts SG (2015) Small-scale characterisation of irradiated nuclear materials: part II nanoindentation and micro-cantilever testing of ion irradiated nuclear materials. J Nucl Mater 462:374–381

Blawert C, Hort N, Kainer KU (2004) Automotive applications of magnesium and its alloys. Trans Indian Inst Metals 57(4):12

Bucci RJ, Warren CJ, Starke EA Jr (2000) Need for new materials in aging aircraft structures. J Aircr 37(1):122–129

Dimiduk DM, Uchic MD, Parthasarathy TA (2005) Size-affected single-slip behavior of pure nickel microcrystals. Acta Mater 53 (15):4065–4077

Dunn BD (1987) Eur Space Agency (ESA) J 11:1

Fukuchi M, Watanabe K (1980) Tensile behavior of γ-phase in Al-Mg system at elevated temperatures. J Japan Inst Light Metals 30 (5):253–257

Galyon GT (2005) Annotated tin whisker bibliography and anthology. IEEE Trans Electron Pack Manuf 28(1):94–122

Gianolaet DS (2011) In situ nanomechanical testing in focused ion beam and scanning electron microscopes. Rev Sci Instrum 82 (6):063901

Guo E-Y, Singh SS, Xie H, Williams JJ, Jing T, Chawla N (2014) Microstructure-based modeling of deformation in steels based on constitutive relationships from micropillar compression. Steel Res Int 85(6):946–953

Han JH, Saif MTA (2006) In-situ microtensile stage for electromechanical characterization of nanoscale freestanding films. Rev Sci Instrum 77(4):045102

Han JH, Rajagopalan J, Saif MTA (2007) MEMS-based testing stage to study electrical and mechanical properties of nanocrystalline metal films. In: MEMS/MOEMS components and their applications IV, vol 6464, p 64640C

Kim J, Plancher E, Tasan CC (2020) Hydrogenation-induced lattice expansion and its effects on hydrogen diffusion and damage in Ti–6Al–4V. Acta Mater 188:686–696

Korte S, Clegg WJ (2011) Discussion of the dependence of the effect of size on the yield stress in hard materials studied by microcompression of MgO. Phil Mag 91(7–9):1150–1162

Kulekci MK (2008) Magnesium and its alloys applications in automotive industry. Int J Adv Manuf Technol 39(9–10):851–865

Laplanche G, Bonneville J, Joulain A, Gauthier-Brunet V, Dubois S (2014) Mechanical properties of Al-Cu-Fe quasi crystalline and crystalline phases: an analogy. Intermetallics 50:54–58

Legros M, Gianola DS, Motz C (2010) Quantitative in-situ mechanical testing in electron microscopes. MRS Bull 35:354–360

Lü YZ, Wang QD, Ding WJ, Zeng XQ, Zhu YP (2000) Fracture behavior of AZ91 magnesium alloy. Mater Lett 44(5):265–268

Lugo M, Jordon JB, Horstemeyer MF, Tschopp MA, Harris J, Gokhale AM (2011) Quantification of damage evolution in a 7075 aluminum alloy using an acoustic emission technique. Mater Sci Eng A 528(22–23):6708–6714

Maire E, Zhou S, Adrien J, Dimichiel M (2011) Damage quantification in aluminium alloys using in situ tensile tests in X-ray tomography. Eng Fract Mech 78(15):2679–2690

Mathew S, Osterman M, Pecht M, Dunlevey F (2009) Evaluation of pure tin plated copper alloy substrates for tin whiskers. Circuit World 35(1):3–8

Michler J, Wasmer K, Meier S, Östlund F, Leifer K (2007) Plastic deformation of gallium arsenide micropillars under uniaxial compression at room temperature. Appl Phys Lett 90(4):043123

Muñoz-Palos JM, del Cristina MC, Adeva P (1996) Synthesis of Mg_2Si powder by mechanical alloying and its consolidation. Mater Trans Japan Inst Metals Mater 37(10):1602–1606

Östlund F (2011) Ductile-brittle transition in micropillar compression of GaAs at room temperature. Phil Mag 91(7–9):1190–1199

Östlundet F (2009) Brittle-to-ductile transition in uniaxial compression of silicon pillars at room temperature. Adv Func Mater 19 (15):2439–2444

Oswald LE (2003) Effects of microstructure on high-cycle fatigue of an Al-Zn-Mg-Cu Alloy (Al-7055). Masters thesis, School of Engineering, University of Pittsburgh, Pittsburgh, PA

Payne J, Welsh G, Christ RJ Jr, Nardiello J, Papazian JM (2010) Observations of fatigue crack initiation in 7075–T651. Int J Fatigue 32(2):247–255

Pearson S (1975) Initiation of fatigue cracks in commercial aluminium alloys and the subsequent propagation of very short cracks. Eng Fract Mech 7(2):235–240

Powell BE, Skove MJ (2004) Elastic strength of tin whiskers in tensile tests. J Appl Phys 36(4):1495

Proff C, Abolhassani S, Dadras MM, Lemaignan C (2010) In-situ oxidation of zirconium binary alloys by environmental SEM and analysis by AFM, FIB, and TEM. J Nucl Mater 404(2):97–108

Ragani J, Donnadieu P, Tassin C, Blandin JJ (2011) High-temperature deformation of the γ-$Mg_{17}Al_{12}$ complex metallic alloy. Scripta Mater 65(3):253–256

Sarvesha R, Ghori U-R, Chiu YL, Jones IP, Singh SS, Jain J (2020) Mechanical property evaluation of second phase particles in a Mg-8Al-0.5Zn alloy using micropillar compression. Mater Sci Eng A 775:138973

Sarvesha R, Chalapathi D, Yadava M, Singh SS (2021) *In-situ* studies on deformation and fracture characteristics of AZ91 Mg alloy. Materialia 18:101177. https://doi.org/10.1016/j.mtla.2021.101177

Schneider AS, Kiener D, Yakacki CM, Maier HJ, Gruber PA, Tamura N, Kunz M, Minor AM, Frick CP (2013) Influence of bulk pre-straining on the size effect in nickel compression pillars. Mater Sci Eng A 559:147–158

Singh SS, Sarkar R, Xie H-X, Mayer Rajagopalan CJ, Chawla N (2014) Tensile behavior of single-crystal tin whiskers. J Electron Mater 43 (4):978–982

Singh SS, Williams JJ, Hruby P, Xiao X, De Carlo F, Chawla N (2014) In-situ experimental techniques to study the mechanical behavior of materials using X-ray synchrotron tomography. Integr Mater Manuf Innov 3(1):109–122

Singh SS, Schwartzstein C, Williams JJ, Xiao X, De Carlo F, Chawla N (2014c) 3D microstructural characterization and mechanical properties of constituent particles in Al 7075 alloys using X-ray synchrotron tomography and nanoindentation. J Alloy Compd 602:163–174

Singh SS, Guo E, Xie H, Chawla N (2015) Mechanical properties of intermetallic inclusions in Al 7075 alloys by micropillar compression. Intermetallics 62:69–75

Singh SS, Williams JJ, Stannard TJ, Xiao X, Carlo FD, Chawla N (2016) Measurement of localized corrosion rates at inclusion particles in AA7075 by In-Situ three-dimensional (3D) X-ray synchrotron tomography. Corros Sci 104:330–335

Singh SS, Stannard TJ, Xiao X, Chawla N (2017) In Situ X-ray microtomography of stress corrosion cracking and corrosion fatigue in aluminum alloys. JOM 69(8):1404–1414

Slama MBH, Maloufi N, Guyon J, Bahi S, Weiss L, Guitton A (2019) In-Situ macroscopic tensile testing in SEM and electron channeling contrast imaging: pencil glide evidenced in a bulk β-$Ti_2$1S polycrystal. Material 12(15):2479

Song G, Kong T, Dusoe KJ, Canfield PC, Lee S-W (2018) Shear localization and size-dependent strength of YCd_6 quasicrystal approximant at the micrometer length scale. J Mater Sci 53 (9):6980–6990

Starke EA, Staley JT (2011) 24—application of modern aluminium alloys to aircraft. In: Lumley R (ed) Fundamentals of aluminium metallurgy. Woodhead Publishing, pp 747–783

Takeuchi S, Hashimoto T, Suzuki K (1996) Plastic deformation of Mg_2Si with the C1 structure. Intermetallics 4(Suppl. 1):S147–S150

Uchic MD, Dimiduk DM, Florando JN, Nix WD (2004) Sample dimensions influence strength and crystal plasticity. Science 305 (5686):986–989

Volkert CA, Donohue A, Spaepen F (2008) Effect of sample size on deformation in amorphous metals. J Appl Phys 103:083539

Wang L, Qin XY, Xiong W, Zhu XG (2007) Fabrication and mechanical properties of bulk nanocrystalline intermetallic Mg_2Si. Mater Sci Eng A 459(1–2):216–222

Weiland H, Nardiello J, Zaefferer S, Cheong S, Papazian J, Raabe D (2009) Microstructural aspects of crack nucleation during cyclic loading of AA7075-T651. Eng Fract Mech 76(5):709–714

Wisner B, Cabal M, Vanniamparambil PA, Hochhalter J, Leser WP, Kontsos A (2015) In-situ microscopic investigation to validate acoustic emission monitoring. Exp Mech 55(9):1705–1715

Xue Y, El Kadiri H, Horstemeyer MF, Jordon JB, Weiland H (2007) Micromechanisms of multistage fatigue crack growth in a high-strength aluminum alloy. Acta Mater 55(6):1975–1984

Yakubtsov IA, Diak BJ, Sager CA, Bhattacharya B, MacDonald WD, Niewczas M (2008) Effects of heat treatment on microstructure and tensile deformation of Mg AZ80 alloy at room temperature. Mater Sci Eng A 496(1–2):247–255

Zeng G, Xian JW, Gourlay CM (2018) Nucleation and growth crystallography of Al_8Mn_5 on B_2-Al(Mn, Fe) in AZ91 magnesium alloys. Acta Mater 153:364–376

Zindal A, Jain J, Prasad R, Singh SS, Cizek P (2017) Correlation of grain boundary precipitate characteristics with fracture and fracture toughness in an Mg-8Al-0.5 Zn alloy. Mater Sci Eng A 706:192–200

Zindal A, Jain J, Prasad R, Singh SS, Sarvesha R, Cizek P, Barnett MR (2018) Effect of heat treatment variables on the formation of precipitate free zones (PFZs) in Mg-8Al-0.5Zn alloy. Mater Charact 136:175–182

Exploring Carbon Surface Using Electron Microscopy: Applications to Energy, Environment, and Health

Priyanka Gupta and Nishith Verma

1 Introduction

Carbon is undoubtedly one of the most versatile elements known to mankind. The ability of the material to form a diverse hybridization and bonding with different elements gives rise to its excellent chemical and physical properties such as high thermal and chemical stabilities, good electrical and thermal conductivities, and a high surface area. Carbon can also bind with itself in different ways, forming various nanostructures. The unique and tuneable characteristics of carbon nanomaterials have provided us an opportunity to use them in many areas, for example, energy storage devices, wastewater remediation, biofertilizers, biosensors, biomedical devices, and air pollution control.

Carbon fibers are a relatively newer material and show various interesting morphologies at micron and nanoscales. In recent times, activated carbon microfiber (ACF) has drawn attention of research community because of the microporous structure of the material possessing a high surface area (1200–1800 m^2/g). Additionally, the narrow diameters (usually 10–20 μm) of the fibers exert a negligible external mass transfer diffusion resistance, when the material is used under practical (flow) conditions. Various functional groups such as ketonic, carboxylic, and hydroxyl present on the ACF surface are also responsible for the high catalytic activity of the material. Furthermore, the catalytic activity of ACF can be enhanced by functionalizing it with various metals.

Recent studies have introduced carbon nanofibers (CNFs) grown on the ACF substrate using catalytic chemical vapor deposition (CVD) (Yadav and Verma 2017; Kumar et al. 2020; Bairagi and Verma 2018; Ashfaq et al. 2017). The CNFs are cylindrical-shaped nanostructures with stacked graphene layers. Such nanostructures with extraordinary chemical and physical properties have been efficiently used as adsorbents and catalysts. The multiscale structured composite of ACFs and the graphitic CNFs has found applications in H_2-storage, plant growth, biosensors, and medical treatments.

Electron microscopy has emerged as a powerful tool for examining the material surface morphologies. Scanning electron microscopy (SEM) can provide information about the texture of carbonaceous materials, including macropores, shape of nanostructures, grain size, and the presence of metal nanoparticles (NPs) dispersed in the ACFs/CNFs. The high-resolution, and low and high magnification SEM images can be used for visually examining the samples. Transmission electron microscopy (TEM) is another analytical tool to examine the material surface, especially its internal texture. TEM can provide the size and shape of micro-nanofibers along with the other micro-nanostructures present in the material. High-resolution (HR) TEM can be used to provide information about the diffraction patterns, crystal planes, fringe width, graphitic characteristics, and different phases present in the carbonaceous materials. We first showcase the different applications of the ACF/CNF-based materials developed in our research laboratory and then discuss the material texture recorded using electron microscopy, and how the SEM/TEM images are extremely useful in understanding the carbon surface.

2 ACF/CNF as a H_2-storage Material

Recent research on energy has primarily focused on finding non-conventional sources of energy because of continuous depletion of fossil fuels globally. Hydrogen is a clean, renewable, and an abundantly available source of energy. Its efficient and safe storage is, however, a concern. Recently, Yadav and Verma (2017) have developed an efficient H_2-storage material based on the multiscale structured

P. Gupta · N. Verma (✉)
Department of Chemical Engineering and Centre for Environmental Science and Engineering, Indian Institute of Technology Kanpur, Kanpur, 208016, India
e-mail: nishith@iitk.ac.in

K. Biswas et al. (eds.), *Electron Microscopy in Science and Engineering*, IITK Directions 6,
https://doi.org/10.1007/978-981-16-5101-4_3

composite of ACF and CNF. The composite is dispersed with the nickel (Ni) and ceria (CeO_2) NPs. Briefly, the acid-pretreated ACF samples are impregnated using an aqueous solution of $Ni(NO_3)_2$ and $Ce(NO_3)_3$. The bimetals-impregnated ACFs are subjected to calcination and H_2-reduction, followed by CVD. The prepared Ni-CeO_2-ACF/CNF show a remarkable H_2-adsorption capacity of 1.36% (w/w) at 200 °C and 1 bar (Fig. 1). Furthermore, complete desorption of H_2 is possible at 300 °C, indicating regeneration of the proposed H_2 storage material to be energy-efficient.

3 Carbon Nanofibrous Beads for Desulfurization

Combustion of diesel, used as a fuel in transportation, generates a significant amount of SO_2, a major atmospheric air pollutants Decomposition of the sulfur (S) containing compounds, viz. thiophene and dibenzothiophene (DBT), also deactivates the catalyst used in the catalytic converters of automobiles, thereby decreasing its overall life (Ai et al. 2012). Recently, carbon nanofibrous beads have emerged as a promising material for the adsorptive desulfurization (ADS) process (Prajapati and Verma 2017). Micron-sized materials of ~0.8 mm size can serve as an efficient packed bed material, without channeling or maldistribution in flow of the liquid to be treated, unlike their counterpart powdery materials. The beads also allow an easy recovery and regeneration post-treatment. Prajapati and Verma (2017) have synthesized the activated carbon beads (ACBs) decorated with Ni-CNF as an efficient adsorbent for ADS. Figure 2 shows a schematics of the experimental setup used for ADS, along with the representative batch adsorption data for thiophene and DBT on NiO/ACBs and Ni-CNF/ACBs. The data shows dependence of the adsorption capacities of the materials on their pore volumes. Ni-CNF/ACBs show a higher adsorption capacity for thiophene, compared to NiO/ACBs. Ni-CNF/ACBs with small pore volume allow adsorption of the relatively smaller-sized thiophene molecules. On the other hand, adsorption of DBT is found to be higher in NiO/ACBs. The relatively small pore volume in Ni-CNF/ACB is inadequate for adsorption of the large-sized DBT molecules, whereas NiO/ACBs having a large pore volume show a high adsorption capacity for DBT.

4 Cu-CNF/ACF as an Adsorbent for Cr(VI) and Micronutrient for Plants

Agricultural fields and water bodies are gradually contaminated by industrial effluents despite stringent regulations in place globally. Toxic metals such as As(III), As(V), Cr(VI), Pb(II), and Cd(II) are common aqueous pollutants. Uptake of the metals from soil by plants can interfere with their physiological processes, adversely affecting their growth. A physical mixture of carbon micro- and nanofibers-based materials has been indicated to be an efficient adsorbent or scavenger of metals in soil, besides a good translocator of the micronutrients including Cu from soil to plant roots and shoots (Kumar et al. 2020; Bairagi and Verma 2018). Kumar et al. (2020) prepared Cu-CNFs grown over the ACFs to scavenge Cr(VI) in soil and simultaneously supply essential nutrients (Cu in this case) to the chickpea plant (Fig. 3). The prepared materials also increased root and shoot lengths significantly. As shown in the figure, Cu-CNF/ACF was ball milled to separate Cu-CNF from ACF. An aqueous dispersion of Cu-CNF and ACF was then mixed in a Cr-stressed medium for germination of chickpea seeds. Plant growth was monitored, and it was found that Cr(VI) was adsorbed on ACF, while the nanosized Cu-CNFs were translocated from soil to the plant roots and shoots, supplying essential micronutrients to the plants.

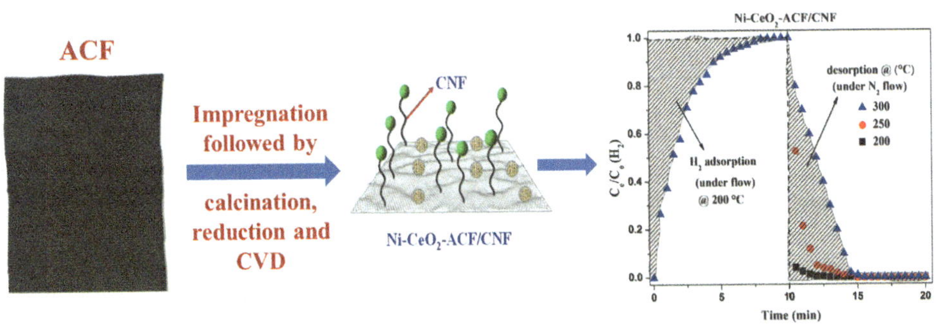

Fig. 1 Schematic representation of the Ni-CeO_2-ACF/CNF storage material and its H_2-adsorption/H_2-desorption characteristics under flow conditions (Yadav and Verma 2017)

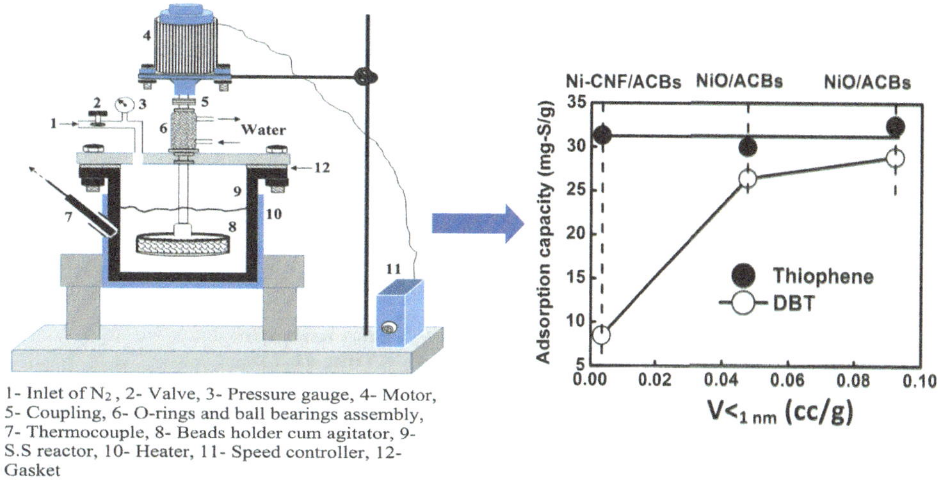

Fig. 2 Schematic illustration of the experimental setup used for the ADS tests and the adsorption capacities (mg S/g) of NiO/ACBs and Ni-CNF/ACBs determined for thiophene and DBT (Prajapati and Verma 2017)

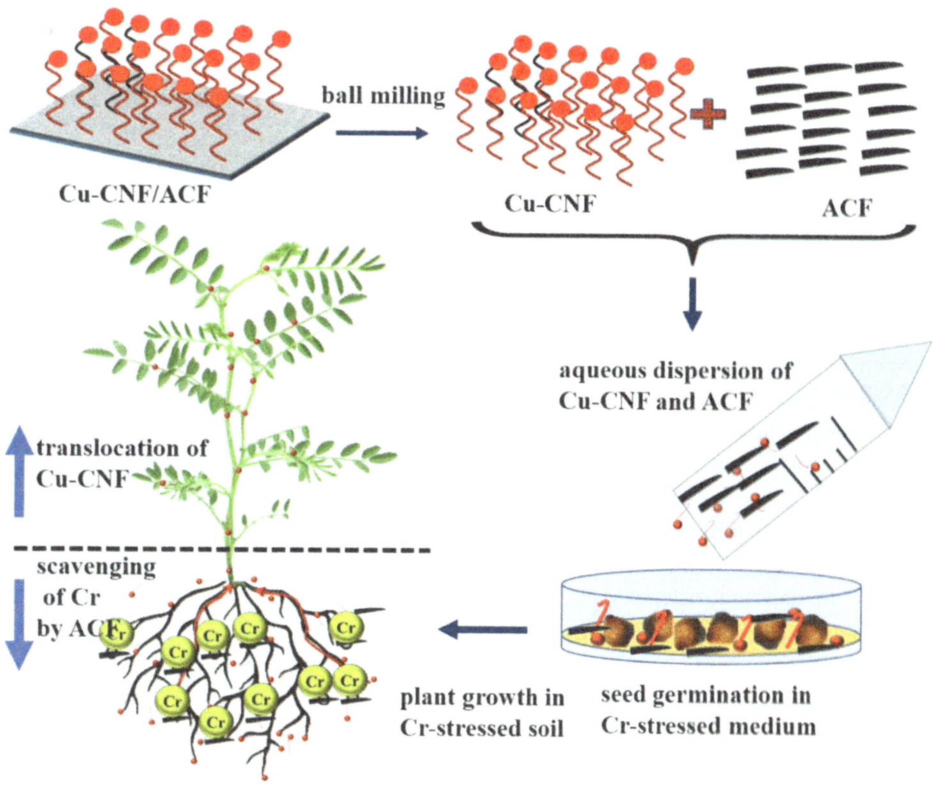

Fig. 3 Graphical representation showing the working principle of a physical mixture of Cu-CNF and ACF for growth of plants with simultaneous removal of Cr (VI) from aqueous soil (Kumar et al. 2020)

5 Cu/Ni-CNF as an Electrochemical Sensor for Cholesterol

Development of a sensor for detecting various biomarkers in blood, with a fast response, good reproducibility, and high sensitivity and selectivity is challenging (Li et al. 2010). Interestingly, Bairagi and Verma (2018) have successfully synthesized the dendritic nanofibers of polymethyl orange (PMO) over Cu/Ni-CNF, as the BMCP electrode, to measure cholesterol in human blood (Fig. 4). PMO, electropolymerized on BMCP using the methyl orange (MO) monomer, serves as the recognition element for cholesterol. Electropolymerization was performed using cyclic voltammetry from −1.0 to 1.0 V. Differential pulse voltammetry (DPV) was used to measure response of the prepared biosensor. The calibration plot (currents vs. cholesterol concentrations) showed a remarkable linearity ($R^2 = 0.999$) over a large concentration range (0.04–600 mg/dL).

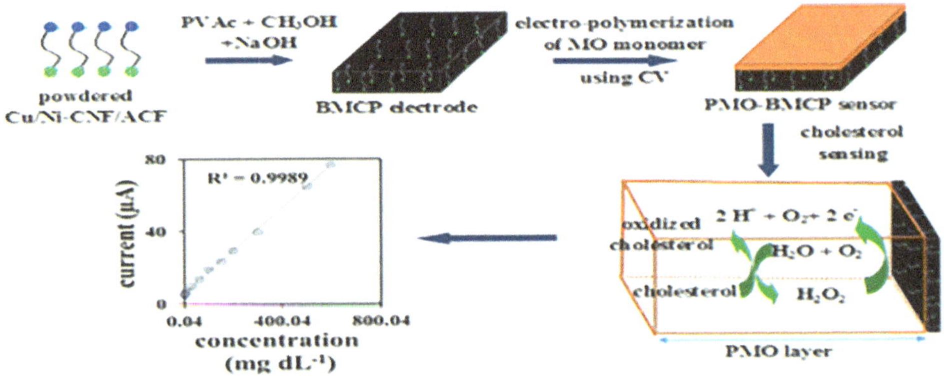

Fig. 4 Schematic illustration of the preparation steps for the BMCP sensor and the calibration plot for cholesterol sensing (Bairagi and Verma 2018)

6 Cu/Zn-ACF/CNF as a Wound Dressing Material

Growing resistance of wound bacteria toward clinical drugs has prompted the development of an effective and site-specific antibacterial therapy or dressing. The Cu and Zn metal NPs, well recognized for their antibacterial properties, can be used for wound treatment with effective deployment techniques. Ashaq et al. (2017) have prepared an efficient wound dressing biomaterial to cure bacterial infections caused by burn, surgery, and injuries. A polyvinyl alcohol (PVA) and cellulose acetate phthalate (CAP) precursor-based polymeric composite film was prepared using suspension polymerization. Cu/Zn-ACF/CNF was separately prepared. The ball-milled Cu/Zn-ACF/CNF was dispersed in an aqueous solution of CAP, and the prepared slurry was added to the polymerization reaction mixture of PVA at incipience of the gel formation (Fig. 5). The prepared polymer–metal–carbon (PMC) composite was mixed with DI water, and the mixture was cast on a Teflon sheet to prepare the dressing material. The material was found to be effective against bacterial dissemination by disrupting the bacterial cell membrane, besides enhancing platelet activation and the blood clotting abilities leading to rapid wound healing.

7 Materials Synthesis

The phenolic resin precursor-based ACF, procured from Kynol, Japan, is pretreated using 0.05 M HNO_3 at 80 °C for 2 h. The acid treatment removes impurities such as chlorides and nitrates, if any, from the ACF surface. The acid-treated ACFs are washed multiple times with DI water until pH of the ACF surface is ~7. Next, the ACF samples are dried in a vacuum oven at 200 °C for 12 h to remove moisture and any trapped gases. The ACFs are impregnated with the aqueous solutions of different metal salts, viz. $Ni(NO_3)_2$, $Ce(NO_3)_3$, $Cu(NO_3)_2$, and $Zn(NO_3)_2$, depending upon the applications. The salt-impregnated ACF samples are dried overnight at room temperature (~30 °C). The dried samples are calcined at 400 °C in an inert atmosphere (N_2) to convert the metal nitrates to metal oxides. The calcined samples are

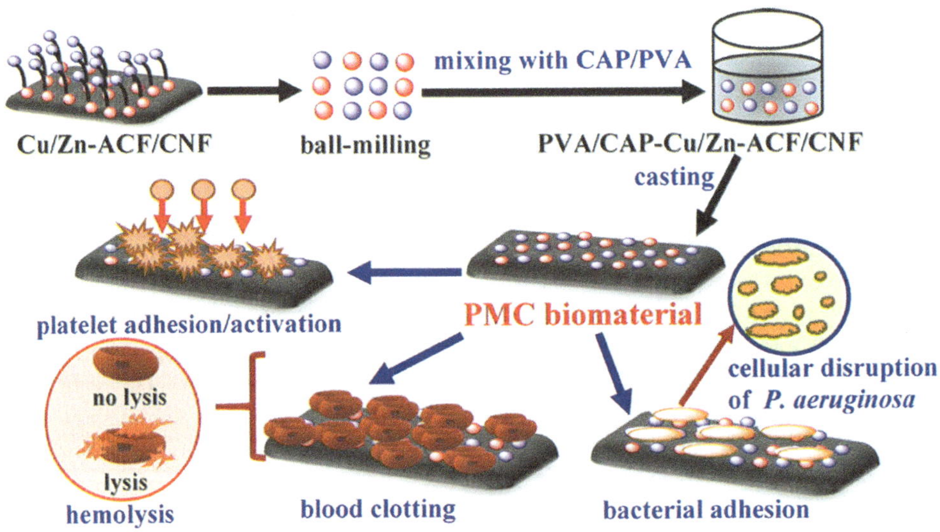

Fig. 5 Schematic representation of the preparation steps for the PMC wound dressing material and its application (Ashfaq et al. 2017)

subjected to the H_2-reduction at suitable temperatures, depending on the types of the impregnated metal salts. The reduction step results in conversion of metal oxides to their elemental form. CNFs are grown on the metal–ACF samples using CVD with acetylene as the carbon source and the metal NPs dispersed in the ACFs acting as the CVD catalyst.

The phenolic resin beads are synthesized using suspension polymerization. The reaction mixture includes 50 mL phenol as the monomer, 63 mL formaldehyde as the solvent, and 2 mL triethylamine (TEA) as the catalyst. Hexamethylenetetramine (HMTA) is used as the cross-linking agent, and PVA is added as the suspension stabilizing agent. The metal salts are added to the reaction mixture at incipience of the bead formation. The phenolic beads are subjected to carbonization and steam activation at 900 °C for 2 and 1 h, respectively, in N_2 atmosphere. The activation step creates porosity in the material. The activated beads are subjected to the H_2-reduction, and CNFs are grown over the porous activated beads by the CVD process. The detailed procedure is described in our study (Prajapati and Verma 2017).

8 Material Surface Characterization (SEM/TEM)

Surface morphology of the prepared materials was examined using the field emission scanning electron microscope (FE-SEM–MIRA3 series, TESCAN). The SEM images were captured using an in-lens detector at the accelerating voltage of 10 kV, filament current of 2.37 A, and working distance of 2–4 mm.

Figure 6 shows the SEM images of the materials tested for H_2-storage: ACF, Ni-CeO_2/ACF, and Ni-CeO_2-ACF/CNF. The low magnification image shows ACF fibers to be cylindrically shaped (Fig. 6a). Approximately uniform-sized micropores can be seen in the high magnification image (Fig. 6b). Figure 6 shows the shiny Ni and CeO_2 nanoparticles in the micropores of the ACF surface. An approximately uniform and dense growth of CNFs can be seen in Fig. 6c, c′. Shiny metal NPs located at the tips of CNFs corroborate the tip growth mechanism of the material (Zheng et al. 2004). The CNFs augment exposure of the metal NPs to the surrounding medium. The increased exposure enhances the H_2-adsorption capacity of Ni-CeO_2-ACF/CNF.

Figure 7 presents the HR-TEM images of Ni-CeO_2-ACF/CNF. The TEM image shows metal NP (dark spot) at the tips of CNFs (Fig. 7a). Figure 7b shows the selected area diffraction pattern of the Ni NP. The three distinct diffraction rings represent the (1 1 1), (2 0 0), and (2 2 0) crystal planes in the Ni NP. Crystallinity of the Ni NP and graphitic characteristics of the CNFs were confirmed by the presence of fringes (Fig. 7c). The fringe width was calculated to be 0.176 and 0.334 nm corresponding to the (2 0 0) crystal plane of Ni and (1 1 1) plane of carbon, respectively (Fig. 7d). The metal NPs catalytically dissociate H_2 to H atoms at the CNF edges, which migrate and diffuse into the porous carbon substrate. Therefore, the spillover effect results in the enhanced adsorption of H_2 in Ni-CeO_2-ACF/CNF (Kim et al. 2008).

The SEM images of Ni-CNF/ACB, used as an adsorbent in ADS, are presented in Fig. 8. Figure 8a shows an approximately dense and uniform growth of CNFs over the Ni-CNF/ACB bead. The average size of Ni-CNF/ACB is measured to be ~0.8 mm. The CNFs are cylindrically shaped structures. The average diameter of the CNFs was measured to be 70 nm. Shiny dots at the tips of CNFs represent a Ni NP (Fig. 8b), which also indicates the tip growth mechanism during CVD. Ni NPs plays an important role in desulfurization via direct Ni-S interaction. A graphitic characteristic of CNFs enhances adsorption capacity of the material via π-π and/or hydrophobic interactions between the graphitic planes of CNFs and the thiophene molecules. The porous Ni-CNF/ACBs with an augmented exposure of Ni adsorb thiophene and DBT in diesel efficiently, with the adsorption capacities determined to be 62.3 and 8.1 mg S/g, respectively. Approximately dense growth of the CNFs over ACB and the location of Ni NPs at the tips of CNFs can be confirmed from the SEM analysis. Clearly, the images provide a visual understanding of how the CNFs augment the exposure of the Ni NPs, enhancing the interactions of the thiophene and DBT molecules with the Ni NPs.

Figure 9 shows the SEM images of Cu-CNF/ACF. As mentioned earlier, the material was used in its dual role: as a provider of the Cu micronutrient to plant and a scavenger of Cr(VI) in soil. Figure 9a corroborates the micron-sized ACF substrate containing micropores. Figure 9b corroborates an approximately uniform growth of CNFs on ACF using Cu as the CVD catalyst. The CNF growth using Cu as the CVD catalyst also followed the tip growth mechanism with the Cu NPs located at the tips of the CNFs, similar to the earlier case using Ni as the catalyst (Fig. 6c'). A small size and the negatively charged surface of CNFs facilitated their translocation in plant shoots through xylem. Broken cell compartments were clearly observed in the shoots of plant grown in Cr environment without providing any treatment (Fig. 9d). The intact cellular structure observed in Fig. 9e implies that ACF effectively scavenged Cr by adsorption and prevented it from disrupting the plasma cell membrane of plant. Figure 9f, g confirms that the CNFs and Cu NPs were efficiently translocated to the plant shoots, which acted as the micronutrient and promoted plant growth. Effectiveness of Cu-CNF and ACF can be directly gauged by monitoring plant growth, while the SEM analysis clearly provides an explanation for the plant growth on cellular level (Gupta et al. 2019).

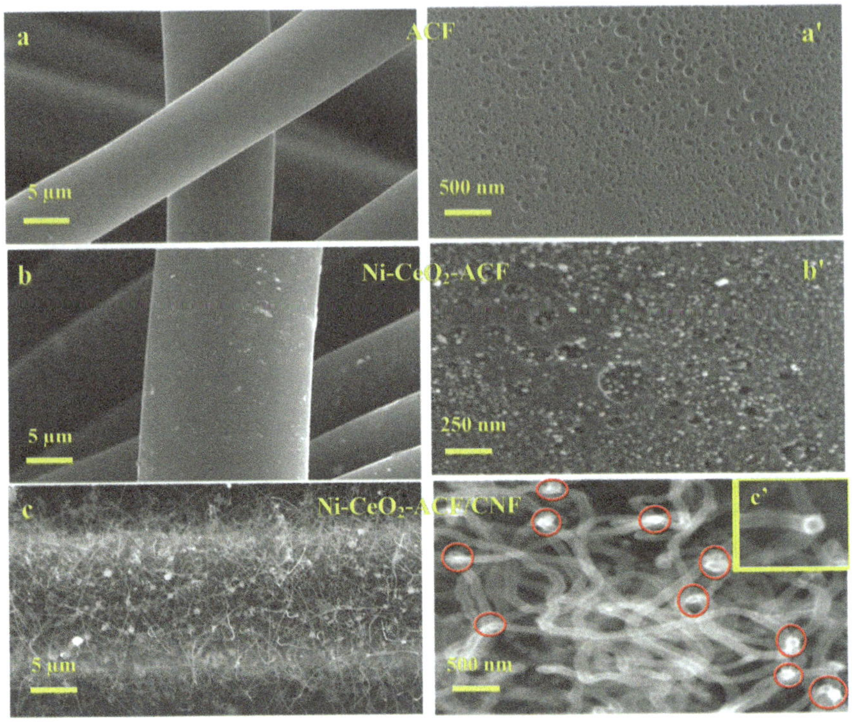

Fig. 6 SEM images at low and high magnifications of **a**, **a′** ACF, **b**, **b′** Ni-CeO_2/ACF, and **c**, **c′** Ni-CeO_2-ACF/CNF (Yadav and Verma 2017)

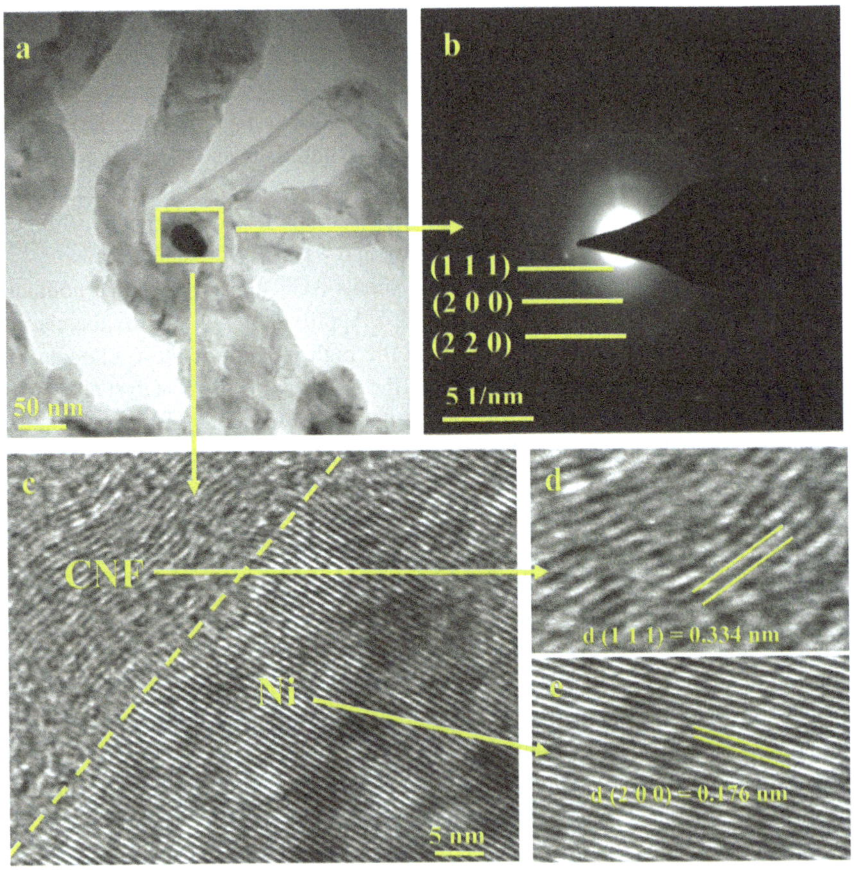

Fig. 7 **a** TEM image of CNF, **b** selected area diffraction pattern of Ni crystal, **c**, **d** fringes present in Ni NPs and CNFs and their corresponding fringe widths (Yadav and Verma 2017)

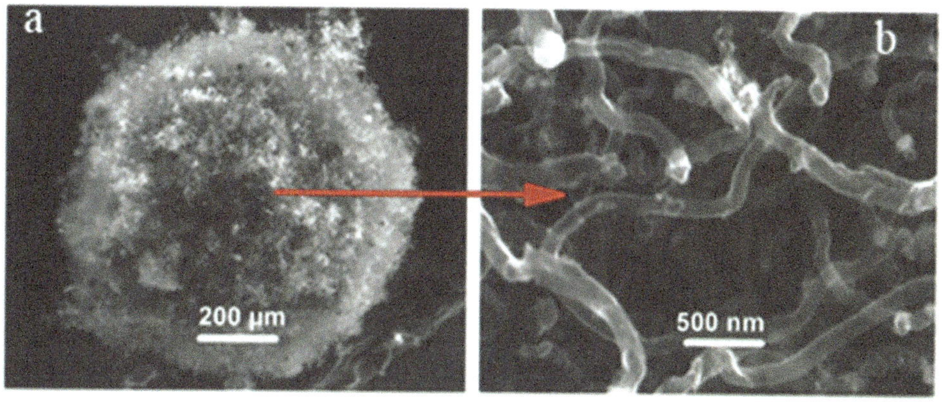

Fig. 8 SEM images of Ni-CNF/ACB at **a** low and **b** high magnifications (Prajapati and Verma 2017)

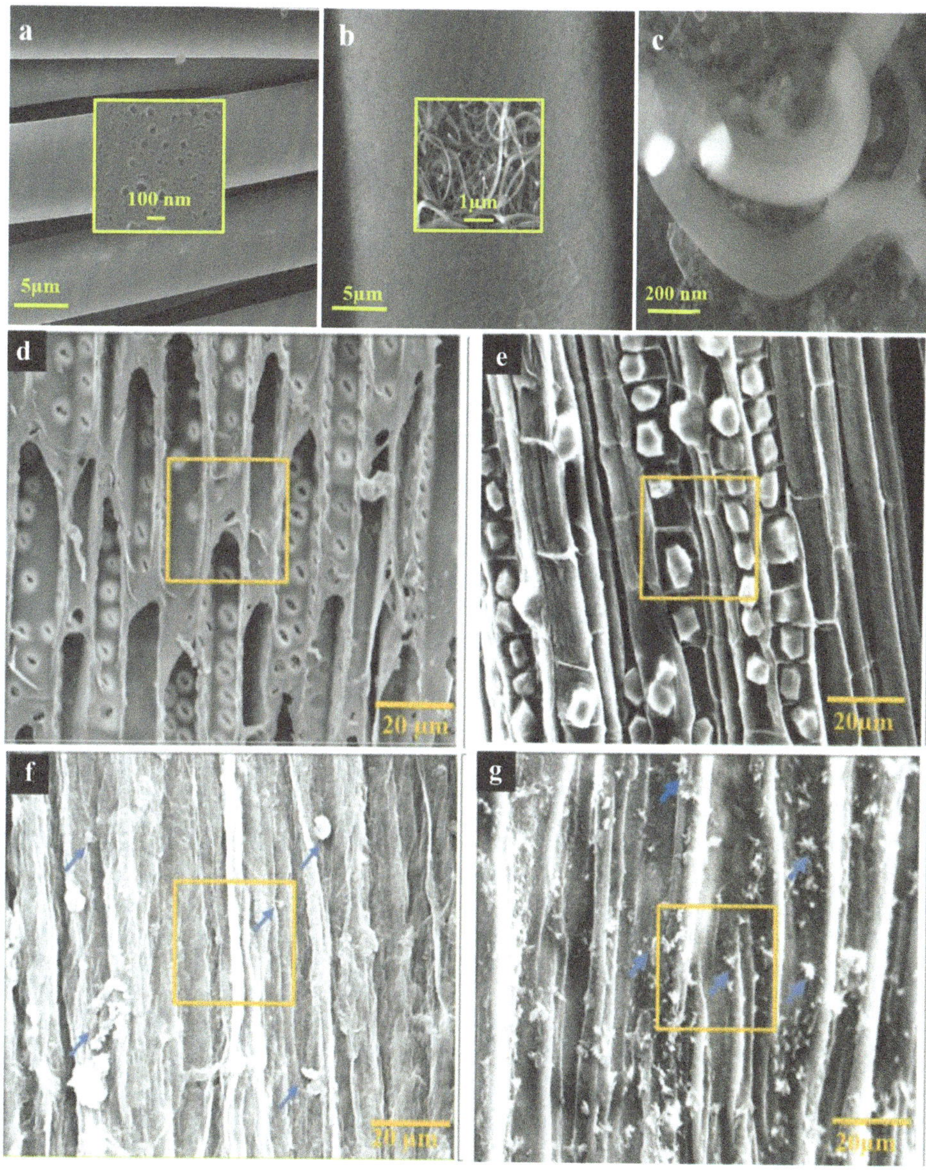

Fig. 9 SEM images at low and high (in inset) magnifications of **a** ACF, **b** Cu-CNF/ACF, **c** Cu-CNF; SEM images of plant shoots grown in Cr-stressed environment and treated with **d** control, **e** ACF, **f** Cu-CNF, and **g** mixture of ACF and Cu-CNF (the arrows point to CNFs) (Kumar et al. 2020)

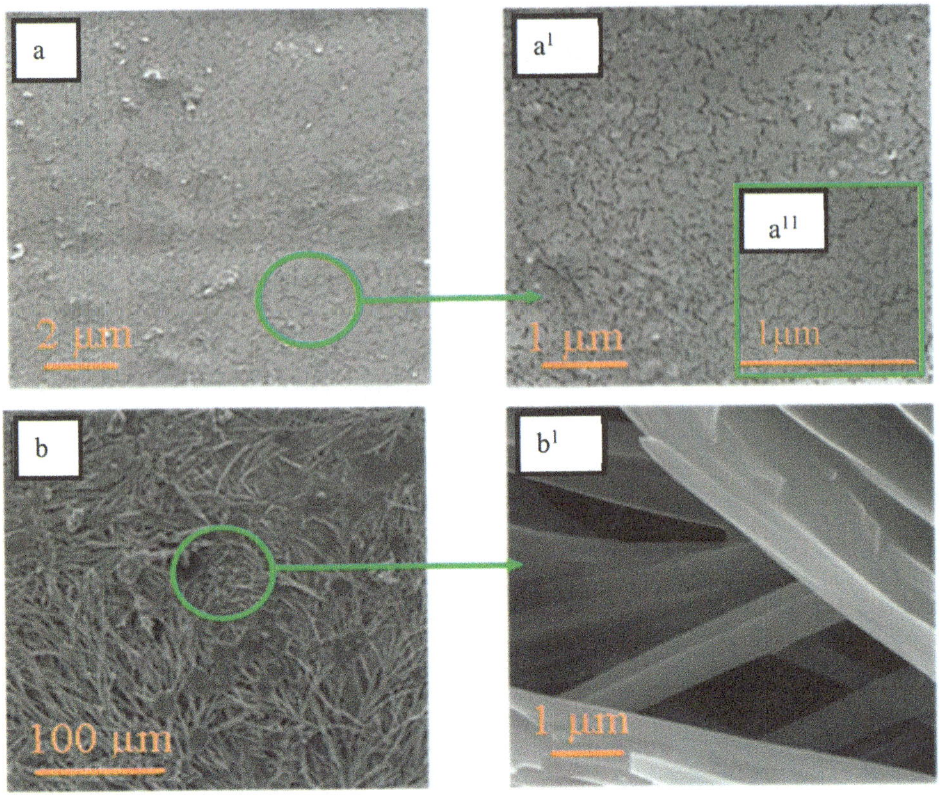

Fig. 10 SEM images at low and high magnifications of **a**, **a**^{1}, **a**^{11} BMCP and **b**, **b**^{1} PMO-BMCP (Bairagi and Verma 2018)

Surface morphology of the BMCP cholesterol sensor can be examined using the SEM images shown in Fig. 10. A smooth surface of BMCP is clearly visible in the low magnification image, whereas roughness in the surface, caused by the CNF growth, can be seen in the high magnification image (Fig. 10a, a^1). The inset figure (a^{11}) confirms a uniform and dense growth of the CNFs in the PVAc polymeric matrix. The SEM images of the electropolymerized PMO over BMCP show a uniform growth of the dendritic PMO fibers (Fig. 10b). The high magnification image clearly shows the porous structure of PMO (Fig. 10b^1). The dendritic-like structure facilitates binding of the PMO recognition element with the cholesterol molecule and sensing of the analyte.

PMC exposed to red blood cells (RBCs), platelets, and bacterial strains was examined by observing any morphological change of the material surface, using the SEM images. During the synthesis stage, loading of Cu-Zn-ACF/CNF in the electrode material was optimized at a concentration level where the carbon fibers started protruding out of the film, creating a rough surface (Fig. 11a) that was suitable for adhesion of RBCs without causing any damage to the cells (Fig. 11b). The quiescent platelets resting on a silicon wafer are shown in Fig. 11b, which on exposure to PMC became activated with formation of a long-spider-like structure (Fig. 11b^1). A control sample of *P. aeruginosa* bacteria is shown in Fig. 11c. On exposure to PMC, the bacterial structure was observed to be distorted (Fig. 11c^1) confirming lysis of the bacteria. Thus, it was possible to gather critical information such as surface roughness of the dressing material, RBC adhesion, platelet activation, and bacterial lysis using the SEM analysis, which helped to optimize the synthesis conditions and determine suitability of the material for wound dressing.

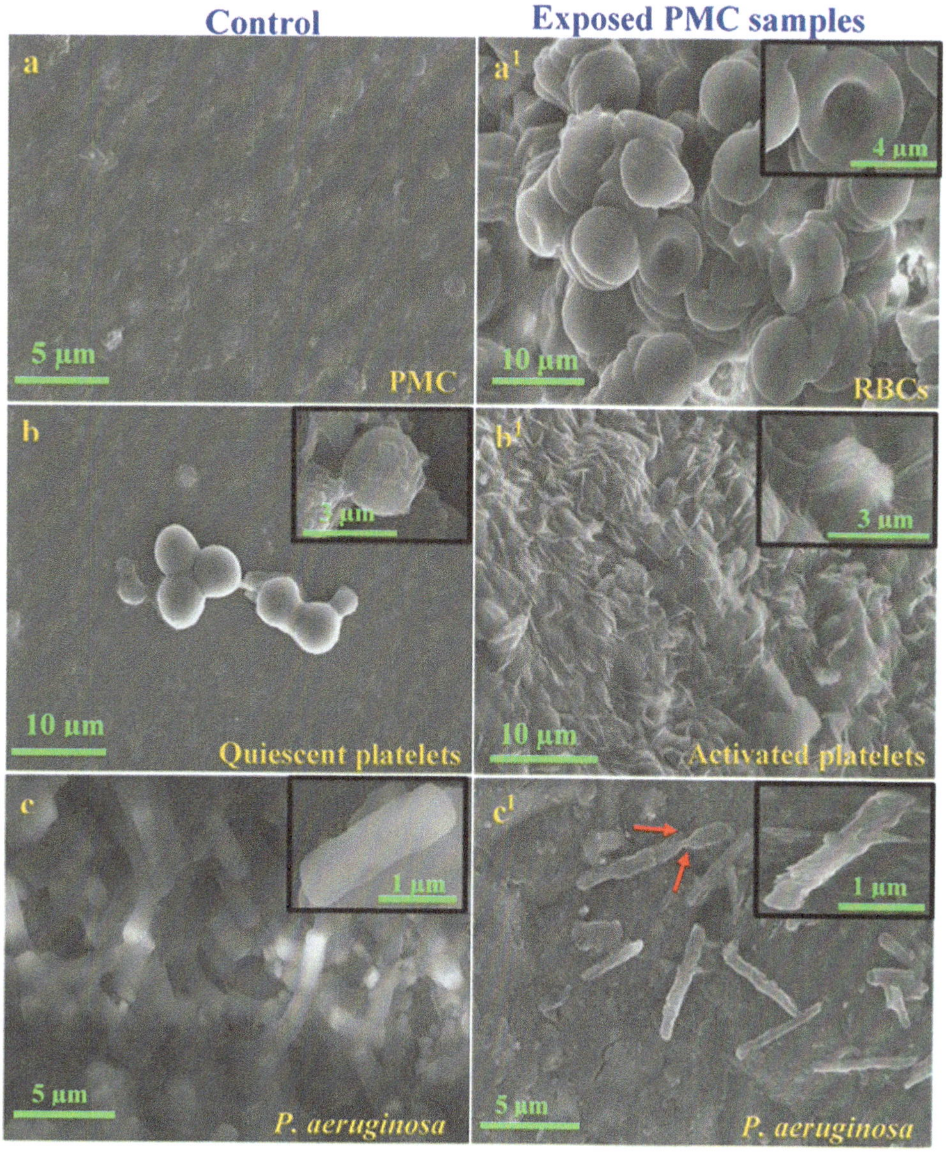

Fig. 11 SEM images of **a** PMC surface with optimized loading of fillers (Cu-Zn-ACF/CNF) as control, **a**[1] RBC-exposed PMC surface, **b** quiescent platelets on silicon wafer as a control, **b**[1] platelet-exposed PMC, **c** *P. aeruginosa* bacteria as a control, **c**[1] P. aeruginosa-exposed PMC (Ashfaq et al. 2017)

Acknowledgements The authors are thankful to the Centre for Environmental Science and Engineering, IIT Kanpur, for providing various research facilities. Contribution of the past and present graduate students studying various aspects of the carbon-based materials is highly acknowledged. Research grants from various government agencies including SERB (DST), DBT, and CSIR are also acknowledged.

References

Ai S, Sui H, Li H (2012) Ind Eng Chem Res 51:2337–2343
Ashfaq M, Verma N, Khan S (2017) Mater Sci Eng C 77:630–641
Bairagi P, Verma N (2018) J Electroanal Chem 814:134–143
Gupta GS, Kumar A, Verma N (2019) Env Sci Nano 6:1246–1258
Kim B-J, Lee Y-S, Park S-J (2008) Int J Hydrogen Energ 33:4112–4115
Kumar A, Gahoi P, Verma N (2020) Chemosphere 239:124760
Li Y, Bai H, Liu Q, Bao J, Han M, Dai Z (2010) Biosens Bioelectron 25:2356–2360
Prajapati YN, Verma N (2017) Fuel 189:186–194
Yadav A, Verma N (2017) Int J Hydrog Energ 42:27139–27153
Zheng G, Kouda K, Sano H, Uchiyama Y, Shi Y, Quan H (2004) Carbon 42:635–640

Electron Backscatter Diffraction Technique: Fundamentals to Applications

Shashank Shekhar, Nitin Kumar Sharma, Sandeep Sahu, and Santanu Misra

1 Introduction

Orientation imaging microscopy (OIM) has long been the quest of material scientists and microscopists, as it provides an immense amount of quantitative data about the microstructure of a material, which can then be related to its processing and also to the performance of the component. There are several techniques which can provide orientation information, some of which are electron channeling contrast imaging (ECCI) in SEM to convergent beam electron diffraction (CBED) and selected area diffraction (SAD) in transmission electron microscope (TEM). Each of these techniques is good in themselves in providing orientation; however, each of them is beset by some drawbacks which have subdued their utilization. A major limitation of these techniques is that they are not suitable for automation which allows to obtain orientation data from various points on a large scanned area. However, it must be pointed out that TEM-based EBSD has also now gained traction and it is gaining applicability among researchers.

In simple terms, electron channeling contrast is obtained due to difference in density of atoms along different directions, which results in varied intensity of backscattered electrons (BSEs) (Joy et al. 1982; Wilkinson and Hirsch 1997; Zaefferer and Elhami 2014). A schematic to explain this effect is shown in Fig. 1. If the electron beam is rastered in two-dimensional space of the sample surface, then one can expect that several lattice planes would together contribute to the electron contrast. One can expect high contrast from planes which are close to normal to the surface, while those away from the normal would show low contrast. Overall, backscattered beam would have a contrast in the form of bands, which carry information about orientation and lattice defects. The bands reflect the inherent symmetry of the orientation of the point, while local features reflect defects in the lattice. Coates was the first person to obtain patterns based on this technique (Coates 1967). This technique is not easy to automate because accurate and automated rocking of beam is not allowed in most electron microscopes. Moreover, the beam rocking process is very slow, and hence getting scans from a large number of points makes the process tedious (Kamaladasa and Picard 2010). Nonetheless, this process has been very successful in understanding lattice defects (Zaefferer and Elhami 2014; Ahmed et al. 1997).

In TEM, when thin foils are subjected to high-energy parallel beam, it leads to diffraction due to lattice points. If the beam illuminates a single crystal, then various planes of the crystal diffract to produce pattern of points. The symmetry and orientation of these points can be directly related to the orientation of the crystal and hence can be used for orientation imaging microscopy. A schematic of the process and the pattern obtained is shown in Fig. 2. Another related technique is convergent electron beam diffraction, which utilizes convergent beam, instead of parallel beam, and results in disks, instead of points in the diffraction pattern. This, too, can be used for understanding the orientation of the crystal.

Orientation recognition from SAD pattern has been commercialized, and it has also become a good tool for orientation imaging microscopy, particularly when the grains or precipitates are small in size.

S. Shekhar (✉) · S. Sahu
Grain Boundary Engineering Lab, Materials Science and Engineering, IIT Kanpur, Kanpur, UP 208016, India
e-mail: shashank@iitk.ac.in

N. K. Sharma
Chemical and Materials Engineering, University of Alberta, Edmonton, AB T6G 21, Canada

S. Misra
Department of Earth Sciences, IIT Kanpur, Kanpur, UP 208016, India

K. Biswas et al. (eds.), *Electron Microscopy in Science and Engineering*, IITK Directions 6,
https://doi.org/10.1007/978-981-16-5101-4_4

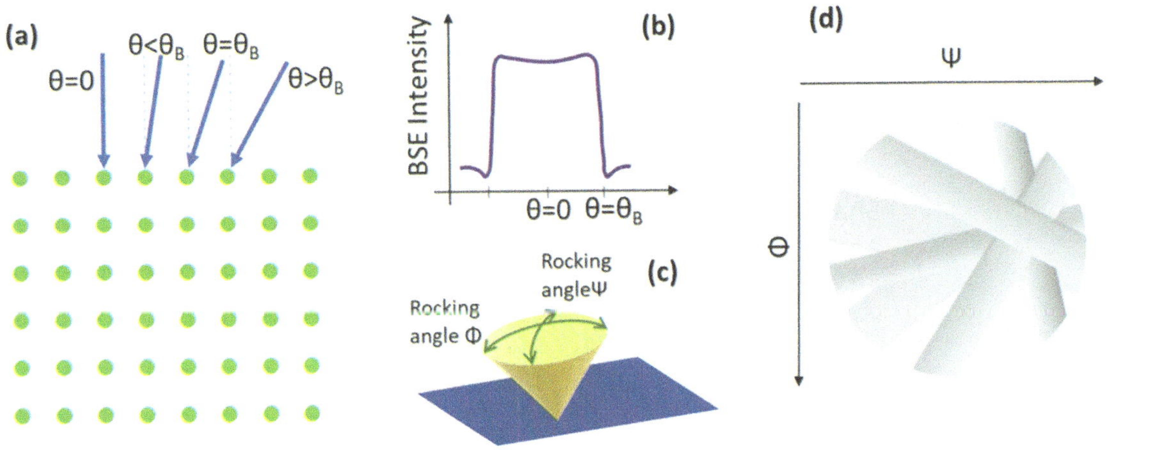

Fig. 1 **a** Orientation variation of incoming beam. **b** Its effect on BSE intensity. **c** Rocking of beam in 2 directions. **d** Schematic of the generated ECCI pattern. **a** and **b** adapted from Wilkinson and Hirsch (1997)

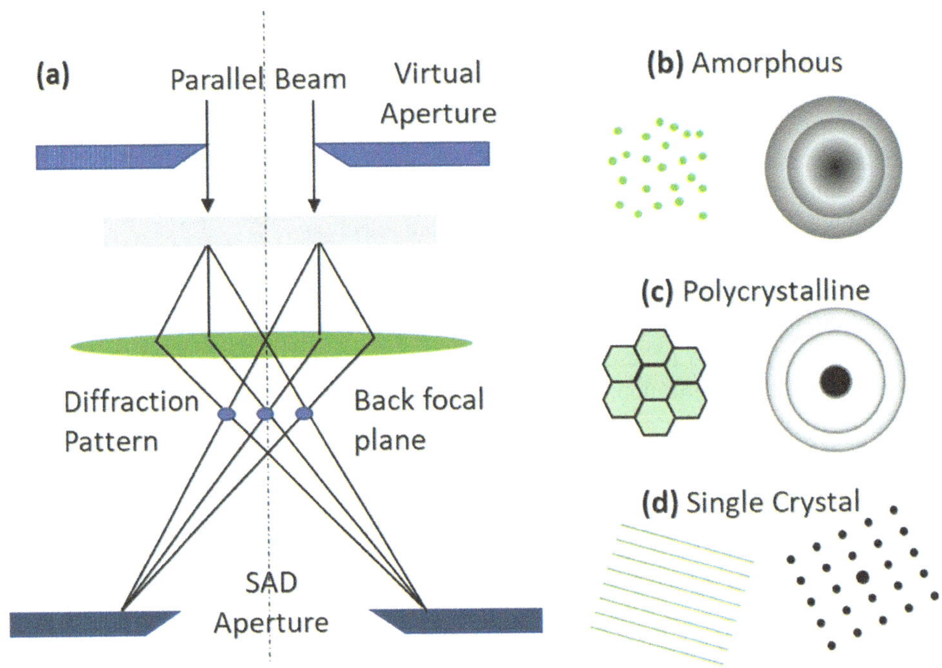

Fig. 2 **a** Schematic of the SAD pattern generation in TEM and the diffraction pattern corresponding to **b** amorphous material. **c** Polycrystalline material. **d** Single crystalline material

2 Origin of Kikuchi Pattern

Kikuchi pattern was first observed by S. Nishikawa and S. Kikuchi in 1928 during diffraction of cathode rays by calcite (Nishikawa and Kikuchi 1928a,b). In one of these publications, they presented transmission Kikuchi patterns (TKPs) (Nishikawa and Kikuchi 1928b), and in the other, they presented backscatter Kikuchi patterns (BKPs) (Nishikawa and Kikuchi 1928a). While most of the work in the early phase was concentrated on transmission Kikuchi diffraction (TKD), last three decades have seen a lot of attention being given to SEM-based backscatter Kikuchi diffraction, which has widely come to be known as electron backscatter diffraction (EBSD). It has further gained prominence due to automation and improvement in hardware which have accelerated acquiring and analyzing speed of these Kikuchi patterns (Kunze et al. 1993).

Kikuchi patterns are formed by the backscattered electrons that satisfy the diffraction condition for a given set of planes. A schematic of the same is shown in Fig. 3. When the electron beam falls on the material, interaction of electron and atoms takes place, and scattering of the incoming electrons occurs. The point of scatter becomes the source of secondary waves which has varying intensity at different orientations. Now, these secondary waves of electrons can

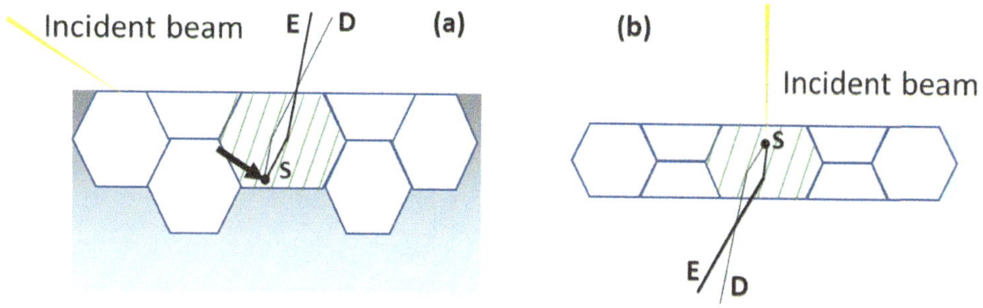

Fig. 3 Schematic showing generation of **a** backscatter Kikuchi diffraction in a bulk sample and **b** transmission Kikuchi diffraction in a thin foil ('S' is the scattering event which acts as source, 'D' is part of the defect cone, and 'E' is part of the excess cone)

further interact with the lattice points and result in diffraction, very similar to that in X-ray diffraction. One major difference with X-ray diffraction, however, is that wavelength of the electron waves is very small, leading to a very small Bragg's angle (θ) in Bragg's equation, $n\lambda = 2d \sin \theta$. For the sake of comparison, wavelength of K_α radiation originating from Cu source during *X*-ray diffraction is ~ 1.54 Å. On the other hand, wavelength of electron at 10 kV accelerating voltage is ~ 0.12 Å. Since the wavelength of these electron waves is an order of magnitude smaller than that of *X*-rays, Bragg's angles also come out to be much smaller than that obtained in X-ray diffraction.

Another major difference with X-ray diffraction is that since the 'source' of electrons is inside the material, diffraction may take place in 'forward' as well as 'backward direction,' as depicted in the schematic. Thus, in this diffraction, there is always a pair of diffracted cones. When these cones intersect with a planar detector, we observe a pair of hyperbolae. But due to the small values of Bragg angles, the curvatures of these hyperbolae are so small that they appear as parallel lines. These parallel lines are known as Kikuchi lines or Kikuchi bands. Because of the nature of its origin, one of the cones has higher intensity than the background, while the one which diffracted from the backward moving waves has intensity lower than the background. Thus, we obtain what are called as 'defect cone' and 'excess cone.' These cones and corresponding Kikuchi lines are formed in both transmission mode and backscatter mode. The geometry of the two modes is somewhat different and would be discussed in next section.

Since the Kikuchi patterns are formed by a fundamental phenomenon of diffraction, they show certain characteristics that help in understanding the structure and orientation of material. Each band in the Kikuchi pattern represents diffraction from a family of planes. Thus, each band has a one-to-one relation with family of planes. This, in turn, implies that intersection of these bands represents intersection of planes, viz. zone axes. Moreover, angle between the bands represents angle between planes. These characteristics of the Kikuchi pattern are exploited to identify the orientation of the individual point of the sample. In scanning electron microscope (SEM), the beam rasters over a region, moving from point to point in a serpentine fashion. Thus, one can obtain orientation of each of these points and recreate a micrograph representing the orientation map of the scanned region. Another important characteristic of these patterns is that the width of each of the bands is proportional to the spacing of the planes of that family. It can be easily shown that the angular separation between the two parallel lines of the Kikuchi band is twice the Bragg angle. From this, it can be extrapolated that if there are defects in the material which can cause variation in the average planar spacing, then it would reflect in the bands. This characteristic has also been exploited in EBSD to quantify the strain in the lattice (Wilkinson and Britton 2012).

3 Automated Indexing of Kikuchi Patterns

We pointed out earlier that application of EBSD has seen an exponential growth in last two decades. This is driven primarily by automation of pattern indexing across a selected grid in the scan area. This automation has allowed indexing of patterns from area as large as several 100 μm along both the directions. Automatic indexing has been achieved on the foundation of improvement in software as well as hardware capabilities. On the hardware front, there is a phosphor screen on which the Kikuchi patterns are formed, and the illuminated pattern is captured by a camera that is located behind this screen. The capabilities of the camera and screen have improved immensely over the years, so that the screen capturing rate has reached in excess of 2500 frames per second. Faster scanning rate has resulted in obtaining large maps in very short times. Once the images are captured, they are analyzed to identify the orientation and phase of the given point. In the next few paragraphs, we explain the method of recognition of Kikuchi pattern and indexing of the orientation of a given point from the obtained Kikuchi pattern.

Once the camera captures the Kikuchi pattern, identification of various lines from the Kikuchi pattern is carried out

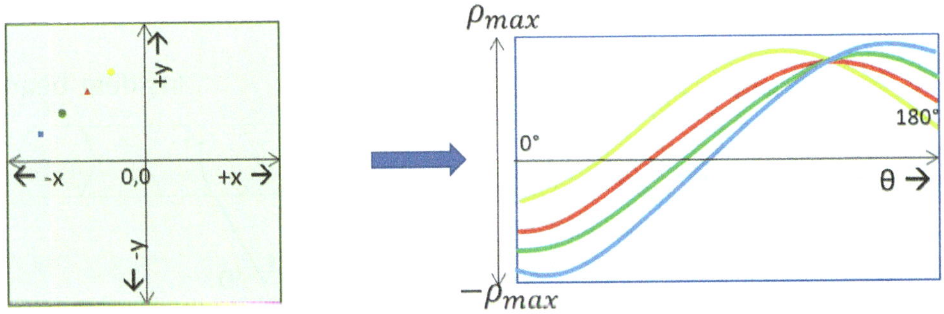

Fig. 4 Hough transformation translates each pixel in image space to a curve in the 'ρ–θ' space, and consequently, a line in the image space appears as an intersection of several of these curves in the 'ρ–θ' space

using Hough transform. In this technique, the line is transformed from Cartesian coordinate to a space where it is represented only by its length 'ρ' and angle 'θ'. To understand this, let us imagine a square image containing just one line. If we want to transform each pixel of this image space into 'ρ' and 'θ' parameter space, then each pixel on the image would transform to a sinusoidal curve in the 'ρ–θ' space. This is because each pixel can be imagined to be a part of infinite number of straight lines passing through it. Set of these straight lines would form a curve as represented in Fig. 4 (left). Now, wherever a line exists in image space, it will be represented as intersection of several of these sinusoidal curves at one point, as shown in Fig. 4 (right). This intersection point in the 'ρ–θ' space has value of 'ρ_i' and 'θ_i' which represents the given line in the image space. In the present context, 'ρ' varies from '$-\rho_{\max}$' to '$\rho_{\max}$' and 'θ' varies from 0 to 180°. Now, if we assign intensity value to each of these pixels in image space, then the intensity value of this particular 'ρ_i' and 'θ_i' would be much higher than that of its neighborhood. When all of Kikuchi pattern is transformed into 'ρ–θ' space, this is called Hough transformation. In the Hough transformed image, third direction represents the intensity, and each straight line in image space is represented by a 'Hough' or a mound, which has relatively higher intensity value compared to its neighbor. The bright lines can be easily identified by the relatively large peaks in the Hough transform space. Once these lines are identified, calculating the angle between the planes is much easier in this 'ρ–θ' space, as one can easily identify the equation for each and every line which is given as: $\rho_i = x\cos\theta_i + y\sin\theta_i$.

Kikuchi pattern is a set of bands with parallel lines, and each of these bands represents a family of planes of the crystal structure of the given phase. The centerline of each of these bands represents the trace of orientation of the given family of planes. Hence, by identifying the lines, as described in the previous paragraph, and by calculating the angle between any pair of bands, we are essentially calculating the angle between corresponding pair of family of planes. This angle between various sets of planes can be compared to the reference values of the crystal structure of the possible phases. At least 3 different sets of mutually intersecting lines and their corresponding angles must match, to uniquely identify the phase and define the crystal orientation of the point on the crystal. In general, 5 to 8 bands or reflectors need to be matched to get confidence in the result and to improve the accuracy of the orientation.

4 Geometry of EBSD Setup

In EBSD, it is very important to understand the geometry of the setup so that appropriate corrections can be made for the geometry during analysis. Intensity of the backscattered electrons has an angular distribution, and this angular distribution is also dependent upon the angle of incidence of the electron beam on the sample (Berger and Niedrig 1999). When the electron beam falls normally to the sample surface, highest intensity of the backscattered electrons lies normal to the plane. However, this distribution is very different when the electron beam has an acute incidence angle. A schematic of the angular density of the backscattered electrons in these two cases is shown in Fig. 5. In general, it is found that maximum intensity is found at an angle which is equal to the angle of incidence of the beam on the sample, as shown in the schematic (Berger and Niedrig 1999). Ideally, one would like to keep the sample normal and the detector right at the pole piece. However, due to constraints of space this is not feasible, and the next best configuration is to keep the sample oriented at some steep angle and keep the detector where one can get the maximum intensity of backscattered electrons. EBSD researchers have found that yield of the backscattered electron is highest at 70° tilt. The overall geometry of the sample with respect to the EBSD detector and the pole piece is shown in Fig. 6a. Figure 6b shows a typical Kikuchi pattern. This particular pattern was obtained from a single-phase material with FCC crystal structure at an accelerating voltage of 20 kV.

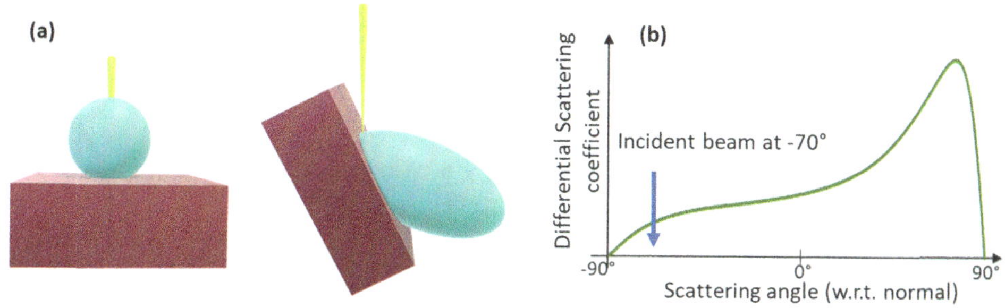

Fig. 5 **a** Schematic representation of the three-dimensional angular distribution of backscatter electrons. **b** Schematic representation of variation of differential scattering coefficient with scattering angle, assuming sample has a 70° tilt. Adapted from Berger and Niedrig (1999)

The tilted sample geometry has a significant role on the overall spatial resolution and also the fact that the lateral resolution is different from the longitudinal resolution of the scanned sample. Figure 7a shows the schematic interaction of the beam with the sample. The depth from which backscattered electrons can escape the surface to reach the detector is denoted by d_z. Its absolute value depends on the accelerating voltage and the atomic number of the given material. In general, its value ranges from 50 to 100 nm, which is a very small depth. This also implies that the surface must be polished and must be free of any asperities at least up to this depth. If there are any remnant strains or scratches due to polishing which are of this order, then obtaining Kikuchi pattern is not possible. This also explains why sample preparation is a very delicate and dedicated step for EBSD. There is dedicated equipment that has been designed in the past few decades, particularly for the preparation of the samples for EBSD. Some of the dedicated equipment is vibratory polishing machine and electropolishing machine.

In Fig. 7a, the largest cross section of the teardrop interactive volume represents the spatial resolution in lateral and longitudinal directions. It is obvious from the figure that this cross-sectional area is much larger than the spot size of the beam. A larger cross section also suggests that the yield of the backscattered electrons would be high. Secondly, it is also clear that due to the tilt of the sample, longitudinal resolution d_y is much larger (poorer) than the lateral resolution d_x. On a first order of approximation, it can be said that $d_y = d_x/\cos\theta$, based on the geometry of the sample, which is tilted at an angle θ from the direction of the electron beam. A schematic of the variation of lateral and longitudinal resolution with change in accelerating voltage is shown in Fig. 7b. The absolute values of resolution can range from 50 nm to few μm. By applying very low accelerating voltages, researchers have achieved resolution as low (good) as 10 nm (Dingley et al. 2005; Chen et al. 2011). This improvement is achieved as the interaction volume decreases with decrease in accelerating voltage.

The fact that resolution is dependent upon the geometry of sample and the interaction volume has been exploited for transmission Kikuchi diffraction in SEM. Here, like in TEM, a thin foil is used whose interaction volume is very small, and thus, the resolution is also small (better). A schematic of the same is shown in Fig. 8. In effect, the resolution is as good as the spot size of the beam falling on the sample can be obtained using this geometry. Resolution up to a few nm can be obtained using this technique (Wang et al. 2016).

5 Data Acquisition Parameters

Previous sections clearly outline the theory that lies behind EBSD-based OIM. Like any experimental technique, there are several other parameters related to hardware and software that need to be optimized in order to obtain good-quality data. In this section, we will discuss some of these important parameters and what points to keep in mind when acquiring data. First and foremost step in good-quality data acquisition is sample preparation. As pointed out earlier, during EBSD, data is acquired from only up to a depth of 50–100 nm from sample surface. This puts a huge obligation of preparing a surface that is free from any polishing artifacts up to a depth of few 10's of nm. However, we will not delve into sample preparation here, and readers are directed to read some of these in-depth studies on sample preparation for EBSD (Wang et al. 2016; Nowell et al. 2005; Michael and Giannuzzi 2007).

Once the Kikuchi patterns from a well-prepared sample are discernible, then the objectives of the users are to obtain high accuracy data and at high frame rate. High accuracy refers to high probability of getting correct identification of the orientation, and high frame rate refers to acquisition of a large number of frames and its analysis per unit time. Both these sets of objectives require different sets of parameters, and hence, there is a need to optimize them. The SEM operating condition should be set such that the current in the SEM is on the higher side. This is particularly true for FESEMs as the total

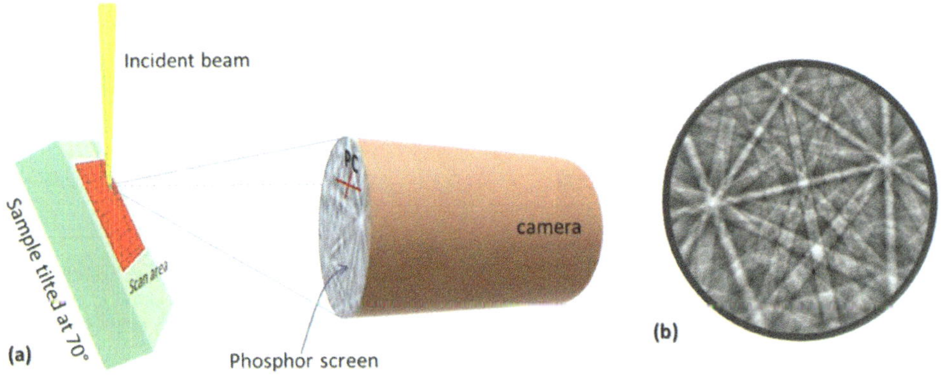

Fig. 6 **a** Geometry of the sample with respect to the incident beam and the EBSD detector (PC refers to pattern center). **b** A Kikuchi pattern obtained from a single-phase FCC crystal

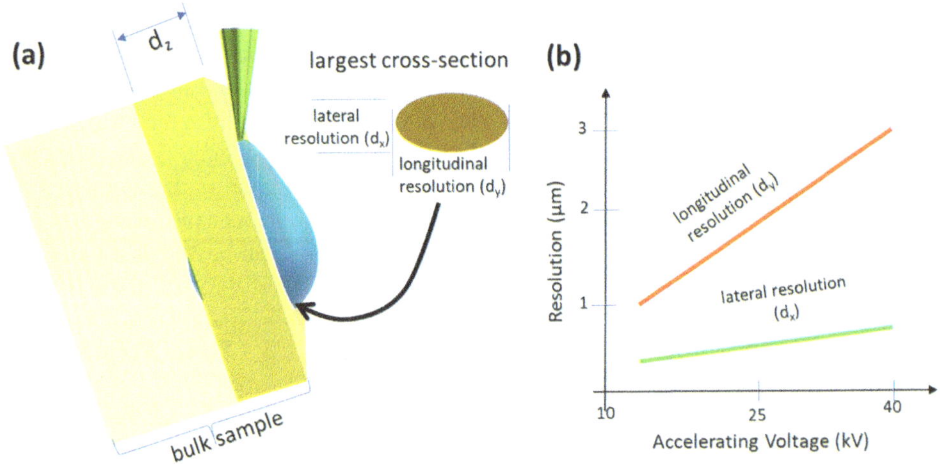

Fig. 7 **a** Schematic representation of interaction of beam with the sample in backscatter diffraction mode, also showing the largest cross section from which backscatter electrons escape. **b** Schematic of the variation of lateral and longitudinal resolution with change in accelerating voltage

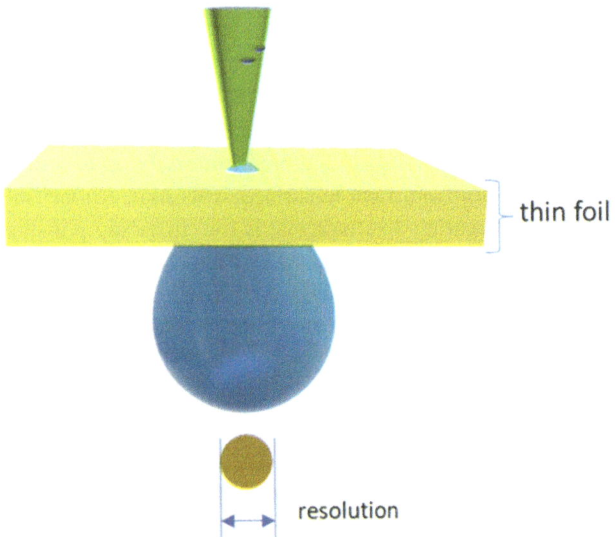

Fig. 8 Schematic representation of interaction of beam with thin foil in transmission Kikuchi diffraction mode. Also showing the large cross section, which represents the resolution of the geometry

current in field emission SEMs is quite low. Good current is necessary for obtaining high-contrast diffraction bands. The accelerating voltage has direct implication on the resolution of data, and it is usually kept at 10 kV. For resolving small particles, one may need to reduce the accelerating voltage to much lower values (Singh et al. 2018).

In the data acquisition window, we get to optimize the contrast of the patterns again, using gain and exposure time. Increasing the gain improves the signal, but the signal-to-noise ratio also deteriorates. On the other hand, increasing the exposure time improves signal as well as signal-to-noise ratio, but the acquisition rate goes down. Additionally, the gain needs to be just sufficient so that there is no saturation in the signal. Another important parameter that affects pattern quality and image acquisition rate is the binning size of the Kikuchi pattern. Usually, the Kikuchi pattern is obtained as a high-resolution image (e.g., 1024 × 1024 pixels). The binning size refers to the number of pixels that would be averaged when analyzing the Kikuchi pattern. Thus, a 1 × 1 binning would imply that all the 1024 × 1024 pixels (1,048,576 pixels) would be analyzed. However, a 4 × 4 binning would imply that only 65,536 pixels would be analyzed. This greatly reduces the analysis time, and hence, the acquisition rate increases drastically. The downside is that this also leads to reduced resolution of the Kikuchi pattern, and hence, it may

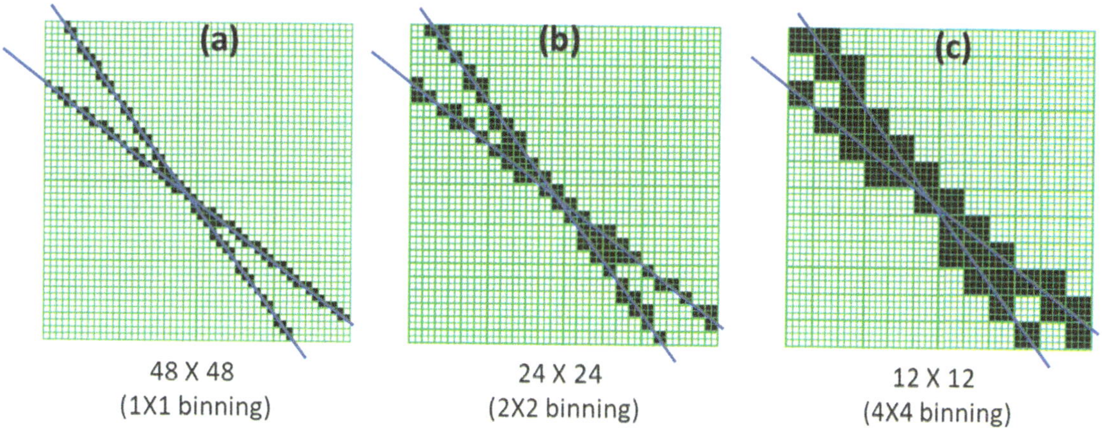

Fig. 9 Effect of binning size on the resolution of the image: Two straight lines are drawn on a grid of 48 × 48 at three different binning sizes. **a** 1 × 1 binning. **b** 2 × 2 binning. **c** 4 × 4 binning

deteriorate the accuracy. This is explained schematically in Fig. 9. Depending on the material and the polishing condition, one needs to identify the highest binning that can give accurate results and thus improve the acquisition rate. Data acquisition software also allows the user to improve the image contrast by subtracting background signal. Background signal refers to the signal being received from several other neighboring grains that can reduce the overall image contrast. By subtracting or dividing this background signal from the obtained signal, the contrast of the pattern obtained from the immediate point is improved significantly.

Once the pattern acquisition parameters are set, the user needs to define the step size for the scan area. Step size is the distance between two consecutive points from which orientation is obtained and thus defines the total number of points that will be acquired in a given scan area. If the step size is very small, one would be able to get very high-resolution micrograph with no visible jig-jag-type structure in the grain boundary; however, this also implies a significantly longer time to acquire the image. Usually, the electron beam inside the SEM has a gradual drift, and for very large scans, the total beam drift may be too large, and the OIM micrograph would yield elongated structures. On the other hand, using a very large step size takes very short time, albeit it sacrifices resolution. In fact, some very small grains may not get detected if the step size is too large. Hence, it is imperative to select an optimal step size. As a rule of thumb, step size should be taken as grain size divided by 10. This would yield on an average 100 points per grain, and the scan speed would also not be compromised. However, if the micrograph consists of very fine grains, then one has to ensure that all these grains are captured. Another rule of thumb is that at least 10 pixels should be present in a region for it to be defined as grain. So, this serves as another guide in selecting the step size. The users should also be aware of the smallest step size that yields meaningful result in their respective SEM. As a point of reference, the smallest step size that gives meaningful result using the Oxford Instruments' Nordlys EBSD detector installed in the FESEM JEOL JSM-7100F in the ACMS facility at IIT Kanpur is 50 nm. This would imply that the smallest grain that can be detected would have an area of 10 pixels × $(0.05\ \mu m)^2$, which is approximately 0.025 μm^2 or a square with ~158 nm length.

6 Data Analysis

In the earlier sections, we discussed the theory of electron backscatter diffraction, and then we discussed the data acquisition process and the important parameters to keep in mind in order to obtain high-quality data at fast scan rates. Next, we need to understand how to interpret this data so that quantitative microstructural information can be extracted. Later, we will provide some case studies where these analyses are put in application. Data that is acquired from the EBSD acquisition software is simply the crystal orientation data for each and every point. Next few paragraphs will elaborate how this information alone is sufficient to extract quantitative information about several microstructural parameters. Some additional data is also collected at each point, which aids in analyzing and quantifying results. EBSD pattern at each point can also be saved, and these are used in special cases to analyze the results to a greater depth. First and foremost, we need to understand what is the mathematical form of these orientations and what is the reference frame with respect to which this orientation data is gathered.

6.1 Orientation Analysis

Orientation is always defined with respect to some reference coordinate. In this sense, orientation is the rotation from the

specimen coordinate system to crystal coordinate system. Mathematically, this can be described by rotation vector 'g'. A schematic is shown in Fig. 10a which represents orientation as rotation from specimen coordinate system to crystal coordinate system. Usually, the three primary orientations of sample coordinate system are denoted as 'rolling direction,' 'normal direction,' and 'transverse direction,' and three coordinates of the crystal are defined by < 100 > , < 010 >, and < 001 > . Another way of representing orientation or transformation is using the Euler angles, which is defined in terms of three angles $(\varphi_1, \emptyset, \varphi_2)$. These sets of angles are also called yaw, pitch, and roll and are explained in Fig. 10b. It can be readily shown that the rotation matrix 'g' and the Euler angles are related by the following equation:

$$g = \begin{vmatrix} \cos\varphi_1\cos\varphi_2 - \sin\varphi_1\sin\varphi_2\cos\emptyset & \sin\varphi_1\cos\varphi_2 + \cos\varphi_1\sin\varphi_2\cos\emptyset & \sin\varphi_2\sin\emptyset \\ -\cos\varphi_1\sin\varphi_2 - \sin\varphi_1\cos\varphi_2\cos\emptyset & -\sin\varphi_1\sin\varphi_2 + \cos\varphi_1\sin\varphi_2\cos\emptyset & \cos\varphi_2\sin\emptyset \\ \sin\varphi_1\sin\emptyset & -\cos\varphi_1\sin\emptyset & \cos\emptyset \end{vmatrix}$$

It is also possible to obtain the Euler angles from the rotation matrix 'g' (Herter and Lott 1993; Shoemake 1994). There are some more mathematical ways of representation of orientation and the misorientation between the points, e.g., Rodrigues vector and quaternions (Heinz and Neumann 1991; Morawiec and Field 1996). We will not get into details of other kinds of representation, and for now, it is sufficient to understand that orientations can be represented in mathematical form and that they can be stored in terms of the above-mentioned parameters. We should also realize that each of these representations is interchangeable, and one can get orientation parameters of one type of representation from other forms of representation.

With orientation data for each point of scan area, one can generate an orientation map giving unique color to each orientation. An easy way to define unique color to each orientation is by using a standard inverse pole figure (IPF) triangle of the crystal structure, with three primary colors (red, green, and blue) at three corners (Nolze and Hielscher 2016). The intermediate points are represented by a mix of these primary colors. Since the IPF represents all the possible orientations of a crystal, the colors provide an easy guide to the orientation of various points in the map. One such pseudo-colored orientation map, where each point was assigned a color based on the color of the corresponding orientation in the inverse pole figure (also shown), is depicted in Fig. 11a. An Inconel-718 sample was taken for this scan, which was found to be single phase. Usually, Inconel contains several precipitates, but this particular sample was processed such that it was mostly single phase. Regions or domains with similar colors depict points with similar orientation and hence represent one crystallite or one grain. Black dots represent points from where Kikuchi pattern could not be obtained or could not be indexed. This scan

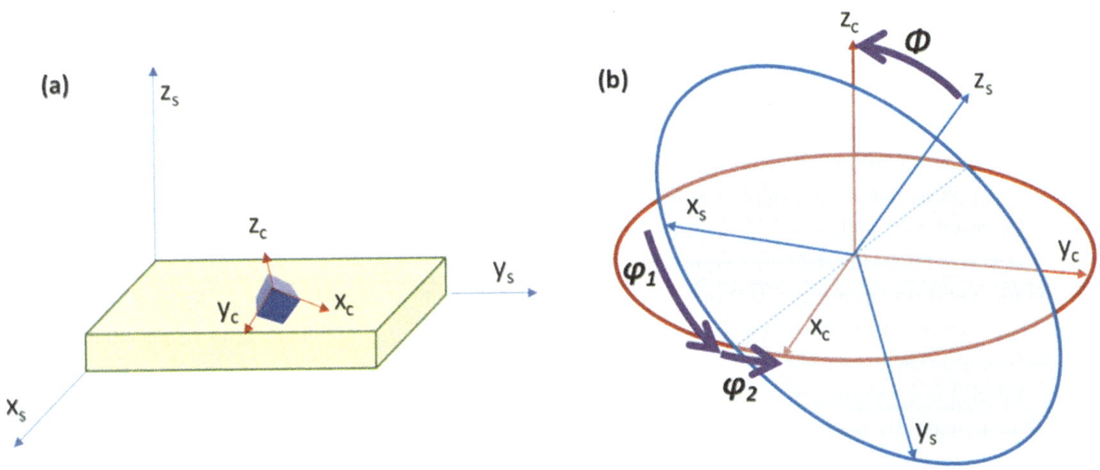

Fig. 10 Orientation of an individual crystal in a sample. **a** Crystal coordinate system (x_c, y_c, z_c) is described with respect to sample coordinate system (x_s, y_z, z_s). **b** This rotation can achieve three consecutive rotations, performed about the z_s-, x'-, and z''-axes by magnitude $\varphi_1, \emptyset$, and φ_2, respectively

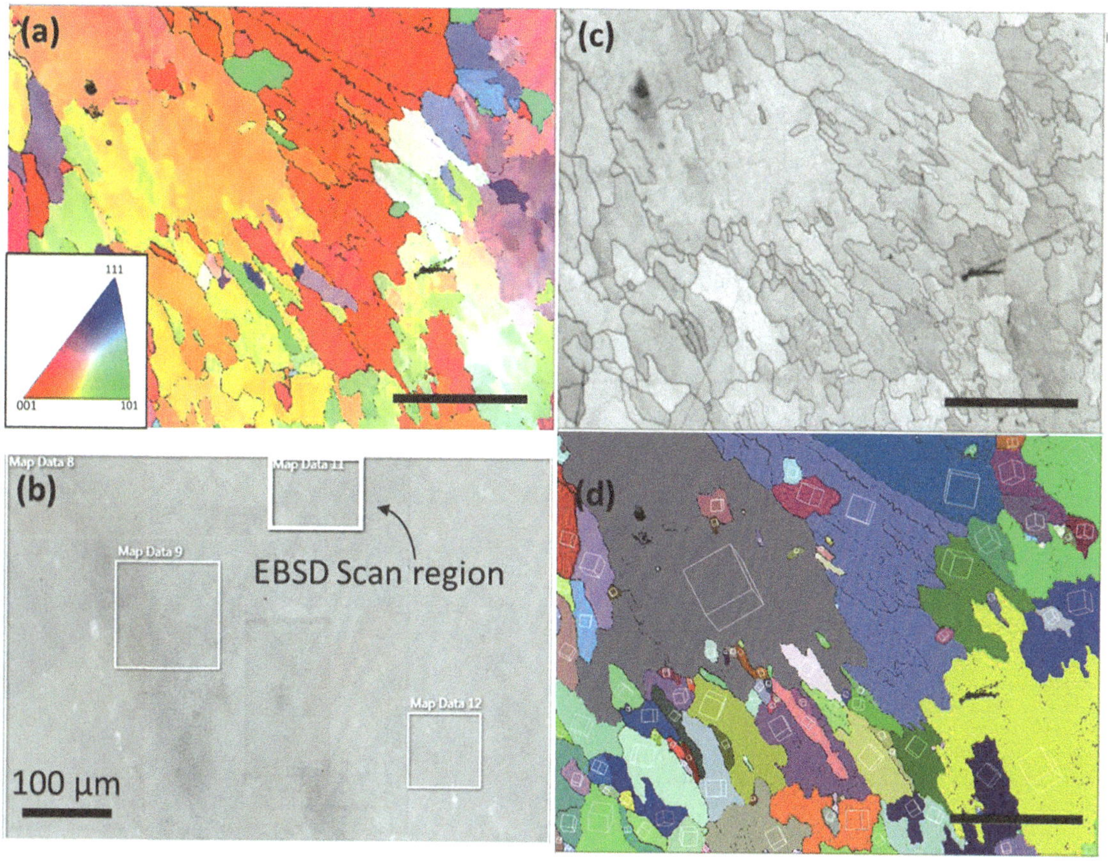

Fig. 11 EBSD of Inconel 718 sample. **a** Orientation map based on pseudo-colors of IPF (shown in inset). **b** SEM micrograph showing the region from where EBSD scan was taken. **c** Band contrast map. **d** Random colored grain map (scale bar = 25 µm, where not mentioned)

was taken with a step size of 150 nm over an area of 100 × 75 µm. This translates to 667 points along the horizontal direction and 500 points along the vertical direction, giving a total of 333,500 points to generate the orientation map. The reference inverse pole figure of cubic crystal structure with its color scheme is also shown in the inset. SEM micrograph of the material is also shown in Fig. 11b for reference, and the region from which scan was taken is marked on the SEM micrograph.

Another very useful map that is almost always generated using EBSD analysis tools is called band contrast map or pattern quality map, depending upon the manufacturer of the instrument. The primary information displayed in these maps is the contrast or average intensity of the Kikuchi bands for each and every point. If the sample is stress-free and generates good Kikuchi pattern, then these points will appear bright. On the other hand, points which are deformed or strained or cannot generate Kikuchi pattern for any other reason appear dark. The map so generated gives an idea about which regions contain defects and which regions are defect-free. Thus, this map can also be equated with the bright field image of TEM where defects usually appear darker relative to the brighter strain-free region. Band contrast map of the above-mentioned sample is also presented in Fig. 11c. Based on similar orientation, grains can be demarcated and random color is assigned to them. This is called random colored grain map, as shown in Fig. 11d.

In microstructural analysis, identification of grains, size, and morphology is a very important parameter. However, orientation map based on IPF color scheme is not sufficient to differentiate between grains. There is a possibility that two grains have similar normal orientation, but they differ in azimuthal orientation; thus, they will be assigned similar colors and hence may seem to be part of the same grain. An example from the EBSD map, discussed above, is shown in Fig. 12. In such cases, Euler maps can be used as a handy tool. Euler maps assign color to different points based on the value of one of the Euler angles. Since there are three different Euler angles to define an orientation, thus there are three different kinds of Euler maps that can be generated. These maps can be used in conjunction with IPF maps to differentiate between grains. However, Euler maps have their own limitations, and other means are needed to identify and quantify information about grains.

Since EBSD is able to extract information about points which have similar orientation and hence form a grain, its

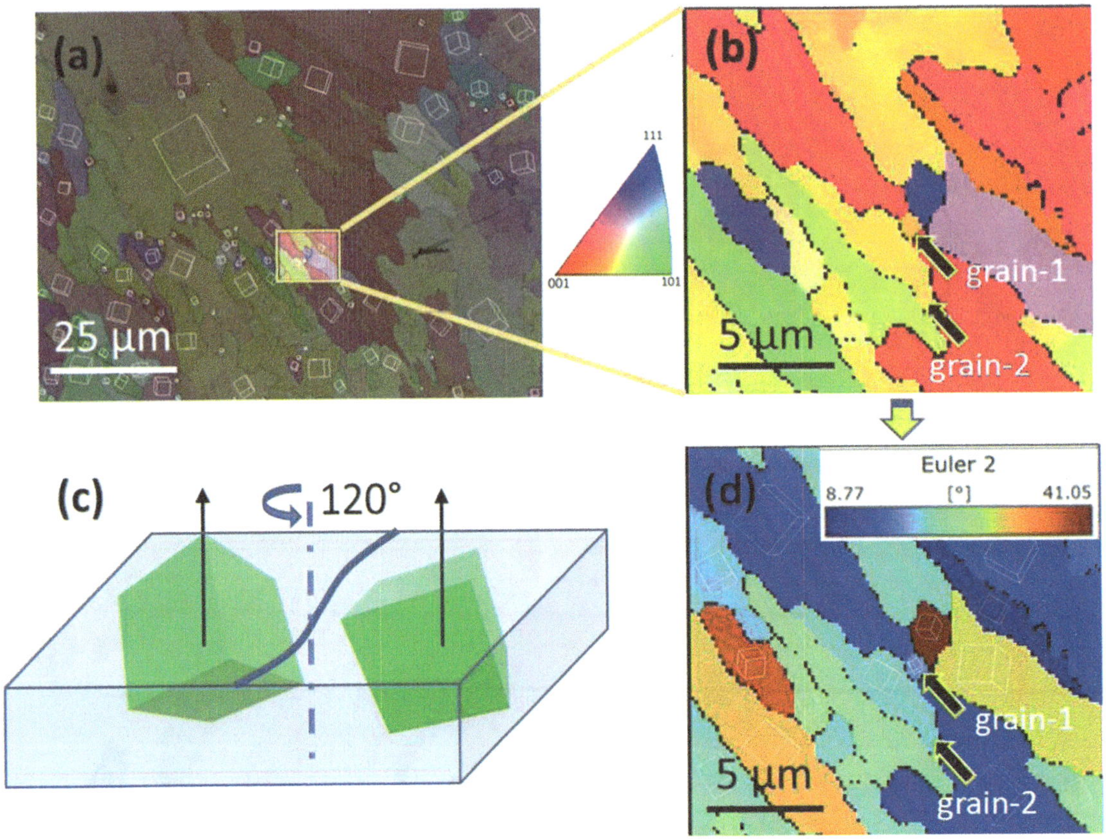

Fig. 12 **a** A small region from the orientation map is highlighted. **b** Orientation map of the highlighted region showing the two grains (grain-1 and grain-2) with similar color. **c** Two different grain scans have same IPF color because they may have same normal orientation, but different azimuthal angles. **d** Additional information from Euler map helps in differentiating between the grains

analysis engine can identify the grains and even add unique random color to each of them. It must be noted that this color is not based on the orientation of the grains or Euler angles, but a random unique color so as to be able to identify them easily. A map with grains in random color is also presented in Fig. 11d. Each of these grains has a particular orientation of the crystallite, and it has been superimposed on the map showing the grains. At this point, it is important to caution the readers that grains in EBSD are not exactly the same as grains understood in metallography. In EBSD, grains are defined mathematically, and hence, one has to define the cutoff misorientation between grains. As long as two neighboring points have misorientation below this critical value, they will be considered part of the same grain, and when they have misorientations greater than this cutoff value, then the two points will be considered as part of two different grains. Usually, this cutoff is taken as 10°, and the random grain map shown in Fig. 11d is based on this definition. A grain may also be composed of some 'sub-grains' where the misorientation between the different parts is less than 10°, and when the grain definition is changed to a small value, say 2°, some of these 'grains' may start to appear. Band contrast map of a selected region of the original map is shown in Fig. 13a. Figure 13b and c shows random grain maps with 10° grain definition and 2° grain definition, respectively. It is obvious from the figure that when the grain definition is reduced, lot more grains 'appear,' and some of these are highlighted in the figure. Grain statistics obtained from the analysis software show that there are 42 grains in Fig. 13b, while there are 83 grains in Fig. 13c. With all the requisite data for individual grains, grain-related parameters like grain size, grain morphology, grain area, etc., are easily quantified by the analysis engines.

Identification of crystal structure and its orientation also allows the EBSD analysis engine to differentiate between various phases. In some cases, where phase differentiation becomes difficult, another SEM-based technique, viz. energy-dispersive spectroscopy (EDS), is brought to use. EDS is another powerful tool which allows one to get quantitative information about composition of a given material along with its spatial distribution. This technique, combined with EBSD, can provide very accurate identification of various phases present in a given material system. Figure 14 shows EBSD maps for duplex steel, which contain both ferrite and austenite phase. Figure 14a shows the IPF map with grain boundaries, while Fig. 14b shows the

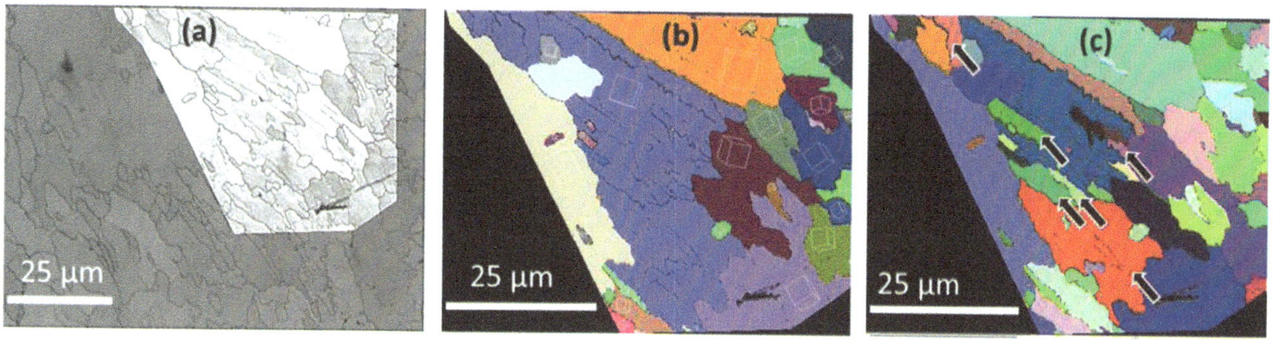

Fig. 13 **a** Region of interest from the original scan is highlighted. **b** Grain map with 10° grain definition. **c** Grain map with 2° grain definition, showing several 'new' grains which have been highlighted by arrow

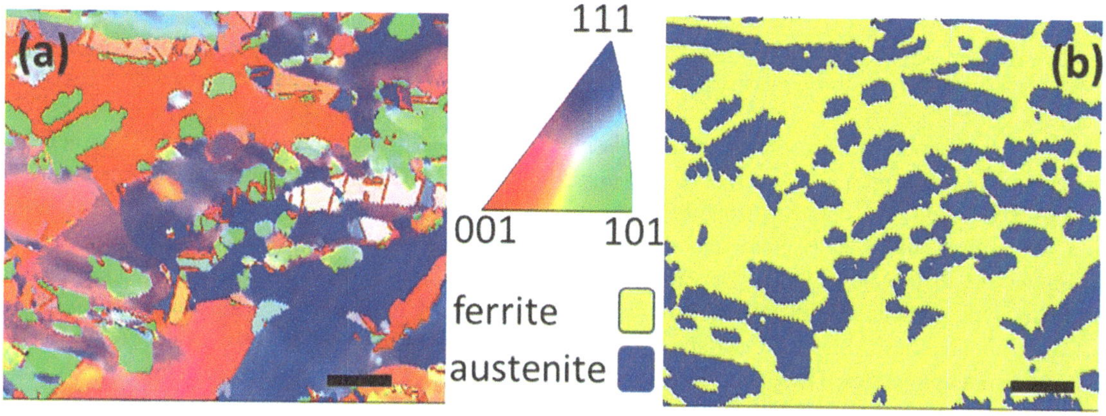

Fig. 14 Duplex steel. **a** Orientation map micrograph based on IPF color (shown here). **b** Corresponding phase map for duplex steel showing austenitic and ferritic phases (scale bar = 100 µm)

phase map of the same region, which differentiates between the two phases present in the material. Based on EBSD, it was determined that this material contained 34% austenite and 66% ferrite. This was also confirmed by ferrite scope study of the material.

6.2 Misorientation Analysis

Once we have the orientation information for each and every point or pixel in the scanned area, we can realize that most other microstructural parameters obtained in EBSD are just a derivative of this data. Since orientation is defined by the rotation matrix 'g', misorientation between two grains inside the same sample whose orientations are defined by rotation matrices 'g_1' and 'g_2', respectively, can be given by: $M = g_1^{-1}g_2$. Thus, misorientation data for any pair of points or pair of grains can be readily calculated. For data on grain boundaries or phase boundaries, misorientation data only from the neighboring points is considered and assigned as interface between the two points. The matrix form of representation of misorientation is very convenient for mathematical transformations and calculation, but misorientations are usually represented as axis–angle pair. Axis–angle pair are not unique, and depending on the symmetry of the crystal, one may obtain several sets of these axis–angle pairs. For instance, for cubic symmetry there are 24 symmetrically equivalent orientations, and this leads to 576 (=24 × 24) symmetrically equivalent misorientations. In such cases, the misorientation with the lowest angle is considered as the misorientation angle or also known as disorientation angle.

One of the simplest representations of misorientation data is the misorientation plot, which presents the frequency of occurrence of various misorientation angles between the neighboring grains of a particular microstructure (Randle et al. 2001). Misorientation plot for the Inconel sample is given in Fig. 15a. As stated earlier, misorientation angle is just one aspect of the misorientation data, and for a complete understanding of the interface between grains, one needs to also identify the misorientation axis and the boundary plane. In general, an interface between two grains is defined by five degrees of freedom. Three of these parameters are associated with misorientation and other two with the interface plane.

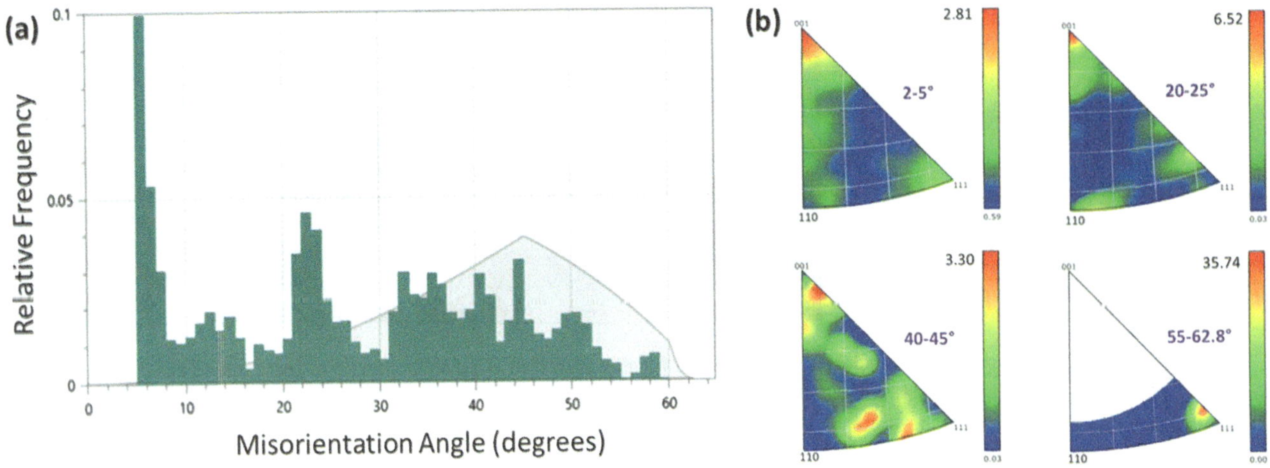

Fig. 15 **a** Misorientation distribution map for Inconel 718 sample. (Gray line indicates theoretical distribution of misorientation for a perfectly random polycrystalline material.) **b** Misorientation axis distribution of the Inconel 718 sample for four different angle ranges

For certain types of boundaries, misorientation angle is not sufficient, and they must be presented in terms of axis–angle pair. A set of axis–angle data obtained from Inconel 600, which is a single-phase material, is presented in Fig. 15b. This data shows the distribution of axis for various angle ranges. Another type of boundary of interest is coincident site lattice (CSL) boundaries, which have certain axis–angle pair that show distinct properties. These boundaries can also be extracted from the orientation and grain data and provide useful information to analyze the microstructure of the material. EBSD has come out as a powerful technique for this field of study, usually called grain boundary engineering. A case study has been provided for appreciation of the utility of EBSD in getting in-depth information about microstructure of material and thereby improving its characteristics.

6.3 Micro-strain Analysis

Residual strain inside the material is an important microstructural parameter that can also be extracted from EBSD data. Plastic strain in the material gets stored as an array of dislocations, which lead to misorientation inside the grain. These misorientations can be calculated in various ways to get different types of information. Some of the most widely used EBSD parameters to represent strain are kernel average misorientation (KAM), grain orientation spread (GOS), and grain reference orientation deviation (GROD). KAM is basically average misorientation of each point with respect to all its neighbors. This parameter is very useful in visualizing localized strains in a sample. Schematic representation of definition of KAM is shown in Fig. 16a.

GOS, on the other hand, represents average spread of the orientation of each grain. This is very useful in understanding average level of strains for individual grains and thus differentiating between the recovered and recrystallized grains from deformed grains. Grains with very low GOS value can be considered as recrystallized grain and free of any strains, while grains with very high GOS value can be considered deformed and still strained. Schematic representation of the definition of GOS and a GOS map for Inconel 718 is shown in Fig. 16b and d, respectively. Another data that is useful in understanding strains inside individual grains is intra-grain misorientation. One way to represent this is by using GROD, where the average misorientation of each point is calculated with respect to the mean orientation of the grain. This is very useful in bringing out the substructures inside a grain. KAM and GROD are similar in character and represent the deviation of individual pixels. The primary difference between the two parameters is that KAM is deviation calculated with respect to immediate neighbor orientations while GROD is deviation calculated with respect to the average orientation of the grain. A GROD map for Inconel 718 is shown in Fig. 16c. Some examples on the use of KAM and GOS to quantify the residual strain present in the material can be found in Sahu et al. 2019; Yadav et al. 2018; Yadav et al. 2019.

6.4 Micro-texture Analysis

We pointed out earlier that a complete understanding of orientation cannot be obtained from the orientation map or any other map for that matter. Maps represent only one parameter of the orientation (e.g., normal direction, Euler angle value, etc.), while orientation has at least three parameters (e.g., three perpendicular orientations or three Euler angles, etc.). It is possible to present the orientation data in three-dimensional space of the Euler angles, and this

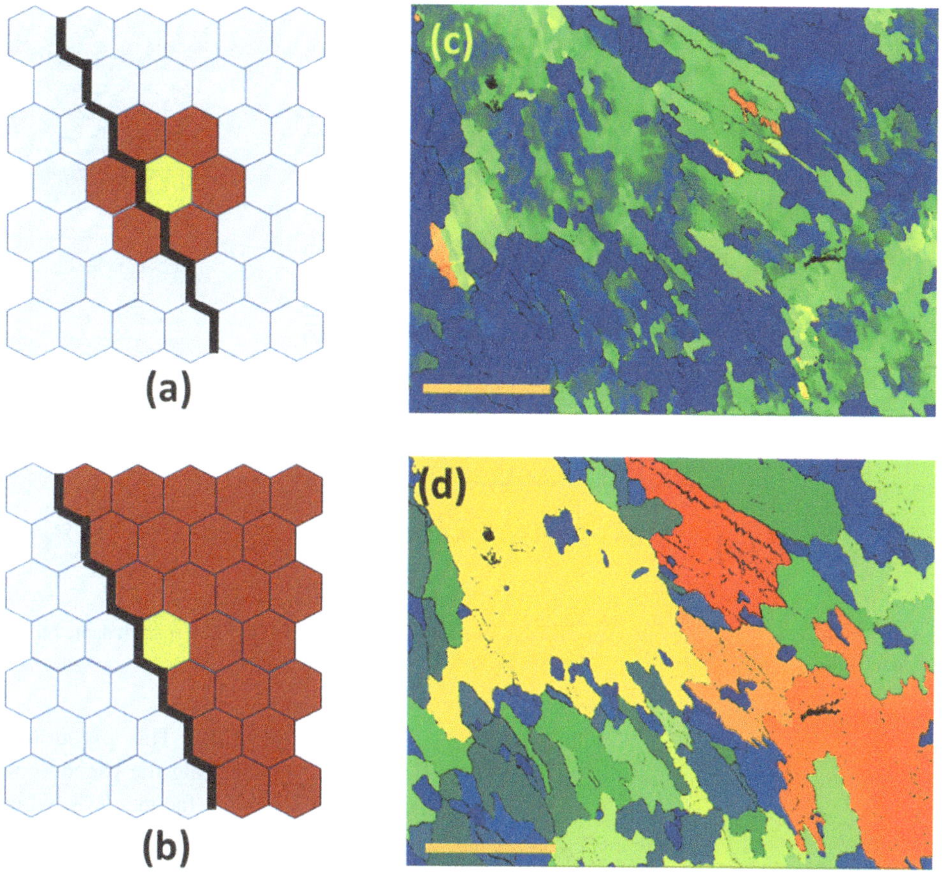

Fig. 16 Schematic explanation of the calculation of **a** KAM and **b** GOS. (Each hexagon represents individual point or pixel of EBSD map.) **c** GROD map and **d** GOS map of Inconel 718 sample

is called orientation distribution (OD). OD does not contain any information on spatial distribution of the pixels, and it only provides information related to density of pixels in this three-dimensional space. It is possible to obtain mathematical probability of orientation distribution, and in that case, it is called orientation distribution function (ODF) (Bunge and Haessner 1968; Bunge 2013). OD and ODF have served as powerful tools in texture analysis of materials. Occurrence of high density of crystal orientations in a particular Euler space denotes particular properties or phenomena in the material. A schematic of various texture components found in the cubic system in Euler space is shown in Fig. 17a (Humphreys 2001). Since plotting and analyzing a 3D information is difficult, this 3D space is cut into slices of 5° along the φ_2-axis. Hence, ODF is a 2D representation of Euler space. Orientation distribution (in 2D) of Inconel 718 sample is presented in Fig. 17b.

Another powerful tool for representation of texture is pole figures and inverse pole figures. Pole figure represents the orientation of a particular crystallographic plane with respect to sample coordinates. It basically shows the alignment of sample coordinates with the crystallographic pole. The term 'pole' refers to the normal of a given crystallographic plane intersecting a hemisphere and projected in two-dimensional plane (see Fig. 18). Pole figures can be generated for any particular crystallographic plane, but are meaningful only for certain low-index planes. Schematic of {111} pole figure of a cubic system giving rise to cube texture, copper texture, and brass texture is shown in Fig. 19. Here, RD, ND, and TD refer to the rolling direction, normal direction, and transverse direction, respectively, of the sample coordinate system. It is useful to recall that pole figures represent data with respect to the sample orientation, and hence, symmetry of the sample will also get reflected in the pole figure.

Inverse pole figure (IPF), as the name suggests, is an inverse representation of data. In IPF, all the crystallographic orientations are represented with respect to a particular sample direction (usually ND). Basically, IPF shows the alignment of crystallographic poles with a specified sample direction. Here too, crystal symmetry is reflected in the inverse pole figure. For cubic systems, we know that there are 24 symmetrically equivalent orientations, which are represented as 24 triangles in the stereographic projection (see Fig. 20a). Hence, for cubic crystal systems, representation of only one standard stereographic triangle is sufficient, shown in Fig. 20b. We can add unique colors to the orientations at the three corners of the triangle, leading to a mix of these colors for all other orientations, as shown in

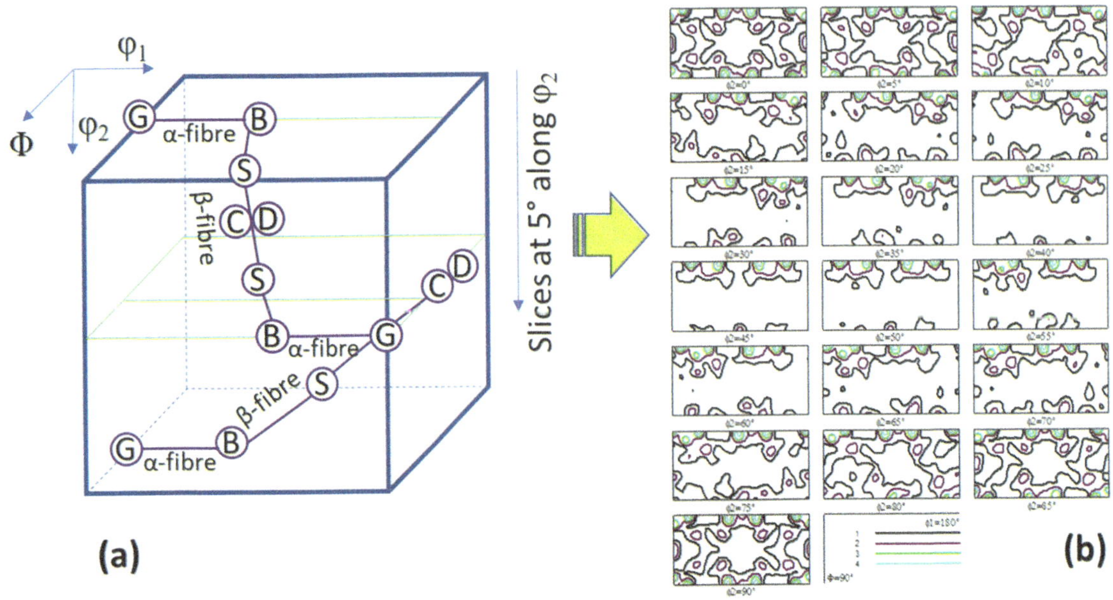

Fig. 17 **a** A schematic of various texture components found in cubic system in Euler space (adapted from ref Humphreys (2001)). **b** ODF map for Inconel 718

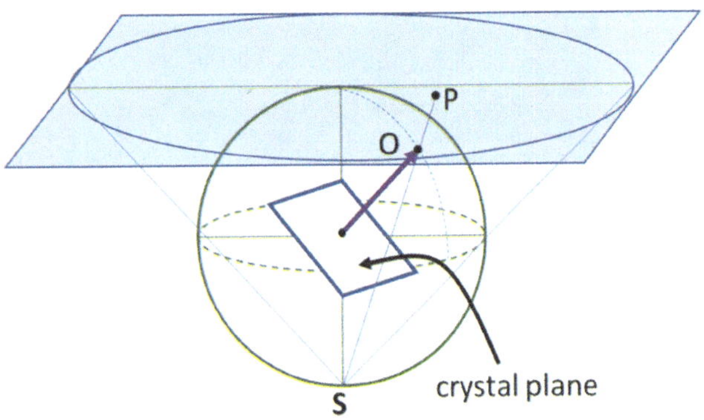

Fig. 18 Origin of pole figure: A crystal plane is shown whose normal intersects with the surface of positive hemisphere at point 'O'. 'S' is the light Source Which when passes through 'O' is projected in 2D plane at 'P', which is called the pole of the crystal plane. Adapted from ref Schwartz et al. 2009

Fig. 20c. This pseudo-colored IPF triangle is utilized for generating the pseudo-colored orientation maps shown earlier for Inconel 718, which has cubic symmetry. For lower symmetry crystal structures, there will be lesser number of the fundamental repeating unit from this stereographic projection, which can be used to add pseudo-color to the orientation map.

7 Case Studies

In the previous section, we gave a brief glimpse of various quantitative analyses that is possible from the data acquired using EBSD-based OIM. In this section, we will showcase some case studies where EBSD analysis is put in application

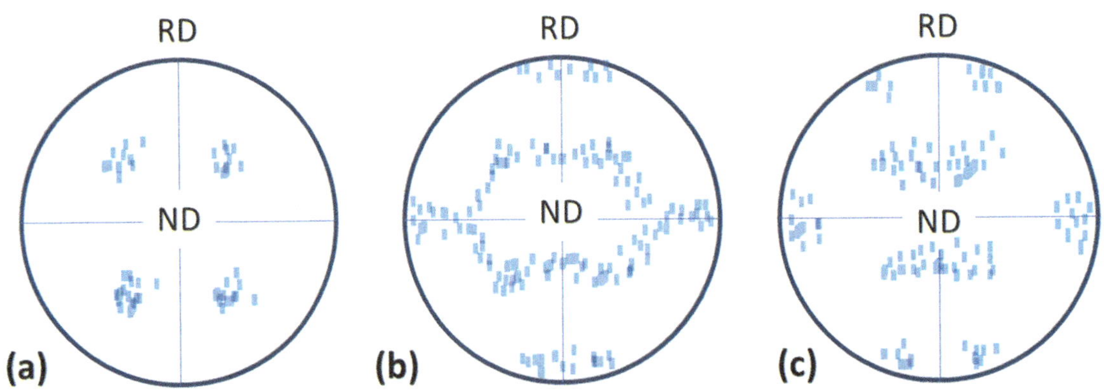

Fig. 19 Schematic of {111} pole figure of a cubic system giving rise to **a** cube texture, **b** copper texture, and **c** brass texture. (RD and ND refer to rolling direction and normal direction of the sample coordinate system.). Adapted from ref Schwartz et al. (2009)

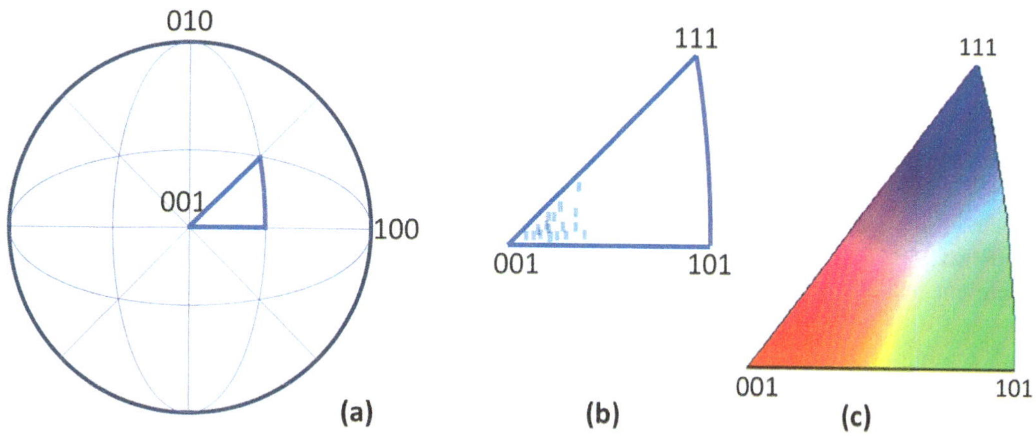

Fig. 20 **a** Stereo net for the representation of inverse pole figure and the standard stereographic triangle for the cubic system is highlighted. **b** Schematic of IPF triangle showing the cube texture. **c** IPF triangle with pseudo-colors which are used for orientation mapping

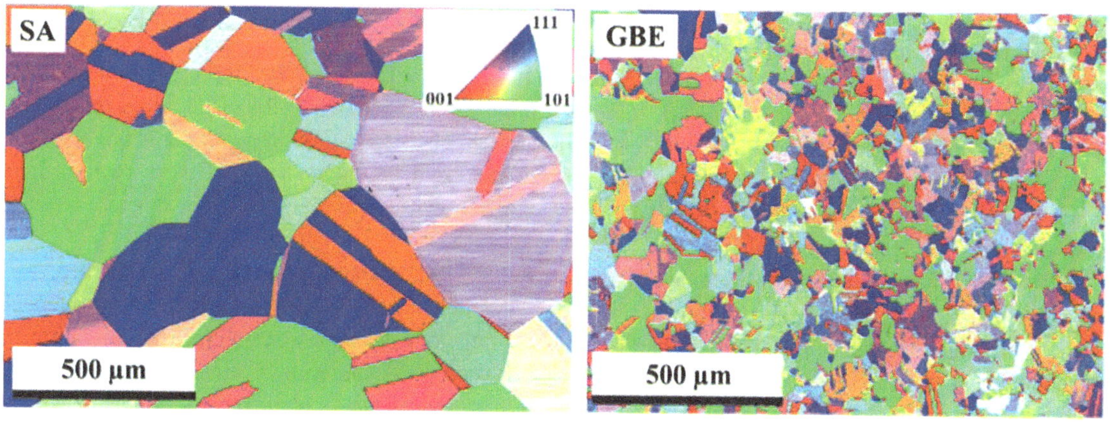

Fig. 21 IPF map of SA and GBE samples

to improve our understanding of the process–structure and structure–property correlation of material.

7.1 Study of Grain Boundary Engineering Using EBSD

EBSD technique is of particular interest, and in fact a necessity, in the field of grain boundary engineering (GBE) (Watanabe 1984; Randle 2004). Specifically, it helps to characterize various interfacial parameters like the fractions of low-Σ coincidence site lattice (CSL) boundaries, grain boundary misorientation deviation, triple junction distribution, and grain boundary connectivity.

The CSL model is used to explain the 'special' properties of some high-angle grain boundaries (HAGBs), which are highly resistant against intergranular degradation than random HAGBs. At some particular misorientation relationships, lattices of the two adjoining grains notionally coincide with each other and give rise to another three-dimensional sub-lattice, known as coincidence site lattice. The degree of coincidence is quantified by a symbol, 'Σ' (sigma), which indicates the reciprocal of the volume density of coinciding lattice sites, without consideration of the grain boundary plane (Brokman and Balluffi 1981). A deviation in the misorientation angle from the exact coincidence is allowed within which the properties of material do not vary much. The most commonly used criterion for the deviation is Brandon criterion (Brandon 1966), given as $\Delta\theta = \theta_m/\Sigma^{1/2}$ where $\Delta\theta$ is the maximum deviation angle allowed from the exact CSL misorientation and $\theta_m = 15°$. The value of low-Σ CSL is taken for $\Sigma \leq 29$, as $\Sigma > 29$ have only a negligible effect on grain boundary characteristics. Σ1 is the same as low-angle grain boundaries. Similar to grain boundaries, triple junctions may also affect intergranular characteristics. Gertsman and Tangri (1995) and Gertsman et al. (1996) classified different types of triple junctions (in 2D) into four kinds, represented as J_i ($i = 0$ to 3), depending upon the number of CSL boundaries they connect. Here, i represents the number of low-Σ CSL boundaries meeting at the triple

junction. Thus, junctions J_2 and J_3 are considered as special/secure junctions for their higher probability to arrest intergranular crack propagation. Junctions J_0 and J_1 are described as non-special/weak junctions for their lower ability in checking the propagation of intergranular degradation. The generation of special triple junctions is also necessary for the effective disruption of the connectivity of random HAGBs networks.

Here, we present a particular case study demonstrating the capabilities of EBSD for the GBE study. In this work, hot rolling and annealing were used as an industrially feasible GBE route to improve the grain boundary structure and, consequently, the functional property (viz. sensitization) of nickel-based superalloy, Alloy 600. Detailed information about this work can be found in Sahu et al. (2019, 2018).

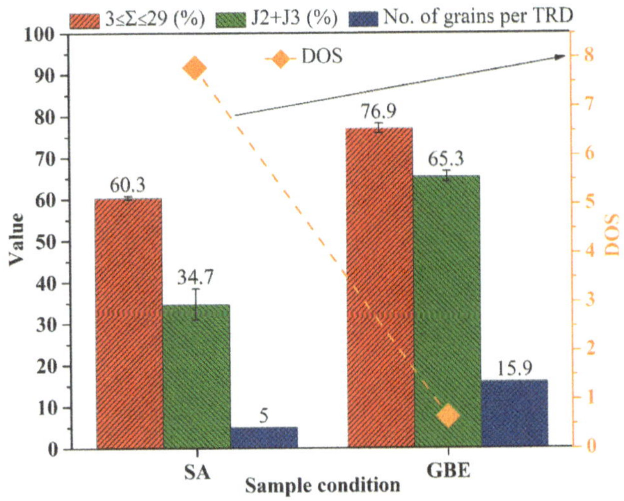

Fig. 22 Effect of thermomechanical processing on the evolution of grain boundary structure and consequently on DOS

7.1.1 Process–Structure Correlation

EBSD was used to understand the effect of thermomechanical processing on the evolution of microstructure and grain boundary structure. Figure 21 shows the IPF map of solution annealed (SA) and GBE sample conditions. It can be observed that thermomechanical processing leads to a large reduction in grain size by dynamic recrystallization. The variation of colors in the IPF maps in both the conditions indicates that there is no strong texture in either the SA condition or after the processing. The effect of processing on grain boundary structure has been quantified by measuring the fractions of special grain boundaries ($3 \leq \Sigma \leq 29$) and special triple junctions ($J_2 + J_3$), and it is shown in Fig. 22. It can be observed that the thermomechanical processing leads to an increase in not only the fraction of special boundaries but also the fraction of special junctions. In other words, this particular processing condition leads to grain boundary engineering as well as triple junction engineering in Alloy 600. This plot also distinguishes the characteristics of solution annealed and grain boundary engineered sample conditions. Even though ~60% special boundaries in the case of solution annealed sample are a fair fraction, a low fraction of special triple junctions makes it unsuitable to be called as grain boundary engineered condition. To further appreciate this effect, information regarding disruption of HAGBs network with the introduction of twin boundaries was collected with the help of twin-related domain (TRD) analysis (Reed and Kumar 2006; Gertsman 2001; Reed et al. 2004). TRD represents a cluster of grains, which are mutually connected by $\Sigma 3^n$ grain boundaries. Thus, a TRD much larger than the grain size would represent extensive multiple-twinning effects leading to high disruption of HAGBs network. The number of grains per TRD for SA and GBE condition has been shown in Fig. 22. This value is very high (15.9) for GBE sample condition in comparison with that of SA (5). Thus, grain boundary map of GBE condition can be expected to show disruption of grain boundaries, while SA condition would show a mutually connected HAGBs network. This is very well reflected in the grain boundary maps of these two particular conditions shown in Fig. 23.

7.1.2 Structure–Properties Correlation

After investigating the effect of thermomechanical processing on grain boundary structure, its correlation with functional property (in terms of sensitization effect) was studied. For it, these two samples were given sensitization heat treatment at 650 °C for 24 h, and the sensitization effect was studied with the help of double loop electrochemical potentio kinetic reactivation (DLEPR) test (Číhal Vr, Štefec R. 2001). Figure 22 shows the DOS values of the two particular conditions. As expected, a modified grain boundary structure after thermomechanical processing led to a sharp decrease in DOS value for GBE condition in comparison with that of SA sample.

The aforementioned results show an unambiguous correlation between grain boundary structure and sensitization effect; however, the role of individual boundaries on chromium carbide ($Cr_{23}C_6$) precipitation is not clear from this experiment. In order to analyze the role of individual boundaries, GBE sample was aged at 704 °C for various times between 0.5 and 100 h, and then, the precipitation of chromium carbides on individual boundaries was studied using EBSD-based OIM map and scanning electron microscopy (SEM) micrograph (showing the distribution of carbides) in the same regions. A typical subset of the EBSD map showing various kinds of boundaries and the corresponding SEM micrograph showing the precipitation of chromium carbides in 0.5 h aged GBE specimen have been demonstrated in Fig. 24. It can be seen that random HAGBs

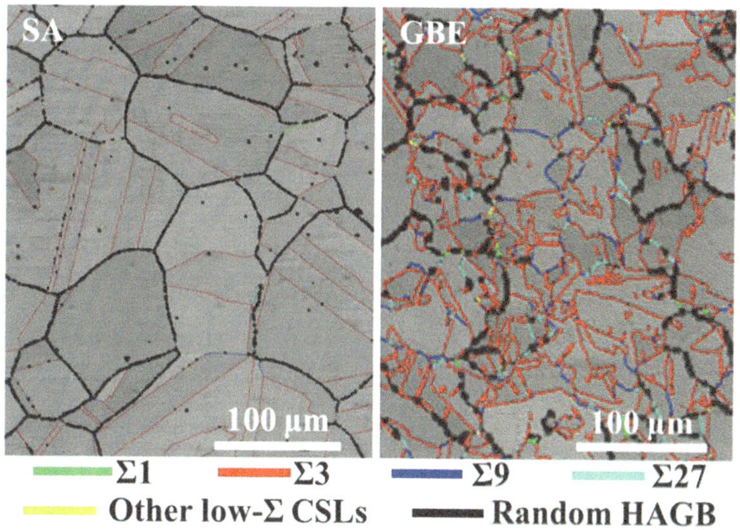

Fig. 23 Band contrast map overlaid with grain boundaries showing the effect of thermomechanical processing on the grain boundary connectivity

are very prone to the precipitation of carbides. On the other hand, low deviation Σ3 boundaries can be viewed to be void of any carbide precipitation. However, with an increase in misorientation deviation (shown by arrows in Fig. 24), even Σ3 boundaries start precipitating chromium carbides. Similarly, Σ9 boundaries are observed to have a low density of carbides.

Some more reports on the application of EBSD to study process–structure and structure–property correlation can be found in Yadav et al. 2016, 2018, 2019; Joham et al. 2017; Sharma and Shekhar 2017; Vaid et al. 2016. In conclusion, this case study showcases the capabilities of EBSD as a powerful quantitative characterization tool.

7.2 Study of Geological Materials Using EBSD

Quartz is one of the most common rock-forming silicate minerals, available in a wide range of crustal rocks, and is an important component to determine the rheology and overall dynamics of the crust. The mineral dominantly occurs in granite and granitoids, sandstones and shales, quartzites and schists. Quartz is also exclusively present in quartz veins and pegmatite dikes. Being a crystalline material, quartz deforms plastically following the laws of dynamic recrystallization under suitable pressure, temperature, and differential stress (Nicolas and Poirier 1976). A typical quartz crystal (right-handed) has several possible slip planes, activation of which is a function of temperature (Fig. 25). The systematic evaluations of such deformation, especially the study of microstructure and texture of the deformed quartz aggregates, provide a series of critical information. This information interprets the ambience, mechanisms, kinematics, and stress magnitude of the overall deformation (Bell and Etheridge 1976; Lloyd and Freeman 1994; Stipp and Tullis 2003; Twiss 1986; Halfpenny et al. 2012; Hunter et al. 2018). Quartz typically deforms maintaining three deformation regimes based on the ambient temperature (Hirth and Tullis 1992)—(i) low temperature (<300 °C); (ii) intermediate temperature (300–600 °C); and (iii) higher temperature (>600 °C). The strain rate is also a crucial factor, which generally decreases at elevated temperatures. Each regime has their characteristic set of microstructures and textures. Optical microscopy with or without universal stage attachment and automated electron backscattered diffraction (EBSD) are two of the most common and popular methods

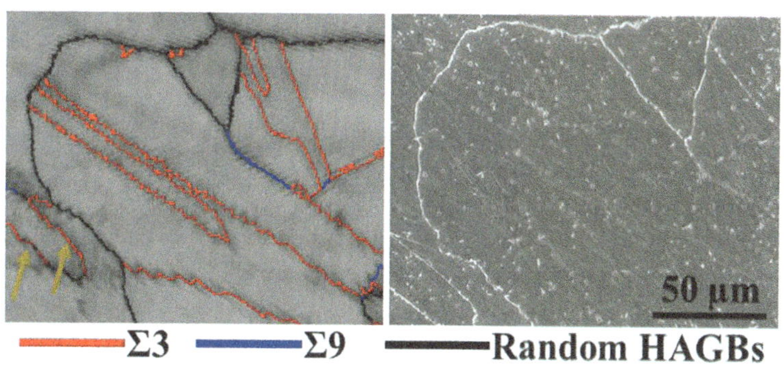

Fig. 24 (Left) Band contrast map and (right) SE image showing the effect of aging time on carbide precipitation on different kinds of boundaries

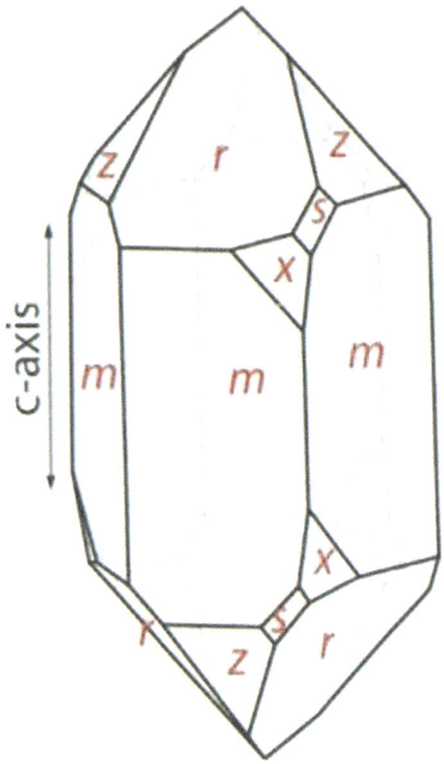

Fig. 25 A typical single quartz crystal (right-handed) showing the different slip planes. The orientation of the *c*-axis is shown by the arrow. The basal plane *a* is orthogonal to the *c*-axis

in order to study the qualitative and quantitative microstructures of quartz.

Here, we present the texture analysis of naturally deformed quartz aggregate. The samples were collected from southern granulite terrain (SGT) in India, and a rock suite underwent metamorphism up to granulite facies (Ghosh et al. 2004). SGT hosts high-grade rocks, like charnockites, khondalites, and other granulite facies metamorphic rocks. The concerned quartz unit typically occurs as discrete stratigraphic unit within the granulites as alternating layers of quartz and iron oxides (magnetite and hematite), popularly referred to as 'banded hematite quartzite' and 'banded magnetite quartzite.' The ultrahigh temperature and pressure granulite facies metamorphism (1000 ± 50 °C/5–9 kbar) in SGT dates back to 2.5 billion years (Raith et al. 1997; Janardhan 1999), which followed a counterclockwise *PTt* path and exhumation processes due to differential upliftment active in recent geological past.

Observations of the samples under a transmitted light optical microscope reveal that quartz (Qtz) grains are dominantly present as elongated thin micro-bands along with opaque minerals (iron oxides, IOx) and pyroxene (Pyx) grains (Fig. 26a). The quartz grains are dynamically recrystallized; in a few places, triple junctions along the grain boundaries are observed, and a large number of grains show undulose extinctions (Fig. 26b). Pyroxene grains remain as porphyroclasts and often show weak shear kinematics (Fig. 26a). Polished sections of the samples observed under the scanning electron microscope in backscatter electron (BSE) mode reveal equant shaped iron oxide grains occurring together in the stretched oxide segments (Fig. 26c).

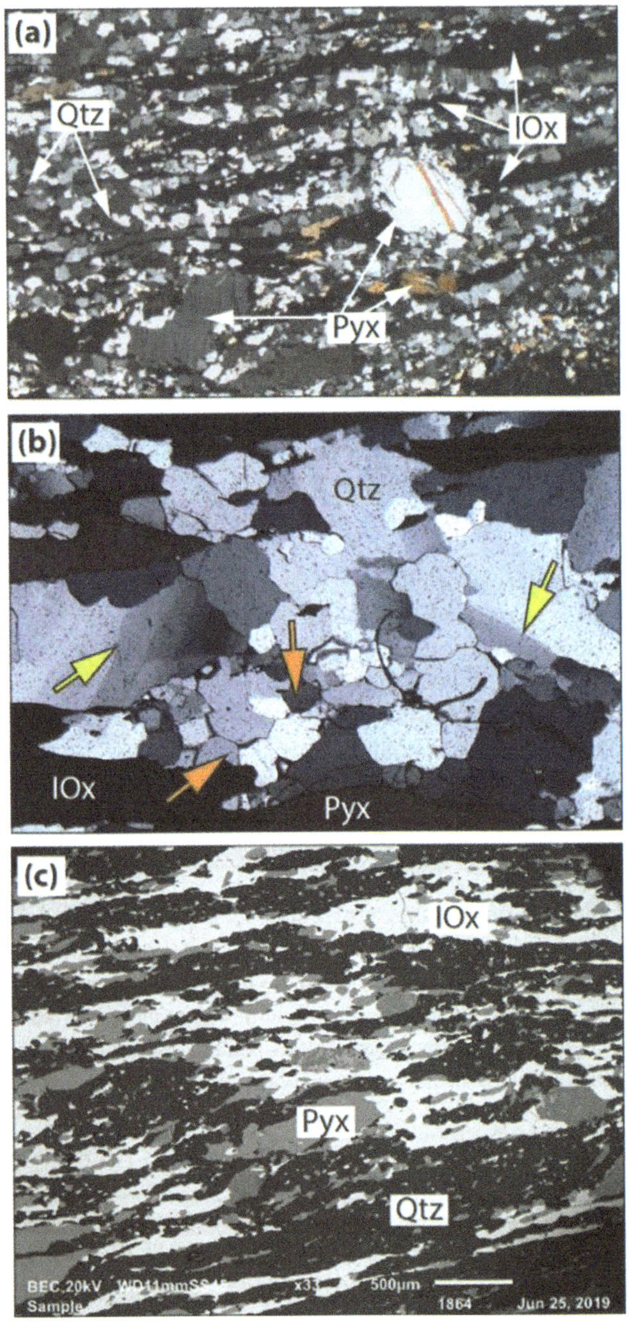

Fig. 26 Transmitted optical (**a**, **b**) and backscatter SEM images of the studied samples observed on the XZ plane of the bulk strain ellipse. In (**b**), the yellow and orange arrowheads point undulose extinctions and triple junctions, respectively, in the quartz grains. Qtz: Quartz; IOx: iron oxides; Pyx: pyroxene. The width of plates **a** and **b** is 10 and 2 mm, respectively

We performed EBSD analysis to study the texture of the quartz grains. A representative sample was cut along the XZ section of the bulk strain ellipsoid and prepared for the analysis following the standard protocols of the EBSD polishing. The EBSD analysis was performed using a field emission scanning electron microscope (JSM 7100F) equipped with an EBSD detector (Oxford Instrument NanoAnalysis, UK) keeping the scan surface of the samples tilted at 70°. The EBSD patterns were collected with 20 mm working distance, 2–5 μm step size, 20 kV accelerating voltage, and ~ 13 nA beam current. Data acquisition from the sample and crystallographic patterns were indexed automatically by Aztec Software (Oxford Instrument NanoAnalysis, UK). MTEX (Mainprice et al. 2011), an open-source MATLAB toolbox (version 5.1.1), was employed to post-process data. Data points with confidence index < 0.1 were removed using the software package. The critical misorientation angle to reconstruct individual quartz grains was chosen to be 10°. The data of the quartz grains is presented in phase map, grain orientation spread (GOS) map, kernel average misorientation (KAM) map, inverse pole figure (IPF) map, and pole figures.

We present the results of EBSD analysis in Fig. 27. The phase map shows that the quartz grains dominate the area with a few smaller hematite and magnetite grains (Fig. 27a). The GOS is noted to be within 5° (Fig. 27b). The IPF map reveals the fact that quartz grains are deformed, and in few, they also show sub-grain boundaries (Fig. 27c). The KAM for majority of the grains lies within 0.004, with few grains characterized by thin bands of high values (>0.016, Fig. 27d). One-point-per-grain pole figures (Fig. 27e–h) are calculated and presented using de la ValléePousin kernel and half width of 15°. The pole figures are contoured to multiples of uniform density (m.u.d). The ⟨c⟩-axis pole figure exhibits a well-defined central girdle. Its obliquity to the XY plane indicates top-to-left sense of shear (Fig. 27e). The cylindricity index (Larson 2018) was calculated to be 0.9, indicating that the quartz grains are highly strained/deformed. Moreover, the maxima of the ⟨c⟩-axis pole figure suggests both rhomb-⟨a⟩ and prism-⟨a⟩ planes were dominantly active, implying deformation within 400–500 °C (Passchier and Trouw 2005). The location of the maxima of the ⟨a⟩-axis pole figure (Fig. 27f) also confirms the same.

7.3 Study of the Effect of Machining Parameters on Subsurface Deformation Using EBSD

Machining is known to make structural changes to not only the surface, but also the subsurface of a machined component (Abolghasem et al. 2012; Shekhar et al. 2012; Wang et al. 2017). The strain, strain rate, and associated temperature rise and eventual microstructural changes in the chip and surface depend largely on the machining configuration. This microstructural transformation leads to change in the functional (Majumdar et al. 2015; Prakash et al. 2015a, b) as well as the mechanical response of the machined component (Gidla 2017; Verma 2014). Surface characteristics like roughness and hardness are known to have an impact on material failure that initiate from the surface such as fatigue failure, fretting fatigue, wear, and stress corrosion cracking as the surface is in contact with the environment (Yuri et al. 2003; Al-Samarai et al. 2012). The surface characteristics of a machined component are also resultant of the machining conditions used during the final shaping operation of the component. Thus, machining parameters affect the surface characteristics as well as the subsurface microstructure of the finished components, which in turn play an important role in deciding the mechanical and functional response of the material.

The overarching goal of this study was to optimize the machining parameters to improve surface characteristics and improve material performance. The specific objective of this work was to understand the effect of machining parameters on the subsurface microstructure and correlate it with surface characteristics. In this regard, simple orthogonal machining of SS316L using tungsten carbide tool was performed on CNC machine. We selected wear volume and hardness as our measure of surface characteristics and microstructure was characterized using EBSD technique. Steel rod was machined at two different speeds (30 and 180 mm/min) for two different feeds (0.05 and 0.2 mm/rev) at two different depths of cut (DOC) (0.1 and 0.5 mm) keeping tool parameters constant, i.e., rake angle (zero degree) and nose radius (0.4). 8-mm disks were taken from the rod, and overall, we had 8 sample conditions as listed in Table 1. Each of these samples was characterized for roughness using optical profilometry. Ball on disk method was used to conduct tribological studies. Tungsten carbide ball has 6-mm diameter, and the sample was made as the disk having diameter 55 mm and thickness 8 mm.

EBSD technique was utilized for characterizing the subsurface microstructure of the machined surface. Small samples from close to the machined surface were taken, and rectangular scans were taken on the transverse region from near the surface toward the inside of the sample. Orientation maps (overlaid on band contrast map and grain boundary map, shown in black) from an area of 120 μm × 40 μm for various sample conditions are presented in Fig. 28. The machined surface is shown by the direction of the arrow. Most of the samples show severe deformation near the surface. The black dots near the surface represent the un-indexed points, which point to some strain in the matrix. The extent of depth of these black dots indicates the extent of subsurface deformation. In some of the conditions, one

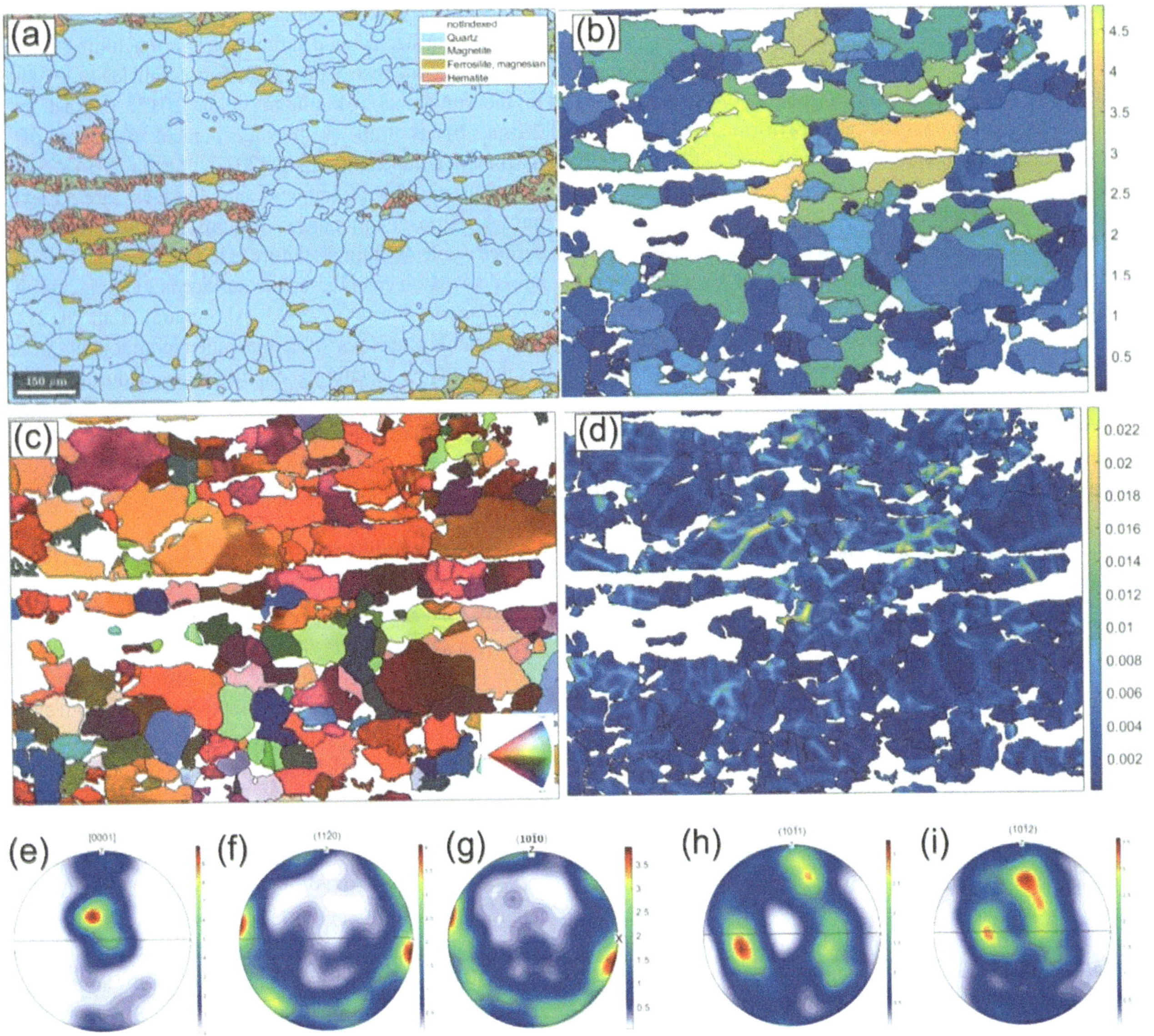

Fig. 27 Selected results of the EBSD analysis. **a** Phase map, **b** grain orientation spread (GOS) map, **c** inverse pole figure (IPF) map along with the key at the inset, **d** kernel average misorientation (KAM) map. One-point-per-grain pole figures of **e** ⟨c⟩-axes, **f** ⟨a⟩-axes, **g** {m}-planes, **h** {r}-planes, and **i** {z}-planes of the quartz grains. The scale is shown only for **a** so as to avoid repetition

Table 1 Details of machining parameters that were selected for machining of SS316L

Sample	Speed (mm/min)	Feed (mm/rev)	Depth of cut (mm)	Rake angle	Nose radius
S1F1D1	30	0.05	0.1	0	0.4
S1F1D2	30	0.05	0.5	0	0.4
S1F2D1	30	0.2	0.1	0	0.4
S1F2D2	30	0.2	0.5	0	0.4
S2F1D1	180	0.05	0.1	0	0.4
S2F1D2	180	0.05	0.5	0	0.4
S2F2D1	180	0.2	0.1	0	0.4
S2F2D2	180	0.2	0.5	0	0.4

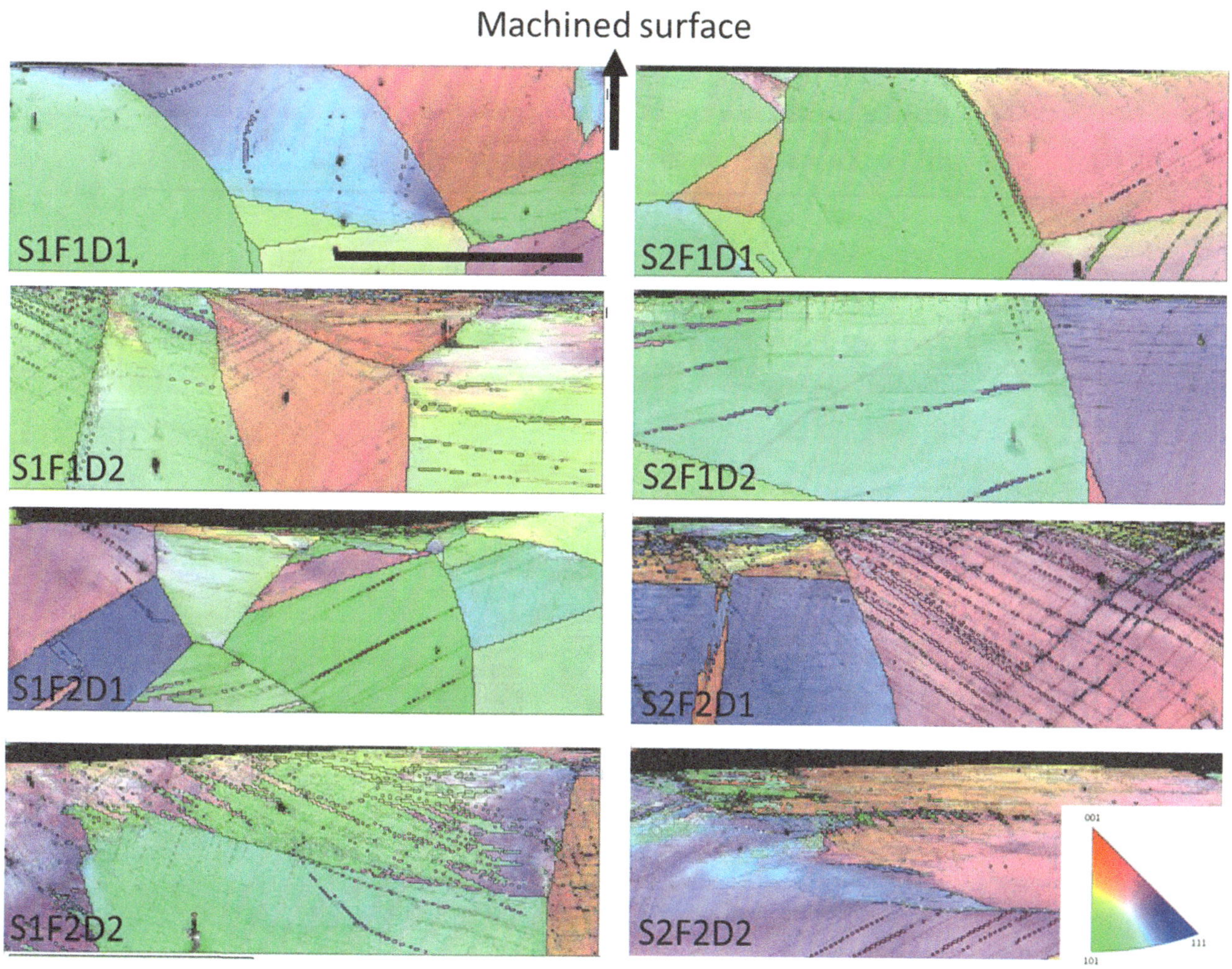

Fig. 28 Orientation maps (overlaid with band contrast map and grain boundary map shown in black) for samples machined under various conditions (scale bar = 50 μm; same for all micrographs)

can see some very refined grains very close to the surface, but it is not there in most of the other conditions. One can conclude that grain refinement, if it happened, was limited to few micrometers near the surface. However, the subsurface deformation does extend much below this. In order to get a better understanding of the subsurface deformation, GROD maps were generated from the EBSD data.

Roughness values and wear volume were plotted for various sample conditions along with the corresponding GROD map in Fig. 29. Here, one can very easily find a correlation between the smaller subsurface deformation and good (low values) roughness condition on the surface (S1F1D1 and S2F1D1). It is likely that subsurface deformation leads to massive slips on various planes, which leads to poor roughness (S1F1D2, S1F2D2, and S2F2D2). On the other hand, best wear resistance is obtained when we have very large subsurface deformation (S1F2D2 and S2F1D2). It is expected as subsurface deformation results in higher hardness near the surface, yielding better wear resistance. However, we found that some sample conditions yield good surface roughness as well as good wear resistance (S2F1D1 and S2F1D2). This most likely happens when there exists a very thin layer of subsurface deformation. A thin layer of subsurface deformation results in minimal upheaval on the surface while still resulting in high hardness for good wear resistance. A closer look at the data also suggests that roughness improves with an increase in speed, decrease in feed, and DOC.

This study clearly establishes that EBSD technique can provide a wealth of information about microstructure. In this work, we were able to relate the surface characteristics to the machining parameters and, in turn, to the subsurface microstructure. This improves our understanding in optimizing the machining parameters to obtain better microstructure as well as better surface characteristics.

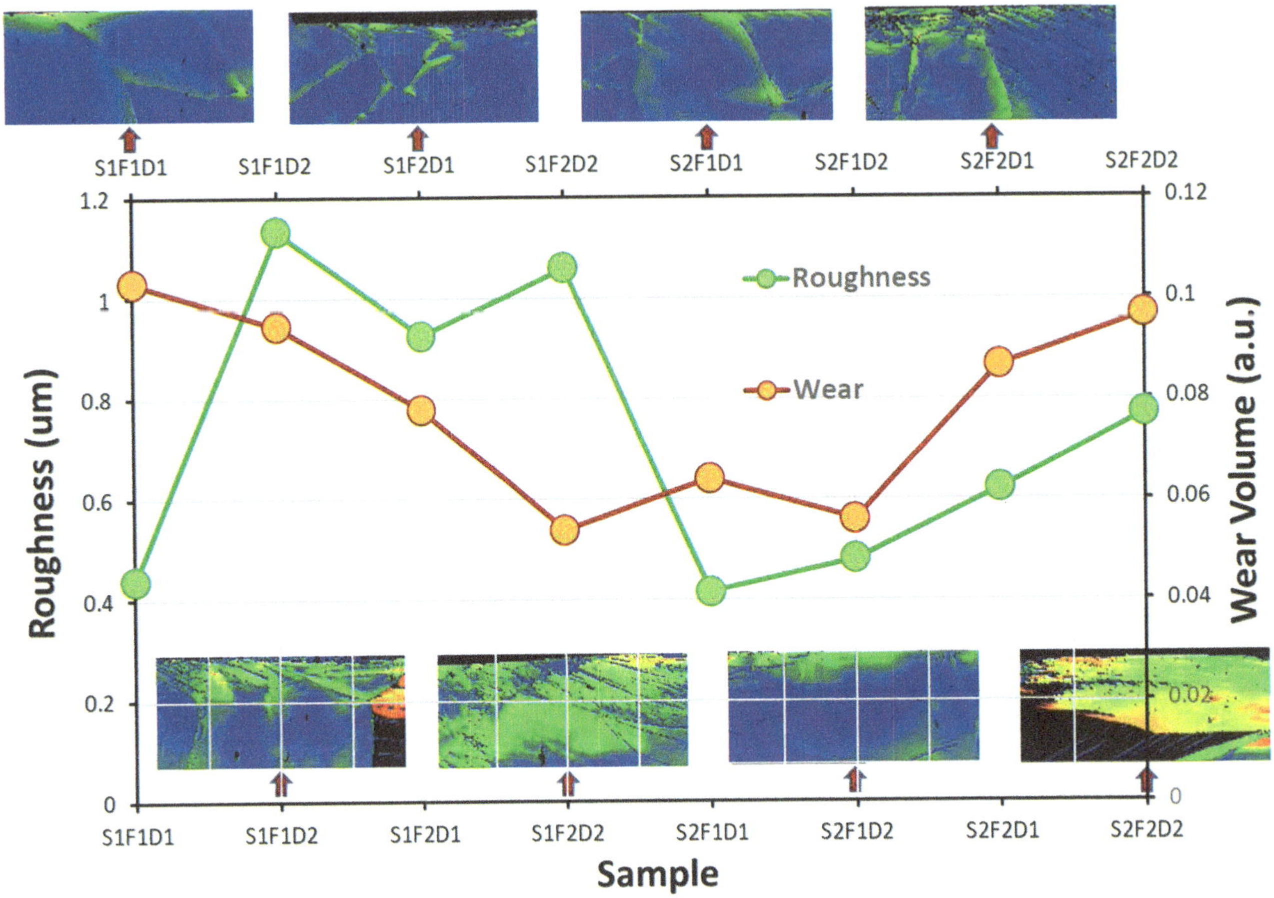

Fig. 29 Variation of roughness and wear volume for various sample conditions (machined surface is toward the top side of each micrograph)

8 Accuracy and Limitations of EBSD

The accuracy with which an absolute orientation of a crystallite can be measured using EBSD is typically ~1° (Humphreys 2001; Schwartz et al. 2009; Humphreys and Brough 1999). This value is dependent on the EBSD acquisition parameters, calibration of the EBSD system, and sample alignment conditions. Although the accuracy of the measurement of an orientation is an important factor in determining the usefulness of EBSD, applications of EBSD in the characterization of grain boundaries and their correlation with properties require very accurate measurement of the relative orientation between the neighboring pixels (Humphreys 2001; Humphreys et al. 1999). Accuracy in the relative orientation becomes even more critical in the case of low-angle grain boundaries, especially the interfaces between sub-grains in the deformed samples (Humphreys et al. 1999; Prior 1999; Wilson and Spanos 2001). Since this relative orientation, or misorientation, is calculated using the absolute orientation data, the accuracy of the measurement of misorientation is related to the precision with which the absolute orientation of individual crystallites can be obtained.

Ideally, all the absolute orientations within a same crystallite should be same, and there should not be any scatter in the orientation data. However, due to the inherent limitations of EBSD, there is a definite value of this orientation noise, ranging from 0.5 to 1° (Wilkinson 2001). These limitations include various factors such as accuracy of pattern solving using Hough transform, CCD camera settings, detector calibrations, accuracy of band detection, and sample alignment. This orientation noise also creates a scatter in the measured data of misorientation between the individual orientations. While this scatter in misorientation data is relatively smaller (~0.2° for misorientation angles higher than 2°) for higher angle grain boundaries, scatters even higher than the actual misorientation for low-angle grain boundaries make an accurate determination of small misorientation angles very difficult (Wilkinson 2001). This further inhibits the study of finer details of a microstructure using misorientation-based parameters like grain average misorientation (GAM), grain orientation spread (GOS), and kernel average misorientation (KAM). Similar to misorientation angles, accurate

Table 2 Typical angular resolution of EBSD in the form of scatter in the measured orientation data (Wilkinson 2001)

Scatter type	Average scatter	Maximum scatter
Absolute orientation	0.5°	1.4°

determination of the misorientation axis also poses certain challenges and is also dependent on the noise of absolute orientation data. Scatter in misorientation axis is not significant for higher misorientation angles. However, the measured misorientation axis for low misorientation angles (<5°) can cover almost complete inverse pole figure, hence making the accurate determination practically impossible (Wilkinson 2001).

Tables 2 and 3 provide a summary of the values of the scatter in the measured orientation and misorientation data, respectively. Average and maximum scatters in the measured orientation data are 0.5 and 1.4°. This scatter is a result of the low precision in the measurement of an individual orientation. As discussed earlier, this precision in the measurement of absolute crystal orientation becomes a limiting factor in the estimation of relative crystal orientation and hence in the characterization of very low-angle grain boundaries. It also makes the application of conventional EBSD potentially inadequate for the characterization of microstructures having deformation features.

Misorientation data is tabulated for 3 different actual misorientation angles, viz. 20, 2, and 0.2°. Maximum scatter in the data of misorientation angles is the standard deviation of the data for each case. It can be seen that for very small misorientation angles such as 0.2°, the scatter in misorientation angle is 0.4°, which is even higher than the actual misorientation angle, and hence, the accurate determination of small misorientation angle is very difficult. In the case of misorientation axis, angles between the measured misorientation axis and the actual misorientation axis are first calculated. Mean scatter and maximum scatter for the misorientation axis are then the mean and maximum value of this data set. Maximum scatter in the misorientation axis for very small misorientation angles reaches such a high value that it becomes practically indefinite, hence written as 'indefinite' in the table.

Improvement in the overall angular resolution of the EBSD technique requires the minimization of the scatter in misorientation data generated. This can ensure the routine and more reliable characterization of very small misorientation angles (<2°). One of the ways to minimize the scatter is either by statistically averaging the orientation data (Humphreys 2001; Wright et al. 2015) or by subtracting a Gaussian-type noise function (Humphreys 1999; Sharma and Shekhar 2018). Although this approach can lead to an improvement in misorientation angle distribution at smaller misorientation angles, improvement in the individual misorientation is not achieved. Changing the operating conditions such as probe current to enhance the quality of backscattered patterns is yet another way to improve the angular resolution (Humphreys and Brough 1999). However, this approach would lead to a decrease in the pattern collection speed and hence will be limited for very smaller area maps. Another approach is to improve the fundamental pattern detection, matching, and solving techniques, including cross-correlation (Bate et al. 2005; Brough et al. 2006; El-Dasher et al. 2003; Wright et al. 2017). These methods are essentially based on the recording of small changes in the absolute positions of similar features in the two patterns from adjacent pixels.

Since this method improves the angular resolution significantly, the EBSD technique with the improved pattern solving method is also known as high-resolution electron backscatter diffraction (HR-EBSD) (Schwartz et al. 2009). Table 4 shows the typical scatter values obtained using a routine HR-EBSD technique. It can be seen that maximum scatter in misorientation angle is only 0.02° even for misorientation angles as small as 0.2°. Maximum scatter in the misorientation axis is also lowered to a definite value of ~14°. This data shows that the EBSD technique with these improved pattern-solving capabilities can be confidently utilized for the routine characterization of deformation

Table 3 Typical angular resolution of EBSD in the form of scatter in the measured misorientation data (Wilkinson 2001)

Actual misorientation	20°	2°	0.2°
Misorientation angle (maximum scatter)	0.2°	0.25°	0.4°
Misorientation axis (mean scatter)	2°	15°	50°
Misorientation axis (maximum scatter)	5°	40°	-Indefinite-

Table 4 Typical angular resolution of HR-EBSD in the form of scatter in the measured misorientation data (Wilkinson 2001)

Actual misorientation	0.2°
Misorientation angle (maximum scatter)	0.02°
Misorientation axis (mean scatter)	5.7°
Misorientation axis (maximum scatter)	13.9°

constituents. This way, the HR-EBSD technique has proved to be pathbreaking in the characterization of localized strains with high resolution (Wilkinson et al. 2014).

It should also be noted that these methods are quite resource-intensive and require a lot of computer space for storing all the electron backscatter pattern (EBSP) data and, in turn, resulting in the increased cost for overall EBSD characterization. However, such limitations are gradually waning with the improvement in computing and storage capabilities.

9 Summary

It is clearly established that EBSD is a very powerful technique that can be applied to all types of crystallographic materials, ranging from metals to ceramics to semiconductors. We provided fundamentals on the origin of Kikuchi pattern and how this data is acquired by the hardware to identifying the orientation of a given material. We have also provided a glimpse of various fundamental analyses that can be carried out with the data extracted using EBSD. Analysis of the data can provide various in-depth understandings of the microstructure and its properties, and this was clearly brought out with the help of some of the case studies discussed here. Toward the latter part, we have also discussed the limitations of this instrument, particularly in terms of the accuracy of the data obtained. This must be kept in mind when interpreting the results and deriving conclusions. It should also be noted that there are several journal articles and books available on the topics listed above, which discuss at length each of these issues. The purpose of this article is to provide the beginners all the necessary information at one place, without getting distracted by great many details. Readers who are looking to gain an in-depth understanding of the subject are directed to the references cited in this article.

Acknowledgements All the EBSD data was generated using the facilities in the Advanced Centre for Material Sciences (ACMS) of IIT Kanpur. Mr. Sivakumar assisted in EBSD data acquisition for the Inconel 718 sample. EBSD of duplex steel was acquired by Prince Setia. Saquib Abdullah, Dripta Dutta, and R. Sarvesha assisted in the EBSD data acquisition and analysis of quartz in case study (B). A part of the work in case study (B) is supported by a DST Swarnajayanti Fellowship (DST/SJF/E&ASA-01/2015-16), awarded to Santanu Misra. Case study (C) is part of the project funded by BRNS, under sanction No. 36(2)/14/39/2016-BRNS/6047.

References

Abolghasem S, Basu S, Shekhar S, Cai J, Shankar M (2012) Mapping subgrain sizes resulting from severe simple shear deformation. Acta Mater 60(1):376–386

Ahmed J, Wilkinson AJ, Roberts SG (1997) Characterizing dislocation structures in bulk fatigued copper single crystals using electron channelling contrast imaging (ECCI). Philos Mag Lett 76(4):237–246

Al-Samarai RA, Haftirman KRA, Al-Douri Y (2012) The influence of roughness on the wear and friction coefficient under dry and lubricated sliding. Int J Sci Eng Res 3(4):1–6

Bate PS, Knutsen RD, Brough I, Humphreys FJ (2005) The characterization of low-angle boundaries by EBSD. J Microsc 220(1):36–46

Bell TH, Etheridge MA (1976) The deformation and recrystallization of quartz in a mylonite zone. Cent Aust Tectonophysics 32(3):235–267

Berger D, Niedrig H (1999) Complete angular distribution of electrons backscattered from tilted multicomponent specimens. Scanning 21 (3):187–190

Brandon D (1966) The structure of high-angle grain boundaries. Acta Metall 14(11):1479–1484

Brokman A, Balluffi RW (1981) Coincidence lattice model for the structure and energy of grain boundaries. Acta Metall 29(10):1703–1719

Brough I, Bate PS, Humphreys FJ (2006) Optimising the angular resolution of EBSD. Mater Sci Technol 22(11):1279–1286

Bunge HJ, Haessner F (1968) Three-dimensional orientation distribution function of crystals in cold-rolled copper. J Appl Phys 39 (12):5503–5514

Bunge HJ (2013) Texture analysis in materials science: mathematical methods. Elsevier

Chen D, Kuo J-C, Wu W-T (2011) Effect of microscopic parameters on EBSD spatial resolution. Ultramicroscopy 111(9):1488–1494

Číhal Vr, Štefec R (2001) On the development of the electrochemical potentiokinetic method. Electrochimica Acta 46(24):3867–3877

Coates DG (1967) Kikuchi-like reflection patterns obtained with the scanning electron microscope. Philos Mag: J Theor Exp Appl Phys 16(144):1179–1184

Dingley DJ, Wright SI, Nowell MM (2005) Dynamic background correction of electron backscatter diffraction patterns. Microsc Microanal 11(S02):528–529

El-Dasher BS, Adams BL, Rollett AD (2003) Viewpoint: experimental recovery of geometrically necessary dislocation density in polycrystals. Scripta Mater 48(2):141–145

Gertsman V (2001) Coincidence site lattice theory of multicrystalline ensembles. Acta Crystallogr A 57(6):649–655

Gertsman VY, Janecek M, Tangri K (1996) Grain boundary ensembles in polycrystals. Acta Mater 44(7):2869–2882

Gertsman VY, Tangri K (1995) Computer simulation study of grain boundary and triple junction distributions in microstructures formed by multiple twinning. Acta Metall Mater 43(6):2317–2324

Ghosh JG, de Wit MJ, Zartman RE (2004) Age and tectonic evolution of Neoproterozoic ductile shear zones in the Southern Granulite Terrain of India, with implications for Gondwana studies. Tectonics 23(3):TC3006

Gidla MR (2017) Effect of machining on mechanical, tribological and functional properties of mild steel, M.Tech. thesis at IIT Kanpur

Halfpenny A, Prior DJ, Wheeler J (2012) Electron backscatter diffraction analysis to determine the mechanisms that operated during dynamic recrystallisation of quartz-rich rocks. J Struct Geol 36:2–15

Heinz A, Neumann P (1991) Representation of orientation and disorientation data for cubic, hexagonal, tetragonal and orthorhombic crystals. Acta Crystallogr A 47(6):780–789

Herter T, Lott K (1993) Algorithms for decomposing 3-D orthogonal matrices into primitive rotations. Comput Graph 17(5):517–527

Hirth G, Tullis J (1992) Dislocation creep regimes in quartz aggregates. J Struct Geol 14(2):145–159

Humphreys FJ (1999) Quantitative metallography by electron backscattered diffraction. J Microsc 195(3):170–185
Humphreys FJ (2001) Review grain and subgrain characterisation by electron backscatter diffraction. J Mater Sci 36(16):3833–3854
Humphreys FJ, Brough I (1999) High resolution electron backscatter diffraction with a field emission gun scanning electron microscope. J Microsc 195(Pt 1):6–9
Humphreys FJ, Huang Y, Brough I, Harris C (1999) Electron backscatter diffraction of grain and subgrain structures—resolution considerations. J Microsc 195(3):212–216
Hunter NJR, Weinberg RF, Wilson CJL, Luzin V, Misra S (2018) Microscopic anatomy of a "hot-on-cold" shear zone: insights from quartzites of the Main Central Thrust in the Alaknanda region (Garhwal Himalaya). GSA Bull 130(9–10):1519–1539
Janardhan AS (1999) Southern granulite terrain, south of the palghat-cauvery shear zone: implications for India-madagascar connection. Gondwana Res 2(3):463–469
Joham R, Sharma NK, Mondal K, Shekhar S (2017) Low temperature cross-rolling to modify grain boundary character distribution and its effect on sensitization of SS304. J Mater Process Technol 240:324–331
Joy DC, Newbury DE, Davidson DL (1982) Electron channeling patterns in the scanning electron microscope. J Appl Phys 53(8): R81–R122
Kamaladasa R, Picard Y (2010) Basic principles and application of electron channeling in a scanning electron microscope for dislocation analysis. Microsc: Sci Technol Appl Educ 3:1583–1590
Kunze K, Wright SI, Adams BL, Dingley DJ (1993) Advances in automatic EBSP single orientation measurements. Textures Microstruct 20:589659
Larson KP (2018) Refining the structural framework of the Khimti Khola region, east-central Nepal Himalaya, using quartz textures and c-axis fabrics. J Struct Geol 107:142–152
Lloyd GE, Freeman B (1994) Dynamic recrystallization of quartz under greenschist conditions. J Struct Geol 16(6):867–881
Mainprice D, Hielscher R, Schaeben H (2011) Calculating anisotropic physical properties from texture data using the MTEX open-source package. Geolog Soc, London, Spec Publ 360(1):175–192
Majumdar P, Shekhar S, Mondal K (2015) Effect of machining parameters on oxidation behavior of mild steel. J Mater Eng Perform 24(1):484–498
Michael J, Giannuzzi L (2007) Improved EBSD sample preparation via low energy Ga + FIB Ion milling. Microsc Microanal 13(S02):926–927
Morawiec A, Field DP (1996) Rodrigues parameterization for orientation and misorientation distributions. Philos Mag A 73(4):1113–1130
Nicolas A, Poirier J-P (1976) Crystalline plasticity and solid state flow in metamorphic rocks. Jokn Wiley & Sons, London, p 444
Nishikawa S, Kikuchi S (1928a) Diffraction of cathode rays by calcite. Nature 122(3080):726–726
Nishikawa S, Kikuchi S (1928b) Diffraction of cathode rays by mica. Nature 121(3061):1019–1020
Nolze G, Hielscher R (2016) IPF coloring of crystal orientation data. Preprint Technische Universität Chemnitz
Nowell MM, Witt RA, True B (2005) EBSD sample preparation: techniques, tips, and tricks. Microsc Microanal 11(S02):504–505
Passchier CW, Trouw RA (2005) Microtectonics, 2nd edn. Springer, Heidelberg
Prakash M, Moon AP, Mondal K, Shekhar S (2015a) Effect of machining configurations on the electrochemical response of mild steel in 3.5% NaCl solution. J Mater Eng Perform 24(9):3643–3650
Prakash M, Shekhar S, Moon A, Mondal K (2015b) Effect of machining configuration on the corrosion of mild steel. J Mater Process Technol 219:70–83
Prior DJ (1999) Problems in determining the misorientation axes, for small angular misorientations, using electron backscatter diffraction in the SEM. J Microsc 195(3):217–225
Raith M, Karmakar S, Brown M (1997) Ultra-high-temperature metamorphism and multistage decompressional evolution of sapphirine granulites from the Palni Hill Ranges, southern India. J Metamorph Geol 15(3):379–399
Randle V (2004) Twinning-related grain boundary engineering. Acta Mater 52(14):4067–4081
Randle V, Davies H, Cross I (2001) Grain boundary misorientation distributions. Curr Opin Solid State Mater Sci 5(1):3–8
Reed BW, Kumar M (2006) Mathematical methods for analyzing highly-twinned grain boundary networks. Scripta Mater 54 (6):1029–1033
Reed BW, Minich RW, Rudd RE, Kumar M (2004) The structure of the cubic coincident site lattice rotation group. Acta Crystallogr A 60 (3):263–277
Sahu S, Sharma NK, Patel SK, Mondal K, Shekhar S (2019) The effect of grain boundary structure on sensitization behavior in a nickel-based superalloy. J Mater Sci 54:1797–1818
Sahu S, Yadav PC, Shekhar S (2018) Use of hot rolling for generating low deviation twins and a disconnected random boundary network in inconel 600 alloy. Metall Mater Trans A 49(2):628–643
Schwartz AJ, Kumar M, Adams BL, Field DP (eds) (2009) Electron backscatter diffraction in materials science, 2nd edn. Springer, US, Boston, MA, pp 21–143
Sharma NK, Shekhar S (2017) Microstructure and property evolution for hot-rolled and cold-rolled austenitic stainless steel 316L. Trans Indian Inst Met 70(5):1277–1284
Sharma NK, Shekhar S (2018) Deconvoluting error in measurement of low angle misorientation distribution. Micron 107:28–34
Shekhar S, Abolghasem S, Basu S, Cai J, Shankar M (2012) Effect of severe plastic deformation in machining elucidated via rate-strain-microstructure mappings. J Manuf Sci Eng 134 (3):031008
Shoemake K (1994) III.5.—Euler angle conversion. In: Heckbert PS (ed) Graphics gems, vol 4. Elsevier Inc, London, pp 222–229
Singh S, Guo Y, Winiarski B, Burnett TL, Withers PJ, De Graef M (2018) High resolution low kV EBSD of heavily deformed and nanocrystalline Aluminium by dictionary-based indexing. Sci Rep 8 (1):10991
Stipp M, Tullis J (2003) The recrystallized grain size piezometer for quartz. Geophys Res Lett 30(21):2088
Twiss RJ (1986) Variable sensitivity piezometric equations for dislocation density and subgrain diameter and their relevance to olivine and quartz. Min Rock Deformation: Lab Stud, AGU Geophys Monogr 36:247–263
Vaid A, Mittal K, Sahu S, Shekhar S (2016) Controlled evolution of coincidence site lattice related grain boundaries. Trans Indian Inst Met 69(9):1745–1753
Verma M (2014) Effect of machining configurations on the mechanical properties of SS316L, M.Tech. thesis at IIT Kanpur
Wang YZ, Kong MG, Liu ZW, Lin CC, Zeng Y (2016) Effect of microscope parameter and specimen thickness of spatial resolution of transmission electron backscatter diffraction. J Microsc 264 (1):34–40
Wang Z, Saldana C, Basu S (2017) Subsurface microstructure and crystallographic texture in surface severe plastic deformation processes. In: International manufacturing science and engineering conference. American Society of Mechanical Engineers
Watanabe T (1984) An approach to grain boundary design for strong and ductile polycrystals. Res Mechanica 11(1):47–84
Wilkinson AJ (2001) A new method for determining small misorientations from electron back scatter diffraction patterns. Scripta Mater 44(10):2379–2385

Wilkinson AJ, Britton TB (2012) Strains, planes, and EBSD in materials science. Mater Today 15(9):366–376

Wilkinson AJ, Britton TB, Jiang J, Karamched PS (2014) A review of advances and challenges in EBSD strain mapping. IOP Conf Ser: Mater Sci Eng 55:012020

Wilkinson AJ, Hirsch PB (1997) Electron diffraction based techniques in scanning electron microscopy of bulk materials. Micron 28 (4):279–308

Wilson AW, Spanos G (2001) Application of orientation imaging microscopy to study phase transformations in steels. Mater Charact 46(5):407–418

Wright SI, Field DP, Nowell MM (2015) Post processing effects on GND calculations from EBSD-based orientation measurements. IOP Conf Ser: Mater Sci Eng 89:012049

Wright S, Nowell M, Basinger J (2017) Precision of EBSD based orientation measurements. Microsc Microanal 17(S2):406–407

Yadav PC, Sahu S, Subramaniam A, Shekhar S (2018) Effect of heat-treatment on microstructural evolution and mechanical behaviour of severely deformed Inconel 718. Mater Sci Eng, A 715:295–306

Yadav PC, Sharma NK, Sahu S, Shekhar S (2019) Influence of short heat-treatment on microstructural and mechanical inhomogeneity of constrained groove pressed Cu-Zn alloy. Mater Chem Phys 238:121912

Yadav PC, Sinhal A, Sahu S, Roy A, Shekhar S (2016) Microstructural inhomogeneity in constrained groove pressed Cu-Zn alloy sheet. J Mater Eng Perform 25(7):2604–2614

Yuri T, Ono Y, Ogata T (2003) Effects of surface roughness and notch on fatigue properties for Ti–5Al–2.5Sn ELI alloy at cryogenic temperatures. Sci Technol Adv Mater 4(4):291–299

Zaefferer S, Elhami N-N (2014) Theory and application of electron channelling contrast imaging under controlled diffraction conditions. Acta Mater 75:20–50

Application of Electron Backscatter Diffraction (EBSD) Method in Earth Sciences

Dripta Dutta, Vikram Maji, Saquib Abdullah, and Santanu Misra

1 Introduction

The electron backscatter diffraction (EBSD) has developed into a powerful tool for acquisition of micro-scale crystallographic information since its emergence in the 1970s. The applications of the EBSD are primarily in the field of material sciences (Schwarzer et al. 2009). Since early 1990s, the geoscientists, particularly from the field of rock deformation, geodynamics and seismic anisotropy, started using this technique as one of the essential tools and also contributing in the development and fine-tuning the method (Prior et al. 2009). Today, the application of texture analysis has considerably expanded due to an increasing diversity of high performance sources for electron, high-intensity X-ray and neutron diffraction, using field emission gun scanning electron microscopy (FEG-SEM), synchrotron and nuclear reactors, respectively.

Rocks are polycrystalline materials and consist of small crystals (grains) of varying compositions. The grains may or may not belong to the same crystallographic systems. The overall arrangement of the grains within the rocks also defines their characteristic microstructures. Under suitable temperature and differential stress, the individual crystals deform by bending and/or distorting their lattices following their rheology, compatibility constraints, and earlier deformation history (Vernon 2018). Such deformations give rise to typical textures of the deformed rocks, quantification of which provides information related to the prevailing conditions of deformation and underlying mechanisms (Fossen 2016). The texture encompasses the overall microstructures of the polycrystalline rocks and also the crystallographic preferred orientation (CPO). The intensity of CPO controls the first-order anisotropy of the rock aggregates, being isotropic for uniform orientation and close to the single-crystal anisotropy for a very strong preferred orientation (Almqvist and Mainprice 2017). The arrangements of the crystals and their shapes also have some influence of the material properties (Almqvist and Mainprice 2017; Passchier and Trouw 2005). Glide and climb of dislocations on slip systems are responsible for the CPO patterns exhibited by the minerals (Maitland et al. 2006). The activation of particular slip systems in a specific mineral is pressure and temperature-dependent. For example, in omphacite (a high-pressure silicate of pyroxene group), the mechanical twinning is identified on (100) and (001), and dislocation glide on the [001](100) slip system at low to intermediate temperatures and high strain rates (Boland et al. 1986). At high temperatures ($T > 500$ °C) and low strain rates, the mineral deforms with multiple slip systems [001](100), [001]{110}, $1/2 < 110 >$ {110} (Zhang et al. 2006). Microstructural characterization by EBSD on both naturally and experimentally deformed geomaterials can reveal different deformation mechanisms, viz. dynamic recrystallization, static recrystallization, and recovery (Prior et al. 2009). The data can also quantify the misorientations within and across the boundaries of the neighboring grains and differentiate between relict and recrystallized grains (Halfpenny et al. 2006). Additionally, calculations of elastic properties of the crystals are possible with the help of EBSD data. The elastic constants then are used to determine the seismic anisotropy, which originates from the anisotropic minerals (phyllosilicates, pyroxenes, olivine, serpentine, etc.) and their orientations in the crust and deep earth (Almqvist and Mainprice 2017).

EBSD is a scanning electron microscope (SEM)-based technique that provides quantitative microstructural, crystallographic, and textural information of the crystalline materials such as rocks, metals, alloys, semiconductors, and ceramics (Prior et al. 2009; Almqvist and Mainprice 2017). The post-processing of raw EBSD data yields quantitative information about the grains (size, shape, and crystallographic orientations), the grain boundaries (low- or

D. Dutta · V. Maji · S. Abdullah · S. Misra (✉)
Department of Earth Sciences, Indian Institute of Technology Kanpur, Kanpur, Uttar Pradesh 208016, India
e-mail: smisra@iitk.ac.in

K. Biswas et al. (eds.), *Electron Microscopy in Science and Engineering*, IITK Directions 6,
https://doi.org/10.1007/978-981-16-5101-4_5

high-angular contrast), and the crystal structures. The SEM system equipped with energy dispersive X-ray spectrometry (EDS) can also identify the different phases (minerals) in a rock sample (Prior et al. 2009; Almqvist and Mainprice 2017). However, the method has its limitation for minerals with solid solutions, which are structurally identical (i.e., the unit cell parameters are same), but they are compositionally different (Prior et al. 2009). In general, for earth scientists, the EBSD technique is an excellent and quick tool to investigate the crystal-scale mechanisms of ductile deformation, which dominates at mid-lower crustal levels, and the upper mantle (Prior et al. 2009).

In this article, we present a comprehensive review of the EBSD techniques and its applications in Earth Sciences. Brief discussions on the working principles of the EBSD instrument, followed by data acquisition, processing and analysis, sample preparation methods for geological samples are presented at the beginning. We then discuss in detail the applications of EBSD in Earth Sciences and how the processed grain-scale data could be utilized in understanding the large-scale geodynamics.

2 Background of EBSD Analysis

2.1 Acquisition Protocol and Background Physics

EBSD is a powerful non-destructive tool for quantifying crystallographic information from a small volume of material using an additional charge coupled device (CCD) camera and detector in a scanning electron microscope (SEM) set up (Karato et al. 2008). High energy stationary electron beam is projected on the prepared sample surface (Fig. 1a), which is kept inclined (~70° to horizontal) toward the detector. Such an arrangement enhances the quality of the diffraction pattern (Cao et al. 2013). The electrons either interact with the nucleus (high angle scattering) or interact with the inter-nucleic electron cloud (low angular deviation) (Venables and Harland 1973). The diameter (1 nm, lowest) of the incident electron beam ensures all possible combinations of interactions.

Part of the incident electrons, after one or more scattering events at varying depths (mostly ~ 20–40 nm), exits the sample and constitutes the back scattered electron (BSE) source (Fig. 1b). The BSEs then encounter a scintillator/phosphor screen (~5 cm in diameter and kept ~ 2 cm away from the specimen), coupled with a lens (sometimes with fiber-optic bundle) that converts the projected BSEs into light. Subsequently, the light energy is captured and processed by a photon-sensitive imaging detector, typically a CCD camera. The diffracted pattern, also known as the Kikuchi pattern (Alam et al. 1954), is the 'gnomic projection' of the lattice planes on to the screen. It consists of linear Kikuchi bands, which are the edges of the two diffracted cones (Fig. 1c, d). The angular width of any Kikuchi band is twice the Bragg angle, and thus related to the interplanar lattice distance of the crystal by Bragg's law. The intensity of the Kikuchi pattern is inversely proportional to the square of the distance between the specimen and the phosphor screen. Intersecting Kikuchi bands form a bright spot and correspond to a zone axis (Fig. 1e), surrounded by higher-order Laue zone (HOLZ) lines.

2.2 Data Processing and Analysis

Electron backscatter patterns (EBSP), captured by the camera, are transferred to the processing computer for further reconstruction. The width, contrast, and sharpness of the Kikuchi bands are primarily controlled by the accelerating voltage (in kV) used for the acquisition (Loretto 2012). Polychromatic source and variations in BSE intensities associated with varying scattering angles introduce significant background component in the data set. Such background noises are typically normalized using a filter of adequate geometry by assigning mean value in the central pixel (Nishikawa and Kikuchi 1928). EBSP with poor contrast can further be enhanced and fine-tuned after background signal subtraction or division from the total signal. This protocol is particularly useful for materials with low atomic numbers.

Crystallographic orientations at the source point are estimated using ESBP of known materials or minerals by indexing. In practice, Hough transform algorithm (Hough 1962) is extensively used for transforming the Kikuchi bands from lines to points (Fig. 2). This step is important for identification of crystallographic orientation, as points can easily be spotted in the Hough space. The peak locations are restored in a sequence of interplanar angles and are compared with the look up table for matching of expected angles to identify the phases present in the sample. The complexity associated with indexing often leads to misorientation of reference points than the actual solution within the error window—generally a degree—of indexing protocols (Schwarzer et al. 2009). *Misindexing* refers to the points in the EBSD map (Fig. 3) with incorrect orientation information. '*Non-indexed*' points are the ones without any optimum solution. The problems associated with indexing are eminent for geomaterials than metals due to low signal level and the fact that minerals with lower symmetry emits continuous spectrum of inter-band angles. This typical property of minerals makes it difficult to find the exact match from the pre-calibrated library as the signal can correspond to more than one set of lattice planes (Prior et al. 2009). Positioning of the camera close to the sample for producing high-quality

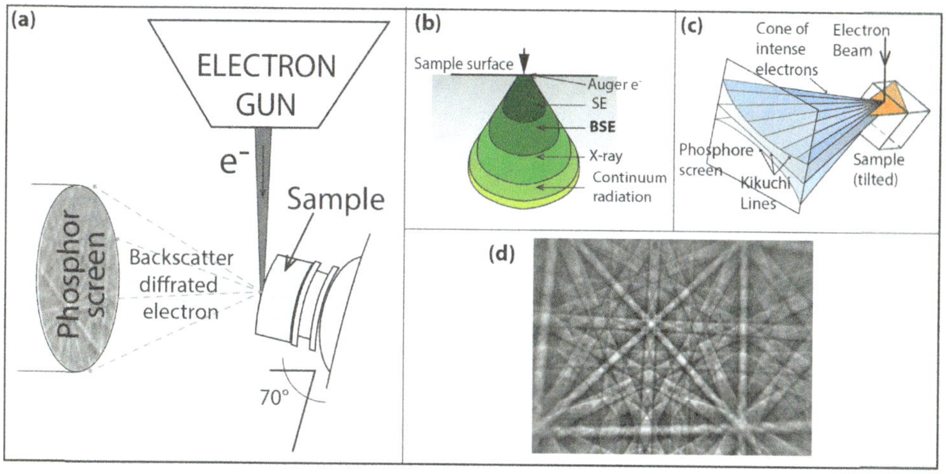

Fig. 1 Various components of the EBSD acquisition method are shown along with the background mechanisms and final outcome. **a** Illustration showing the electron source, sample, and detector with phosphor screen. **b** Diagram, showing the interaction of the electron beam with the sample. The depth of penetration determines the characteristics. **c** Three-dimensional (3D) illustration for formation of diffraction cone when electron beam interacts with a lattice plane to produce Kikuchi lines. **d** EBSP showing Kikuchi bands formed after BSE interact with the detector screen (image from Oxford Instruments)

Fig. 2 Different stages of indexing method are shown to identify CPO from EBSP. **a** SEM image with a cross mark showing the location of incident electron beam. **b** EBSP showing Kikuchi bands. **c** and **d** illustrates Hough transformation from a straight line into a point. **e** Hough 'space' as simplified in (**d**). **f** The peaks are identified as points in Hough 'space.' **g** and **h** The Kikuchi bands shown in (**b**) are identified with their actual crystallographic orientation. (i) CPO of the material at incident point (**a**) with the figure in inset showing the orientation in 3D. *Source* Oxford Instruments

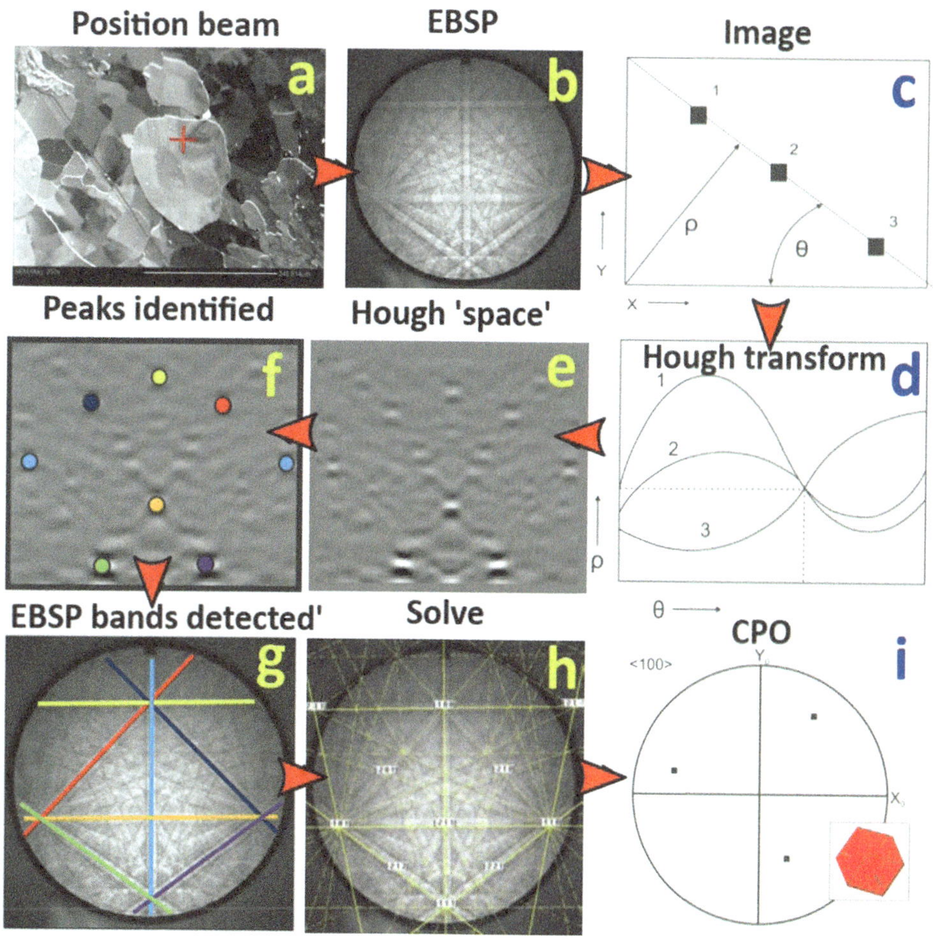

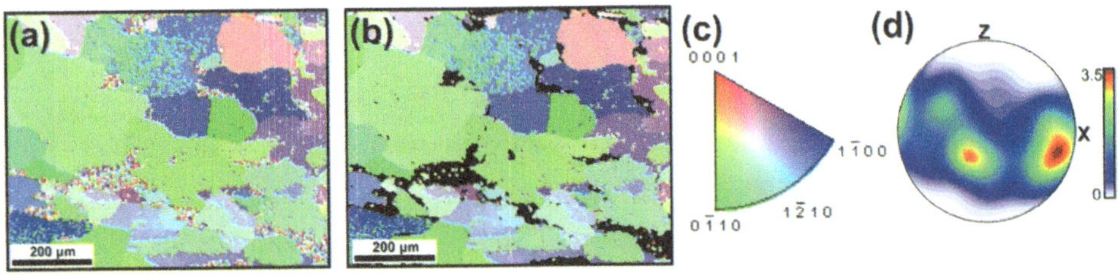

Fig. 3 Typical **a** and **b** orientation maps, the corresponding **c** color key, and **d** pole figure plot. The poorly indexed data points in (**a**) were removed to produce the map in (**b**). This was done in EDAX OIM v8. The pole figure is an equal area, lower hemisphere stereographic projection that is contoured to multiples of uniform density using MTEX v5.2. The sample is a gneiss from the Trans-Himalayan terrane, near Puga (Ladakh Union Territory, India). All the grains in **a** and **b** are of quartz

patterns and maintaining reasonable numbers of index points are often useful to reduce the indexing-induced glitches. Enhanced beam current and longer acquisition time are also good practice to improve the ESBP quality. Modern acquisition systems are capable of EBSP capturing and indexing very rapidly (~100 s of EBSPs per second), and reproducing EBSD map with detailed information on crystal types, orientations, etc.

Once the acquisition and the necessary corrections are performed, and the artifacts are minimized, the processed data can then be further analyzed using both commercially available and open-source software packages. Among them, MTEX (Bachmann et al. 2010) is an open-source user-friendly MATLAB toolbox. The EBSD data is normally visualized based on the orientations and shape of the crystals, phase contrasts, grain boundary contrasts (boundaries are defined with deviation in orientation angles) for both mono-and poly-mineralic assemblages. The CPO is generally displayed as pole figures which consist of poles of lattice planes on a stereonet that corresponds to the sample reference frame. The realtive differences in the orientations of the structural elements (e.g., lineation and/or foliation) and the crystallographic reference axes can also be inferred from inverse pole figures (IPF). Individual crystallographic orientations are plotted as single points using orientation distribution function (ODF) method (Bunge 1981).

2.3 Sample Preparation

There are no definite guidelines with suitable information for adequate sample preparation, and therefore, though the principles remain same, the protocols vary for specific geological sample and available instruments. A deformed sample is generally observed along the *XZ* plane of the strain ellipsoid, where *X* represents the stretching direction (equivalent to rolling direction, RD), identified by the lineation and *Z*-direction is orthogonal to the foliation plane (equivalent to normal direction, ND) (Fig. 4). A careful observation, sample collection and cutting the samples along

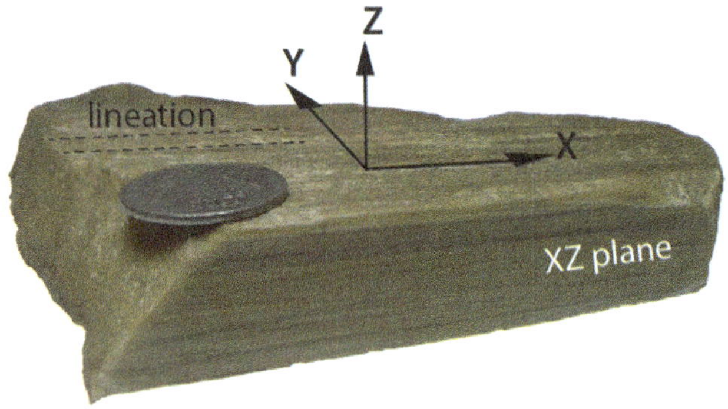

Fig. 4 Illustration to show the sections at which the EBSD data should be collected from a deformed rock. The sample is a naturally sheared quartzite, collected from Singhbhum Shear Zone, India. The top surface is parallel to the foliation plane (*XY*), and *X* is the stretching direction which is identified by the lineation observed on the *XY* plane. The cut surface (*XZ* plane) is the key surface, which should be processed to collect the EBSD data. (The sample is from the personal collection of S. Misra)

the *XZ* plane, are very important for extracting representative EBSD data (Fig. 4). Standard mechanical processes of initial grinding and polishing are the primary starting points but often damages the soft minerals at the sample surface. One has to take special care for soft and flaky minerals, while polishing. For porous and/or fragile samples, resin impregnation in vacuum is recommended. After the initial polishing, a combination of chemical–mechanical polishing (colloidal silica, electropolishing, ion milling, and chemical or plasma etching) ensures damage-/scratch-free surface for common rock forming minerals (Koll et al. 2011). After the final polishing, the quality of the polishing can be checked with a reflected light microscope. It is worthwhile to have a quick, manual 'point and click' investigation with the sample in the SEM chamber to ensure good-quality polishing; otherwise, preparation procedures may possibly require revisiting. After the satisfactory level of polishing, the nonconductive (non-metallic) samples are lightly sputter coated with carbon, unless the samples are being analyzed in low vacuum. A conductive circuit must be ensured between the sample and the stage.

Backscatter and/or secondary electron imaging are useful guidelines for selection of initial area and the step size to be used. However, the selection of step size is objective dependent. For instance, if overall texture estimation is the primary aim, then using relatively coarse step size is relevant, whereas for investigating localized/intragranular deformation, a finer step size is recommended.

3 Applications in Earth Sciences

Although EBSD had emerged as a useful technique back in the 1970s, it was not until the 1990s when geologists started utilizing it. A common and useful technique before the EBSD era was fitting a universal-stage (*U*-stage) attachment in the transmitted light microscope, the data processing of which used a FORTRAN-based program (Mainprice 1990) at the later times. A number of pioneering work unraveled the deformation mechanisms and CPOs of quartz from various tectonic settings (Schmid et al. 1986). Although *U*-stage measurements for quartz are easier to obtain, the presence of strong undulose extinctions in the crystals can distort the results, and hence, necessary precautions must be taken beforehand. Moreover, it can only measure *c*-axis orientations, which are sufficient in most of the cases but not always (Passchier and Trouw 2005). Automated microscopic fabric analyser (MiFA) is also another useful instrument, which measures the orientation of the *c*-axis of the crystals; limited again for uniaxial minerals (Wilson et al. 2007). Geologists also used few other instruments in order to determine the crystallographic orientations, including *X*-ray goniometry (Schmid et al. 1986) and computer-integrated polarization microscopy (CIP) (Heilbronner and Tullis 2006). Even though, the outcomes from the methods are well comparable with each other, but have certain advantages and disadvantages.

The SEM-based EBSD remains the most widely used method to extract crystallographic information from the minerals to date. In comparison with the other techniques, listed above, the advantages include higher spatial and angular resolution, ability to determine the complete CPO including Dauphine twins and faster speed of data acquisition (Peternell et al. 2010). There has been a surge in EBSD-centric articles since the late 1990s (Prior et al. 2009), and these works were not restricted only to quartz. The results discussed CPOs of important earth forming minerals, such as feldspar (Prior and Wheeler 1999), olivine (Zhang et al. 2000), garnet (Mainprice et al. 2004), pyroxene (Tommasi et al. 2006), mica (Abdullah et al. 2020; Lloyd et al. 2009), calcite (Barnhoorn et al. 2004), amphibole group of minerals (Abdullah et al. 2020; Ko and Jung 2015), and chromite (Ghosh et al. 2017). EBSD, along with numerical modeling, simulations, and deformation experiments at elevated pressure and temperature, has significantly improved our understanding of the physical processes and deformation mechanisms prevailing in the Earth's interior.

The EBSD technique is primarily used by structural geologists and solid earth geophysicists to infer the (i) deformation mechanism and slip system (Passchier and Trouw 2005), (ii) deformation temperature (Law 2014), (iii) shear kinematics (Passchier and Trouw 2005), and (iv) kinematic vorticity number (Xypolias 2010), to name a few. Crystallographic vorticity axis (CVA) analysis (Michels et al. 2015) and seismic anisotropic studies (Almqvist and Mainprice 2017) are some of the recent applications of EBSD in geosciences. Moreover, if the EBSD data is integrated with *X*-ray energy dispersive spectroscopy (XEDS), the phases present in the sample can also be differentiated based on their chemical composition. In the following sections, we discuss some of the applications of EBSD in geosciences.

3.1 Deformation Sense, Mechanism, and Temperature

When rocks undergo plastic deformation, the lattices of the constituent grains are distorted and their corresponding crystallographic axes tend to align themselves in accordance to the deforming forces. This is called crystallographic preferred orientation or CPO (Schmid et al. 1986). The obliquity of the central girdle of the mineral CPO (particularly quartz) plots on the pole figures has been widely used to infer the sense of shear (Fig. 5, Passchier and Trouw (2005)). Moreover, this also provides a qualitative estimate about the amount of non-coaxiality. The CPO fabric skeleton reflects the active slip system, which in turn depends upon the temperature at which those grains deformed (Fig. 6, Passchier and Trouw (2005)). The opening angle (*OA*, in degrees) of the quartz CPO fabric (Hunter et al. 2018) also varies with temperature, and thus acts as a proxy for the same (Law 2014). Also, (Faleiros et al. 2016) reported two mathematical equations depicting the relationship between the opening angle and the deformation temperature (T):

$$T(^{\circ}\mathrm{C}) = 6.9 \times OA + 48 (OA \leq 87^{\circ}) \quad (1)$$

$$T(^{\circ}\mathrm{C}) = 4.6 \times OA + 258 (OA \geq 87^{\circ}) \quad (2)$$

3.2 Kinematic Vorticity Number

Understanding the kinematics of deformation is crucial to decipher the geodynamic evolution of a terrain. Natural deformations are never perfectly coaxial or non-coaxial, but

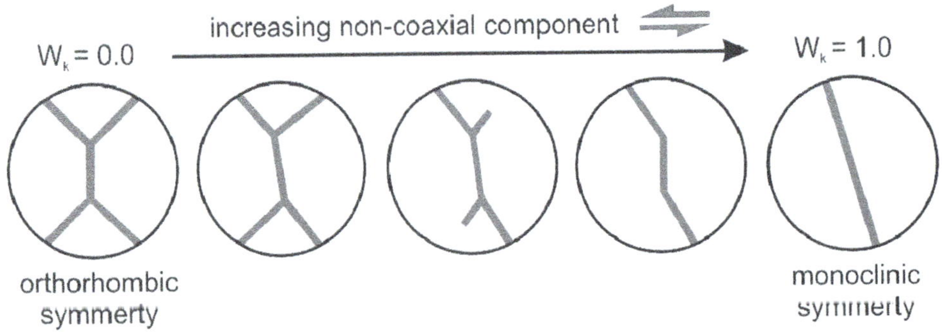

Fig. 5 Schematic illustration showing the variation in quartz CPO fabric skeleton with increasing simple shear component of deformation. Shear sense: sinistral. Modified after Fig. 1c of (Hunter et al. 2018). W_k = Kinematic vorticity number

Fig. 6 Temperature dependency of quartz CPO fabric. Reproduced from Passchier and Trouw (2005). BLG: Bulging recrystallization, SGR: Sub-grain rotation, GBM: Grain boundary migration

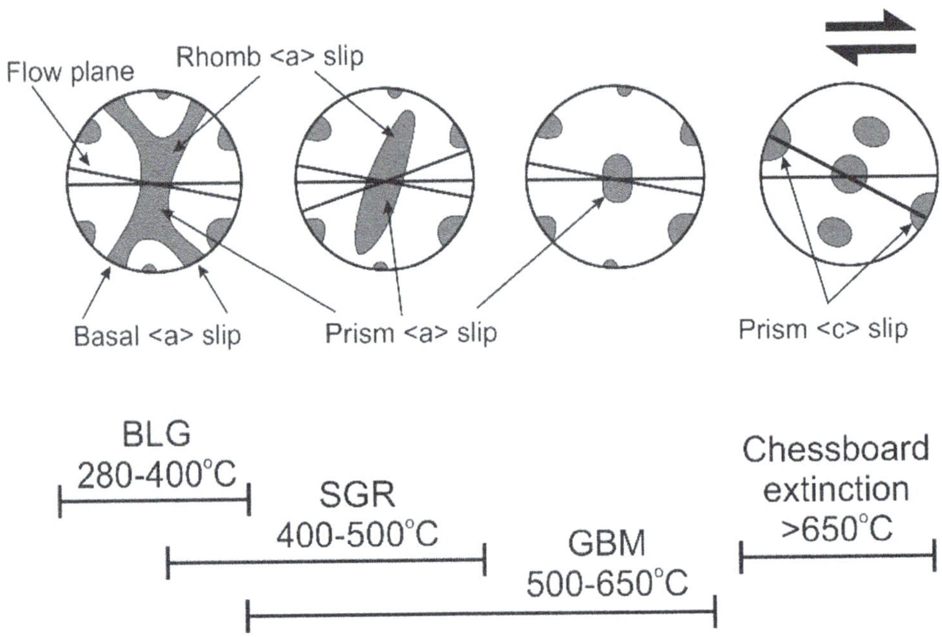

are combinations of the two aforementioned extremities. The proportion of each component is quantified by the kinematic vorticity number (KVN or W_k), and the number may vary within a single terrain or shear zone (Tikoff and Fossen 1995). Over the years, several techniques have been reported to derive the KVN (Xypolias 2010). EBSD-derived quartz petrofabric data is also useful in this regard and has been utilized by several geologists (Xypolias 2010). This technique is also known as the R_{XZ}/δ method, wherein R_{XZ} is the strain ration and δ is the angle between the foliation and the perpendicular to the central girdle in the quartz CPO (Fig. 7).

Fig. 7 Schematic illustration of a CPO fabric with the foliation (SA) and the angle β. The dotted line marks the perpendicular to the central girdle. Adopted after (Sarkarinejad et al. 2010)

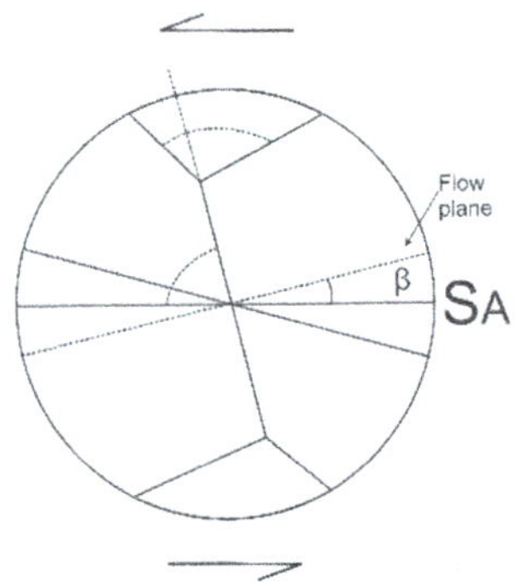

3.3 Crystallographic Vorticity Axis Analysis

Plastic deformation rotates minerals with respect to an axis called the bulk vorticity axis (BVA). Consequently, all the intragranular crystallographic axes get reoriented such that they lie along a girdle in a stereoplot. The pole to the girdle denotes the vorticity axis for that particular grain. Michels et al. (2015) utilized this concept and applied rotational statistics on a deformed grain population to deduce the orientation of BVA from EBSD-based petrofabric data. The

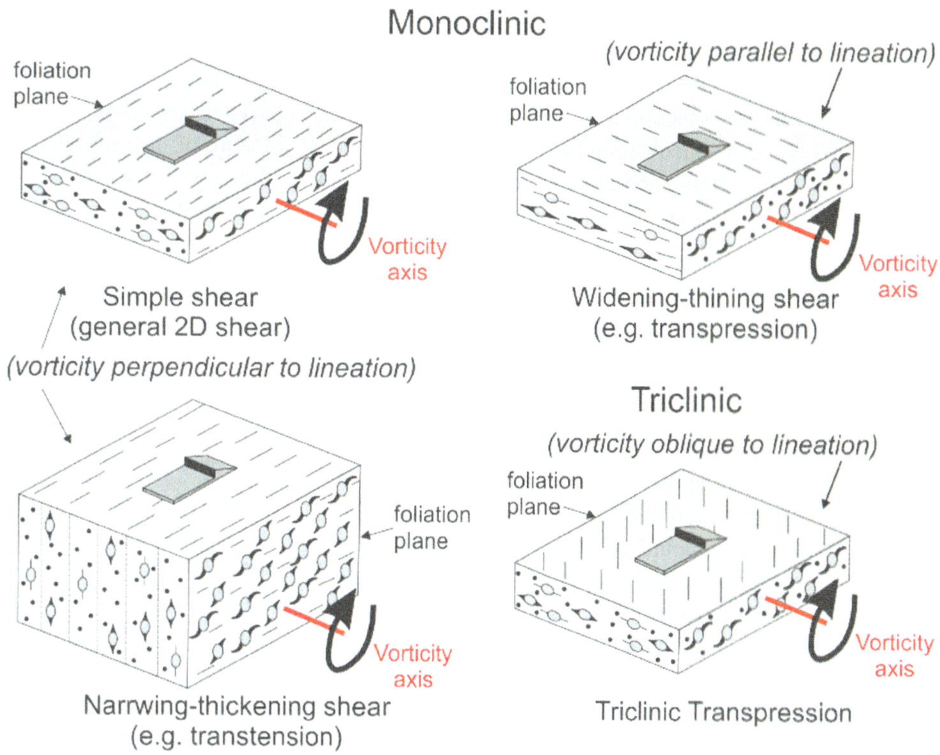

Fig. 8 Schematic figure illustrating types of kinematic flows and the angular relationships between the meso-fabrics to the vorticity axes. Reproduced from fig. DR1 of (Michels et al. 2015)

outcome when compared with the meso-fabric (e.g., lineation and foliation) orientations helps to comment on the symmetry (monoclinic or triclinic, Fig. 8) nature of deformation (transpressional or transtensional; Díaz-Azpiroz et al. (2019)). Once the orientation of the BVA is estimated, one can derive the same for the vorticity normal section (VNS) that is normal to the BVA. The VNS may not be parallel to the lineation (Díaz-Azpiroz et al. 2019) and is the most appropriate section to determine the kinematics of the deformation (Passchier and Trouw 2005).

3.4 Seismic Anisotropic Studies

While the heterogeneity is a crucial factor in controlling the subsurface dynamics, mechanical, thermal, and seismic anisotropy play significant role to manifest the deep-earth mechanisms at surface. Anisotropy in rocks results from a regular arrangement of atomic bonds in a crystal or, at a larger scale, the repetition of layers of rocks with different compositions or structures and varying elastic properties (Mainprice 1990). Though elastic anisotropy develops at crystal scale, its affects can pass on to larger scales when the anisotropic objects are arranged in a systematic way. Anisotropy of physical properties is a 2nd rank tensor and changes the characteristic strain fields produced by an applied stress, since some directions are easier to deform than others. It may therefore localize strain, the mechanism that initiates plate tectonics (Bercovici 2003). The term 'seismic anisotropy' refers to the directional variation in seismic velocities, which in turn depend on the elastic properties of the crystals (Almqvist and Mainprice 2017). Deformation-induced preferred alignment of crystallographic axes is considered to be one of the reasons for such elastic anisotropies, which could also be imparted due to the presence of melt networks, fractures, or variations in chemical compositions (Almqvist and Mainprice 2017; Almqvist et al. 2015). Fouch and Rondenay (2006) reported the upper crust to be seismically anisotropic. However, previously (Hirn et al. 1987) had advocated the opposite.

The effect of crystallographic arrangement on the velocity was noted in the 1940s. However, it was the work of Hess (1964), where the shear-induced olivine CPO was reported to be the cause of seismic anisotropy in the upper mantle. Since 1970s, several research works have been published on predicting seismic properties from the CPO data (Peselnick et al. 1974; Mainprice 2007). The FORTRAN script in Mainprice (1990) is one of the most widely used codes to deduce seismic anisotropies and plot the pole figures. Recently, these codes have been rewritten in the MATLAB programming language and included into the MTEX toolbox package. Although majority of the seismic anisotropic studies have been carried out on olivine CPOs from peridotites and serpentinites (Ben Ismail , Mainprice 1998), interests in subduction zone geodynamics have led geoscientists to study seismic properties of exhumed eclogites too (Mainprice et al. 2004; Abdullah et al. 2020; Almqvist et al. 2015).

4 Future Directions

Future research with the EBSD data may include comparative studies of the seismic properties derived from the petrofabric data obtained through the field geophysical measurements, ultrasonic laboratory experiments of the rock samples, and/or well-logs. Techniques to identify vorticity normal sections (VNS) from oriented drill cores have also been developed recently (Blenkinsop et al. 2015). We believe this could further help in deriving elastic properties from the same core using different techniques.

Moreover, the applications of machine learning (ML) and artificial neural network could also be implemented on EBSD data. A few very recent works showed that material scientists have embarked on that journey already (Kaufmann et al. 2020a, b). Furthermore, the link between petrofabric data and deformation could also be evaluated and approached utilizing ML techniques that would include training the algorithm using published database. These algorithms could then serve to predict outcomes from future data sets.

5 Summary and Conclusions

The article briefly reviews the working principles of the EBSD technique and its major applications in Earth Sciences. The EBSD technique had developed back in the 1970s, but geoscientists started to implement the method since 1990s onwards. *U*-stage, MiFA, X-ray goniometry, CIP were some of the instruments extensively used in the pre-EBSD era. Kikuchi patterns are the primary outcome of the EBSD method when BSEs interact with the detector/phosphor screen. Hough's algorithm is the key fundamental transformation used for extracting the indexing information of crystals from the Kikuchi patterns. During the reconstruction phase, different case-specific protocols are followed to eliminate the background noise. The major challenges encountered during post-processing of the EBSD data are the misindexing- and nonindexing-induced errors. The post-processing is performed using commercially available software packages; however, numerous researchers are now using the open-source MTEX toolbox that can be run on the MATLAB platform.

Deformation temperatures can be estimated from the opening angles derived from the pole figures and also by identifying the slip systems from inverse pole figures. The obliquity of CPO skeleton to the foliation can be utilized to infer the shear sense and calculate the KVN. Recently devised CVA analysis can help in estimating the orientation of the bulk vorticity axis from the EBSD-derived petrofabric data. Anisotropy in seismic velocities in the crust and upper mantle is primarily controlled by the elastic properties of the constituent material phases, and significant breakthroughs were established by assessing olivine CPOs from peridotites and serpentinites specimens. Future research in this field may incorporate the applications of machine learning, big data analytics, and artificial neural networks for faster processing of data and better accuracy of the results.

Acknowledgements The authors thank the editors for an invitation to write this article. The financial supports from SERB (ECR/2016/001988) and DST Swarnajayanti Fellowship (DST/SJF/E&ASA-01/2015-16) are greatly acknowledged.

References

Abdullah S, Misra S, Sarvesha R, Ghosh B (2020) Resurfacing of deeply buried oceanic crust in Naga Hills Ophiolite, North-East India: petrofabric, microstructure and seismic properties. J Struct Geol 139. https://doi.org/10.1016/j.jsg.2020.104141

Alam MN, Blackman M, Pashley DW (1954) High-angle Kikuchi patterns. Proc R Soc Lond Ser Math Phys Sci 221:224–242. https://doi.org/10.1098/rspa.1954.0017

Almqvist BS, Mainprice D (2017) Seismic properties and anisotropy of the continental crust: predictions based on mineral texture and rock microstructure. Rev Geophys 55:367–433. https://doi.org/10.1002/2016RG000552

Almqvist BSG, Misra S, Klonowska I et al (2015) Ultrasonic velocity drops and anisotropy reduction in mica-schist analogues due to melting with implications for seismic imaging of continental crust. Earth Planet Sci Lett 425:24–33. https://doi.org/10.1016/j.epsl.2015.05.039

Bachmann F, Hielscher R, Schaeben H (2010) Texture analysis with MTEX – free and open source software toolbox. Solid State Phenom 160:63–68. https://doi.org/10.4028/www.scientific.net/SSP.160.63

Barnhoorn A, Bystricky M, Burlini L, Kunze K (2004) The role of recrystallisation on the deformation behaviour of calcite rocks: large strain torsion experiments on Carrara marble. J Struct Geol 26:885–903. https://doi.org/10.1016/j.jsg.2003.11.024

Ismail WB, Mainprice D (1998) An olivine fabric database: an overview of upper mantle fabrics and seismic anisotropy. Tectonophysics 296:145–157. https://doi.org/10.1016/S0040-1951(98)00141-3

Bercovici D (2003) The generation of plate tectonics from mantle convection. Earth Planet Sci Lett 205:107–121. https://doi.org/10.1016/S0012-821X(02)01009-9

Blenkinsop T, Doyle M, Nugus M (2015) A unified approach to measuring structures in orientated drill core. In: Richards FL, Richardson NJ, Rippington SJ et al (eds) Industrial structural geology: principles. Geological Society of London, Techniques and Integration, pp 99–108

Boland JN, Tullis TE (1986) Deformation behavior of wet and dry clinopyroxenite in the brittle to ductile transition region. In: Hobbs BE, Heard HC (eds) Geophysical monograph series. American Geophysical Union, Washington, D. C., pp 35–49

Bunge HJ (1981) Fabric analysis by orientation distribution functions. Tectonophysics 78:1–21. https://doi.org/10.1016/0040-1951(81)90003-2

Cao Y, Jung H, Song S (2013) Petro-fabrics and seismic properties of blueschist and eclogite in the North Qilian suture zone, NW China: implications for the low-velocity upper layer in subducting slab, trench-parallel seismic anisotropy, and eclogite detectability in the subduction. J Geophys Res Solid Earth 118:3037–3058. https://doi.org/10.1002/jgrb.50212

Díaz-Azpiroz M, Fernández C, Czeck DM (2019) Are we studying deformed rocks in the right sections? best practices in the kinematic analysis of 3D deformation zones. J Struct Geol 125:218–225. https://doi.org/10.1016/j.jsg.2018.03.005

Faleiros FM, Moraes R, Pavan M, Campanha GAC (2016) A new empirical calibration of the quartz c-axis fabric opening-angle deformation thermometer. Tectonophysics 671:173–182. https://doi.org/10.1016/j.tecto.2016.01.014

Fossen H (2016) Structural geology, 2nd edn. Cambridge University Press, Cambridge, United Kingdom

Fouch MJ, Rondenay S (2006) Seismic anisotropy beneath stable continental interiors. Phys Earth Planet Inter 158:292–320. https://doi.org/10.1016/j.pepi.2006.03.024

Ghosh B, Morishita T, Ray J et al (2017) A new occurrence of titanian (hydro) andradite from the Nagaland ophiolite, India: Implications for element mobility in hydrothermal environments. Chem Geol 457:47–60. https://doi.org/10.1016/j.chemgeo.2017.03.012

Halfpenny A, Prior DJ, Wheeler J (2006) Analysis of dynamic recrystallization and nucleation in a quartzite mylonite. Tectonophysics 427:3–14. https://doi.org/10.1016/j.tecto.2006.05.016

Heilbronner R, Tullis J (2006) Evolution of c axis pole figures and grain size during dynamic recrystallization: results from experimentally sheared quartzite. J Geophys Res 111:B10202. https://doi.org/10.1029/2005JB004194

Hess HH (1964) Seismic anisotropy of the uppermost mantle under oceans. Nature 203:629–631

Hirn A, Damotte B, Torreilles G, Party ES (1987) Crustal reflection seismics: the contributions of oblique, low frequency and shear wave illuminations. Geophys J Int 89:287–296. https://doi.org/10.1111/j.1365-246X.1987.tb04421.x

Hough PVC (1962) Method and means for recognizing complex patterns

Hunter NJR, Weinberg RF, Wilson CJL, Law RD (2018) A new technique for quantifying symmetry and opening angles in quartz c-axis pole figures: implications for interpreting the kinematic and thermal properties of rocks. J Struct Geol 112:1–6. https://doi.org/10.1016/j.jsg.2018.04.006

Karato S, Jung H, Katayama I, Skemer P (2008) Geodynamic significance of seismic anisotropy of the upper mantle: new insights from laboratory studies. Annu Rev Earth Planet Sci 36:59–95. https://doi.org/10.1146/annurev.earth.36.031207.124120

Kaufmann K, Maryanovsky D, Mellor WM et al (2020a) Discovery of high-entropy ceramics via machine learning. Npj Comput Mater 6:1–9. https://doi.org/10.1038/s41524-020-0317-6

Kaufmann K, Zhu C, Rosengarten AS et al (2020b) Crystal symmetry determination in electron diffraction using machine learning. Science 367:564–568. https://doi.org/10.1126/science.aay3062

Ko B, Jung H (2015) Crystal preferred orientation of an amphibole experimentally deformed by simple shear. Nat Commun 6:6586. https://doi.org/10.1038/ncomms7586

Koll L, Tsipouridis P, Werner EA (2011) Preparation of metallic samples for electron backscatter diffraction and its influence on measured misorientation. J Microsc 243:206–219. https://doi.org/10.1111/j.1365-2818.2011.03495.x

Law RD (2014) Deformation thermometry based on quartz c-axis fabrics and recrystallization microstructures: a review. J Struct Geol 66:129–161. https://doi.org/10.1016/j.jsg.2014.05.023

Lloyd GE, Butler RWH, Casey M, Mainprice D (2009) Mica, deformation fabrics and the seismic properties of the continental crust. Earth Planet Sci Lett 288:320–328. https://doi.org/10.1016/j.epsl.2009.09.035

Loretto MH (2012) Electron beam analysis of materials. Springer Science & Business Media

Mainprice D (1990) A FORTRAN program to calculate seismic anisotropy from the lattice preferred orientation of minerals. Comput Geosci 16:385–393. https://doi.org/10.1016/0098-3004(90)90072-2

Mainprice D (2007) Seismic anisotropy of the deep earth from a mineral and rock physics perspective. In: Vol 2: Mineral Physics. Elsevier, pp 437–491

Mainprice D, Bascou J, Cordier P, Tommasi A (2004) Crystal preferred orientations of garnet: comparison between numerical simulations and electron back-scattered diffraction (EBSD) measurements in naturally deformed eclogites. J Struct Geol 26:2089–2102. https://doi.org/10.1016/j.jsg.2004.04.008

Mainprice D, Hielscher R, Schaeben H (2011) Calculating anisotropic physical properties from texture data using the MTEX open-source package. In: Prior DJ, Rutter EH, Tatham DJ (eds) Deformation mechanisms, rheology and tectonics: microstructures. Geological Society of London, Mechanics and Anisotropy, pp 175–192

Maitland T, Sitzman S (2006) Backscattering Detector and EBSD in Nanomaterials Characterization. In: Zhou W, Wang ZL (eds) Scanning microscopy for nanotechnology. Springer, New York, New York, NY, pp 41–75

Michels ZD, Kruckenberg SC, Davis JR, Tikoff B (2015) Determining vorticity axes from grain-scale dispersion of crystallographic orientations. Geology 43:803–806. https://doi.org/10.1130/G36868.1

Nishikawa S, Kikuchi S (1928) Diffraction of cathode rays by Calcite. Nature 122:726–726. https://doi.org/10.1038/122726a0

Passchier CW, Trouw RAJ (2005) Microtectonics, 2nd edn. Springer, Berlin, Heidelberg

Peselnick L, Nicolas A, Stevenson PR (1974) Velocity anisotropy in a mantle peridotite from the Ivrea Zone: application to upper mantle anisotropy. J Geophys Res 79:1175–1182. https://doi.org/10.1029/JB079i008p01175

Peternell M, Bitencourt MdeF, Kruhl JH, Stäb C (2010) Macro and microstructures as indicators of the development of syntectonic granitoids and host rocks in the Camboriú region, Santa Catarina, Brazil. J South Am Earth Sci 29:738–750. https://doi.org/10.1016/j.jsames.2009.11.006

Prior DJ, Wheeler J (1999) Feldspar fabrics in a greenschist facies albite-rich mylonite from electron backscatter diffraction. Tectonophysics 303:29–49. https://doi.org/10.1016/S0040-1951(98)00257-1

Prior DJ, Boyle AP, Brenker F, Cheadle MC, Day A, Lopez G, Peruzzi L, Potts G, Reddy S, Spiess R, Timms NE, Trimby P, Wheeler J, Zetterstrom L (1999) The application of electron backscatter diffraction and orientation contrast imaging in the SEM to textural problems in rocks. Am. Mineral. 84(11–12):1741–1759. https://doi.org/10.2138/am-1999-11-1204

Prior DJ, Mariani E, Wheeler J (2009) EBSD in the earth sciences: applications, common practice, and challenges. In: Schwartz AJ, Kumar M, Adams BL, Field DP (eds) Electron backscatter diffraction in materials science. Springer, pp 345–360

Sarkarinejad K, Samani B, Faghih A et al (2010) Implications of strain and vorticity of flow analyses to interpret the kinematics of an oblique convergence event (Zagros Mountains, Iran). J Asian Earth Sci 38:34–43. https://doi.org/10.1016/j.jseaes.2009.12.015

Schmid SM, Casey M (1986) Complete fabric analysis of some commonly observed quartz C-axis patterns. In: Hobbs BE, Heard HC (eds) Geophysical monograph series. American Geophysical Union, Washington, D. C., pp 263–286

Schwarzer RA, Field DP, Adams BL, et al (2009) Present state of electron backscatter diffraction and prospective developments. In: Schwartz AJ, Kumar M, Adams BL, Field DP (eds) Electron backscatter diffraction in materials science. Springer, pp 1–20

Tikoff B, Fossen H (1995) The limitations of three-dimensional kinematic vorticity analysis. J Struct Geol 17:1771–1784. https://doi.org/10.1016/0191-8141(95)00069-P

Tommasi A, Vauchez A, Godard M, Belley F (2006) Deformation and melt transport in a highly depleted peridotite massif from the Canadian Cordillera: implications to seismic anisotropy above subduction zones. Earth Planet Sci Lett 252:245–259. https://doi.org/10.1016/j.epsl.2006.09.042

Venables JA, Harland CJ (1973) Electron back-scattering patterns—a new technique for obtaining crystallographic information in the scanning electron microscope. Philos Mag J Theor Exp Appl Phys 27:1193–1200. https://doi.org/10.1080/14786437308225827

Vernon RH (2018) A practical guide to rock microstructure, 2nd edn. Cambridge University Press, Cambridge, United Kingdom

Wilson CJL, Russell-Head DS, Kunze K, Viola G (2007) The analysis of quartz c-axis fabrics using a modified optical microscope. J Microsc 227:30–41. https://doi.org/10.1111/j.1365-2818.2007.01784.x

Xypolias P (2010) Vorticity analysis in shear zones: A review of methods and applications. J Struct Geol 32:2072–2092. https://doi.org/10.1016/j.jsg.2010.08.009

Zhang S, Karato S, Gerald JF et al (2000) Simple shear deformation of olivine aggregates. Tectonophysics 316:133–152. https://doi.org/10.1016/S0040-1951(99)00229-2

Zhang J, Greenii H, Bozhilov K (2006) Rheology of omphacite at high temperature and pressure and significance of its lattice preferred orientations. Earth Planet Sci Lett 246:432–443. https://doi.org/10.1016/j.epsl.2006.04.006

Electron Probe Micro-Analyzer: An Equipment for Accurate and Precise Micro-Composition Analysis

Kaustubh N. Kulkarni, Aparna Tripathi, Abhinav Varshney, Jyoti Chandra, Siva Kumar, Sandeep Sangal, Debajyoti Paul, and Kallol Mondal

1 Introduction

An electron microscope is probably the most versatile characterization equipment that a materials scientist is blessed with. The generation of several different types of signals from the interactions of the primary electron beam with the sample gives access to analysis of multitude of the sample characteristics. Two most important of them are the topographical imaging and the micro-composition analysis; the latter being the topic of focus here. An electron probe micro-analyzer (EPMA) is essentially an electron microscope dedicated mainly for micro-compositional analysis, and it is equipped with certain additional features to serve this purpose. Examples of such additional features are the multiple channels for separating and counting specifically chosen characteristic X-rays, and an electron beam optics designed to give much higher beam stability and beam currents than usually available with typical electron microscopes. Depending upon the way X-ray signals are analyzed, micro-compositional analysis can be classified into two types, namely energy dispersive spectroscopy (EDS) and wavelength dispersive spectroscopy (WDS). In the former, the characteristic X-rays generated from the sample are collected all together, and their counts are recorded based on their energies. In the latter, user-selected characteristic X-rays are collected and counted; all other X-rays are filtered out as they are made incident on a pre-set Bragg diffractor. Thus, WDS is a batch-processing technique that analyzes desired X-ray wavelengths one by one. Although most EPMAs can be fitted with an EDS detector, the EPMA is meant primarily for WDS. Hence, in this article, we will focus on WDS, with EDS being discussed elsewhere in this book.

EPMA is probably the most accurate and precise tool for micro-composition analysis. However, the user needs to be aware of the right procedures of operation and data analysis in order to fetch the desired accuracy from the tool. This combined with inherent slow nature of the batch processing of X-rays often leads to long analysis times. Hence, EPMA often remains an under-utilized instrument despite of its unmatched accuracy and precision as well as its potential of usage in diverse applications. Hence, the main objective of this article is to introduce EPMA to a general materials researcher interested in accurate and precise compositional analysis on microscale. In order to keep it simple, to serve this purpose, detailed review of various concepts is intentionally avoided, and the stress is given more on explaining in simple language the important technical aspects of WDS analysis including the way various corrections are applied to the raw intensity data collected from the instrument.

The article starts with a brief history of EPMA followed by a discussion of its working principle. This is followed by a very short description of construction of EPMA. The various corrections applied to the raw data collected and their application procedures are then explained in some details. At the end, several case studies are discussed based on the state-of-the art research published from IIT Kanpur that essentially involved major usage of EPMA. It is expected that this discussion along with the various case studies will encourage many more researchers to find applications of EPMA in their research.

K. N. Kulkarni (✉) · A. Tripathi · A. Varshney · S. Sangal · K. Mondal
Department of Materials Science and Engineering, IIT Kanpur, Kanpur, India
e-mail: kkaustub@iitk.ac.in

A. Varshney
Department of Mechanical Engineering, Maulana Azad National Institute of Technology, Bhopal, 462003, India

J. Chandra
CSIR—National Geophysical Research Institute, Hyderabad, Telangana 500 007, India

J. Chandra · D. Paul
Department of Earth Sciences, IIT Kanpur, Kanpur, India

S. Kumar
Advanced Center for Materials Sciences, IIT Kanpur, Kanpur, India

K. Biswas et al. (eds.), *Electron Microscopy in Science and Engineering*, IITK Directions 6,
https://doi.org/10.1007/978-981-16-5101-4_6

2 A Brief History of EPMA

The first instrument making use of electron probe for compositional analysis was reported by Hillier and Baker in 1944 (Hillier and Baker 1944). In their instrument, they measured the energy lost by the primary electrons due to inelastic collisions with the atoms of the specimen being analyzed. The energy lost was correlated with the characteristic X-rays of the elements present. The first EPMA based on the analysis of characteristic X-rays generated due to collisions of primary electrons with sample atoms is credited to Raymond Castaing who developed this equipment as a part of his Ph.D. thesis (Castaing 1952). Castaing and Guinier first presented the concept of EPMA in an Electron Microscopy conference held in Delft in 1949 (Cosslet 1948). In 1953, they presented the first application of EPMA by point-by-point analysis of the diffusion profiles between copper and zinc (Caistaing and Guinier 1953). Castaing also established the approximation of proportionality between the intensity of characteristic X-rays emitted by an element and its concentration in the alloy sample after accounting for the matrix effects. CAMECA manufactured the first commercial EPMA prototype in the year 1956. Several manufacturers later came up, but currently, to the authors' knowledge, there are only two other commercial manufacturers of EPMA in addition to CAMECA, viz. JEOL and Shimadzu. Improvement in technology and analytical framework has been going on since then. Detection limits are continuously being improved due to higher probe currents (up to $10\mu A$), counting times, and larger surface of the analyzing crystal along with better background correction strategies. With more upcoming challenges, developments in EPMA will continue in coming years as well.

3 Working Principle of EPMA

When an electron beam irradiates a sample, a variety of signals are generated, some of which are characteristic X-rays, secondary electrons, backscattered electrons, and cathodoluminescence. These signals can be used to characterize the sample in terms of its composition and microstructure. The electron from the primary beam (incident beam) interacting inelastically with the sample can knock off an electron from the inner most orbitals of a sample atom resulting in its ionization. The unstable atom can return back to the ground state only after an electron from an outer shell falls into the inner shell, releasing the energy in the form of a characteristic X-ray photon. This energy is the difference between the energy levels of the two orbitals involved and is unique to an element. This characteristic X-ray photon can be used to identify the element present in an unknown sample. Energy and wavelength of the characteristic X-rays are related by

$$\lambda = \frac{12.3985}{E} \tag{1}$$

where λ is in Angstrom, and the energy E has the unit of keV. The X-ray generated due to falling of an electron from L-shell to K-shell is denoted as K_α whereas that due to transition of an electron from M-shell to K-shell is denoted as K_β. Similarly, falling of an electron from M-shell to L-shell gives rise to an L_α and from N-shell to L-shell gives rise to an L_β X-ray. Transition from N-shell to M-shell would generate an M_α X-ray and so on.

An EPMA is equipped with multiple spectrometers each of which can be preset to collect the desired wavelengths of X-rays and record their intensities. The X-rays are emitted from the sample in all the directions. Only small fraction of X-rays with a certain take-off angle can enter a given WDS spectrometer for detection. For WDS analysis, all the X-ray wavelengths other than the selected one should be filtered out before reaching the detector. For this purpose, each spectrometer channel can have one or more analyzing crystals, called Bragg diffractors or reflectors, each with a particular interplanar spacing d. At a given angle of incidence θ, a crystal will diffract X-rays of a specific wavelength when Bragg's law of diffraction is satisfied:

$$n\lambda = 2d \sin\theta \tag{2}$$

In order to reflect the sufficient intensity of the X-rays onto the detector, area of the specimen under observation, the reflector, and the detector (proportional counter) all should lie on one circle of a fixed radius called Rowland circle. Since sample remains fixed in its position, motion of the remaining two components, the reflector and the detector, should be synchronized so as to focus the desired wavelength onto the detector by satisfying the Bragg's law, Eq. (2). A typical arrangement of the reflector and the detector with respect to the stationary source (i.e., the sample here), called Johannsson geometry, is schematically illustrated in Fig. 1. Each crystal in a spectrometer channel moves on a linear trajectory inside the channel (shown by the blue dashed line in Fig. 1) and at the same time be tilted by certain angle so that θ can acquire a range of values and the crystal can diffract a range of wavelengths. This is the reason why in usual EPMA communications, the specific X-rays to be detected with a given crystal are identified with a macro-linear dimension (on the linear trajectory of the reflector) rather than in the form of its wavelength in nm or energy in keV. Due to the predefined coordinated movements of the reflector and the detector, it is easy to convert these linear dimensions to the wavelength or energy by knowing the geometry of the particular spectrometer.

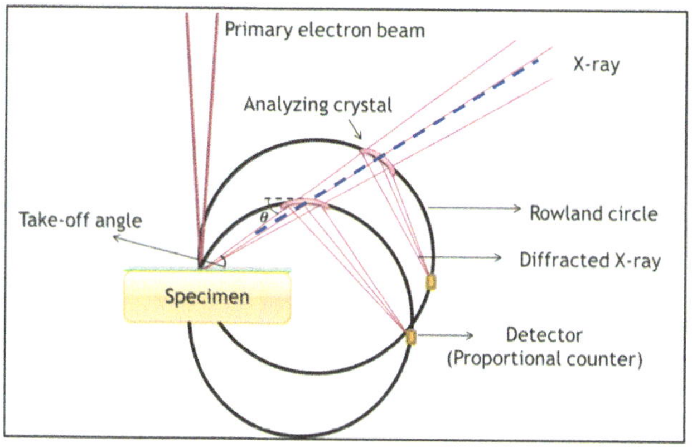

Fig. 1 Working principle of WDS spectrometer showing the observation field of the specimen, the reflecting crystal, and the detector lying on a common Rowland circle

The EPMAs typically give the options to represent the obtained WDS spectra in the form of intensity versus the linear dimension or, versus wavelength or energy.

Upon diffraction, the X-rays of the selected specific wavelength enter the detector, which is a proportional counter filled with either Xenon or Argon inert gas along with methane. The gas ionizes upon interacting with incident X-rays and releases photoelectrons. This signal is further sent to amplifiers and analog-to-digital converter for recording the X-ray intensity. Corrections for dead time and background have to be applied to the raw intensity data before further processing. Matrix corrections are applied to the X-ray counts using established algorithms, the basics of which are covered in a later section. Finally, the corrected intensities are converted to concentration of the element present in the unknown sample which is displayed on screen.

WDS has the capability to detect composition of elements present in trace amounts (as low as 100 ppm). Energy resolution (5 eV) is also better than that by EDS technique (about 100 eV). With reduced beam size, spatial resolution in an EPMA can reach below $1 \mu m$.

4 Basic Construction

The basic functioning of an EPMA is similar to a scanning electron microscope (SEM) in that a focused high energy electron beam is bombarded onto the sample being studied and the various signals generated from the interactions of the electron beam with the samples are analyzed for imaging and micro-composition analysis. Hence, the EPMA and SEM share most of the components. However, since EPMA is primarily meant for WDS analysis of X-rays, multiple spectrometer channels are provided to serve this purpose. The main components of the EPMA thus include a source for primary electron beam, magnetic lenses for focusing and guiding the electron beam onto the sample, an optical microscope for accurate positioning of the sample, and the WDS spectrometers housing the Bragg reflectors and X-ray detectors.

4.1 Emission Source (Reed 2005; Akhtar et al. 2018)

W-filament, lanthanum hexaboride (LaB_6) or field emission gun (FEG) can be used as a source of primary electron beam. The first two emitters work on the principle of thermionic emission, in which the electron source is heated to a temperature that is high enough for the electrons to overcome work function of the material. FEG which is a tungsten rod with very sharp tip (<100 nm) does not require heating and is therefore referred to as cold cathode. Electrons are extracted by applying a high voltage of 3–5 kV near the tip. Due to nonthermal functioning, FEG guns have a longer lifetime (1–5 years) as compared to the other two sources. Moreover, much larger current density ($1,00,000A/cm^2$) or brightness can be obtained in FEG as compared to tungsten filament ($3A/cm^2$). This results in higher current in the same beam size or the same current at a smaller beam size (submicron) for FEG filament. Therefore, FEG gives increased spatial resolution and signal-to-noise ratio as compared to *W*-filament. FEG has a disadvantage of being very expensive as compared to LaB_6 or *W*-source. FEG also requires ultrahigh vacuum to prevent poisoning of cathode from trace elements in the chamber (10^{-10} torr). Vacuum requirement for LaB_6 is 10^{-7} torr while that for *W* is 10^{-5} torr. Other than cold cathode, FEG can be Schottky type which requires both heat and external electric fields to overcome the potential barrier. Long-term current stability of thermionic emitters is much better. For comparison, a *W*-based EPMA gives the beam current deviation of less than $\pm 0.05\%/hr$ and $\pm$ 0.3%/12 h, whereas Schottky-based FEG gives about $\pm$ 0.3%/hr and $\pm$ 1%/12 h [*from JEOL data for JXA-iSP100 and JXA-iSP200F*]. LaB_6 gives the beam stability performance that is in between the two. This is the reason why tungsten filaments are preferred source for microanalysis which essentially requires current to be stable for longer times rather than high image resolution. W-filament can also be heated and cooled quickly as compared to LaB_6 filament but at the cost of lower brightness and spatial resolution. FEG is more suited for low voltage applications providing low interaction volume at the same time ensuring good strength of the signal for EDS and WDS analysis. This has specific applications in studying thin films, multilayer assemblies, coatings, and small-sized inclusions (Rinaldi and Llovet 2015).

4.2 Column (Reed 2005; Akhtar et al. 2018)

The column in an EPMA consists of condenser lens, scanning coils, objective lens, apertures, and stigmator coils. Condenser lenses are electromagnetic lenses which converge the electron beam and align it along the optic axis. Current in the lens controls the probe diameter. Smaller the spot size better will be the spatial resolution of the sample. Scanning coils raster the beam on the sample for elemental mapping or imaging. Slow scanning results in a good signal-to-noise ratio and vice-versa. Current in the scanning coil controls the magnification of the image. Objective lenses are closest to the object and are used to focus probe on to the sample. Stigmator coils are used to correct the x and y deflection of the beam to produce beam with rounder shape and clearer image. Apertures are micron size holes in a metal disc which help in reducing the diameter of the beam and sample charging. Choice of aperture size depends completely on the requirement of the sample. The entire column is evacuated typically up to 10^{-5} torr if W-filament is used to avoid electron dispersion and cathode contamination.

4.3 EDS and WDS Spectrometer Channels

An EPMA usually has one to five WDS channels and can also be mounted with an EDS detector. Each WDS spectrometer channel houses one or more Bragg reflectors and a detector. All the channels are usually mounted symmetrically so that the take-off angle remains the same. Multiple wavelength dispersive spectrometers help in parallel analysis of many elements at a time and thus reduce the analysis time for multicomponent samples. For energy dispersive spectrometry, silicon drift detector (SDD) is used to count X-ray signals having an energy resolution of 120 eV, being very close to the theoretical limit. For WDS, gas proportional counter with P10 gas (a mixture of 10% methane and 90% argon) is used as a detector. Argon is ionization gas, while methane acts as a quenching gas to reduce the dead time of the counter. As compared to SDD, energy resolution is much higher in WDS (<10 eV) resulting in precise elemental identification.

The JEOL JXA 8230 EPMA at IIT Kanpur is equipped with one EDS and four WDS channels which facilitate quick as well as accurate compositional analysis. Each of the four spectrometers house two single crystals as given below:

1. Channel 1: LiFH and PETH
2. Channel 2: LDE2 and TAP
3. Channel 3: LiF and PETJ
4. Channel 4: LiF and PETJ.

This EPMA is based on W-gun that gives the highest beam stability and high beam currents (up to 10 μA) for better statistics. If higher resolution is desired, W can be replaced with LaB_6 but at the cost of slightly reduced beam stability and current.

4.4 Optical Microscope

As described in an earlier section, the sample, the reflector, and the detector should lie on a common Rowland circle. Since the spectrometer collects the X-rays at a fixed take-off angle, any slight change in the height of the sample may result into the sample being out of the circle and the subsequent loss of intensity. Hence, for precise and accurate measurement of concentrations, it is necessary to align the sample surface exactly with its position on the Rowland circle. An optical microscope (OM) is invariably used for this purpose due to its very narrow depth of field (less than 1 micron). OM is placed coaxially to the electron beam. The shallow depth of field of the OM helps in accurately aligning the height of the area under observation, and thus, OM is one of the most crucial components of an EPMA for ensuring accuracy and precision of the measurements.

5 WDS Analysis Methodology

The composition analysis with WDS by EPMA can be classified into two types, viz. qualitative analysis and quantitative analysis. Qualitative analysis, as the name suggests, deals with only the identification of elements present in a sample whose composition is unknown. The detectors scan the entire range of elements (in our case boron to uranium), and the elements present in the sample are identified based on the various peaks of characteristic X-ray energies collected by the detectors. Since the entire range of peaks has to be scanned, qualitative analysis usually takes a long time, but the advantage is that it does not miss any elements, which is due to high resolution of WDS. Qualitative analysis is frequently useful for geological samples and minerals.

In quantitative analysis, the composition of a sample is determined in terms of weight fractions of various elements present in the sample. Since WDS is a standard-based analysis technique, one has to a priory know all the elements present in the sample. For composition analysis of a completely unknown sample, i.e., in the absence of a complete knowledge of elements present in the sample, it has to be first subjected to qualitative analysis for identifying the various elements. Once the elements are identified, the

appropriate standards can be selected, and the quantitative analysis can be then carried out on the sample. It should be noted here that EPMA characterizes the elements based on their characteristic X-ray energies or wavelengths and hence, it is incapable of identifying the chemical states of the elements present. This is not an issue in the analysis of metals and alloys, in which it is typically required to know only the weight fractions of individual elements. In case of compounds, as usually encountered in minerals and geological samples, calibration and quantification are usually done based on the knowledge of the oxidation states of the elements or stoichiometry of the compound. EPMA is most frequently used for quantitative analysis. Hence, we will look into the details of the quantitative analysis using WDS.

5.1 Quantitative Analysis by WDS

As mentioned earlier, WDS analysis is a standard-based analysis. Hence, it is first necessary to perform calibration step, in which a reference sample with known concentration is analyzed for each of the elements present in the sample to be characterized. Let us call the sample whose composition has to be quantified as 'unknown sample'. A 'standard' is a sample that contains one or more elements present in the unknown sample and whose composition is already known. Each of the elements present in the unknown sample has to be calibrated with at least one standard. In the analysis of metals and alloys, pure elements are most commonly used as standards, whereas in the analysis of geological samples and minerals, pure compounds or their mixtures are used as standards.

The first step in the analysis is to decide upon the particular characteristic X-ray (K_α, L_α, M_α, etc.) that will be analyzed for each of the elements. The various factors that need to be considered during the selection of the X-ray line are energy of the particular X-ray, intensity of the X-rays desired, possible overlap with peaks of the other elements present in the unknown sample, the accelerating voltage to be used, and the range of scan available on the spectrometer to be used. Out of the five factors, the first three are fundamental in nature, whereas the latter two are more practical, dependent on the equipment being used. Although it is desirable to select K_α lines due to their large intensities, their energies for heavier elements maybe too high to be excited by the given accelerating voltage. A typical rule of thumb is that for using a particular X-ray, numerical value of its energy (in keV) has to be lower than half the accelerating voltage (in kV). Thus, for analyzing copper under 20 kV accelerating voltage, one can use Cu K_α radiation which has an energy of 8.046 keV. However, if the accelerating voltage has to be restricted to below 10 kV, for example, for enhancing the spatial resolution of the image, then one has to analyze Cu L_α with energy of 0.928 keV. Most EPMAs work with highest possible accelerating voltage of 30 kV, and hence, for heavy elements (Yttrium and beyond) one has to settle for L_α or lower energy X-rays. Lower intensities in such cases can be addressed with longer accumulation times to improve the statistics. During the calibration step, each of the standards is first subjected to excitation under fixed accelerating voltage and probe current for sufficient amount of time, and intensity of the desired X-ray from the standard sample (I_{Std}) is recorded in terms of counts per second. Then, the unknown sample is exposed to the same exciting conditions as the standard and the intensity of the desired X-rays collected from the unknown sample (I_{ukn}) are recorded. As per Castaing's first approximation (Castaing 1952), the ratio of the concentrations of an element in the unknown sample to that in the standard is taken as the ratio of intensities of the corresponding X-ray 'generated directly from the primary electrons' in the unknown sample to that in the standard. However, in reality, the intensities of 'collected' signals are modified due to various factors, and a correction coefficient has to be applied for each of these factors. The various corrections to be applied include background correction, atomic number correction (Z), absorption correction (A), and fluorescence correction (F). Of course, the measured intensities are corrected after taking into account the dead time during counting. If I_{Std} and I_{ukn} are the intensities of the X-ray in standard and unknown sample after applying respective background corrections, and if C_{Std} is the concentration (in weight fraction) of the element in the standard, then the concentration (wt. fraction) of the element in the unknown sample (C_{ukn}) is given by

$$C_{\mathrm{ukn}} = C_{\mathrm{Std}} \cdot \frac{I_{\mathrm{ukn}}}{I_{\mathrm{Std}}} \cdot Z \cdot A \cdot F \quad (3)$$

Z, A, and F are commonly referred to as 'matrix corrections' or ZAF corrections (Philibert and Tixier 1968) as they depend upon the type of matrix being analyzed. The various corrections applied to the collected raw intensities are briefly described in the following few sections.

5.1.1 Background Corrections

It is well known that production of any characteristic X-ray is also accompanied by production of a continuous spectrum of X-rays called as Bremsstrahlung. Although the intensity of the Bremsstrahlung is typically low, they do tend to increase the collected intensity of the desired characteristic X-ray, and hence, they add to the background noise. Moreover, the intensity of background is different in different samples including in standard and unknown samples. Hence, the background noise has to be subtracted from the obtained intensity of the characteristic X-ray, before it is

processed further. The background intensity is typically measured at a position, which is sufficiently away from the characteristic peak under consideration so that a part of the peak itself does not get counted in the background. It should be made sure that no other peak from other elements of the sample is at or in the vicinity of the background-collection position. If the background is continuously varying across the peak, the background collections are done at two positions, one lower than the peak position and the other higher than the peak position. The background count at the peak position is then taken as the mean of the two background counts. It is necessary to collect and apply background to standard and unknown samples individually.

5.1.2 Atomic Number Correction (Z)

The depth to which the primary electron beam can penetrate into the sample depends upon the occurrence of inelastic scattering events of the primary electrons as these events tend to slow down and eventually stop the electrons. The spatial distribution of the primary electrons will be guided by the elastic scattering events that tend to deflect the electrons without much loss in their energies. The total interaction volume of primary electrons in the sample depends upon the average atomic number of the sample and the accelerating voltage. The interaction volume in a lighter matrix is higher than that in a heavier one. For example, the interaction volume of the primary electrons in pure aluminum will be much higher than in an alloy of Cu-10 wt% Al. If we are analyzing concentration of aluminum with pure Al as standard, then the production of Al K_α X-rays in pure aluminum standard will be from much higher volume than in Cu-10 wt % Al. Hence, the obtained ratio of intensities of Al K_α in the unknown sample to that in the standard sample will be lesser than 0.1. Moreover, some of the primary electrons would be lost due to their backscattering and subsequent exit from the sample. The backscattering effect also depends upon the average atomic mass. Thus, the energy available for production of X-rays is different in the unknown sample than in the standard (Henrich 1991). Hence, a correction factor has to be applied to account for different interaction volumes and backscattering events in the standard and the unknown samples. This is called atomic number correction, denoted as Z.

Atomic number correction (Z_i) for an element i depends upon two aspects; first, the penetration of the electron into the matrix, which is basically governed by the stopping power (P_i) of the matrix and second, the backscattering of the electron (R_i). The parameters R_i and P_i further depend upon the composition of the alloy, over voltage ratio, i.e., the ratio of accelerating voltage (E_0) to K-shell excitation energy (E_K) of the element, average atomic number of the matrix, and the average atomic weight of the matrix. The Z correction for an element i can be given in terms of stopping power factor (P_i) and backscattering factor (R_i) as

$$Z_i = \frac{R_i^{\mathrm{Std}}}{R_i^{\mathrm{Unk}}} \times \frac{P_i^{\mathrm{Unk}}}{P_i^{\mathrm{Std}}} \quad (4)$$

Since only the energies within accelerating voltage (E_0) and the desired excitation energy (E_{Ki}) are of concern, only the ratio E_0/E_{Ki}, also known as overvoltage potential (U_i), is of significance in evaluating atomic number correction. An expression for the penetration factor (P_i) as derived by Love et al. (Love et al. 1978) for an n-component sample can be given as

$$P_i = \frac{1}{M}\left[1 + 16.05\left(\frac{J}{E_{Ki}}\right)^{1/2}\left(\frac{U_i^{1/2} - 1}{U_i - 1}\right)^{1.07}\right] \quad (5)$$

where J is the mean ionization potential of the sample, and M is evaluated as

$$M = \sum\nolimits_{j=1}^{n} \frac{C_j Z_j}{A_j} \quad (6)$$

J for an n-component system can be evaluated as

$$J = \frac{1}{M}\sum\nolimits_{j=1}^{n}\left(\frac{C_j Z_j}{A_j}\ln J_j\right) \quad (7)$$

The average ionization potential of a pure element j (J_j) is approximately proportional to the atomic number (Bloch 1933), and experimentally, a constant value for the ratio of J/Z of 11.5 eV has been obtained for aluminum (Wilson 1941). More accurate expression for J_j as proposed by Berger and Seltzer (Berger and Seltzer 1964) for $Z \geq 13$ is

$$J_j = 9.76 Z_j + 58.8 \cdot Z_j^{-0.19} \quad (8)$$

The backscattering factor (R) is the fraction of ionization remaining in the target after accounting for loss due to backscattering of primary electrons. It is related to the backscatter coefficient (η) of the electron, which is the fraction of the incident electrons that are backscattered. If all backscattered electrons retain their original energy, then $R = 1-\eta$. However, the BS electrons possess a range of energies as they undergo some inelastic collisions on their way out. As shown by Duncumb and Reed (Duncumb and Reed 1968) based on the data on backscatter coefficients (η) reported by Bishop (Bishop 1967), the backscattering factor (R) can be expressed as a simple function of atomic number (Z) and overvoltage ratio ($U_i = E_0/E_{K(i)}$). Ducumb and Reed (Duncumb and Reed 1968) have tabulated the data for R as function of Z and $1/U_i$. In a multicomponent sample, the backscatter coefficient (R_{ji}) for a given X-ray i of energy $E_{K(i)}$ in a matrix j can be calculated simply by interpolation of

the data with an interpolation error of less than 0.2% (Duncumb and Reed 1968). One equation for R_{ji} obtained by least square method as given in the JEOL's user manual for JXA-8230 (JXA-8230) can be written as

$$\begin{aligned} R_{ji} = 1 - X_j V_i\left[-0.187204 + 1.67366V_i - 1.51187V_i^2 + 0.707063V_i^3\right] \\ + X_j\left(3.63547 - 1.9914V_i - 1.6539V_i^2 + 0.477246V_i^3\right) \\ + X_j^2\left(-4.04514 - 4.11268V_i + 9.26509V_i^2 - 2.79199V_i^3\right) \\ + X_j^3\left(1.54054 - 3.43134V_i - 5.22007V_i^2 - 1.23353V_i^3\right) \end{aligned} \quad (9)$$

where $X_j = Z_j/100$ and $V_i = 1 - 1/U_i$.

The total backscatter factor for i (R_i) in the sample is then evaluated as

$$R_i = \sum_{j=1}^{n} C_j R_{ji} \quad (10)$$

5.1.3 Absorption Correction (A)

X-ray emitted by an atom i in a sample maybe absorbed by another atom j whose absorption edge lies close to the wavelength of the characteristic X-ray of i that we are measuring. There will be continuous mass absorption of the X-ray signals as they are traveling through the sample, which depends upon the mass absorption coefficient (μ/ρ). The X-rays generated at lower depths are more likely to escape and reach the detector than those generated at higher depths. Also, the X-rays traveling at lower angles are less likely to escape than those traveling at higher angles. Thus, the intensity of the X-rays of i observed would be lower than those actually generated because of the absorption effects. Hence, a correction factor needs to be applied to correct for the signals of i lost due to the absorption, which is different in the sample than in the standard. In a multicomponent alloy, the absorption factor for i is most commonly evaluated based on simplified form of Philibert's formula (Philibert 1963), extended to multicomponent system as follows:

$$f_i = \frac{1 + h_i}{\left[1 + \frac{X_i}{\sigma_i}\right]\left\{1 + h_i\left(1 + \frac{X_i}{\sigma_i}\right)\right\}} \quad (11)$$

where h_i is the factor depending upon atomic number and atomic weight of i given by Philibert 1963

$$h_i = 1.2\frac{A_i}{(Z_i)^2} \quad (12)$$

X_i is the factor depending upon mass absorption coefficient for the wavelength being considered, and the take-off angle is given by

$$X_i = \left({}^{\mu}/_{\rho}\right)^i_{\text{Specimen}} \operatorname{cosec}(\theta) \quad (13)$$

and for a multicomponent sample, X_i can be evaluated as (Private communication with JEOL EPMA experts 2019)

$$\left({}^{\mu}/_{\rho}\right)^i_{\text{Specimen}} = \sum_j C_j \left({}^{\mu}/_{\rho}\right)^i_j \quad (14)$$

and σ_i is Lenard's coefficient, which according to Heinrich and Yakowitz (Heinrich and Yakowitz 1975) can be given as

$$\sigma_i = \frac{4.5\text{x}10^5}{E_0^{1.65} - E_{Ki}^{1.65}} \quad (15)$$

Once the factors for standard (f_i^{Std}) and the unknown sample (f_i^{Ukn}) are known, the absorption correction factor for an element i in the sample is given by

$$A_i = \frac{f_i^{Std}}{f_i^{Ukn}} \quad (16)$$

5.1.4 Fluorescence Correction (F)

If the energy of a characteristic X-ray of an element j lies at an absorption edge of the element i, the later would fluoresce by the former. If the fluoresced X-ray is being measured, the apparent intensity would be higher than originally generated by direct excitation. The fluorescence factor for excitation of i by j is given by Reed (2005, 1965)

$$\gamma_{ij} = C_j \cdot J_i \cdot D_{ij} \cdot \frac{\left({}^{\mu}/_{\rho}\right)^j_i}{\left({}^{\mu}/_{\rho}\right)^j_{\text{Specimen}}} \cdot \left\{\frac{\ln(1 + u_{ij})}{u_{ij}} + \frac{\ln(1 + v_{ij})}{v_{ij}}\right\} \quad (17)$$

$$D_{ij} = \left(\frac{U_j - 1}{U_i - 1}\right)^{1.67} \quad (18)$$

$$u_{ij} = \frac{\left({}^{\mu}/_{\rho}\right)^i_{\text{Specimen}}}{\left({}^{\mu}/_{\rho}\right)^j_{\text{Specimen}}} \cdot \operatorname{cosec}(\theta) \quad (19)$$

$$v_{ij} = \frac{\sigma_i}{\left({}^{\mu}/_{\rho}\right)^j_{\text{Specimen}}} \quad (20)$$

and J_i is the coefficient depending upon absorption edge jump ratio of i and the fluorescence yield of j. The values of J_i are tabulated by Reed (Reed 2005, 1965). The fluorescence correction factor is then given by

$$F_i = \frac{1 + \sum_j \gamma_{ij}^{STD}}{1 + \sum_k \gamma_{ik}^{Unk}} \quad (21)$$

5.1.5 Determination of ZAF Corrections

As can be seen from Eqs. (5), (10), (14), and (17), each of the correction factors Z_i, A_i, and F_i is dependent on all the elemental concentrations that we are trying to determine. Hence, the correction factors have to be determined by using iterative algorithms. First the raw intensity ratios (K'_{raw}) are determined for all the elements after correcting the intensities for background and dead time. As a first approximation, the concentration of each element is taken as normalized raw intensity ratio for that element:

$$K_i = \frac{K'_{raw,i}}{\sum_{j=1}^{n} K'_{raw,j}} = C_i \qquad (22)$$

The concentrations C_i are then used for evaluating the three correction factors (Z_i, A_i, F_i) for each element. The new set of concentrations are then obtained by applying the ZAF correction factors based on Eq. (3). In the next iteration, the new concentrations are used to evaluate the set of (Z_i, A_i, F_i), and this process is repeated until all the concentrations converge.

5.1.6 Phi-Rho-Z Correction Method

Castaing in his original work (Castaing 1952) had suggested the expression for intensity of a characteristic X-ray of an element A generated in a sample as

$$I_A^{Unk} = \theta C_A \int_0^{\infty} \phi_s(\rho z)\exp\left(-\mu_S^A \cdot \rho z \cdot \operatorname{cosec}\psi\right)\mathrm{d}(\rho z) \qquad (23)$$

where C_A is the concentration of A in the sample (in weight fraction), ρ is the density of the sample, z is the depth, μ_S^A is the mass absorption coefficient of the X-ray in the sample, ψ is the take-off angle, and θ is a constant depending upon instrumental parameters. ρz is commonly referred to as mass-depth parameter and the function $\phi_s(\rho z)$ is the 'ionization distribution' that gives the number of X-rays generated as a function of penetration of primary electron into the sample.

Similar expression can be written for intensity generated in a pure elemental standard, and since the constant θ is dependent on instrumental parameters, it cancels out upon taking the intensity ratios if the instrumental parameters are kept constant. Thus, the intensity ratio can be written as

$$K_A = C_A \frac{\int_0^{\infty} \phi_s(\rho z)\exp\left(-\mu_S^A \cdot \rho z \cdot \operatorname{cosec}\psi\right)\mathrm{d}\rho z}{\int_0^{\infty} \phi_A(\rho z)\exp\left(-\mu_A \cdot \rho z \cdot \operatorname{cosec}\psi\right)\mathrm{d}\rho z} \qquad (24)$$

where $\phi_A(\rho z)$ is the ionization distribution function in pure A and μ_A is the mass absorption coefficient of the X-ray in pure A. The distribution function $\phi(\rho z)$ is usually determined by tracer method in which a thin layer of element A is sandwiched inside B at a depth z from the surface. $\phi(\rho z)$ for X-rays of A in B is then defined as "the intensity generated by the thin layer of A at the depth z, relative to that generated in an isolated layer of A of the same thickness" (Reed 2005). Packwood and Brown (Packwood and Brown 1982) showed that the $\phi(\rho z)$ function can be accurately modeled with a Gaussian type of function, which combined the atomic number and absorption correction in a single expression (Brown and Packwood 1982). Fluorescence corrections have to be calculated separately. Phi-Rho-Z correction method has been commonly used for analysis of light elements, silicates, and oxides.

5.1.7 Calibration Curve Method

Ziebold and Ogilvie (Ziebold and Ogilvie 1964) empirically observed that intensity ratio versus concentration plots for most binary systems can be fitted with the following relation:

$$\frac{1 - K_i}{K_i} = \alpha_{ij} \frac{1 - C_i}{C_i} \qquad (25)$$

where, C_i is the concentration of i in mass fraction and K_i is the ratio of intensity of characteristic X-ray of i in the sample to that in pure i, after applying the background and dead time corrections. α_{ij} is the fitting constant for the relation for i in binary system i-j. They also proposed that this relation can be extended to multicomponent systems, in which case the fitting parameter for the relation (α_i) can be expressed as

$$\alpha_i = \frac{\sum_{j \neq i} \alpha_{ij} C_j}{\sum_{j \neq i} C_j} \qquad (26)$$

Thus, for multicomponent systems, one needs to know the α_{ij} parameters for each of the binary pair i-j of the system.

The calibration curve method is especially useful while analyzing low concentrations of elements such as carbon in steels. For this, samples of known concentrations are analyzed in a small range typically encountered in the alloys. In such small concentration ranges, the intensity versus concentration can be simply related linearly as

$$I_i = A_i C_i + B_i \qquad (27)$$

where I_i is the absolute intensity for i at a concentration C_i and A_i and B_i are fitting constants. Once the fitting constants are determined over a small concentration range of interest, any sample with C_i lying in the desired range can be determined by just determining the intensities and applying Eq. (27).

The main advantage of calibration curve method is that the application of the complicated ZAF corrections is not required separately.

6 Case Studies

Various case studies in which EPMA has been used as an essential characterization tool are presented in this section. Although the various cases presented here are taken from already published works from our research groups, the focus here is to bring out the relevance of EPMA studies in these research works. Solid–solid diffusion couples are often used in determining interdiffusion coefficients in multicomponent systems. In a diffusion couple, two alloys of different compositions are placed in contact with each other and isothermally annealed at the desired temperature for sufficient time to develop measurable concentration profiles in the diffusion zone. After diffusion annealing, the couple is quenched in order to retain the microstructure and concentration profiles developed at high temperature to room temperature. The quenched couple is then sectioned parallel to the diffusion direction and metallographically polished to observe the microstructure developed across the initial weld plane (the plane at which the two terminal alloys were in contact at the beginning). The concentration profiles developed in a single-phase diffusion couple (the couple having the same phase in the diffusion zone as well as in the two terminal alloys with no phase interface) are further analyzed for obtaining interdiffusion coefficients. Thus, accurate and precise measurements of the concentration profiles are key in determination of interdiffusion coefficients. The diffusion profiles are typically a few hundreds of microns in width. To get a good profile, one needs to measure concentration of each diffusing species at every one or two microns. One may afford to determine concentrations at larger intervals toward the terminals as the concentration profiles tend to become flatter near the terminals. However, determining the entire concentration profiles by such point-by-point analysis takes a few hours of time. Moreover, the intensities of selected X-ray peaks have to be determined first on the standards before starting the analysis of the diffusion profiles. The standard calibration adds to the time of the analysis. However, all this analysis is essential in obtaining accurate and precise concentration profiles using WDS. One of the main advantages of using EPMA is the high stability of the electron beam current that the instrument is designed to give, which is essential to get consistent statistics of the X-rays over the longer length of time. Hence, EPMA is often used in the analysis of the diffusion couples. Two case studies are presented below that illustrate the use of EPMA data for determining interdiffusion coefficients; one in a ternary system and another in a quinary system.

Multiphase diffusion couples are characterized by development of planar or non-planar interfaces and multiphase diffusion zones in the couples. If a planar interface exists between two single-phase regions, local equilibrium can be assumed at the interface. It means that the concentrations on the two sides of the interface correspond to the equilibrium compositions of the phases. Thus, the concentration profiles are characterized by discontinuities at the planar interfaces. By extrapolating the concentration profiles from either side of the interface, one can obtain information of a tie-line. Thus, an accurate determination of concentration profiles can help in determining phase diagrams. One of the case studies presented below illustrates the use of EPMA analysis on multiphase diffusion couples in determining quaternary isotherm of Fe–Ni-Co–Cu system.

The microstructure developed across a joint is crucial in determining the properties and performance of mixed-material joints. Hence, it is important to understand the concentration profiles developed across a joint during the joining process and post-joining heat treatments. Thus, EPMA can be an important tool in studying mixed-material joining. Study of the effect of alloying elements on joining of aluminum alloy to steel is also presented as one of the case studies.

Understanding the partitioning of carbon and other alloying elements in various phase transformations that occur in steels is critical in continual development of new grades of steels. Especially, carbon concentration in steels is typically very low, between 0 to 2 wt%. In this range, use of elemental standard does not yield accurate carbon concentration. Hence, calibration curve method is most often used for microanalysis of carbon contents in steels. This method is illustrated with a case study of development of a new grade of steel.

EPMA is also very critical in analyzing geological samples. Hence, one case study is presented on analysis of geological samples. In the end, a case study on WDS analysis on a Ni-based superalloy is presented, and application of mapping and point-by-point analysis on solidified microstructure is illustrated. The classic case of peak overlaps, and advantage of EPMA in resolving such peaks is also illustrated with this superalloy that contains nine elements.

6.1 Determination of Interdiffusion Coefficients in Ternary Ti–Al-Nb System (Tripathi et al. 2018)

Ti-based alloys are potential lightweight alternatives for steels and other heavy materials used for components in automobile, aerospace, and bio-implant industry. However, their cost is the biggest hurdle in their widespread use. The recent development in extraction of titanium in powder form has enabled the availability of titanium powder at a very low cost (Sachdev et al. 2012). This has led to a rise in interest from industrial and research communities in developing

titanium parts with blended elemental powder metallurgy (BEPM) techniques (Sachdev et al. 2012). For developing and controlling such BEPM processes, in which alloying takes place by solid state diffusion during sintering itself, understanding of diffusion in Ti-based alloys is critical. Hence, our research group has been focusing on investigating interdiffusion in various titanium systems including Ti–Al-Nb (Tripathi et al. 2018), Ti–Al-Mn (Tripathi et al. 2020), and Ti–Al-Mo (Chauhan and Kulkarni 2021). The study in Ti–Al-Nb system is briefly illustrated below.

In this study (Tripathi et al. 2018), several ternary diffusion couples between various Ti–Al-Nb alloys were prepared and isothermally annealed at three different temperatures of 1060, 1100, and 1170 °C for 48 h. The concentration profiles developed within the diffusion zones of the couples were analyzed by point-by-point analysis technique in EPMA using WDS. Two example concentration profiles, one for the diffusion couple between Ti-35Nb and Ti-10Al-8Nb and the other for the couple between Ti-15Al-29Nb and pure Ti (concentrations in at%), both obtained using the JEOL JXA-8230 EPMA in ACMS, IIT Kanpur, are presented in Fig. 2a–b.

Both the couples were diffusion annealed at 1170 °C for 48 h. The profiles shown in Fig. 2a–b were obtained by employing an accelerating voltage of 20 kV and a probe current of 20 nA. The characteristic X-rays used for the analysis were K_α for titanium and aluminum and L_α for niobium. The X-ray intensities were calibrated using pure elemental standards. The collected intensities for both the standards as well as the diffusion couples were corrected by applying ZAF correction algorithm, which is provided by JEOL as a user-selectable inbuilt procedure in the JXA-8230 EPMA.

Based on Kirkaldy's method (Kirkaldy et al. 1963), to determine ternary interdiffusion coefficients at one composition, one needs to set up two independent diffusion couples with their diffusion paths intersecting at least at one composition, i.e., the composition at the intersection point is common to the diffusion zones of both the couples. One can determine the set of four ternary interdiffusion coefficients at this common composition by setting up four independent equations based on the experimental penetration curves of the couples and the interdiffusion fluxes determined from these curves. In Ti–Al-Nb system, several diffusion couples were having their diffusion paths intersecting with other diffusion couples, and hence, the ternary interdiffusion coefficients could be determined in the beta (BCC) phase of the Ti–Al-Nb system at several compositions at the three temperatures studied. The ternary interdiffusion coefficients so determined in the beta (BCC) phase of Ti–Al-Nb system are listed in Table 1. The strong diffusional interactions existing in the Ti–Al-Nb system are highlighted by the large

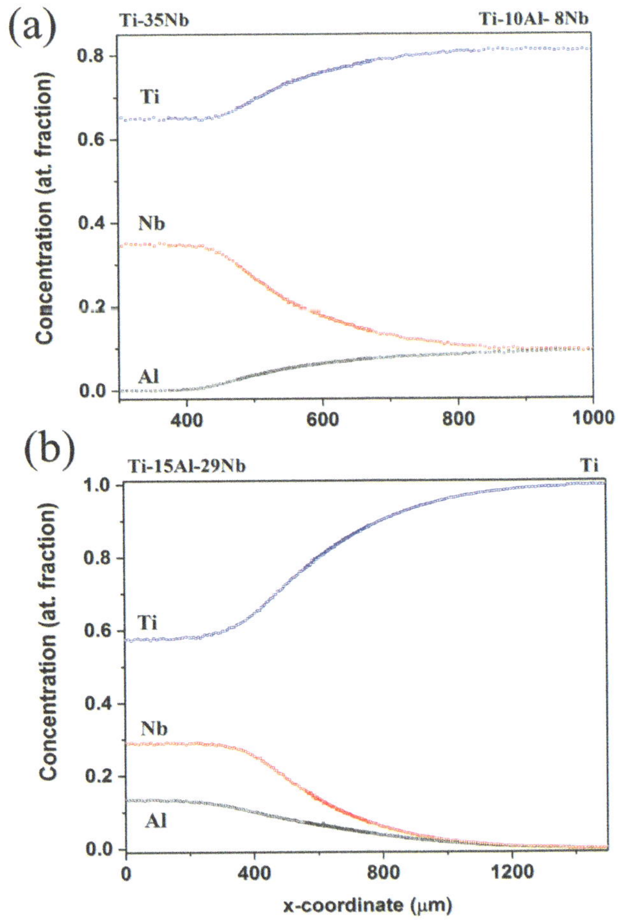

Fig. 2 Experimental concentration profiles developed in the diffusion zones of two Ti–Al-Nb diffusion couples annealed at 1170 °C for 48 h and obtained using point-by-point analysis using WDS in EPMA (Tripathi et al. 2018). **a** Diffusion couple between Ti-35Nb and Ti-10Al-8Nb and **b** Diffusion couple between Ti-15Al-29Nb and pure Ti (concentrations in at%)

magnitudes of cross-interdiffusion coefficients as seen from Table 1. The cross-coefficient $\tilde{D}^{Nb}_{TiAl}$ is negative and comparable in magnitude with the main coefficient, $\tilde{D}^{Nb}_{TiTi}$ which implies that the interdiffusion of titanium is retarded down the concentration gradient of aluminum, while it is enhanced up the gradient of aluminum.

6.2 Interdiffusion in Quinary Fe–Ni-Co-Cr-Mn High-Entropy Alloy (Verma et al. 2020)

High-entropy alloys (HEAs) are emerging as a promising class of new materials due to the various combinations of properties that they offer (Miracle and Senkov 2017). Presence of sluggish diffusion in HEAs has been the most debated topic in the field of HEA materials (Divinski et al. 2018). As far as interdiffusion is considered, flux of a

Table 1 Interdiffusion coefficients in β (BCC) Ti–Al-Nb system experimentally determined at various temperatures and compositions (Tripathi et al. 2018)

Temperature (°C)	Composition (at %)			Interdiffusion Coefficients (10^{-14} m^2/s)			
	Ti	Nb	Al	$\tilde{D}^{Nb}_{TiTi}$	$\tilde{D}^{Nb}_{TiAl}$	$\tilde{D}^{Nb}_{AlTi}$	$\tilde{D}^{Nb}_{AlAl}$
1060	80	14	6	4.2	−2.1	−0.7	5.7
	77	16	7	3.2	−4	−0.7	4.7
	72	20	8	2.6	−2.6	−0.7	3.2
	76	21	3	1.5	−1.4	−0.1	2.0
	73	23	4	1.6	−1.7	−0.3	2.1
	70	24	6	1.6	−2.1	−0.4	2.1
	70	26	4	0.8	−1.0	−0.1	1.3
	69	26	5	0.9	−1.3	−0.3	1.4
	62	27	11	2.1	−0.3	−0.9	1.1
	62	28	10	2.4	0.2	−0.7	1.4
1100	74	22	4	2.5	−2.8	−0.5	3.7
	71	23	6	2.8	−2.8	−0.6	3.9
	77	17	6	4.6	−3.3	−1.0	6.2
	76	21	3	2.7	−2.4	−0.3	3.4
	78	18	4	3.5	−2.3	−0.1	4.8
1170	70	26	4	3.0	−2.9	−0.5	4.4
	73	22	5	4.5	−4.6	−0.9	6.8
	78	15	7	12.9	−18.3	−3.1	16.2

component can be retarded or amplified depending upon the diffusional interactions of the other components, which are in turn guided by the cross-interdiffusivities and relative concentration gradients. In an earlier study conducted in our lab, the significance of diffusional interactions in driving such interdiffusion effects was established through appropriately designed quinary diffusion couples in Fe-Ni-Co-Cr-Mn system (Verma et al. 2017). In order to quantitatively determine the diffusional interactions, however, the knowledge of multicomponent interdiffusion coefficients was necessary. In principle, one could extend Kirkaldy's approach for ternary interdiffusion, to an n-component system. However, it would require preparing ($n-1$) diffusion couples with their diffusion paths intersecting at one composition. Preparing such a set of diffusion couples was unfeasible until recently when Morral (Morral 2018) proposed a 'body diagonal diffusion couples' approach to possibly get a set of required number of diffusion couples having at least one common composition in their diffusion zones. We reported, for the first time in the literature, the entire sets of quaternary and quinary interdiffusion coefficients by applying the body diagonal diffusion couple approach in Fe-Ni-Co-Cr and Fe-Ni-Co-Cr-Mn systems (Verma et al. 2020). In this case study, we shall consider only the quinary Fe-Ni-Co-Cr-Mn system.

One needs sixteen interdiffusion coefficients to define interdiffusion at a given composition of a quinary system. If one can obtain four independent diffusion couples whose diffusion paths intersect at one point in the four-dimensional quinary composition space, the sixteen interdiffusion coefficients could be determined at the composition of the intersection. As per body diagonal diffusion couple approach, we prepared diffusion couples with the terminal alloys selected from ends of body diagonals of a hyper-cube formed in the quinary composition space. For this particular set of couples, the mean composition used was equimolar composition (i.e., 20Fe-20Ni-20Co-20Cr-20Mn), and the composition difference employed was 6 at%. Four such diffusion couples, BD-1–BD-4, annealed at 1000 °C for 100 h were found to have diffusion paths intersecting at one common composition with an uncertainty of less than 1 at%.

The experimental composition profiles for the four quinary diffusion couples are presented in Fig. 3a–d.

These concentration profiles were obtained using WDS analysis in JEOL JXA-8230 EPMA. Accelerating voltage of 25 kV and a probe current of 20 nA were employed for the WDS analysis, which was carried out with pure elemental standards. The intensities of K_α X-rays determined for each of the elements (Fe, Ni, Co, Cr, and Mn) in the couples as well as on standards were corrected by applying ZAF corrections by JEOL's inbuilt program. The concentration profiles were then fitted and analyzed for interdiffusion fluxes by using *Multi*DiFlux program (Day et al. 2005). Sixteen equations were set up at the common compositions

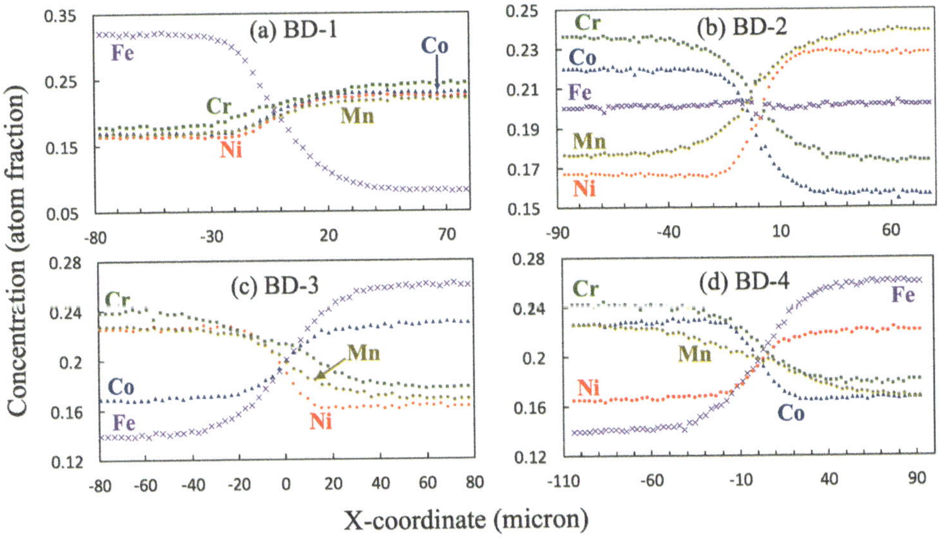

Fig. 3 Experimental concentration profiles developed in the diffusion zones of four quinary diffusion couples annealed at 1000 °C for 100 h, obtained by point-by-point analysis using WDS in EPMA (Verma et al. 2020)

Table 2 Set of sixteen quinary interdiffusion coefficients experimentally determined at the equimolar composition of Fe-Ni-Co-Cr-Mn system at 1000 °C (Verma et al. 2020). The interdiffusion coefficients are reported in 10^{-16} m²/s

$\tilde{D}^{Cr}_{CoCo}$	$\tilde{D}^{Cr}_{CoFe}$	$\tilde{D}^{Cr}_{CoMn}$	$\tilde{D}^{Cr}_{CoNi}$	$\tilde{D}^{Cr}_{FeCo}$	$\tilde{D}^{Cr}_{FeFe}$	$\tilde{D}^{Cr}_{FeMn}$	$\tilde{D}^{Cr}_{FeNi}$
3.2	0.8	−0.1	1.5	2.8	5.5	−1.0	4.1
$\tilde{D}^{Cr}_{MnCo}$	$\tilde{D}^{Cr}_{MnFe}$	$\tilde{D}^{Cr}_{MnMn}$	$\tilde{D}^{Cr}_{MnNi}$	$\tilde{D}^{Cr}_{NiCo}$	$\tilde{D}^{Cr}_{NiFe}$	$\tilde{D}^{Cr}_{NiMn}$	$\tilde{D}^{Cr}_{NiNi}$
−0.5	−0.3	9.1	−3.3	1.4	0.6	−1.9	3.3

based on the four independent fluxes and four independent concentration gradients measured in each of the couples. The equations were then solved simultaneously to get the set of sixteen quinary interdiffusion coefficients at the common composition, which happens to be the equimolar composition within experimental error. The quinary interdiffusion coefficients so determined at the equimolar composition of the Fe-Ni-Co-Cr-Mn system are presented in Table 2.

The values of cross-interdiffusion coefficients in Fe-Ni-Co-Cr-Mn system as listed in Table 2 corroborate the proposed "existence of strong diffusional interactions in HEA" in our earlier studies (Verma et al. 2017). Especially significant are the cross-coefficients $\tilde{D}^{Cr}_{FeNi}$ and $\tilde{D}^{Cr}_{NiMn}$. The former being positive indicates that the interdiffusion of iron is retarded up the concentration gradient of nickel and enhanced down its gradient, whereas the negative value of the latter indicates that the interdiffusion of nickel is enhanced up the gradient of manganese and retarded down its gradient.

6.3 Determination of Quaternary Isotherm of Fe-Ni-Co-Cu at 950 °C (Krishna and Kulkarni 2018)

As mentioned earlier, multiphase diffusion couples can give valuable information about phase diagrams. There are abundant studies reporting experimental phase diagram determination in binary and ternary systems. In a first of its kind study in the literature, we have determined a significant part of the quaternary isotherm of Fe-Ni-Co-Cu system at 950 °C with multiphase diffusion couple experiments (Krishna and Kulkarni 2018). The ternary Fe-Ni-Cu system exhibits a large miscibility gap separating Cu-rich FCC-1 and Fe-rich FCC-2 at 950 °C (Gupta 1990). This miscibility gap is expected to extend into the quaternary Fe-Ni-Co-Cu system, and the purpose of this work (Krishna and Kulkarni 2018) was to determine this quaternary miscibility gap at 950 °C. Since Fe-Ni-Co ternary system is expected to show almost complete miscibility at 950 °C (Guillemet 1989), the diffusion path of a diffusion couple prepared between a ternary Fe-Ni-Co alloy as one terminal and pure copper as another terminal most probably would pass through the miscibility gap. Hence, eleven diffusion couples were prepared between ternary Fe-Ni-Co alloys and pure copper. All 11 couples developed planar interfaces between Cu-rich FCC-1 phase and Fe-rich FCC-2 phase. The concentration profiles in all the couples were determined by point-by-point analysis in WDS mode with JEOL JXA-8230 EPMA using K_α X-rays and pure elemental standards for each of the elements Fe, Ni, Co, and Cu. The micrograph of diffusion zone and the concentration profiles for one of the couples assembled between 10Co-40Fe-50Ni and pure copper are presented in Fig. 4a–b, respectively. The planar interface

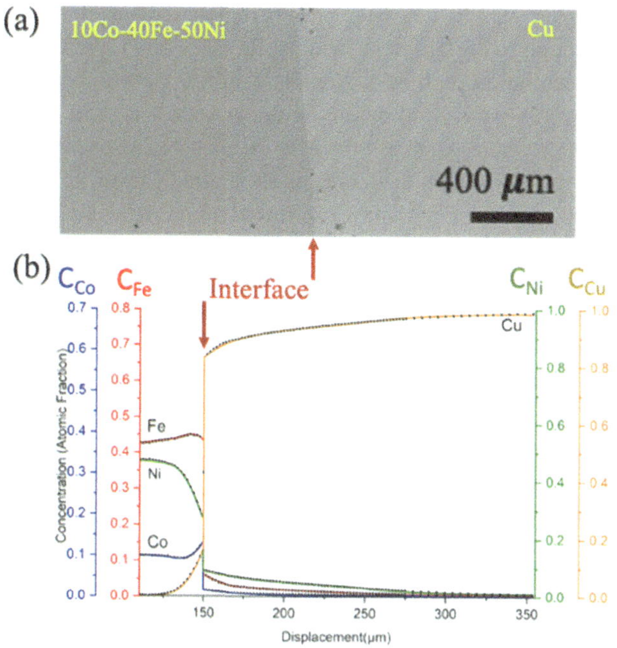

Fig. 4 **a** Microstructure around the interface and **b** concentration profiles in the diffusion zone developed in a diffusion couple between 10Co-40Fe-50Ni and pure copper annealed at 950 ºC for 72 h. The interface position on the micrograph as well as the concentration profiles is marked by red arrows

between FCC-1 and FCC-2 is clearly evident from and marked by the discontinuity in the concentration profiles.

The experimental concentration profiles for all the couples were fitted by interpolation with Cubic Hermite polynomials using *Multi*DiFlux program (Day et al. 2005). It should be noted that if WDS analysis is carried out exactly at a sharp interface, the X-ray signals are generated from both sides of the interface due to large interaction volume (1–2 microns) of primary electrons. Hence, it is recommended to get the concentration data only up to about 2 microns on either side of the interface. The concentrations of the two phases exactly at the interface should then be found out by extrapolation of the concentration profiles from both sides onto the interface position. The equilibrium concentrations of all the constituent elements in both phases at the interface were determined using multiphase module of the *Multi*-DiFlux program for each of the couples studied. Due to long diffusion annealing of the couples, local equilibrium can safely be assumed at the interface. Thus, the extrapolated compositions represent the compositions of the two phases which are in equilibrium at the interface. This enabled not only the determination of the surface enclosing the two-phase region FCC-1 + FCC-2 on the quaternary isotherm of Fe-Ni-Co-Cu system at 950 ºC but also the fixing of tie lines in this two-phase region. For details of the graphical representation of the isotherm and its mathematical equation, the work of A. B. Krishna and K. N. Kulkarni (Krishna and Kulkarni 2018) is referred to.

6.4 Mixed-Materials Joining (Dangi et al. 2018)

With increasing demand for lightweighting, 'mixed-material' or 'hybrid' structures have become need of the hour for automobile industry (Jiangqi et al. 2008; Jennings and Gould 2008). For making the hybrid structures a reality, joining of dissimilar metals becomes essential. However, formation of intermetallics (IM's) at the joint interface is the biggest issue in most of the dissimilar metals joining. Particularly in joining of steel to aluminum alloys, the brittle aluminide-based IM's reduce the performance and life of the joints. As these IMs form by diffusion process, diffusional and thermodynamic interactions among the various elements play a crucial role in deciding the nature and growth rate of the IMs. This case study (Dangi et al. 2018) was undertaken in order to understand the effect of alloying elements that are generally present in commercial steels on the growth rate of IM at the iron/aluminum alloy interface. For this study, various Fe–X alloys (where *X* = Mn, Ni, and Si) were dipped in liquid AA 6061 alloy at 750 °C for various times (Dangi et al. 2018). The growth rates of IMs formed at the interface were measured and compared with those formed at the interface of pure Fe and AA 6061 alloy with similar experiments. The micrographs of the IMs developed for various Fe–X alloys are shown in Fig. 5a–d. The growth constants of the IM layer for pure Fe, Fe–Mn, Fe–Ni, and Fe-Si as determined from the experiments done for various

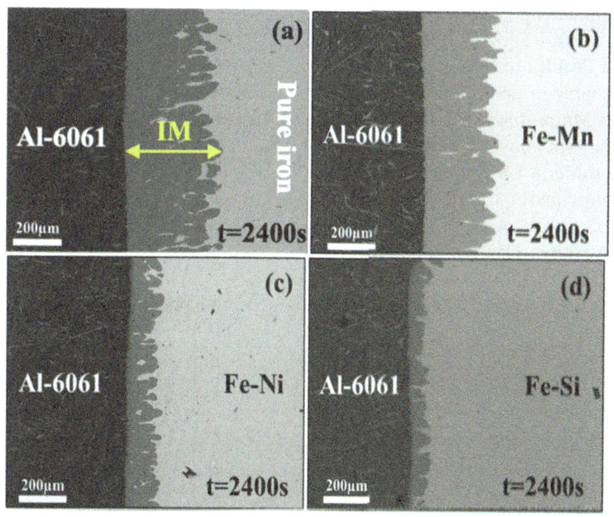

Fig. 5 SEM micrographs of the interfaces developed for various Fe–X alloys dipped in liquid aluminum alloy AA 6061 at 750 °C for 2400 s. **a** pure Fe, **b** Fe-2%Mn, **c** Fe-2%Ni, **d** Fe-2%Si (Dangi et al. 2018)

times were found to be (in 10^{-11} m^2/s) 6.1, 3.3, 0.8, and 0.4, respectively (Dangi et al. 2018). Thus, the presence of each of the three alloying elements in iron helps in reducing the IM growth. However, effect of Si is the strongest followed by Ni and Mn. These effects have been explained based on the diffusional and thermodynamic interactions (Dangi et al. 2018).

Validity of these results for Mn was also obtained by comparing the IM growths observed in the spot welds of IF steel and HSLA 340 with AA 6022 (Tripathi et al. 2017). The joints of IF steel having negligible Mn content (~0.097wt%) display higher IM thickness than that of HSLA having Mn content of 0.7 wt% (Tripathi et al. 2017).

In order to understand the effect of various alloying elements on the IM growth, concentration profiles were determined in the diffusion zones of the LS couples by point-by-point EDS analysis conducted in JEOL JXA-8230 EPMA. The advantage of using EPMA even for EDS analysis in determining these concentration profiles was that the stable beam current could be obtained in EPMA during the entire duration of the long analysis. Concentration profiles of Fe, Al, and Si developed in LS couple formed by dipping pure iron in liquid AA6061 alloy at 750 °C for 1200 s are shown in Fig. 6a. The various phase interfaces developed in the diffusion zone are indicated by dotted lines labeled as IF-1, IF-2, and IF-3 for the interface between Fe and Fe_2Al_3, that between Fe_2Al_3 and $FeAl_3$, and that between $FeAl_3$ and AA6061, respectively. In all other LS couples' studies, same phase regions were developed although with different widths. Figures 6b–d present the concentration profiles of element *X* in LS couples formed by immersing Fe–X alloy in liquid AA6061 at 750 °C for 2400 s where *X* stands for Mn, Ni, and Si, respectively. It can be seen that the concentration gradient of Si is the steepest in the Fe_2Al_3 layer followed by Ni, whereas Mn has almost zero slope in the layer. This indicates that Si is the slowest and Mn is the fastest diffusing species in Fe_2Al_3 layer. Based on this, it could be said that the effect of silicon in restricting the IM growth across the steel/AA6061 interface is due to the reduced diffusivities in the IM layer due to the presence of silicon (Dangi et al. 2018).

6.5 Carbon Concentration in Steel by Calibration Curve Method (Varshney et al. 2016a)

This case study on steels highlights the utility of calibration curve method in determining carbon concentration in steels at micro-level. There are various convenient methods available for accurately determining the carbon concentration in steels at a macro-level. However, macro-level composition is not a true representative of local micro-level composition due to the presence of multiple number of finely distributed phases in the steel. Knowledge of carbon distribution in various phases is of prime significance while

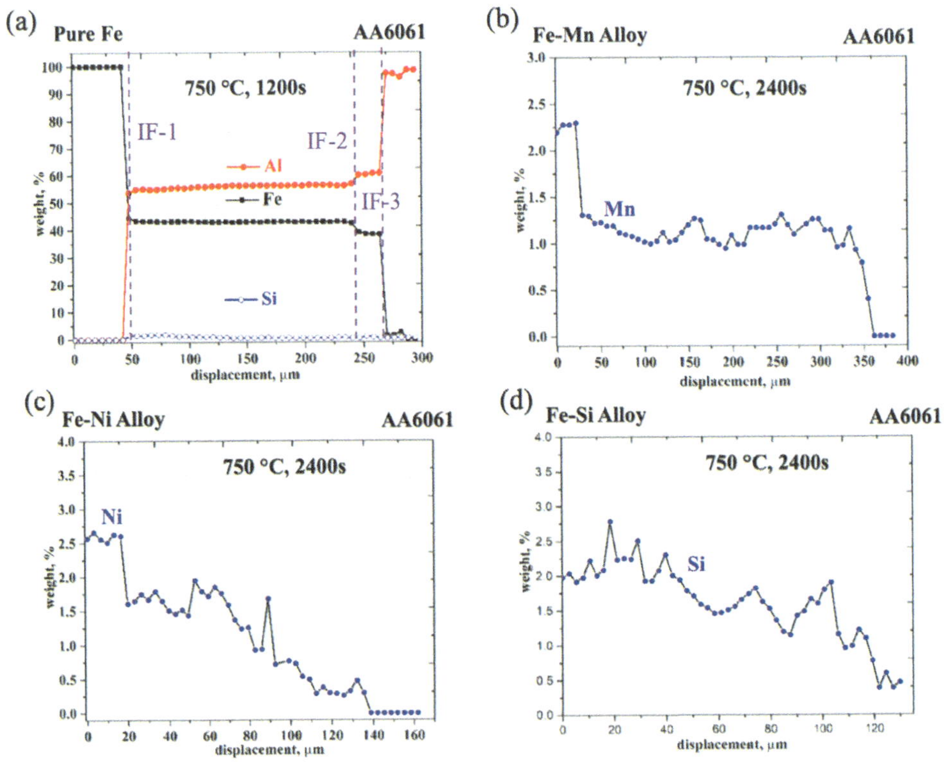

Fig. 6 Experimental concentration profiles developed in various liquid–solid (LS) couples formed by immersing Fe–X alloy in liquid AA6061 alloy at 750 °C. **a** Profiles of Fe, Al, and Si in LS couple of pure iron and AA6061, **b** Mn profile in LS couple of Fe–Mn alloy and AA6061, **c** Ni profile in LS couple of Fe–Ni alloy and AA6061, **d** Si profile in LS couple of Fe-Si alloy and AA6061 (Dangi et al. 2018)

designing various heat treatments. The following discussion presents an example of how EPMA analysis helped in understanding the role of carbon distribution in phase transitions and resultant properties.

A medium carbon high silicon steel with composition 0.61C-1.71Si-0.86Mn (wt%) was austenitized at 1040 °C followed by air cooling for various times from 0 to 40 s. At the end of the air cooling, the steel was austempered at various temperatures of 300, 350, and 400 °C for 10 min followed by quenching in water to room temperature. The purpose of the heat treatment was to design a microstructure comprising multiple phases with varying mechanical properties and to retain large amount of austenite at room temperature so that the best combination of strength and ductility can be obtained in a low alloyed steel. Purpose of the air cooling during heat treatment was to nucleate pro-eutectoid ferrite at the prior austenitic grain boundaries. Temperature of the sample during air cooling (recorded using an Arduino-based data acquisition system) was in the intercritical temperature range, i.e., in ($\alpha + \gamma$) phase field. Due to a large difference in the maximum solubility limit of *C* in ferrite or α (0.02wt.%) as compared to austenite or γ (2.1 w.%), *C* is expected to partition from α to γ during air cooling, resulting in *C*-enriched austenite (γ'). Austempering was then carried out to transform γ' to bainitic ferrite. Due to the presence of high silicon in steels, the inhibition of carbide formation was anticipated. Carbon that could have been utilized in carbide formation would now enrich and stabilize the untransformed austenite, which would then get retained in the microstructure after quenching to room temperature. Thus, after the completion of heat treatment, the microstructure of the steel was expected to comprise pro-eutectoid ferrite at the grain boundaries along with bainite and carbon-enriched retained austenite inside the grains resulting in a multiphase microstructure.

Microstructure of the samples austempered at 350 °C after air cooling for 10–40 s is shown in Fig. 7. Pro-eutectoid ferrite at the grain boundaries and the bainitic ferrite inside the grain can be easily observed in all the samples. In the samples cooled for 30 and 40 s, some pearlite can also be observed. Investigations of mechanical properties of the heat treated steels showed an excellent combination of strength and ductility. The high tensile strength was due to the presence of hard bainite in the microstructure, whereas the high tensile ductility was due to the presence of soft pro-eutectoid ferrite along with the retained austenite (Varshney et al. 2016a).

Content of retained austenite in the present case, as measured from X-ray diffraction analysis, was observed to have reduced after the tensile test. Scanning electron microscopic analysis of gauge lengths of the tensile specimens post-tensile test revealed the presence of martensite in the microstructure (Varshney et al. 2016a, b). Retained austenite under the application of strain tends to transform to martensite which delays necking by suppressing the localized deformation and increasing the work hardening rate resulting in both high ductility and strength (Varshney et al. 2016b, 2017). This is known as the transformation-induced

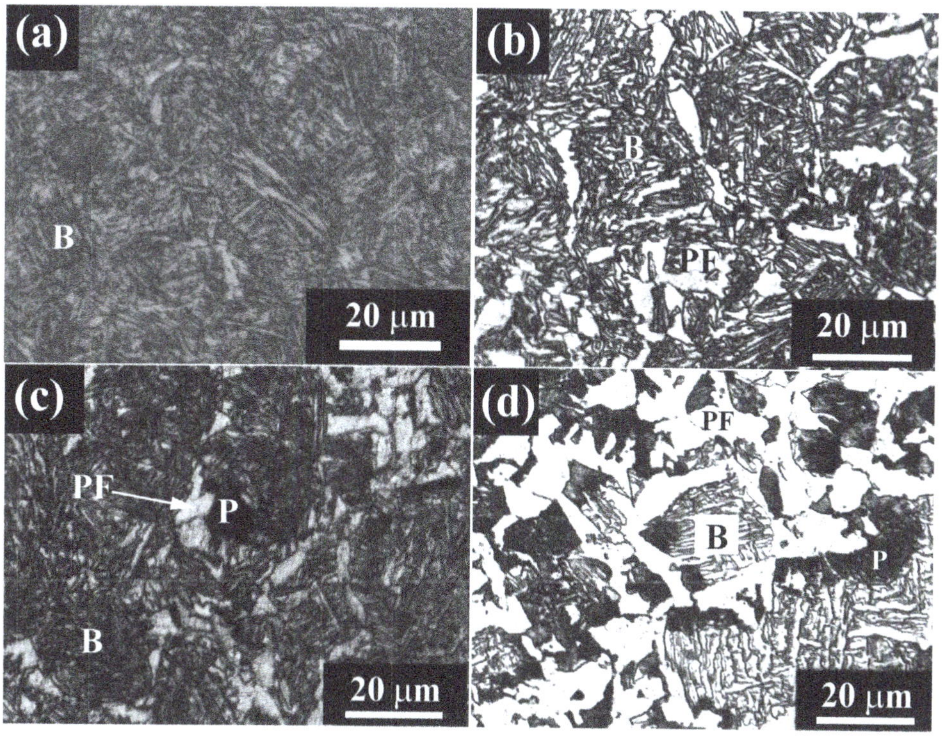

Fig. 7 Optical microstructure of the samples austempered at 350 °C after air cooling for **a** 10 s, **b** 20 s, **c** 30 s, and **d** 40 s. White etched region is the pro-eutectoid ferrite (PF), gray etched region is bainite (*B*), and black etched region is pearlite (*P*) (Varshney et al. 2016a)

plasticity (TRIP) phenomenon. The Ludwigson equation, which accurately predicts the flow behavior of metastable austenitic stainless steels, was found to closely represent the flow behavior of the steels austempered at 350 and 400 °C in this study (Varshney et al. 2016b). Both depletion of austenite during tensile straining and large extent of fitting of the true stress–strain data to the Ludwigson equation indicate that strain-induced transformation of austenite is playing an important role in the deformation of steels. The susceptibility of retained austenite to transform to martensite under the application of strain depends on its M_s (martensitic start) temperature. One of the primary factors that influences the M_s temperature is the carbon content of austenite.

Detailed microstructural examination revealed the presence of carbides in the microstructure of the samples austempered at 350 and 400 °C after air cooling for 30 s (Varshney et al. 2017). Presence of carbides in spite of the large amount of Si content in steels (1.71 wt.%) was surprising. Previous literature suggests high chances of carbide precipitation during austempering when the amount of carbon in the parent austenite is high. As discussed above, bainite transformation in this study initiated in γ'. Thus, it was very important for the investigators to determine the amount of carbon in austenite after air cooling (i.e., in γ') as well as in the retained austenite. Knowledge of the carbon content in γ' may be helpful in understanding the reason for carbide precipitation during austempering, while knowledge of the amount of carbon in retained austenite may aid in explaining the susceptibility of the austenite to undergo the TRIP phenomenon.

Energy dispersive spectroscopic (EDS) analysis determines inaccurate *C* content because of low atomic weight of *C*. Wavelength dispersive spectroscopy (WDS) provides a unique feature to accurately determine the amount of *C* content in submicron region of the specimen. WDS installed in a JEOL make EPMA (JXA-8230) at ACMS, IIT Kanpur, was used to determine the carbon content by generating a calibration curve.

To determine carbon content in the desired phase, the machine was first calibrated with five steel samples of known compositions. Fe-**0.1C**-0.28Si-1.8Mn-1.75Ni-0.3Al-0.027Nb-0.08 N, Fe-**0.41C**-0.313Si-0.750Mn-0.129Cr-0.0038 V-0.119 N, Fe-**0.61C**-1.65Si-0.86Mn-0.1Cr, Fe-**1.03C**-0.215Si-0.408Mn-1.04Cr-0.009Mo-0.06Ni-0.09Cu, and Fe-**2C**-0.481Si-0.375Mn-1.26Cr-0.07Ni-0.016Co-0.012Cu-0.013Ti-0.08 N were the five standard steel specimens used for the study. The compositions of all the standard samples were determined with SPECTROMAXx optical emission spectrometer, which itself was calibrated with certified reference materials provided by MBH Analytical Ltd., England. Uniform martensitic microstructure was obtained in all the standard specimens used for calibration by water quenching the steel sample upon suitable

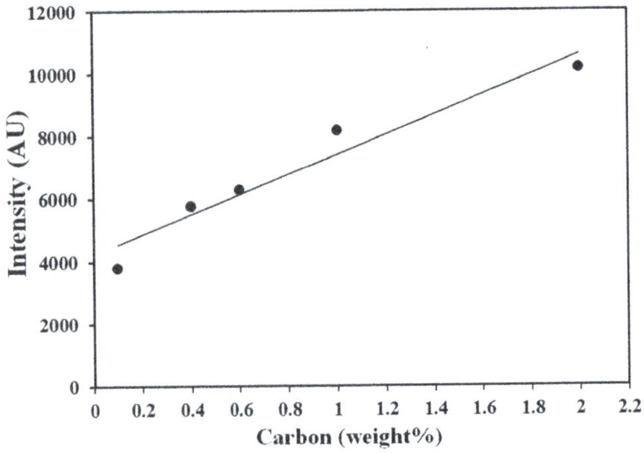

Fig. 8 Calibration curve generated by using various steel compositions of known carbon content (Varshney et al. 2016a)

austenitization prior to calibration procedure. This was done to ensure homogenous composition in a single-phase matrix in the standards. For each specimen, intensities of carbon K_α X-Rays were recorded at the probe condition of 20 kV and 20 nA. A calibration curve was generated by plotting intensities versus carbon content as shown in Fig. 8. Under the similar conditions in which the calibration curve was generated, desired regions of the samples with unknown carbon content were analyzed. The X-ray count from the selected region was noted, and with the help of the previously generated calibration curve, shown in Fig. 8, amount of carbon was determined.

To determine the amount of carbon in γ' after continuous cooling for various durations, the samples air cooled for 0 to 40 s were directly quenched in water to retain the amount of carbon partitioned in austenite during air cooling. The microstructure of the steel samples obtained after water quenching are shown in Fig. 9. Pro-eutectoid ferrite (*F*) and martensite (*M*) can be clearly observed in the microstructures. Due to the fast diffusionless transformation, martensite will have similar carbon content as that in prior austenite after respective air cooling duration. Under the similar conditions in which the calibration curve was determined, X-ray count in the martensitic region of the water quenched sample was measured by impinging the electron beam onto it. X-ray counts measured from the small region were compared with the calibration curve in Fig. 8, and the carbon content of the region was determined.

The variation in carbon content in the untransformed austenite (martensite) with air cooling duration has been shown in Fig. 10. Increase in the carbon content in martensite with increase in air cooling duration till 30 s can be observed. The increase is clearly due to more amount of carbon getting partitioned into austenite, which in turn resulted from increased content of pro-eutectoid ferrite during air cooling. A slight decrease in the carbon content in

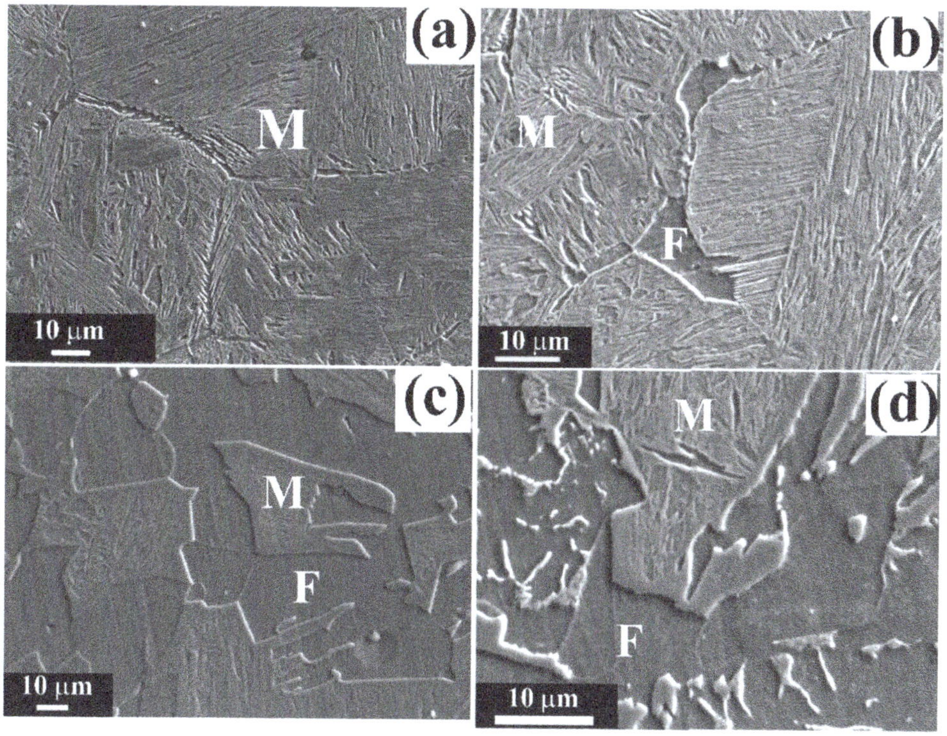

Fig. 9 Microstructure of the water quenched samples air cooled for **a** 10 s, **b** 20 s, **c** 30 s, and **d** 40 s. pro-eutectoid ferrite at the grain boundaries and martensite inside the untransformed austenitic grains can be observed

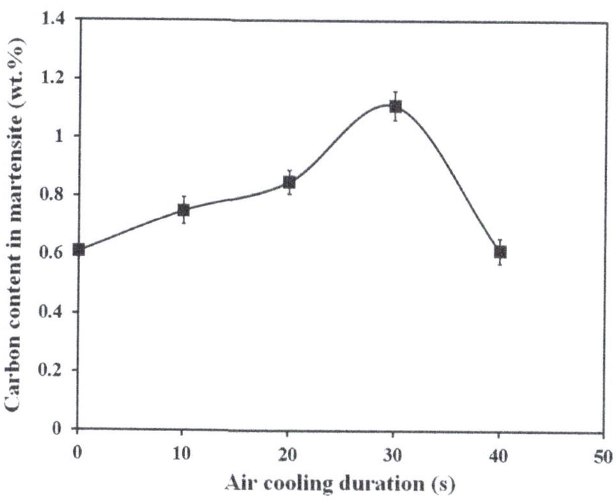

Fig. 10 Variation of carbon content in the martensitic regions with continuous cooling duration (Varshney et al. 2016a)

the samples air cooled for 40 s might be due to nucleation of pearlite in the microstructure. Carbides in pearlite would have consumed some carbon and then reduced the amount of the carbon in the untransformed region.

Previous extensive microstructural examinations revealed the presence of carbides in the samples air cooled for 30 s and austempered at 350 and 400 °C. In the samples air cooled for 0, 10, and 20 s, carbides were not found to be present (Varshney et al. 2017). From Fig. 10, it is clear that high carbon content in austenite in the samples cooled for 30 s led to the precipitation of carbides during austempering. Takahashi and Bhadeshia (Takahashi and HKDH Bhadeshia. 1990) in their theoretical study on the effect of carbon content in parent austenite on the precipitation of carbides in bainite established that probability of the precipitation of carbides inside bainitic ferrite lath increases with increase in the carbon in parent austenite. Thus, measurement of carbon content in austenite after air cooling with EPMA helped to understand the reason for carbide precipitation taking place in spite of high Si content of the steels.

6.6 Application of EPMA in the Field of Earth Sciences/Geosciences

EPMA is an essential research tool routinely used in complex mineralogical and petrological studies of geological (rocks and minerals including ore minerals) and planetary materials. It is routinely used for nondestructive quantitative geochemistry—to precisely determine major oxides and trace element abundances—of in-situ mineral phases such as olivine, pyroxenes, apatite, monazite, uraninite, and thorite, or tiny inclusions in a mineral, at a scale of few microns on the surface of solid samples. Therefore, it is also widely used in experimental petrology with an objective of characterizing phase changes and partition behavior of elements during melting, etc. For petrological investigation, a geological

sample must be in the form of either a thin-polished section mounted on a glass slide (predominantly used) or polished sample in a resin block.

The main advantage of EPMA is its capability to acquire the chemical composition of a targeted small spot (1–2 microns) within a (primary, secondary, or accessory) mineral grain, employing WDS technique. The main applications of EPMA in Earth Sciences/Geology can be summarized as follows.

1. This technique is mainly used to precisely analyze the chemical (major oxides and trace constituents) composition of the mineral grains in geological samples such as rocks, minerals, and glasses by wavelength dispersive spectrometry in a nondestructive way. Many times, the variation in elemental concentrations within a single mineral grain can be determined from the rim to the center, which are used to estimate the temperature and the pressure under which the mineral formed. Detailed mineral chemistry of all mineral phases, particularly tiny melt inclusions, helps to obtain the parental magma composition, which in turn can be linked to the origin of such magma.
2. Chemical composition of small-sized spots (1–2 microns) can be analyzed, which is particularly beneficial in analysis of fluid inclusions or small glass globules trapped within small mineral grains.
3. Elemental mapping, showing false color images characterizing spatial distribution of elements in a sample of interest, is done to identify chemical zoning within a mineral grain, as well as to identify mineral phases.
4. Different images prepared by EPMA technique, particularly, secondary electron images, backscattered electron images (BSE) and cathodoluminescence images reveal the textural (shape, size and orientation of grains, and their relationship) aspects of a geological sample that aid in drawing inferences on magma cooling. For example, high-resolution BSE images of the sample combined with micro-composition analysis obtained from EPMA help to study micro-textures in detail, in-situ characteristics, and resolve complex chemical variations within individual mineral phases; these are often difficult to achieve using an optical microscope.
5. The primary and secondary (or altered) nature of the mineral grain can be determined using probe data, e.g., mantle-derived mineral or crustal-derived mineral, reaction rims, hydrothermal alteration, etc. The presence and identification of mantle and crustal xenoliths (foreign fragments) within the rock sample can be easily identified at a microscopic level.
6. EPMA is useful to analyze the elemental components of sedimentary rocks, including B, Ga, Ba, Sr, Co, V, Cr, Mn, Fe, and Ni. This information helps to evaluate the effect of redox conditions, depth of water column, and salinity on the formation of sedimentary rock in a basin.
7. This technique has been used for geochronology, particularly for U-Th age of monazite, uraninite, thorite, and xenotime minerals. Monazite dating by EPMA is a reliable and powerful dating technique and widely used in the geochronological study of monazite-bearing rocks that does not require measurement of isotope ratios.

A Case Study: Apatite from the Amba Dongar Carbonatite Complex

The Amba Dongar Carbonatite Complex, Gujarat, is a type locality for occurrence of carbonatite rocks (containing more than 50 modal% carbonate minerals) as well as alkaline rocks such as nephelinites. In general, carbonatite has high economic significance, particularly for the rare earth elements (REE), Nb, and phosphates (Simandl 2015). Globally, carbonatite complexes are well known for the largest source of REE deposits (Harmer and Nex 2016); REE-bearing phases are bastnaesite, britholite, and monazite. The mineral apatite (phosphate-bearing phase) commonly occurs as an accessary mineral in both carbonatites and the associated nephelinite rocks. In this regard, apatite chemistry obtained via EPMA analysis can be used to understand genetic relationship between the carbonatites and nephelinites, as well as the origin of the parental magma(s). Chandra et al. (Chandra et al. 2018) reported the mineral chemistry of apatites from three different calciocarbonatites and one nephelinite. The electron probe data for major and trace element compositions of apatite was obtained using a CAMECA SXFive electron probe micro-analyzer (EPMA) at IIT Bombay. Targeted apatite in thin-polished samples were excited with a primary electron beam sourced from lanthanum hexaboride (LaB_6) and operated at 15 kV and 20 nA with a beam of 1 μm diameter. Calibration was done using both natural and synthetic minerals and elemental glass (apatite (F, P), diopside (Ca), albite (Na), $SrSO_4$ (Sr), NaCl (Cl), Th-glass (Si), La-glass (La), Ce-glass (Ce), Pr-glass (Pr), and Nd-glass (Nd).

Considerable compositional variation is observed in the analyzed major oxide and selected trace element compositions of apatites from three calciocarbonatite samples and a nephelinite sample (Chandra et al. 2018). Apatites from both rocks show similar F and FeO contents and REE abundances except for La. These similarities in the elemental abundances indicate a common parental magma and support a genetic relationship between the calciocarbonatites and the associated nephelinite rocks. Also, apatites in carbonatites contain up to 0.4 wt% Na_2O, which indicates a comparatively more volatile content in the original parental carbonate magma. This volatile content of the original parental carbonate

magma might have been lost to the country rocks (or host rock) causing wide spread fenitization, a process of chemical alteration (mainly alkali metasomatism) of country rocks in the form of aureole around carbonatite intrusion by mantle fluids containing Na, K, F, Cl, CO_2, etc.

Backscattered electron images of apatites in calciocarbonatites and nephelinite are presented in Fig. 11a–d. Apatite cumulate in calciocarbonatites has higher CaO content as compared to other forms of apatites. Apatite cumulate is an early formed mineral phase than other forms of apatites identified using these images. Apatite shows various textural features in calciocarbonatites: (1) scattered or disseminated apatites in calcitic groundmass (Fig. 11a), (2) clusters of apatites near calcite boundaries (Fig. 11b), and (3) apatite cumulates (Fig. 11c). Nephelinite contains apatites of varying size and habit (Fig. 11d). Petrography of calciocarbonatites reveals that apatite cumulate is the second most fractionated mineral phase after calcite.

These forms of apatite reflect continuous apatite fractionation with accompanying physicochemical changes during calciocarbonatite formation from the rising carbonatite melt (Chandra et al. 2018). EPMA analyses constrain the composition of SiO_2 (0.01–0.34 wt%) and SrO (0.58–0.95 wt%) contents of apatites in calciocarbonatites, which are comparatively lower than the apatites in nephelinite (SiO_2, 0.69–1.10 wt%; SrO, 1.32–2.6 wt%). In contrast, the P_2O_5 (39.9–41.3 wt%) and Na_2O (0.1–0.38 wt%) contents of apatites in calciocarbonatite are distinctly higher than those in nephelinite (P_2O_5, 38.6–39.6 wt%; and Na_2O, 0.06–0.13 wt%). These variations in major oxides suggest that apatite crystallization may have continued after immiscible separation of the carbonatite melt and the silicate melt from a common parental carbonated silicate magma.

6.7 Microstructure Study of Ni-Based Superalloy

Ni-based superalloys are widely used in aero-engine applications, such as in turbine blades and vanes, due to their exceptional high temperature strength (Schafrik and Sprague 2004; Pollock and Tin 2006). This class of alloys is mainly based on Ni as the principal element, and they obtain their strength on account of the coherent Ni_3Al-based phase having $L1_2$ crystal structure. The refractory alloying elements such as W, Nb, and Mo are added for solid solution strengthening of the matrix (γ) phase, whereas the elements such as Ti, Nb, and Ta assist in the formation and strengthening of the precipitate (γ') phase (Pollock and Tin 2006). In general, Ni-based superalloys contain a large number (8–10) of alloying elements, and their distribution and partitioning during solidification significantly affect the properties of the alloys in as-cast as well as post-processed conditions. EPMA is the most useful tool for experimental investigations of distribution of various alloying elements in a Ni-based superalloy.

Figure 12 presents a BSE micrograph of a directionally solidified Ni-based superalloy provided by GE Research—Bangalore. The dendritic structure is clearly highlighted by light gray contrast (Arrows labeled 1 on Fig. 12), whereas the interdendritic $\gamma + \gamma$' eutectic regions are highlighted by dark gray contrast (Arrow labeled 2 on Fig. 12). The precipitates containing Ti and the refractory elements Ta, W,

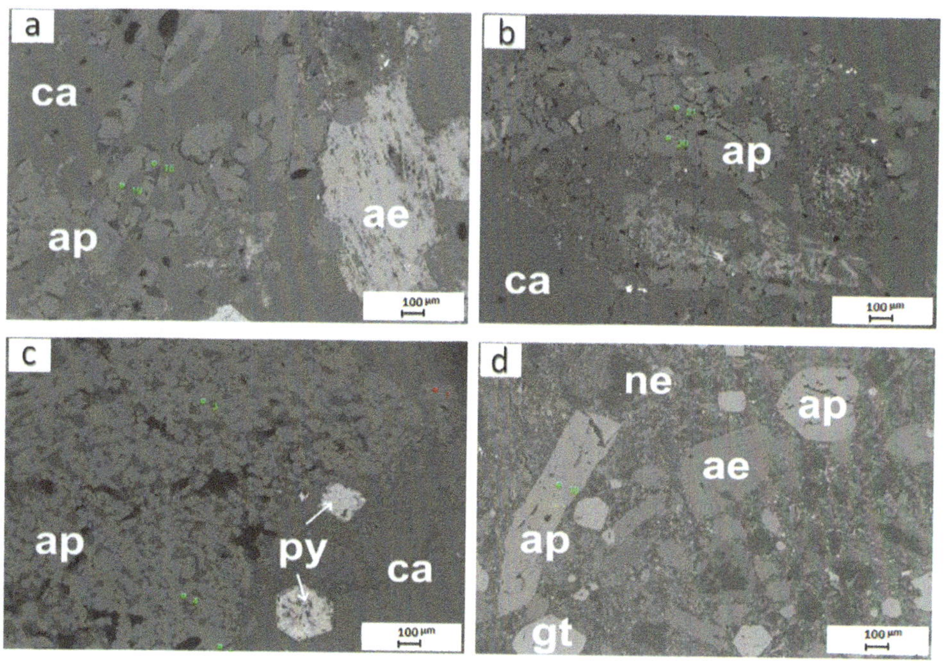

Fig. 11 Photomicrographs of backscattered electron images of various apatite forms from three calciocarbonatites: (a–c) and one nephelinite (d) from the Amba Dongar Carbonatite Complex (Chandra et al. 2018). **a** size variations in apatites with calcitic groundmass, **b** apatite clusters along the boundaries of calcite crystals, **c** apatite cumulate, **d** apatite crystals in nephelinite. Locations of microprobe spots are shown by green dots. Symbols are ca: calcite, ap: apatite, ae: aegirine, py: pyrochlore, ne: nepheline, and gt: garnet

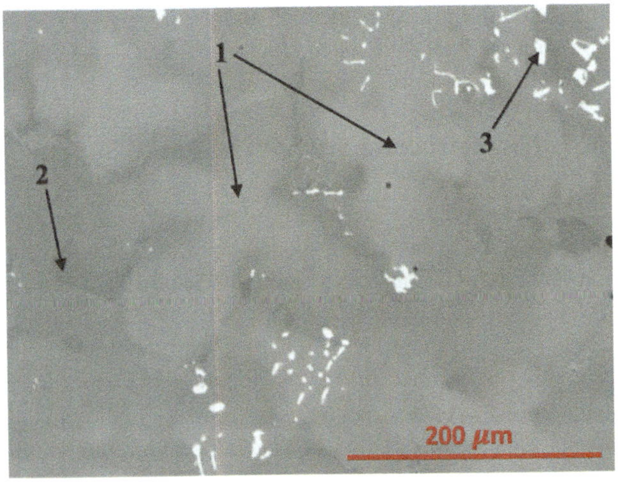

Fig. 12 BSE micrograph of a solidified nickel-based superalloy. Dendritic regions, interdendritic regions, and refractory element-rich precipitates are marked by Arrows 1, 2, and 3, respectively

and Nb are the bright regions on the micrograph (Arrow labeled 3 on Fig. 12).

The areas rich in various elements can be nicely captured in elemental maps prepared by WDS. As examples, the elemental maps collected for Ti (K_α), Ta (L_α), W (L_α), and Mo (L_α) are presented in Fig. 13a–d, respectively. In the Ti-map shown in Fig. 13a, the dendrites are clearly highlighted due to the enrichment of titanium in the interdendritic regions and its gradual deprival toward the center of the dendrite. Maps of Ti and Ta shown in Fig. 13a–b correctly highlight the precipitates rich in them, whereas Fig. 13c–d shows more or less uniform distribution of tungsten and molybdenum in the dendritic regions. Enrichment of interdendritic regions with tungsten and depletion with molybdenum are also clearly visible. The intensity of each pixel in the map can be converted into concentration after applying appropriate ZAF corrections at each pixel, and the intensity maps can be converted into composition maps. Quantitative analysis at each pixel can also be obtained in a tabular form. Such quantitative data is very useful in validating the various solidification models used for simulation of microstructure of as-cast superalloys. Such simulations are routinely performed in industry for design and control of various processing routs, and availability of such quantitative maps from EPMA can be a very valuable resource in such developments.

In order to get an idea about how concentration distribution of various elements varies across a dendrite arm, point-by-point quantitative analysis was conducted across a dendritic arm shown by a yellow dotted line on Fig. 13a. The analysis was carried out using pure elemental standards and with the probe conditions of 25 kV and 20 nA. The X-ray lines used for the WDS analysis were Ni-K_α, Al-K_α, Co-K_α, Cr-K_α, Ti-K_α, Nb-L_α, Mo-L_α, Ta-L_α, and W-L_α. The concentration profiles obtained across the dendritic arm are presented in Fig. 14.

It can be seen that Ti gradually increases from center of the dendrite toward the outer and the interdendritic regions are characterized by higher amount of titanium. Ni and Al are seen to partition in the same way, whereas Co and Cr are partitioning exactly opposite to Ni and Al. Ta, Mo, and Nb seem to be segregated only on the MC intermetallics. Such quantitative data on concentration profiles of a microstructure is essential for modeling certain processes such as homogenization annealing.

Fig. 13 Elemental maps produced by WDS for **a** Titanium, **b** Tantalum, **c** Tungsten, and **d** Molybdenum

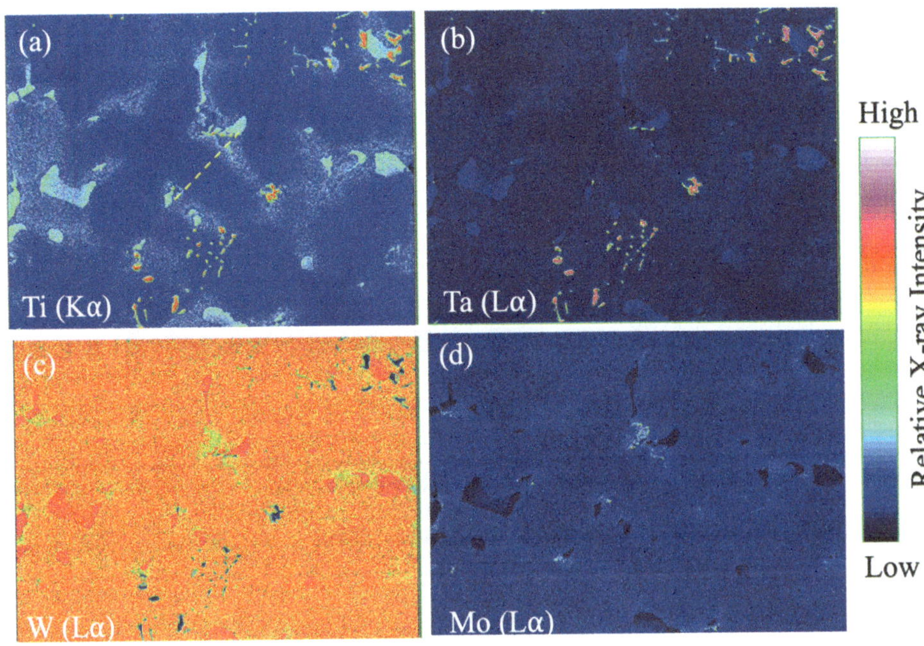

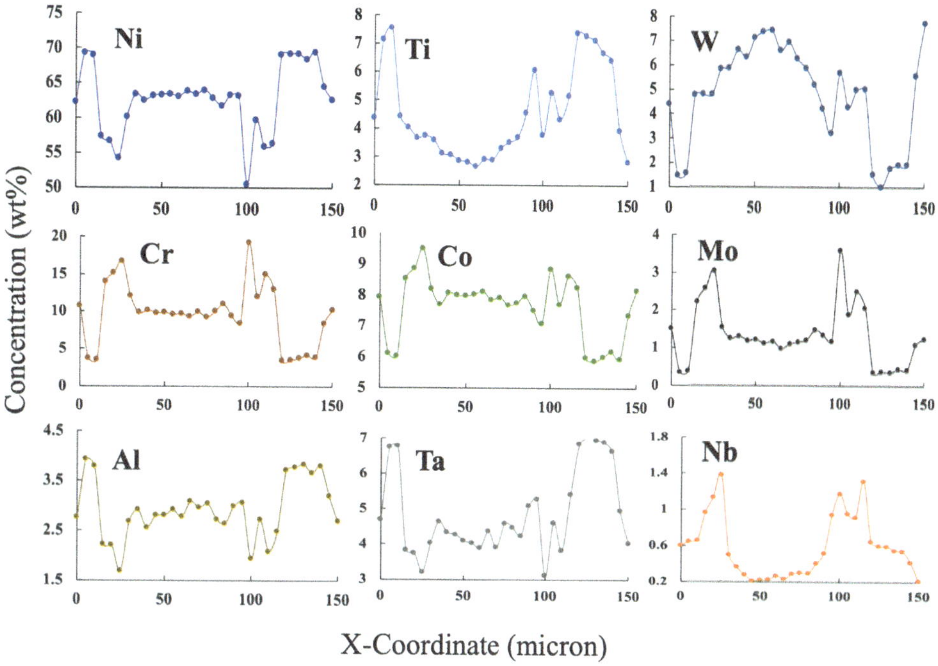

Fig. 14 Concentration profiles of all elements in the Ni-based superalloy analyzed by WDS across a dendritic arm

It should be noted here that while analyzing Ni-based superalloys, there maybe overlap of several peaks from various alloying elements, and hence, WDS with higher energy resolution should be a better choice than EDS. For example, the part of spectra obtained by WDS and EDS on the superalloy used in the present study is presented in Fig. 15a–b. It can be seen that Ni-K_β (8.267 keV), Ta-L_α (8.146 keV), and W-L_α (8.398) peaks are very close to each other. These peaks are overlapping in the EDS spectrum. However, they are clearly resolved in the WDS spectrum. Such a high resolution obtained by WDS increases the accuracy of the quantitative analysis manifold over that done by EDS. Similarly, Ni-K_α (7.48) and Co-K_β (7.649) are very close to each other such that they are not resolved in the EDS spectrum (Fig. 15b) but can be clearly resolved by the WDS spectrum (Fig. 15a).

For quantitative analysis with 25 kV, Ta-L_α (8.146 keV) and W-L_α (8.398) lines can be used. However, the precaution has to be taken while collecting the background intensities, which are usually collected from positions that are close enough to the peak position so as to properly represent the background of the peak and at the same time slightly away enough so as to avoid the interference from the peak width. In case of Ta-L_α and W-L_α, since Ni-K_β is very close to both the peaks, one also has to make sure that the positions for their background collections are not interfered by the peak width of Ni-K_β. Thus, it is necessary to quickly assess the peak positions of all possible characteristic X-rays generated from the sample as they may interfere with the measured peak or background intensities even though these X-rays are not going to be under consideration for analysis.

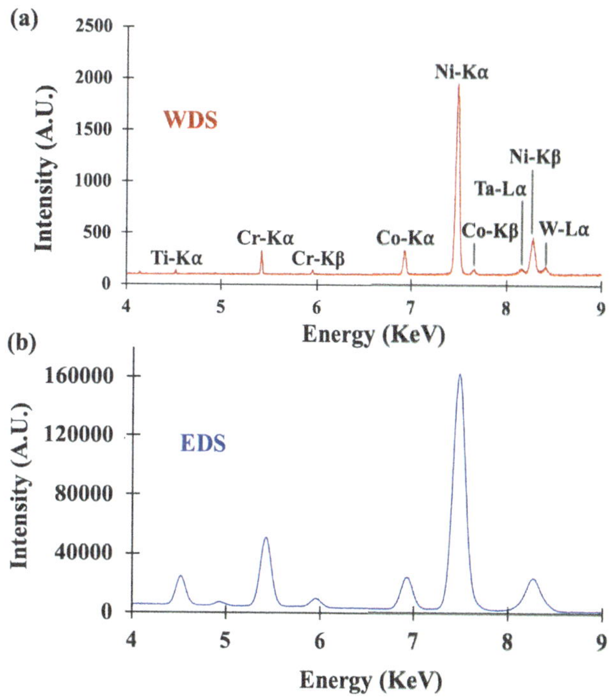

Fig. 15 Part of the X-ray energy spectra obtained by **a** WDS and **b** EDS on the Ni-based superalloy illustrated in the present study

7 Summary

Electron probe micro-analyzer (EPMA) is one of the most accurate and precise tools for micro-composition analysis of multicomponent samples. EPMAs are equipped with an EDS

and multiple WDS channels. However, WDS, due to its better accuracy and energy resolution, should be the preferred choice for both qualitative and quantitative analysis wherever high accuracy and precision are needed. Although the intensities of X-rays collected by detectors are significantly affected by the sample's matrix effects, the various correction methods including ZAF, Phi-Rho-Z, or calibration curves essentially yield quite accurate analysis with the help of standards. The various case studies were discussed that covered the EPMA applications in range of materials including steels, titanium alloys, nickel-based superalloys, high-entropy alloys, and geological materials. The various applications covered in these case studies included determination of interdiffusivities and phase equilibria, understanding of phase transformation during heat treatments, gathering the quantitative microstructure-composition map data for model validation, and understanding the genetic relationship between the geological rock samples. Although only limited cases could be covered in the present article, the utility of EPMA is essentially boundless whenever and wherever accurate and precise micro-composition analysis is desired.

Acknowledgements The authors are grateful for the generous support from various funding agencies and organizations with which the discussed case studies have been conducted: Indian Space Research Organization, General Motors USA, GE Research—Bangalore, GOALI grant from NSF and IIT Kanpur. Thanks to GE Research—Bangalore for providing the Nickel-based superalloy for the case study. The authors are also thankful to JEOL's EPMA experts for useful discussions.

References

Akhtar K, Khan SA, Khan SB, Asiri AM (2018) Scanning electron microscopy: principle and applications in nanomaterials characterization. In: Sharma SK (ed) Handbook of materials characterization. Springer International Publishing AG, pp 113–146

Berger MJ, Seltzer SM (1964) Tables for energy losses and ranges for electrons and positrons. Natl Acad Sci Natl Res Counc Publ 1133:205–268

Bishop HE (1967) Optique des Rayons X et Microanalysis. Hermann, Paris

Bloch F (1933) Bremsvermogen von Atomen mit mehreren Elektronen. Zeitsehrift Fiir Physik. 81:363–376

Brown JD, Packwood RH (1982) Quantitative electron probe microanalysis using Gaussian curves. X-Ray Spectrom 11(4):187–193

Caistaing R, Guinier A (1953) Point-by-point chemical analysis by X-ray spectroscopy: electronic microanalyzer. Anal Chem 25 (5):724–726

Castaing R (1952) Application des sondes electroniques a une methode d'analyse ponctuelle. Office National d'Estudes et Recherches Aeronautiques, paris, France

Chandra J, Paul D, Viladkar SG, Sensarma S (2018) Origin of the Amba Dongar carbonatite complex, India and its possible linkage with the Deccan Large Igneous Province. Geological Society, London, Special Publications, Geological Society of London vol 463. pp 137–169

Chauhan GPS, Kulkarni KN (2021) Investigations of ternary interdiffusion in β (BCC) phase field of Ti-Al-Mo system. Metall Mater Trans A 52A:413–425

Cosslet VE (1949) Conference on electron microscopy. Nature 164:481–483

Dangi B, Brown TW, Kulkarni KN (2018) Effect of silicon, manganese and nickel present in iron on the intermetallic growth at iron-aluminum alloy interface. J Alloys Compd 769:777–787

Day KM, Dayananda MA, Ram-Mohan LR (2005) Determination and assessment of ternary interdiffusion coefficients from individual diffusion couples. J Phase Equilib Diffus 26:579–590

Divinski SV, Pokoev AV, Esakkiraja N, Paul A (2018) A mystery of sluggish diffusion in high-entropy alloys: the truth or a myth. In: Mehrer H (ed) Diffusion foundations, vol 17. pp 69–104

Duncumb P, Reed SJB (1968) The calculation of stopping power and backscatter effects in electron probe microanalysis. In: Heinrich KFJ (ed) Quantitative electron probe microanalysis, vol 298. NBS Special Publication, pp 133–154

Guillemet A (1989) Assessing the thermodynamics of the Fe-Co-Ni system using a CALPHAD predictive technique. CALPHAD; 13 (1):1–22

Gupta KP (1990) The Cu-Fe-Ni (Copper-Iron-Nickel) system. In: Phase diagrams of ternary nickel alloys, Part 1. Indian Institute of Metals, Kolkata, pp 290–315

Harmer RE, Nex PAM (2016) Rare earth deposits of Africa. Episodes 39:381–406

Heinrich KFJ, Yakowitz H (1975) Absorption of primary X Rays in electron probe microanalysis. Anal Chem 47(14):2408–2411

Henrich KF (1991) Strategies of electron probe data reduction. In: Henrich KFJ, Newbury DE (eds) Electron probe quantitation. Springer Science+Business Media, New York, pp 9–18

Hillier J, Baker RF (1944) Microanalysis by means of electrons. J Appl Phys 15:663–675

Jennings J, Gould J (2008) A new road for automotive architectures. Welding J 87(10):26–30

Jiangqi L,Fengchong L, Jiqing C (2008) New technology of lightweight and steel-aluminum hybrid structure car body. Chin J Mech Eng 6:6

JEOL User Manual for JXA-8230

Kirkaldy JS, Lane JE, Mason GR (1963) Diffusion in multicomponent metallic systems: VII solutions of the multicomponent diffusion equations with variable coefficients. Can J Phy 41(12):2174–2186

Krishna AB, Kulkarni KN (2018) Experimental determination of quaternary isotherm of Fe-Ni-Co-Cu at 950 °C by diffusion couple technique. Materialia 4:549–552

Love G, Cox MG, Scott VD (1978) A versatile number correction for electron-probe microanalysis. J Phys D Appl Phys 11:7–21

Takahashi MM, Bhadeshia HKDH (1990) Model for transition from upper to lower bainite, Mater Sci Technol 6:592

Miracle DB, Senkov ON (2017) A critical review of high entropy alloys and related concepts. Acta Mater 122:448–511

Morral JE (2018) Body-diagonal diffusion couples for high entropy alloys. J Phase Equilib Diffus 39:51–56

Packwood RH, Brown JD (1981) A Gaussian expression to describe curves for quantitative electron probe microanalysis. X-Ray Spectrom 10(3):138–146

Philibert J (1963) A method of calculating the absorption correction in electron probe microanalysis. In: Pattee HH, Cosslett VE, Engstrom A (eds) X-ray optics and X-ray microanalysis. Academic Press, New York, pp 379–392

Philibert J, Tixier R (1968) Some problems with quantitative electron probe microanalysis. In: Heinrich KFJ (ed) Quantitative electron

probe microanalysis. NBS Special Publication 298, National Bureau of Standards, Washington, DC, pp 13–34

Pollock TM, Tin S (2006) Nickel-based superalloys for advanced turbine engines: chemistry, microstructure and properties. J Propul Power 22(2):361–374

Private communication with JEOL EPMA experts (2019)

Reed SJB (1965) Characteristic fluorescence corrections in electron-probe microanalysis. Br J Appl Phys 16

Reed SJB (2005) Electron microprobe analysis and scanning electron microscopy. Cambridge University Press, Cambridge

Rinaldi R, Llovet X (2015) Electron probe microanalysis: a review of the past, present, and future. Microsc Microanal 21(5):1053–1069

Sachdev AK, Kulkarni K, Fang ZZ, Yang R, Girshov V (2012) Titanium for automotive applications: challenges and opportunities in materials and processing. JOM 64:553–565

Schafrik R, Sprague R (2004) Saga of gas turbine materials part II. Adv Mater Process 162(4):27–30

Simandl GJ (2015) Carbonatites and related exploration targets. In: Simandl GJ, Neetz M (eds) Symposium on Strategic and Critical Materials Proceedings 13–14 November 2015; Victoria, British Columbia. British Columbia Ministry of Energy and Mines, British Columbia Geological Survey Paper, vol 3. pp 31–37

Tripathi S, Verma V, Brown TW, Kulkarni KN (2017) Effect of small amount of manganese on the interdiffusivities in Fe-Al alloys. J Phase Equilib Diffus 38:135–142

Tripathi A, Middleton S, Lavernia EJ, Sachdev AK, Kulkarni KN (2018) Ternary interdiffusion in β (BCC) phase of the Ti-Al-Nb system. J Phase Equilib Diffus 39(6):841–852

Tripathi A, Kulkarni A, Kulkarni KN (2020) Interdiffusion in β (BCC) phase of Ti-Al-Mn system at 1100 °C. Metall Mater Trans A 51A:1789–1798

Varshney A, Sangal S, Kundu S, Mondal K (2016a) Super strong and highly ductile low alloy multiphase steels consisting of bainite, ferrite and retained austenite. Mater Des 65:75–88

Varshney A, Sangal S, Kundu S, Mondal K (2016b) Superior work hardening behavior of moderately high carbon low alloy super strong and ductile multiphase steels with dispersed retained austenite. Mater Des 99:439–448

Varshney A, Sangal S, Mondal K (2017) Exceptional work-hardening behaviour of medium-carbon high-silicon low-alloy steels. Metall Mater Trans 48:589–593

Varshney A, Sangal S, Gouthama, Pramanick AK, Mondal K (2017) Microstructural evidence of nano-carbides in medium carbon high silicon multiphase steels. Mater Sci Eng A 708:237–247

Verma V, Tripathi A, Kulkarni KN (2017) On interdiffusion in FeNiCoCrMn high entropy alloy. J Phase Equilib Diffus 38(4):445–456

Verma V, Tripathi A, Venkateswaran T, Kulkarni KN (2020) First report on entire sets of experimentally determined interdiffusion coefficients in quaternary and quinary high entropy alloys. J Mater Res 35(2):162–171

Wilson RR (1941) Range and ionization measurements on high speed protons. Phys Rev 60(11):749–753

Ziebold TO, Ogilvie RE (1964) An empirical method for electron microanalysis. Anal Chem 36(2):322–327

Nanosciences and Advanced Imaging Centre: Unravelling Attributes by Electron Microscopy

Rajneesh Kumar Prajapati, Manish Kulkarni, Prabhat K. Dwivedi, and Sri Sivakumar

1 Introduction

The microscope has been emerged as the most fundamental tool for research in diverse fields of science and engineering, owing to limited resolving power of human eye. Resolving power or resolution of an unaided human eye is about 0.2 mm, which refers to the minimum distinguishable distance between two points. In order to see the points closer than that, a lens or a microscope, which is essentially the assembly of lenses is required to magnify the object. Since the dawn of science, there has been a lasting thrust among researchers to get the intricate details of their specimen in increased magnification, which offered substantial impetus to craft a microscope with enhanced resolution.

While relentless efforts for better resolution, it was realized that the resolving power of light microscope was not only limited by the number and quality of the lenses but also by the wavelength of the visible light used for illumination, thus precluding atomic scale imaging. A major breakthrough occurred in 1920s, when de Broglie discovered that accelerated electrons in vacuum behaves as light wave and exhibit wavelength thousands times shorter than that of visible light. Moreover, it was realised that these electrons have similar effect of electric and magnetic field as glass mirrors and lenses have on visible light. It didn't take long to translate these insights in to a microscope based on accelerated electron beam and in 1932 Knoll and Ruska proposed the term electron microscope. They developed the idea of electron lenses in to practical reality and later in 1986 received noble prize for this crucial discovery[1]. Since the development of first transmission electron microscope (TEM), enormous improvements in resolution have occurred over the past few decades which enabled advanced TEM to offer resolution close to 0.1 nm or better. In modern era, TEM has become an indispensible tool for establishing attributes such as particle size, crystalline habit, elemental composition and many more. While, *insitu* TEM provides a deeper insight to material sample under varying heating condition; *cryo* TEM opened newer paradigms towards imaging of diverse biological and other beam sensitive samples. Moreover, recent developments in tomography and quantitative scanning TEM (STEM) have further expanded the abilities of TEM by allowing three-dimensional (3D) reconstructions at nanoscale instead of only two-dimensional (2D) projections.

In this diverse and fast changing arena of nanosciences and nanoengineering, an analytical facility equipped with advanced electron microscopes and specimen preparation tools is highly desirable for sustainable research. In this milieu, Nanosciences (CNS) and Advanced Imaging Centre (AIC) at IIT Kanpur, has been established to disrupt the stratification of discipline in the characterization of materials (Fig. 1).It is among the eight centres supported by the Department of Science and Technology (DST) across India with the objectives of providing state of the art imaging facility and resources for research and development activities. These centres offer a critical mass and outstanding expertise in the wide range of electron microscopy techniques available for materials characterisation down to atomic scale. This facility is intended to bring together multidisciplinary expertise to drive synergy and amplify our characterization capabilities which support continuous fundamental research, innovations, brain storming and global interactions with academia as well as industry. Over the past few years Nanosciences and Advanced Imaging Centre has became the materials characterization hub for the academic institution, research centre and industry.

2 Electron Microscopes at CNS and AIC

Nanosciences and Advanced Imaging Centre offers two main types of electron microscope, namely, the transmission electron microscope (TEM) and the scanning electron

R. K. Prajapati · M. Kulkarni · P. K. Dwivedi · S. Sivakumar (✉)
Center for Nanosciences and Advanced Imaging Center,
IIT Kanpur, Kanpur, UP 208016, India
e-mail: srisiva@iitk.ac.in

K. Biswas et al. (eds.), *Electron Microscopy in Science and Engineering*, IITK Directions 6,
https://doi.org/10.1007/978-981-16-5101-4_7

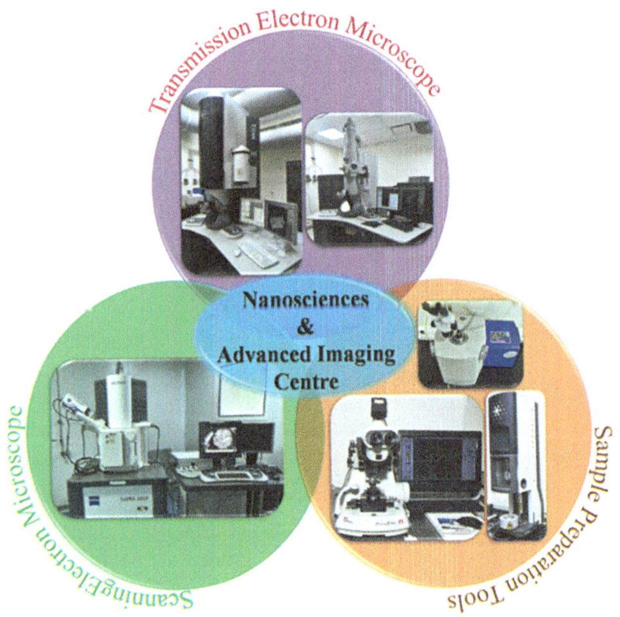

Fig. 1 Schematic overview of imaging facilities at nanosciences and advanced imaging centre

microscope (SEM). A transmission electron microscope produces an image by passing a high voltage electron beam through a very thin specimen that is transparent/semi-transparent to electrons. The beam that is transmitted through the specimen carries structural information about the specimen, which can then be magnified by the microscope. In stark contrast, a scanning electron microscope detects secondary and backscattered electrons that arise from the surface as a result of excitation by the original electron beam.[2]

The scanning electron microscope does produce lower resolution images than the transmission electron microscope, but since it uses surface electron interactions, it can image bulk samples which enable scientists to achieve 3D information about the physical features of the specimen.

Additionally, Scanning transmission electron microscopy (STEM) invoked the technology of both the scanning electron microscope and the transmission electron microscope. Major advantage of STEM imaging is that the signal is generated by the electrons scattered out at high angles and collected by high-angle annular dark field detector (HAADF), known for its intuitive atomic number contrast (Z-contrast imaging), which led to characteristic elemental mapping of the specimen (Fig. 2). Moreover, similar to TEM, STEM also requires very thin samples, as the technique mainly involves looking at the electron beam transmitted through and emerging from the specimen.

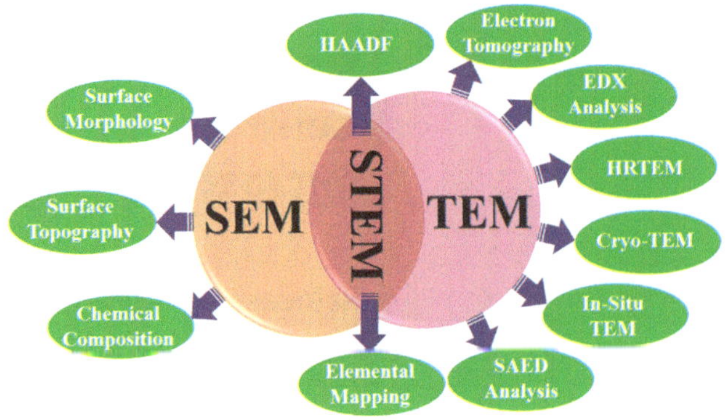

Fig. 2 Schematic representation of analytical abilities of SEM and TEM at nanoscience and advanced imaging centre IIT Kanpur

3 Scanning Electron Microscope

Center for Nanosciences (CNS) offers Zeiss Supra 40VP Field Emission Scanning Electron Microscope (FESEM), suitable for observing structures as small as 1 nm on the surface of the material with three-dimensional appearance. It is equipped with a field emission cathode as electron source and three different detectors namely In-lens SE, SE2 detectors and variable pressure secondary electrons detector (VPSE). In order to be observed with an SEM, objects are preferably made conductive for currents. This could be achieved by coating them with an extremely thin layer (1.5–3.0 nm) of gold or gold–palladium by using sputter coater available at the centre (Fig. 3).

4 Transmission Electron Microscope

TEM facility is present at Advanced Imaging Centre, comprised of two transmission electron microscopes, operating at different acceleration voltage and is meant for imaging diverse samples ranging from nanomaterials to biological samples.

4.1 FEI-Titan G2 60–300 kV TEM

The FEI Titan G2 60–300 scanning transmission electron microscope (STEM/TEM) is an advanced analytical field emission scanning transmission electron microscope for the characterization and chemical analysis of wide range of materials and nanostructures, down to the atomic level. It is equipped with a high-brightness Schottky-field emission electron source, a high-resolution Gatan Imaging Filter

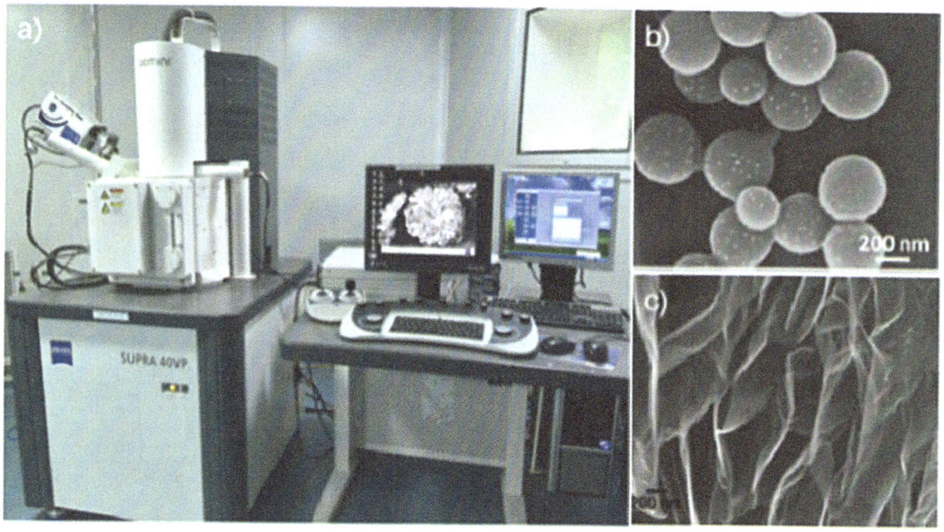

Fig. 3 **a** FESEM at the centre for Nanosciences; SEM image of **b** peptide soft structure decorated with Au nano particles(Reproduced from ref. 3 with permission from The Royal Society of Chemistry); **c** Graphine sheets (Reproduced from ref. 4 with permission)

(GIF), and X-ray energy dispersive spectrometer (EDS) for elemental and chemical analysis of materials at high spatial resolution. The microscope system also includes a high angle annular dark field detector (HAADF) for scanning transmission electron microscopy (STEM) and for chemical analysis of very small volumes. This instrument permits access to get critical information during imaging by exploiting diverse range of analytical, heating, cooling, and double tilt specimen holders (Figs. 4 and 5).

4.2 FEI-Tecnai G2 12 Twin 120 kV TEM

The Tecnai is an efficient and easy operation microscope with excellent analytical capabilities. It uses LaB_6 filament as electron source and could be exploited for the analysis of wide variety of samples ranging from materials to soft biological samples at room temperature as well as cryo-temperature. Moreover, it is compatible with tomography which could be useful in determining localization, orientation, shape and distribution.

5 Sample Preparation Lab

Unlike SEM, TEM does not offer a lot space for specimen. Additionally, specimen needs to be very thin so that electron can penetrate from the sample and form an image. This requires critical efforts to prepare quality samples for TEM as the results are strongly influenced by the quality of thin specimen.The imaging and analytical facilities at AIC are complimented by extensive sample preparation facilities for TEM and the preparation equipment covers a wide range of techniques to handle the large variety of samples brought

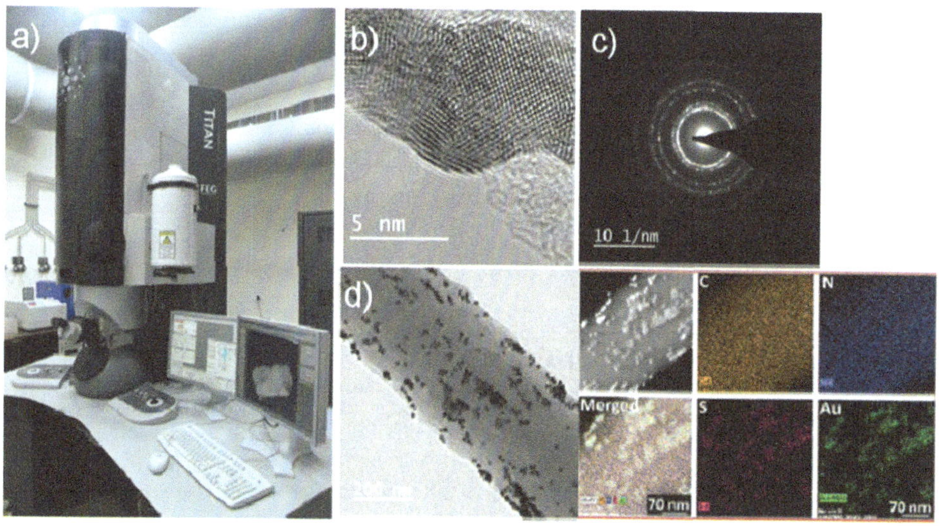

Fig. 4 **a** FEI-Titan G2 60–300 kV TEM, **b** HRTEM image, **c** SAED pattern of standard gold cross grating sample, **d** Elemental mapping of gold coated nanofibres (Reproduced from ref. 5 with permission from The Royal Society of Chemistry)

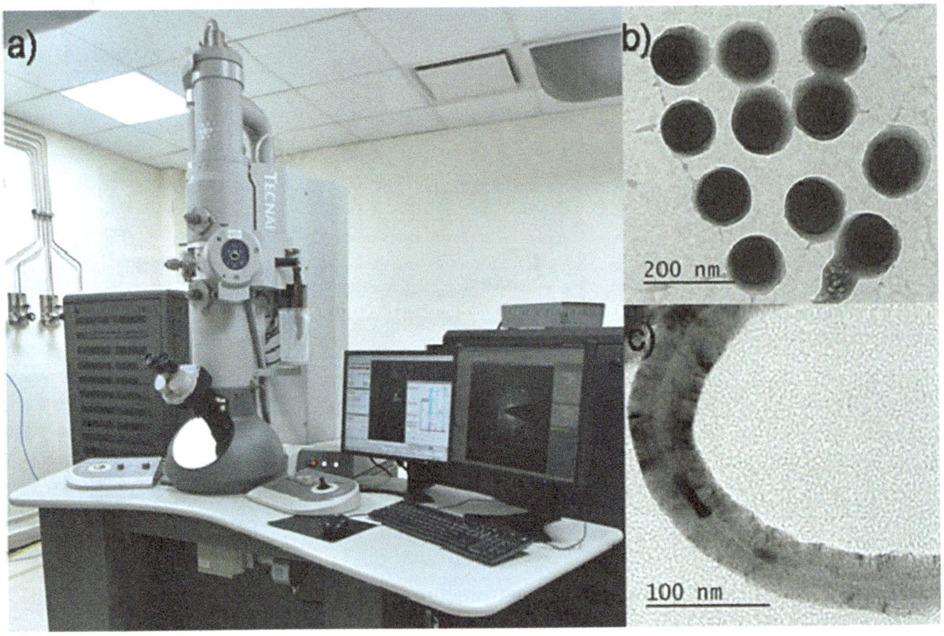

Fig. 5 **a** FEI-Tecnai G2 12 Twin 120 kV TEM; **b** TEM image of paint samples with core–shell structure; **c** TEM image of carbon nanotube

into the facility.While powdered sample can be dissolves/dispersed in an appropriate solvent followed by drop-casting over a supporting copper grid of 3 mm width; bulk samples require specific tools for cutting, grinding, dimpling, electropolishing and ion milling. For SEM preparation, there are carbon and gold sputter coaters, which can also be used for replica techniques. Moreover, centre is equipped with instruments required to proceed with soft material samples as well as biological samples, both at room and cryo temperature. Detailed description of tools available at the center has been discussed.

6 Precision Low Speed Saw

The TechCut-4 is a compact, multipurpose precision low speed saw designed to cut wide variety of small or delicate samples which cannot sustain at elevated temperature generated due to friction caused by high speed sectioning. The pivoting cutting arm has adjustable weights to apply or counterbalance downward force to the sample during sectioning. Cutting fluid is drawn from the reservoir by the blade to cool the sample. Samples up to 2" thickness can be sectioned by using a 3' to 6" blade range.

7 Variable Speed Polisher/Grinder

The MetPrep-1 grinding/polishing machine is excellent for polishing delicate samples using handheld tools with lapping films (Fig. 6b). It features digital control of all operations including run/stop, platen speed, platen direction and coolant flow. It includes 8' or 10" platens with rotation speed ranges from 5–350 RPM, in either clockwise or counterclockwise direction, with smooth, consistent low-end torque.

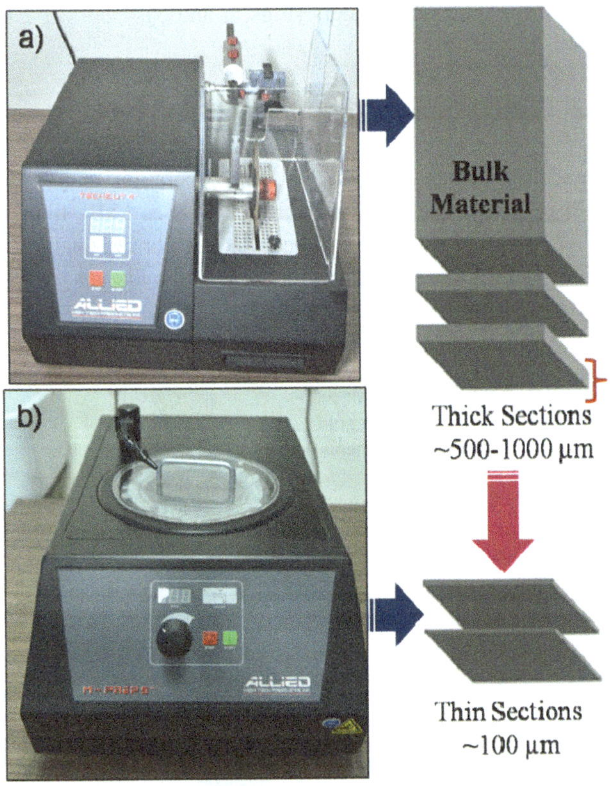

Fig. 6 **a** precision low speed saw; **b** Variable speed polisher and grinder and schematics of their capabilities

8 Ultrasonic Disk Cutter

The Ultrasonic Disk Cutter readily cuts transmission electron microscopy (TEM) specimens from hard, brittle materials without mechanical or thermal damage. It produces disk specimens as thin as 10 μm or cylindrical rods up to 10 mm length from bulk samples or rectangular wafers, which are subsequently being used in the preparation of cross-section TEM specimens. The cutting tool movement is governed by the excitation of lead zirconate titanate crystals oscillating at a frequency of 26 kHz. The cutting medium is abrasive slurry of either boron nitride or silicon carbide.

9 Dimpling Grinder

Dimpling Grinder is a state-of-the-art mechanical grinder required for prethining of specimens for ion milling while preparing electron microscopy samples. Dimpling is a rapid technique that involves rotating both the grinding wheel and the specimen, produces a specimen with only its central area reduced to a thickness of a few microns. The dimpling grinder features grinding rate control, a precise indication of specimen thickness, and an easy-to-use interface. The specimen can be accurately positioned using an optical microscope with transmitted and/or reflected light. The final specimen thickness is readily programmed for accurate, unattended operation (Fig. 7).

10 TEM Mill

TEM Mill is a sophisticated ion milling and polishing system offering reliable, high performance specimen preparation. It is compact, precise, and consistently produces high-quality transmission electron microscopy (TEM) specimens with large electron transparent areas from a wide variety of materials. It is equipped with two independently adjustable TrueFocus ion sources working over a wide range of operating energies (100 eV to 10 keV) and adjustable milling angle range of −10 to + 10°. These variables could be exploited for the rapid milling and slow specimen polishing of TEM specimens (Fig. 8).

11 PowerTome PC Ultramicrotome

PowerTome Ultramicrotome (including Cryo-ultramicrotome) is a computer controlled ultramicrotome used for the preparation of ultrathin/semi-thin sections as well as very flat

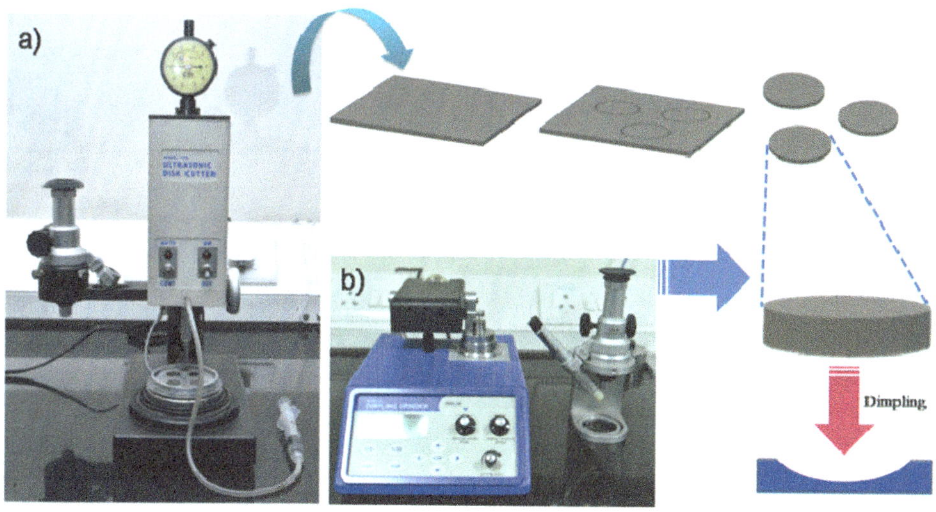

Fig. 7 **a** ultrasonic disc cutter; **b** Dimpling grinder and workflow scheme

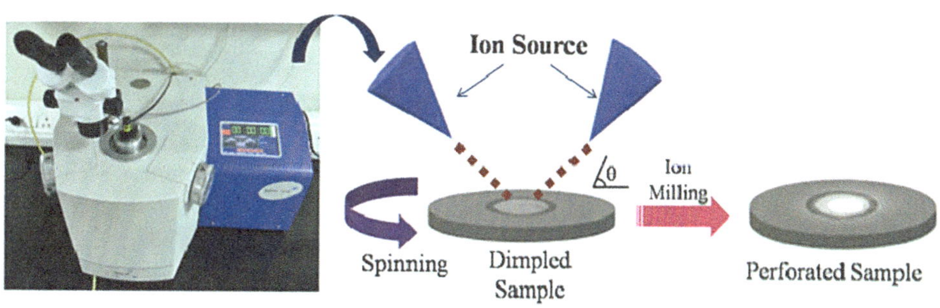

Fig. 8 Ion milling and its working scheme

surfaces of plastics, biological and biomedical objects for various microscopic investigations. This machine offers automatic sectioning range from 5 nm to 15 µm with cutting speed range from 0.1 to 100 mm/sec and there is a digital section counter and feed totaliser.

12 Vitrobot

The Vitrobot is a semi automated device for vitrification (plunge freezing) of aqueous samples. Critical vitrification parameters, such as temperature, relative humidity, blotting pressure and time, can be precisely controlled. A simple touch-screen user interface and programmable process control allow for consistent and high-yield sample output (Fig. 9).

13 Plasma Cleaner

Plasma cleaner automatically and quickly removes organic contamination (hydrocarbon) from electron microscopy specimens and specimen holders. A low energy, reactive gas plasma cleans without changing the specimen's elemental composition or structural characteristics. The Plasma Cleaner features easy-to-use front panel controls and an oil-free vacuum system for optimal processing.

14 Automatic Twin-Jet Electropolisher

Electrolytic thinning of conductive materials is an effective method of quickly producing specimens for transmission electron microscopy (TEM) without any induced artifacts. In Twin-Jet Electropolisher, twin jets simultaneously polish both sides of the sample, creating electron transparent specimens within a few minutes. The electropolisher features easily adjustable electrolyte flow, polishing voltage, termination detection sensitivity, and jet and specimen holder positions (Fig. 10).

15 Conclusions

In the current era of scientific research where chemistry, biology, material science, engineering, medicine and other disciplines are converging, comprehensive material characterization facility are essential to overcome the delay in

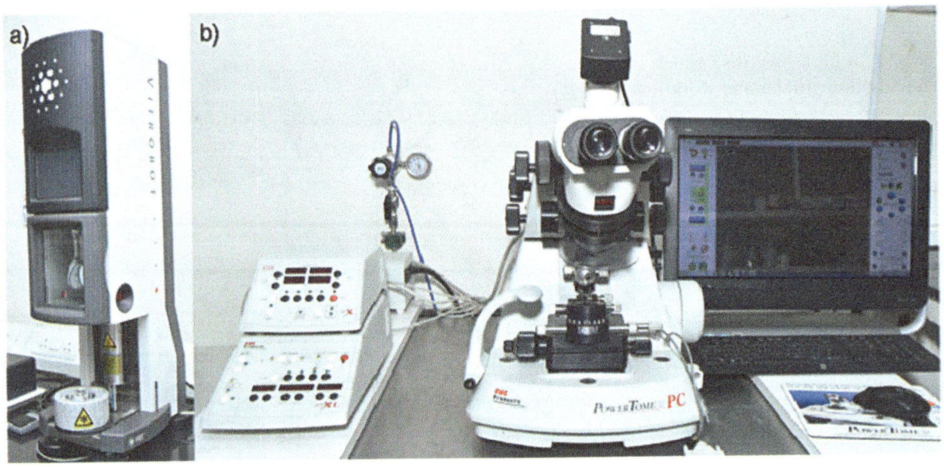

Fig. 9 **a** Vitrobot for plunge freezing, **b** Ultramicrotome for sectioning of samples

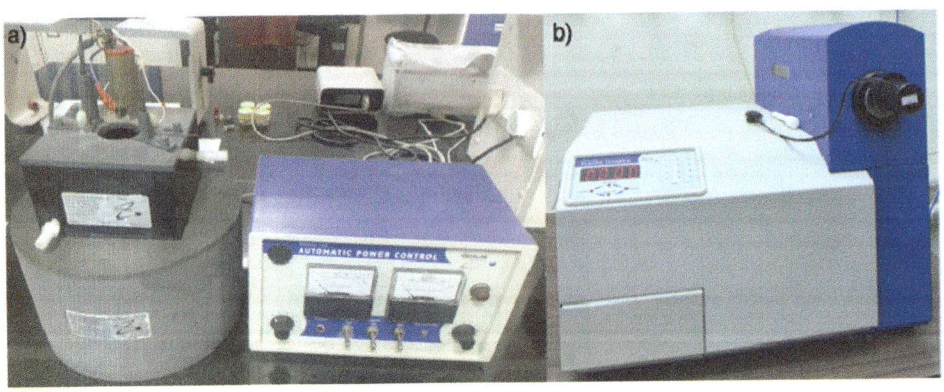

Fig. 10 **a** Automatic Twin-Jet Electropolisher; **b** Plasma cleaner

scientific discoveries. From the past few years, Nanosciences and Advances Imaging Centre are operating as a central facilities with users from inside the institute as well as access to local industry and outside universities.We are the centre which evolved as expert base breaking through the current characterization limitations in nanotechnology, medicine, environmental science, energy materials, and beyond.

Acknowledgements We gratefully acknowledge IITK grant for establishing electron microscopy facilities and providing infrastructural and recurring support for maintenance of the facilities. All authors are specially thankful to Profs. Ashutosh Sharma and Sandeep Verma for their efforts in establishment of CNS and AIC facilities.

Notes and References

Williams DB, Carter CB (1996) Transmission electron microscopy: a textbook for materials science. Plenum Press, New York

Zhou W, Wang ZL (eds) (2006) Scanning microscopy for nanotechnology. Springer, New York

Barman AK, Verma S (2010) Chem Commun 46:6992–6994

Naqvi TK, Srivastava AK, Kulkarni MM, Siddiqui AM, Dwivedi PK (2019) Silver nanoparticles decorated reduced graphene oxide (rGO) SERS sensor for multiple analytes. Appl Surf Sci 478:887–895

Saravanan RK, Naqvi TK, Patil S, Dwivedi PK, Verma S (2020) Purine-blended nanofiber woven flexible nanomats for SERS-based analyte detection. Chem Commun (Camb) 56(43):5795–5798

In-Situ Transmission Electron Microscopy Investigation of Phase Transformation Behavior of Alloy Nanoparticles

Khushubo Tiwari and Krishanu Biswas

1 Introduction

In every basic nanoscale science, research and commercial production of nanotechnologies entirely rely upon the potential of instruments and methodologies to determine, fabricate, sensitize, and manipulate the system at the nanoscale. Over the past decades, microscopy has gained advantages as compared to other characterization tools. Since it is more descriptive, the producing micrographs of objects that are directly associated to their morphology, shape, structure, and composition and thus it reveals spatial heterogeneities (Sinclair 2013). Recently, high-resolution transmission electron microscopy (TEM) is routinely utilized to acquired lattice high-resolution images of nanocrystalline materials through conventional TEM optics. However, in recent times, the state of the art has to turn to the sub-Angstroms high-resolution imaging and investigation attained using the images or examine aberration-corrected TEM instrument (Urban 2009; Krivanek et al. 2010).

Observing the physical process 'on-site' as they are arising and under many external stimuli is the dominant goal of the *in-situ* time-resolved technique. *In-situ* transmission electron microscopy (TEM) recently has drawn extraordinary attention from several fields ranging from chemistry, biology, and material science (Dehm et al. 2012; Banhart 2008). Since *in-situ* TEM is an essential and powerful tool for the nanomaterial depiction, it provides significant opportunities to probe the dynamic change in chemical composition, size, shape, and interface structure of nanoscale materials. At present, it is possible to acquire images at the atomic scale of materials in real time under several external stimuli to assessing relevant properties. Different kinds of *in-situ* TEM holders have been developed with the potential of capturing images and measurements under stress, optical excitation, heat, magnetic, and electric fields (Zewail 2010; Butler and Hale 1981).

Further, the advancement of environmental cells permits an investigation to be performed in different liquid and gaseous environments (Boyes and Gai 1997). Besides, the processing system and data acquisition improved temporal resolution and are capable of handling extensive data set generation. In the recent time, the motivation of *in-situ* TEM is to match scientific challenges, e.g., explaining synthesis route, nanoscale property, chemical activity measurement of nanoparticle, and mechanism of atomic scale failure; all these lead to the establishment of more explicit fabrication/synthesis–structure relationship properties (as shown in Fig. 1).

In this present article, we will illustrate some of the interpretation and understanding that has been attained by examples depicted from our work and experimental investigations of nanoalloy materials.

2 *In-Situ* TEM Instrumentation and Operation

In the past few years, various developments and modifications have been carried out in the dedicated design of electron microscopy columns. The vast advancement of auxiliary attachments, for example, stages, *in-situ* reaction process. At present, accessories and instruments for *in-situ* microscopy are not limited only for laboratory-made purposes but also crucial in commercially available. In this part of the section, a brief review of the modern or advance instrumentation for *in-situ* TEM will be discussed.

Typically, the microscope and specimen requirement for performing *in-situ* TEM or STEM (Scanning Transmission Electron Microscopy) experiments rarely not different from conventional TEM of STEM operation. Only the significant change is in the ability to employ external conditions and a few methods of analyzing as well as recording the resulting

K. Tiwari · K. Biswas (✉)
Department of Material Science and Engineering, Indian Institute of Technology, Kanpur, 208016, India
e-mail: kbiswas@iitk.ac.in

K. Biswas et al. (eds.), *Electron Microscopy in Science and Engineering*, IITK Directions 6,
https://doi.org/10.1007/978-981-16-5101-4_8

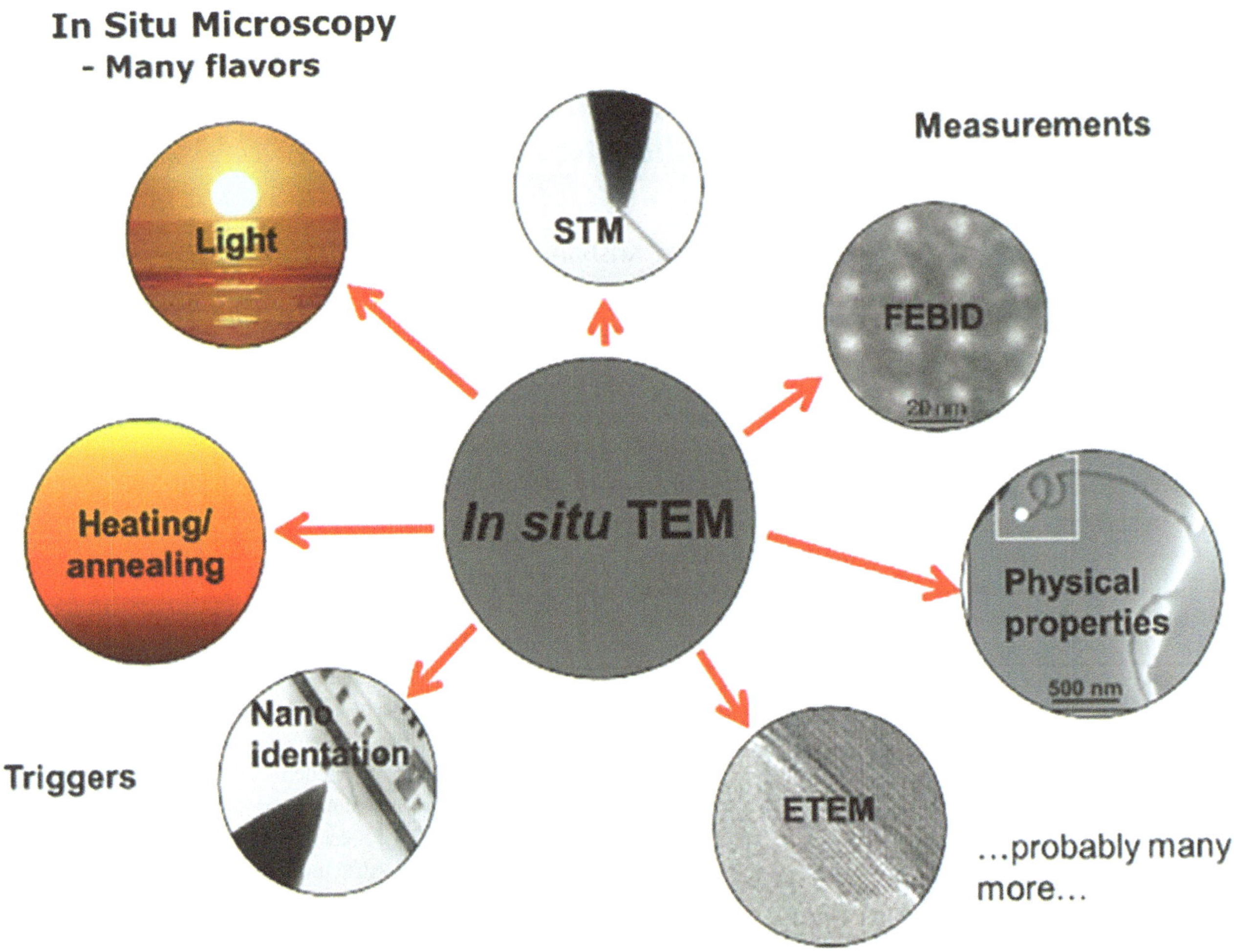

Fig. 1 External stimuli currently used for *in-situ* observations on TEM platform (Sinclair 2013)

dynamic reactions. Nowadays, the majority of the TEM systems are connected with charge-coupled devices (CCDs), which can function at ultrafast rates and with the television (TV) rate cameras. These attachments can record images within tens of milliseconds. Few significant drawbacks have been observed while recording images like considerable drift, tilting, and bending of the specimen. Thus, it is utmost to optimize the stability of the sample, stage, holder, and electron optics to the most satisfaction of our ability. These limitations can be reduced by recording images at ultrafast acquisition rates as inside the ultrafast electron microscope (UFEM). The operation and various examples of employing UFEM, including many benefits of using aberration-corrected TEM optics, for exploring nano-millisecond dynamics of many experiments have already been described and reviewed in the literature (LaGrange et al. 2008; Zewail and Thomas 2010). It is worth mentioning that this technique establishes an exciting opportunity of studying reactions and transformations that occur at the femtosecond time scale.

2.1 *In-Situ* Stages and Holders

In recent years, custom-made stages or modified sample arm has received a lot of attention due to the possibility to change materials by utilizing external influences inside the TEM (Han et al. 2007; Chen and Peng 2011). There are several types of TEM sample holders' ability of heating/cooling, specimen arms, evaporation/deposition of materials, and straining and lasing that are commonly available commercially or easily can be manufactured without much problem in the laboratory. In this section, we will briefly only discuss two modes of operations we widely used for our investigation.

I. ***Heating Stages:*** Many phenomena such as transformation or reactions such as recrystallization, growth, and phase transformation in materials occur at increasing temperature. *In-situ* heating holders for TEM are generally incorporated of the specimen arm and employ accurate Joule heating and heat dissipation

to acquire stable and tuneable samples at elevated temperatures. Gatan has manufactured the *in-situ* heating holder employed at IIT Kanpur with model number 652. This holder can be used up to a temperature of 1000 °C in the Tantalum furnace. The specimen is secured inside the holder using a beryllium hex ring mechanism and can be tilted up to $\alpha = \pm 45°$ and $\beta = \pm 30°$. The mechanical link between the heater and the stage of this model is made of a material with a near-zero coefficient of expansion to minimize thermal drift. Moreover, the temperature at the specimen holder tip is maintained near the heat of the specimen stage using a water-cooled specimen rod, thereby allowing for the least thermal loss. Figure 2 shows a schematic diagram of a Gatan single tilt heating holder that can adapt a 3-mm disk sample and can go 1000 °C while using a Tantalum furnace (https://www.gatan.com/products/tem-specimen-holders/heating-situ-holders; Idrees 2013).To perform high-resolution imaging at high temperatures, it is substantial to obtain stability at high temperatures and extremely low specimen drift. But these factors are difficult to attain due to a large specimen stage that has large thermal mass and thus contribute to gradual temperature response. To overcome these issues, the micro-fabricated heating holder has been assembled and is commercially available by DENs solution (https://www.denssolutions.com/en/our-products/sample-heat-ing-systems) and Protochips Inc. (http://www.protochips.com/products/aduro.html). Figure 3 shows the photograph of the *in-situ* heating holder of the Gatan model no. 652 available at the advance imaging center of IIT Kanpur. In these particular holders, integrated circuitry is commonly used to develop localized resistive heating instantly on the specimen support. These stages depict very low thermal mass and extremely high thermal stability that permits high-resolution imaging at high temperatures.

II. ***Cooling Stages:*** TEM cooling holders are used for applications which necessitate low-temperature observations of *in-situ* phase transformations and to reduce contamination due to carbon migration. They can also be used to reduce unwanted thermal effects in various analytical techniques such as energy-dispersive X-ray spectroscopy (EDS) by reducing contamination and mass loss. Typically, such holders are cooled via a well-insulated, bubble-free cryogen dewar. The high mechanical stability of the dewar helps to minimize drift during use. Precise temperature control of the specimen is achieved through a conductor rod connecting the specimen holder to the cryogen dewar, which contains an electric heater to control the specimen temperature. The temperature of the holder is monitored by a calibrated silicon diode that provides a sensitive response for precise temperature control of the specimen. The holder also provides a robust mechanism for tilting the sample with the β-tilt maximum of ± 30°. Figure 4 presents the photograph of the *in-situ* cooling stage (Gatan Inc.) available at IIT Kanpur for investigation.

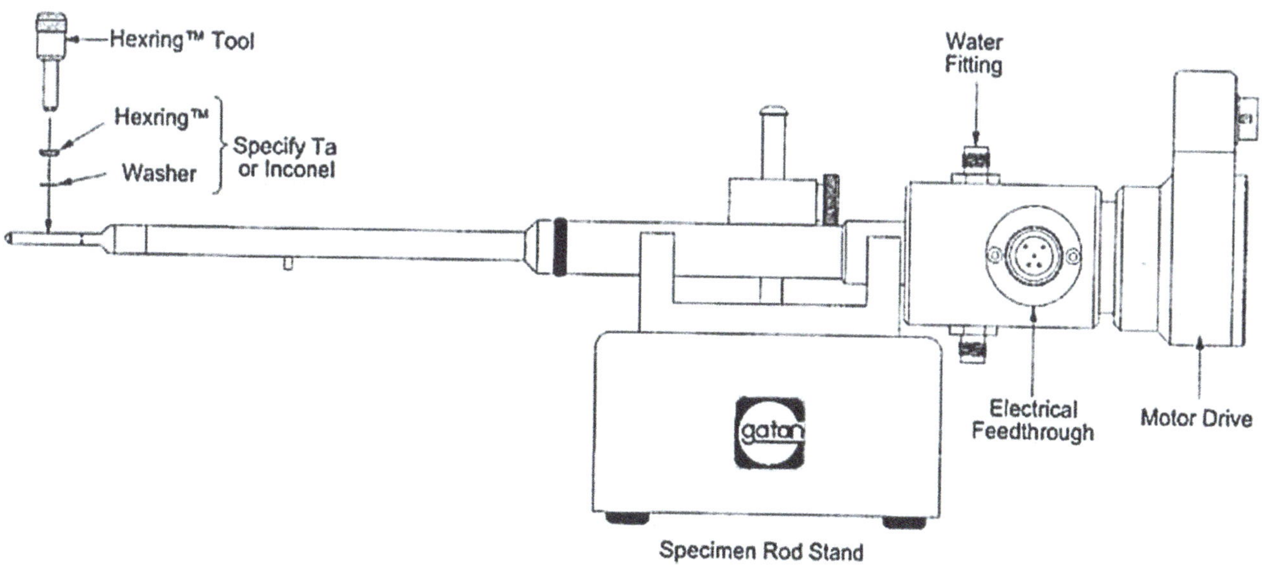

Fig. 2 Schematic figure of the Gatan single tilt heating holder (https://www.gatan.com/products/tem-specimen-holders/heating-situ-holders)

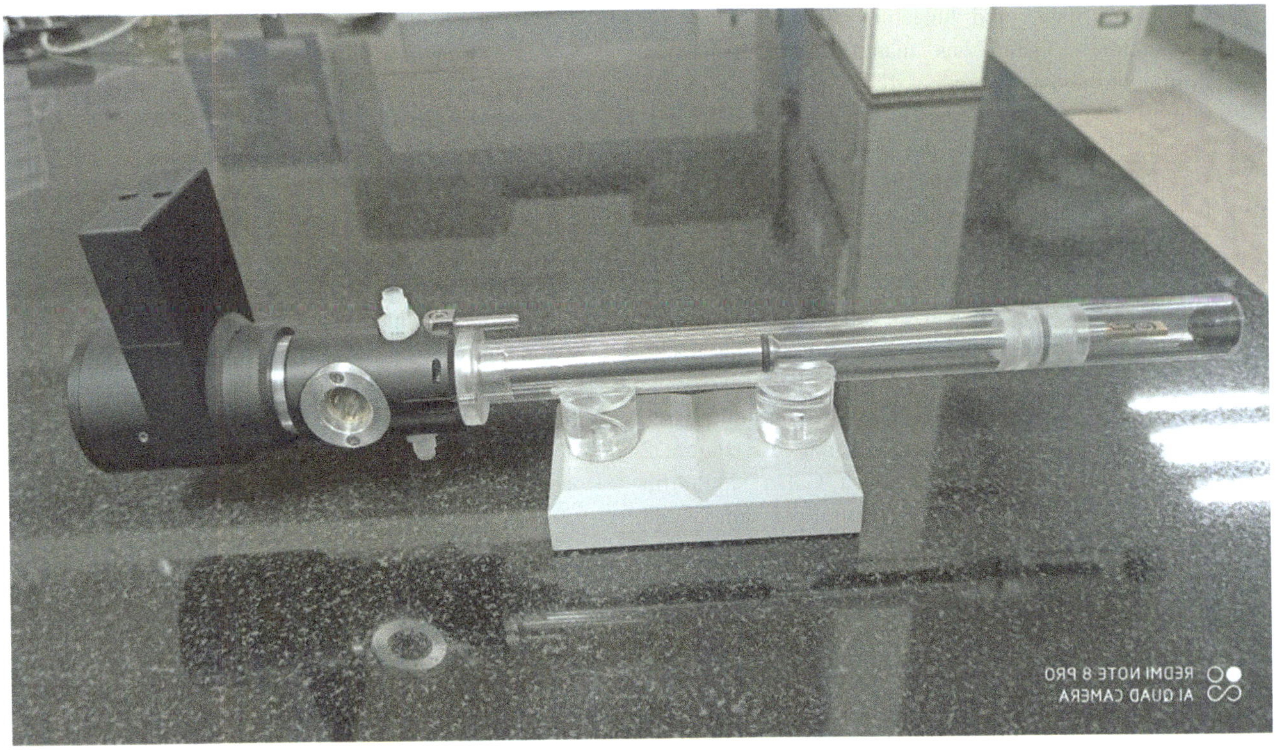

Fig. 3 Photograph of the *in-situ* heating holder of the Gatan model no. 652 available at advance imaging centre of IIT K

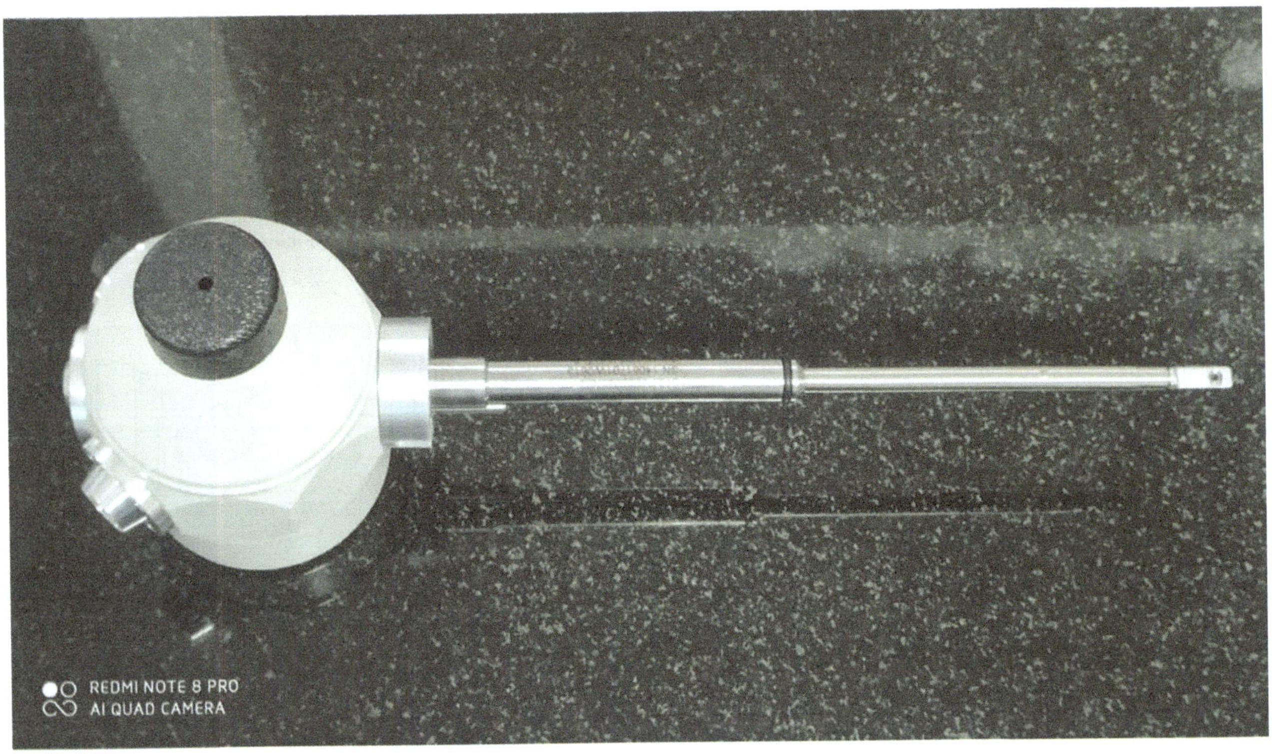

Fig. 4 Photograph of the *in-situ* cooling holder (Gatan Inc.) available at advance imaging centre of IIT K

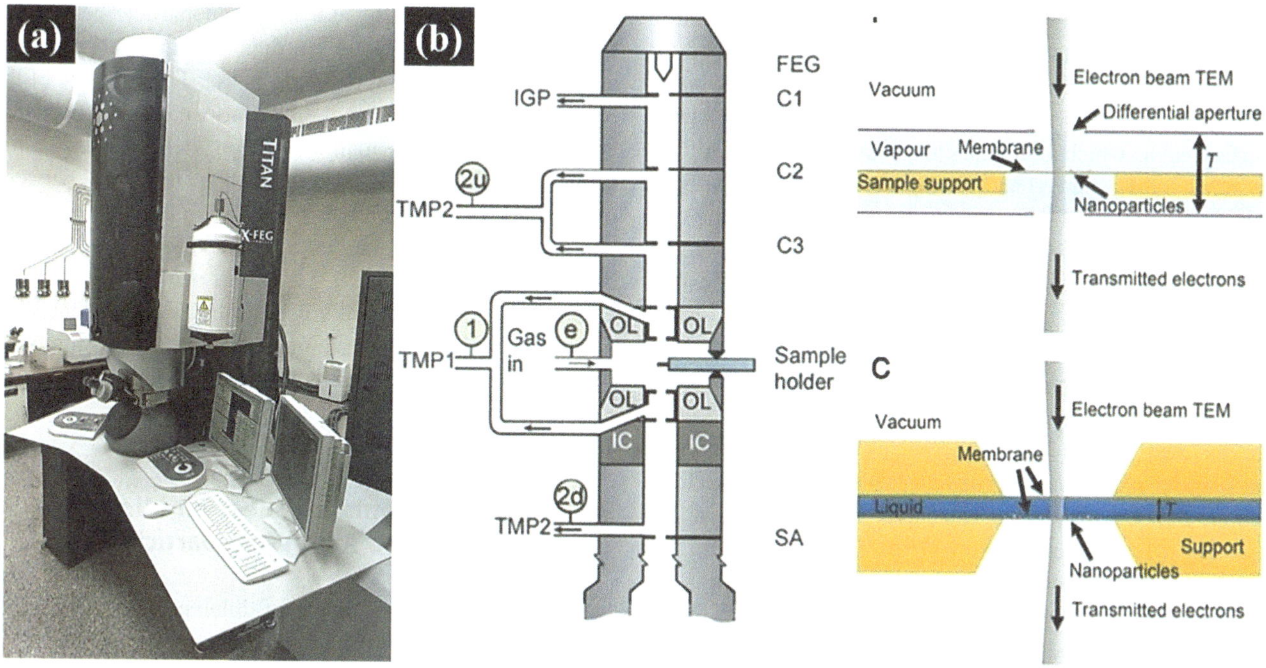

Fig. 5 **a** Photograph of FEI Titan 80–300 field emission scanning transmission electron microscope (**b**). **a** A diagram of a typical in-situ TEM with a differential pumping system, indicating the ultra-HV system, the pressure-limiting apertures and two sets of the differential pumping systems (He et al. 2020)

2.2 Advanced Transmission Electron Microscopy

The FEI Titan 80–300 STEM is an advanced analytical field emission scanning transmission electron microscope competent of atomic-level imaging and analysis on a wide range of materials and nanostructures (as shown in Fig. 5a–b) (He et al. 2020). The Titan is equipped with an electron energy loss spectrometer and X-ray energy-dispersive spectrometer for elemental and chemical analysis of materials at high spatial resolution. The microscope system comprises a scanning module and a high-angle annular dark-field detector for scanning transmission electron microscopy (STEM) and chemical analysis of minimal quantities. Aberration-corrected STEM/TEM is proficient at producing images with 0.07 nm resolution with Cs correction. It is equipped with a high-brightness Schottky field emission electron source with a high maximum beam current (>100 mA), a high-resolution Gatan imaging filter (GIF) Tridiem energy filter, and with third-order spectrometer aberration correctors. The imaging aberration corrector can entirely correct for coherent axial aberrations up to third order and partially compensates for fourth- and fifth-order aberrations. The microscope has two 2048 × 2048 slow-scan CCD cameras; one is bottom-mounted, and one is the GIF camera. The maximum tilt angle for the STEM with a double-tilt holder is ± 40°, whereas the maximum tilt angle with tomography holder is ± 80°.

3 Phase Transformations in Nanostructured Materials Using *In-Situ* Electron Microscopy

Nanotechnology has become a rapidly emerging field in recent times. Nanomaterials often show an effective and drastic change in physical, chemical, mechanical, electronic properties as compared to their bulk counterparts (Calvo 2013). The most typical characteristic observed in nanosized materials is the size dependence of several properties, including electrical, catalytic, magnetic, thermal, and optical (Jellinek 2008; Ferrando et al. 2008). It reveals that these properties strongly depend on grain size or crystallite size. Therefore, extraordinary and novel properties showed by the nanomaterials have attracted the researchers. From the last two decades, nanoalloys have developed as a unique field to enhance the properties of the materials. In general, nanoalloys are commonly referred to as multimetallic nanoparticles, without chemical ordering inside the alloy (Calvo 2015). Considerable researches have been reported in the literature based on the various properties and structural complexity originating due to shape, size, and composition effects (Calvo 2015; Ferrando 2016). The principle of phase transformation of nanoalloys necessitates being investigated to comprehend the size-dependent effect in the properties of nanoalloys, e.g., melting temperature, the thermal stability of different phases, alloying at the nanosized particle, order–

disorder transformation, etc. These nanomaterials can be in the form of free-standing (without matrix) or embedded (encapsulated in the matrix) nanoparticles. In free-standing nanoparticle, the surface energy is created due to the large surface area, which dominates the total free energy of the system. On the other hand, in the embedded nanoparticle, the additional interfacial energy is created due to the formation of an interface between particle and matrix. This interfacial energy can be altered by embedding the nanosized particle in different matrices (Chattopadhyay and Bhattacharya 2004; 2003).

From the last two decades, the phase transformation study of pure metal nanoparticles embedded in amorphous, crystalline, and quasicrystalline matrices has been extensively investigated (Mei and Lu 2007; Chattopadhyay and Goswami 1997). From these extensive studies led to a fair understanding of the phase transformation (i.e., melting and solidification) behavior and morphological evolution of nanoparticle embedded in various matrices. The alloy nanoparticles can be further classified based on their morphology into two distinct categories: single and multiphase alloy nanoparticles (shown in Fig. 6). In the case of multiphase nanoalloy particle forms, additional interfaces between phases exhibit in the alloy nanoparticle as compared to the single-phase nanoalloy particle and pure metal nanoparticle (Chattopadhyay and Bhattacharya 2004). Biphasic alloy nanoparticle comprises two different phases, and triphasic alloy can have three distinct phases (shown in Fig. 6 with a research example). The existence of an additional interface constitutes between phases that are the same for both the free and embedded alloy nanoparticles. Interfacial energy comprises both chemical and structural contributions.

From the last two decades, extensive researches have been carried out on the phase transformation of single-phase nanoalloys (Khan and Biswas 2015; Siem* and Johnson 2005). Recently, multiphase alloy nanoparticle has gained tremendous attention due to their distinct properties as compared to pure metal or single phase. The majority of the research work focused on multiphase nanoalloy particles embedded in various matrixes. From these studies, it has been categorically indicated that the interface between matrix and nanoparticle plays a vital role in the melting behavior and thermal stability of nanoalloys (Chattopadhyay and Bhattacharya 2004, 2003,2009). It is also noted that the effect of matrix on the melting and solidification behavior of embedded nanoparticles cannot be decoupled. This limits the possibility of understanding the intrinsic phase transformation behavior of alloy nanoparticle.

3.1 *In-Situ* Transmission Electron Microscopy of Multiphase Alloy Nanoparticle

In this section, we will dwell on different aspects of phase transformation of multiphase nanoalloy particles. In particular, melting and solidification of free and embedded multiphase alloy nanoparticle will be discussed. In the following, we will discuss some of the investigations achieved from our research work carried out in our laboratory at IIT Kanpur.

3.2 Method and Materials

It is important to note that in general, the behavior is often shown by free nanoparticles are not same what observed in embedded nanoalloy particle. The properties altogether depend on the methodology that has been utilized to prepare the nanomaterials. In the following section, we will first briefly discuss the synthesis route of nanoparticle.

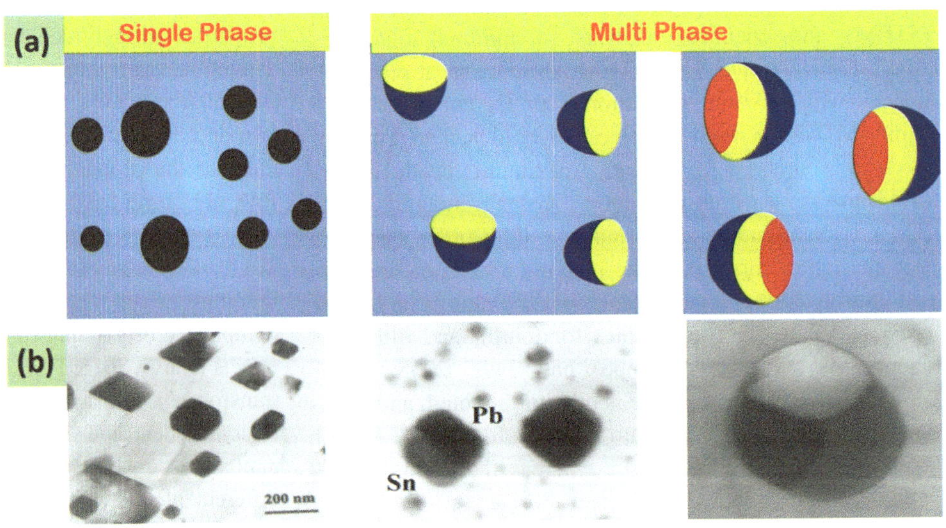

Fig. 6 **a** Schematic representation of distinct categories of alloy nanoparticles: single and multiphase **b** the examples of each category from the research work

I. ***Synthesis of free alloy nanoparticles***

To synthesize the free alloy nanoparticle, several facile chemical synthesis routes have been adopted. The chemical route has been reported to be an effective route due to the controlled synthesis of the particle with desirable shape, size, and composition. Several routes have been employed to synthesize free nanoalloy particles. In this section, we will only discuss the most popular route in the trend for preparing these nanomaterials.

First is the solgel process; this route is widely used to synthesize free alloy nanoparticles. The solgel process has two approaches: hydrolysis and condensation. This process is initiated with the formation of a concentrated mixture containing hydroxide or metallic oxide by hydrolysis (Jones 1990; Brinker and Scherer 2013). The next route is micro-emulsion method or reverses micellar route; in this route, hydrophilic head and hydrophobic tailor of the surfactant are conducted inward and outward, which ensues into the formation of the internal core holding water (Garcia Esparza 2011). Therefore, reverse micelle is regarded to be the nanoreactors because the reaction occurs in its inner core. In addition to this route, the solvothermal or hydrothermal method is very commonly used for preparing free nanoparticle. The fundamental principle of this route is that when the solvent is heated in a closed vessel, the temperature increases much above the ideal boiling point, which further leads to self-generated pressure exceeding higher than the ambient pressure, and this raises the boiling point of the solvent much above the vital temperature and pressure. Later, the solvent behaves like a supercritical liquid (Byrappa and Adschiri 2007).

II. ***Synthesis of nanoembedded particles***

In recent times, the most popular synthesis route for preparing embedded nanoparticle is melt spinning (rapid solidification route) and ion implantation. These processes are very competent when the embedded nanoparticle makes the immiscible system with the matrix. Rapid solidification is associated with a distinctive cooling rate of the order of 10^6K/s, in which the cooling rate is attained by a conductive heat transfer process (Suryanarayana 1991). On rapid cooling a melt by an immiscible realm, the liquid phase separates and makes an emulsion of clear liquids. Later on, the significant fraction of melts solidifies as the matrix, thereby developing a distribution of small packet liquid particle dispersed in the matrix. Eventually, the liquid particles get solidified to provide final nanomaterials, whereas, in the case ion implantation process, high-energy ions generate the energy contributed to local altering or disordering of the matrix of the materials (Ziegler 2012). This process encounters in the solid state and is substantially dominated by the crystal orientation of the matrix. Therefore, it often observes an epitaxial orientation relationship between the matrix and nanoparticles. Further, the mechanical alloying route is also utilized for the formation of nanoembedded particles, which includes breaking down both embedded nanoparticle and matrix by continuous fracturing and re-welding process in the solid state (Suryanarayana 2001).

3.3 Results and Discussion

In the following section, the experimental results on several alloy systems will be deliberated and discussed. Primary interest will be given to the melting of the alloy nanoparticles. We will start presenting with the melting behavior of free nanoalloy, followed by the embedded nanoparticle.

In order to understand the intrinsic melting behavior of an alloy nanoparticle, the nanoalloy should not be confined by matrix; i.e., the nanoparticle needs to be free surfaces. In this respect, some studies have been carried out on free single and multiphase nanoalloy particles (Khan and Biswas 2015; Bhattacharya and Chattopadhyay 2007; Johnson et al. 2000; Khan et al. 2015). Recently, we have attempted an effort to investigate the size effect on the melting behavior of the multiphase Pb-Sb alloy nanoparticle by extensive use of *in-situ* TEM. From the equilibrium phase diagram, the binary system Pb-Sb shows a two-terminal solid solution of FCC (Pb) and rhombohedral (Sb) and exhibits eutectic reaction at the temperature of 251.4 °C for the composition of Pb-17.5 at.%Sb (Massalski 1992). The composition was chosen for study the multiphase free alloy nanoparticle was Pb-17.5 at.%Sb. Free nanoalloy particles were synthesized by the solvothermal route (Devi and Biswas 2015; Devi et al. 2019). During *in-situ* studies, a sequence of video of the heating experiment was recorded and further analyzed to acquire the melting behavior of individual nanoalloy particles. Thermocouple made up of a Chromel–Alumel was attached to the specimen holder to record the temperature, and the temperature was calibrated (± 2 °C). Figure 7 indicates the heating sequence of the two-phase alloy nanoparticle. Up to the temperature of 234 °C, no considerable change in the shape of nanoparticle has been observed, whereas the relative area fractions and their facets of phases present in the nanoparticle undergo alteration while heating. As the temperature rises and reaches 239 °C, an abrupt change appeared at the triple junction of the outer surface and interface between (Pb)/(Sb), which suggests the initiation of melting. The onset melting temperature of Pb-Sb alloy nanoparticle (239 °C) is lower (13.5 °C) than the

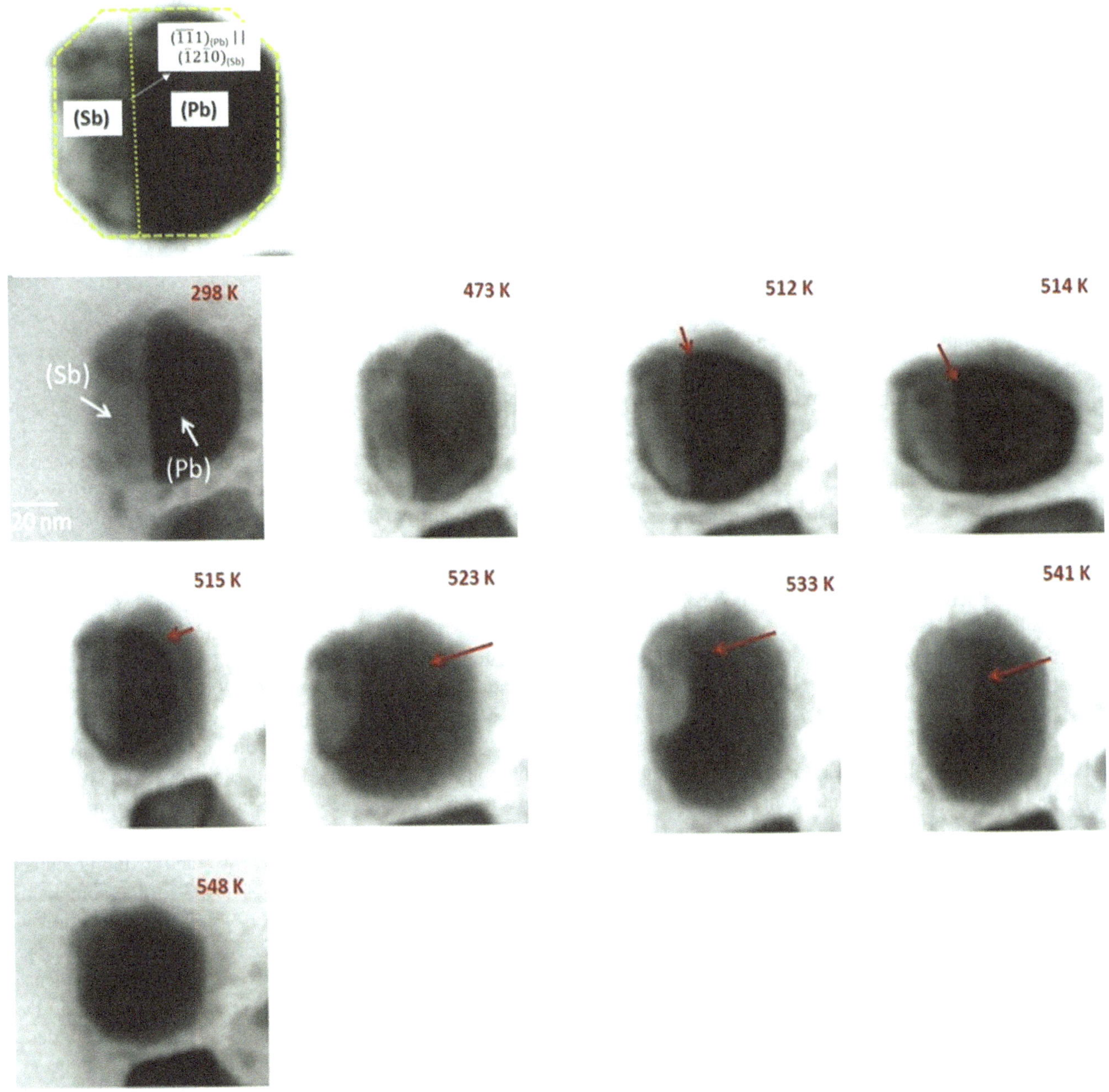

Fig. 7 A series of TEM micrographs showing melting within a Pb-Sb nanoparticle during the in situ heating experiment (Devi et al. 2019)

equilibrium eutectic temperature (252 °C). As the temperature rises further, initially, the liquid front spread along the (Pb) surface boundary instead of spreading along with the interface between (Sb)/(Pb). At the temperature of 250 °C, the (Pb) phase entirely melts; subsequently, the liquid front propagates along (Sb) phase, and the whole nanoparticle became molten (at 275 °C).

As we have stated earlier, the embedded nanoparticle can constitute multiple phases having different shapes and sizes, with a common interface. In the case of two-phase embedded nanoparticle, they comprise three interfaces: the interphase interface between two phases and interfaces among matrix and two phases of the nanoparticle. These interfacial energies have a key role in determining the phase transformation behavior of multiphase embedded nanoparticles. Therefore, it provides lots of opportunities to change the interface between the phases in the nanoalloy particle and matrix (Chattopadhyay and Bhattacharya 2004; Chattopadhyay 2005). In this regard, we have investigated to understand the phase transformation of multiphase embedded Pb–Sn nanoalloy particles *via* a melt spinning route. Earlier extensive investigations have been reported on

literature (Bhattacharya et al. 2002; Fecht and Perepezko 1989; Fecht et al. 1989; Johnson et al. 2001). Johnson et al. depicted the formation of a single phase of (Pb) solid solution before the melting of the nanoalloy particle embedded in the Al matrix prepared by ion implantation (Johnson et al. 2001). Subsequently, Bhattacharya et al. performed an *in-situ* heating experiment to probe the melting behavior of Pb–Sn (1:1) nanoparticle embedded in the Al matrix via melt spinning (Bhattacharya et al. 2002). Therefore, it shows some ambiguity in the understanding of the melting behavior of the Pb–Sn nanoalloy particle. Thus, to investigate the existence of exact melting behavior, an attempt has been made to carry out an in-depth investigation of $Pb_{26.1}Sn_{73.9}$nanoparticles embedded in two different matrices: Al (crystalline) and Al-Cu-Fe (quasicrystals) via melt spinning. While the presence of Pb–Sn nanoinclusions in the Aluminium matrix, synthesized through rapid solidification route, leads to the formation of two-phase nanoparticles consisting of (Pb) (FCC) and β-Sn (Tetragonal). Taking this into account, a detailed investigation has been carried out on the melting and solidification behavior of the Pb–Sn biphasic embedded alloy inclusions using *in-situ* TEM investigation tools. The subsequent discussion involves the phase transformation behavior of biphasic Pb–Sn alloy nanoparticles embedded in the crystalline (aluminum) and the quasicrystalline ($Al_{65}Cu_{20}Fe_{15}$) matrices. Particularly, $Pb_{26.1}Sn_{73.9}$ alloy undertakes eutectic solidification (L → Pb + β-Sn) through regular lamellar morphology at 183 °C. Detailed in-situ heating stage experiment has been performed inside the TEM column in both cases. The evolution of the melting event is depicted by a set of dark-field images (as shown in Fig. 8a–g). Preliminary heating (much below 171 °C) changes the area of the illuminated (Pb) phase. This shows that there is the tuning of the volume fraction of (Pb) and β-(Sn) phases in the nanoparticle as a function of the temperature. The assessment *via* the dark-field images indicates that the relative volume fraction of (Pb) declines as the temperature rises. However, Sn from (β-Sn) segment dissolves into the (Pb) segment at 171 °C. It can be clearly seen that the biphasic particle changes into metastable single-phase FCC (Pb) at the corresponding temperature followed by the melting of the particle at about 182 °C, which is almost the bulk melting temperature (183 °C) of the alloy particles. This is the first such clear indication showing transformation during an in-situ TEM study. The results of the in-situ cooling of an alloy nanoparticle embedded in the QC matrix from the liquid state are shown in Fig. 9b. The bright field micrograph of the biphasic particle is shown in Fig. 9a, showing β-(Sn) and (Pb) regions. The figure illustrates the completely molten state of the particle. The figure shows that a small portion of the particle has been solidified. In-depth diffraction experiment shows the solidified portion as FCC (Pb). At about 150 °C (Fig. 9d), complete solidification occurs for the particle into metastable FCC (Pb). Upon subsequent cooling while in the solid state, the metastable phase separates into (Pb) and (Sn) lamellae. The particle achieves a morphology similar to a eutectic particle consisting of FCC (Pb) and BCT β-(Sn) at room temperature.

Since multiphase embedded nanoalloys are noticeably different and complex in comparison with single-phase nanoalloys, the total Gibbs free energy increases due to the presence of additional interface within the nanoparticles. This sequentially can change the melting and alloying behavior of nanoparticles. Hence, an in-depth understanding of the thermal stability of the multiphase embedded nanoparticles is imperative. To investigate the thermal stability of the multiphasic nanoparticles, triphasic alloy nanoparticles have been selected. It becomes more cumbersome to understand the triphasic embedded alloy nanoparticles because of the presence of three distinct phases and a large number of interfaces between matrix and phases in addition to the internal interphase interface within the nanoparticles. Nevertheless, the embedded triphasic alloy nanoparticles offer the best possible scenario to understand the nanoscale alloying. Thus, to understand the melting behavior of triphasic nanoparticles, we have chosen Bi-In-Sn alloy nanoparticle embedded in the icosahedral quasicrystalline (IQC) matrix (Tiwari et al. 2020). The calculated phase diagram demonstrates the two invariant eutectic reactions E1 and E2 at the temperature of 76.08 and 58.73 °C, respectively. For the present investigation, a ternary eutectic reaction (E1) present in the bismuth-rich region of the phase diagram has been selected. The eutectic reaction is associated with the transformation of liquid to three solid phases; (Bi), BiIn, and (β-Sn). Triphasic $Bi_{44}In_{32}Sn_{23}$ nanoalloy embedded in IQC ($Al_{65}Cu_{20}Fe_{15}$) matrix was synthesized *via* the melt spinning route. An *in-situ* heating experiment has been performed inside the TEM column for a detailed investigation of the melting behavior of the nanoparticles. Figure 10a shows the sequence of the micrographs, revealing the melting of the nanoparticle. A set of bright field images depicts the progression of the melting event. Initially, the heating up to 40 °C shows no substantial change in the nanoparticle. At 45 °C, the transformation of (γ-Sn) to (β-Sn) and at 70 °C, the whole (γ-Sn) region completely transforms into (β-Sn). Concurrently, there is an initiation of melting at the triple junction of BiIn, (Bi), and IQC matrix. BiIn melts at 77 °C and melts transverse along with the interphase interface. As the temperature increases, the propagation of the melt front initiates along (β Sn), and the matrix interface and (Bi) phase melt abruptly once the temperature reaches 100 °C. The schematic illustration of the melting of triphasic Bi-In-Sn embedded nanoparticle is shown in Fig. 10b.

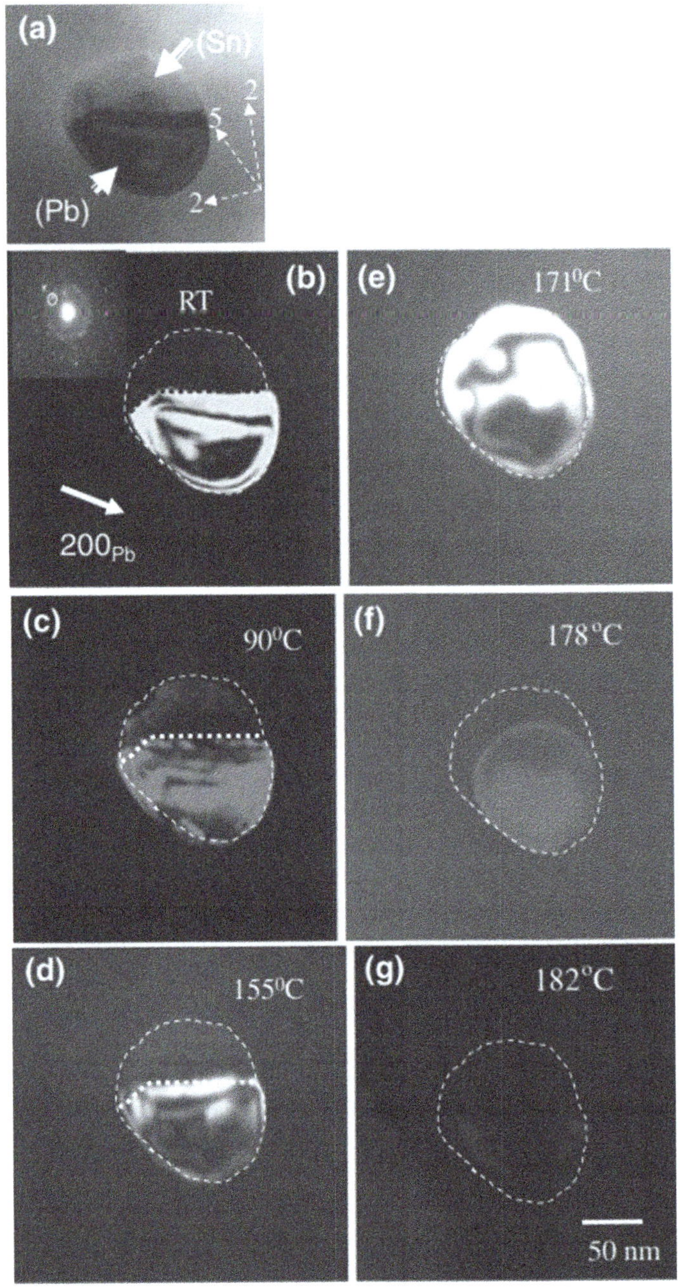

Fig. 8 Dark-field images obtained using in situ melting TEM study of **a** Pb–Sn eutectic biphasic particle within a matrix grain: a bright field micrograph; **b** RT; **c** 90 °C; **d** 157 °C; **e** 171 °C; **f** 178 °C and **g** 182 °C (Tiwari et al. 2020)

4 Other Kind of *In-Situ* Holder and Their Applications

I. **Environmental *In-situ* TEM**

A conventional TEM requires a high vacuum (order of 10^{-6} tor or higher) inside the specimen chamber to yield the operation of electron source as well as to minimize scattering apart from the sample (Boyes and Gai 1997; Gai et al. 2008), whereas various processes with primary importance in material science, for example, catalytic reactions or crystal growth, are participating in high gas pressure or atmospheric pressures. A detailed characterization procedure for understanding the kinetics of these processes by electron microscopy is to sample, *ex-situ* at various reaction times. On the other hand, accurate dynamics information of the complete transformation during, such as gas-phase catalytic process or vapor–liquid–solid growth is merely possible to acquire by carrying out *in-situ* reaction inside the TEM. Thus, the further led to the development of dedicated TEM and a representing technique known as environmental electron microscopy (Boyes and Gai 1997; Gai et al. 2008).

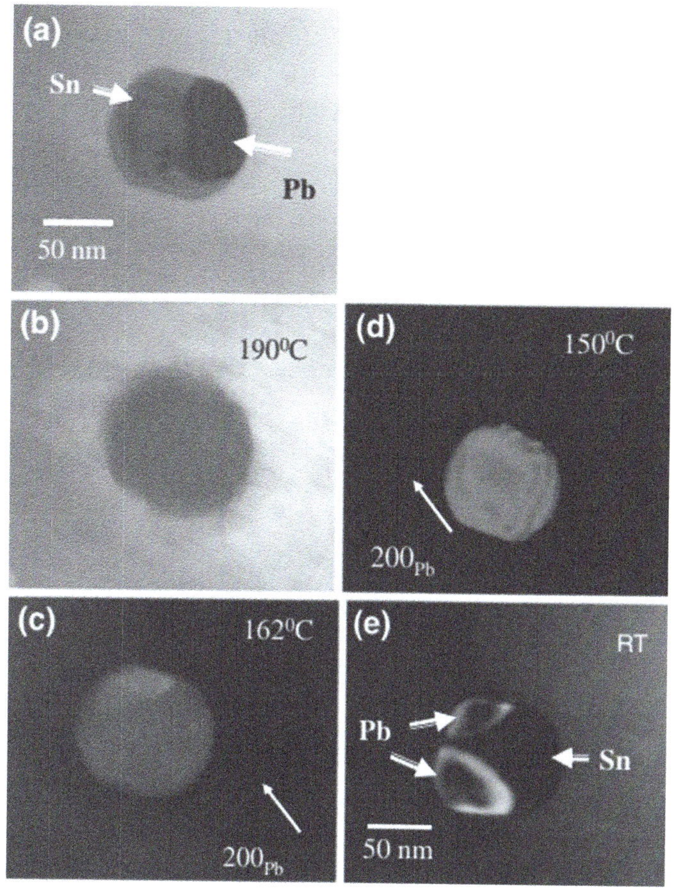

Fig. 9 **a** Bright-field image of the biphasic particle at room temperature; **b** at 190 °C, Dark-field images obtained using in situ TEM study of the biphasic particle within a matrix grain: **c** 162 °C; **d** 150 °C and **e** room temperature (Tiwari et al. 2020)

High-resolution environmental electron microscopy was developed in 1997 by Boyes and Gai (1997), which was built by few modifications of the electron chamber of a company Philips CM30 electron microscopy (Gai et al. 1995). Figure 11 shows the schematic representation of environmental electron microscopy setup. In the environmental TEM setup, differential pumping is attached by turbomolecular pumps (TMOs) or molecular drag pumps (MDPs) among the apertures. Subsequently, Hitachi (https://hitachi-hta.com/products/electron-ion-and-probe-microscopy/transmission-electron-microscopes/h-9500-300kv-te), FEI (https://www.fei.com/products/transmission-electron-micro-scopes/titan/etem.aspx), and JEOL (https://www.jeolusa.com/PRODUCTS/Transmission-Electron-Microscopes-TEM/Analytical-Data-Optimization/Practical-Remote-In-Situ-Microscopy-PRISM) all developed customized environmental TEM equipment based on the same approach. Despite the fact that these TEMs are more costly than the conventional electron microscopy, these instruments are going more accessible to the scientific community as well as acquiring many attentions and popularities. Most importantly, when environmental TEM module is attached to an aberration-corrected optics, instruments develop extremely powerful in probing any transformation behavior at very high resolution, underneath varying gas atmosphere and high temperature. The greater advantage of having aberration-corrected optics is in the potential to acquire high atomic resolution images in a single exposure (Gai et al. 2010). Recently, a method has been developed where gas is introduced around the sample through a gas injection nozzle, which is equipped on a sample heating holder. In this modified assembly, other components like objective lens pole pieces, specimen chamber, and the vacuum system are remained unaltered. These electron microscopies are relatively less complicated and expensive, which permits imaging of gas *in-situ* processes at an atomic resolution at room temperature (RT).

II. **Electrical Holders**

Electrical transport measurements of single or array of 1D nanostructures are generally determine by employing electrical probing stations with subsequently developing interaction *via* electron or optical beam lithography (Gai et al. 2008). Nowadays, TEM has improved and developed in terms of electrical

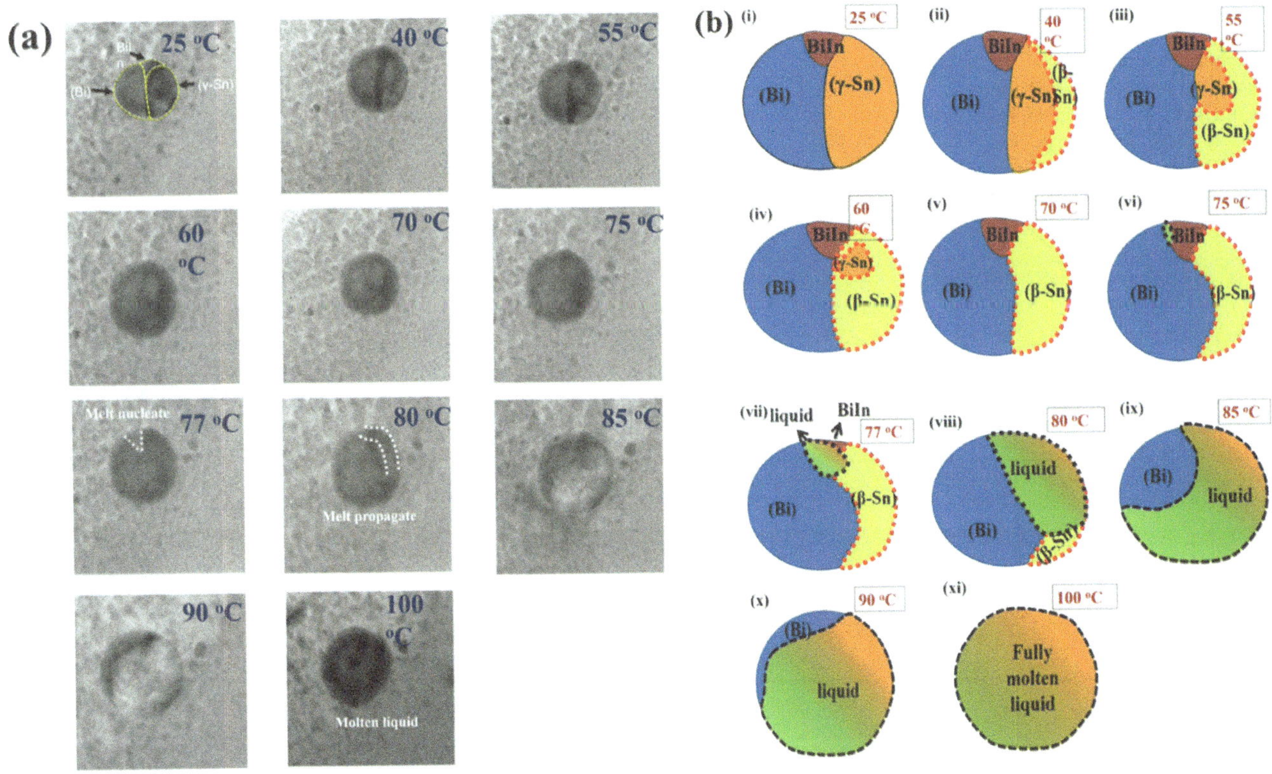

Fig. 10 **a** A series of bright field micrographs showing the melting sequence of tri-phasic Nanoparticles in IQC matrix at different temperature; **b** (i–xi) Schematic illustration of the melting process of tri-phasic Bi-In-Sn alloy Nanoparticles (Gai et al. 2008)

transport measurements. Several suppliers are available in the market, such as Gatan, Hummingbird, Ab, and Nanofactory Instruments. Generally, there are two types of the electrical holder, first, with integrated circuitry for adjoining micro-fabricated chips. This approach utilizes prefabricated circuitry prepared by lithography on Si chips comprising thin silicon nitride membranes. Few more forms of TEM holders are commercially available from Nanofactory Instruments AB using micro-fabricated circuitry. Second is with piezo-driven nanoprobe contact. In this approach, there is a large investment for buying a completely dedicated piezo-driven stage. However, both types of holders are equally important, and they can also be utilized for the selective heating experiment of nanoscale materials (Mølhave et al. 2006).

III. **Mechanical Stages**

These kinds of stages are specifically used for atomic force microscopy (AFM) and nanoindentation techniques. They are commonly utilized to probe the mechanical properties of nanomaterials. In this technique, it uses fine tips (probes) interacting with the specimen surface. However this tip/specimen interaction does not provide any visualized independently except inferred only. These are based on two general approaches: (a) micro-fabricated microelectromechanical system (MEMS) that are equipped inside TEM sample arm (Peng et al. 2008) and (b) assigned nanoindentation holder including piezo-driven probes incorporated with the specimen arm (Tang et al. 2012). In this, the load is employed using a thermal actuator on one end of the free-standing sample and is determined on the other end, utilizing a differential capacitive load sensor. Similarly, in electrical probing, AFM or piezo-driven nanoindenter specimen holders are frequently employed to investigate the mechanical properties of growth of nanowires (Zhu and Espinosa 2005).

IV. **Liquid Cells**

It remained a challenge for decades for the microscopy community to observe a liquid sample under an electron microscope due to lots of problems in sustaining a large volume of the liquid sample inside the electron column (Ruska 1942). From the last decade, 'liquid cells' design has overcome all the limitations for high-resolution electron microscopy (Williamson et al. 2003). This gained immediate attention in the bio and life sciences community at the same time it opened the vast possibility in the material science

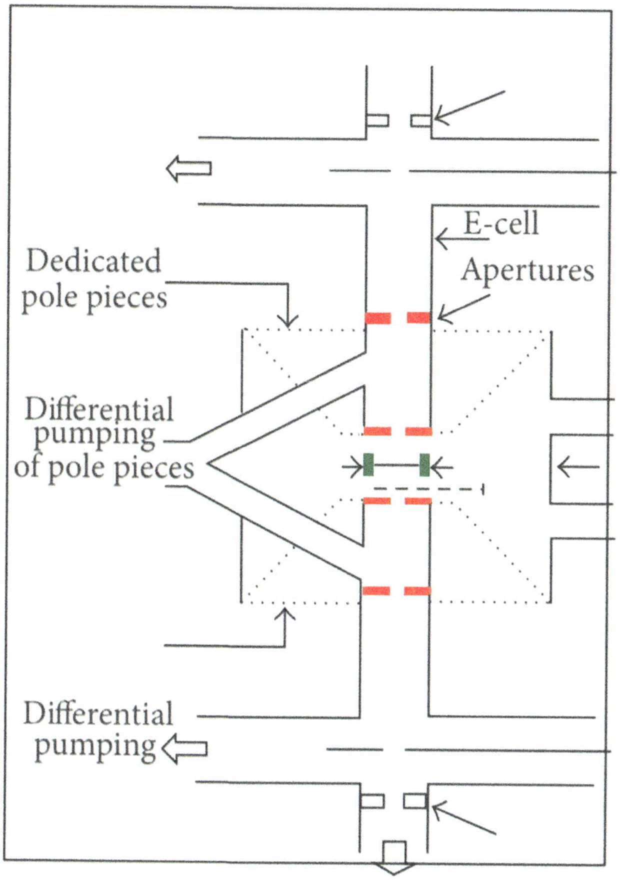

Fig. 11 Schematics of environmental TEM set-up featuring differential pumping, dedicated apertures, and pole piece, 1997 adapted from Boyes and Gai (1997)

community. The liquid cell setup is remarkably distinct from the environmental *in-situ* electron microscopy in that it has the potential to support stable and thin liquid layers. The design of liquid cell shows a hermetically completely sealed that confines the liquid into a layer of micrometer thick inside the thin electron transparent window. The electron transparent window is prepared by silica or silicon nitride (Grogan et al. 2011). Recently, an approach has been developed using single-layered graphene sheets to hold small pockets of liquid. The significant advantage of this method is that due to very less electron scattering volume as compared to silicon nitride or silica-based liquid cell, it contributes to good lattice resolution imaging.

V. **Lasers and Ion Beam Irradiation**

In general, laser or ion sources are integrated part of the electron column of scanning electron microscopy (SEM) because of large specimen column. At present, all the important producers of microscopes have systems named MultiBeam (JEOL), Crossbeam (Carl Zeiss), and Dual Beam (FEI) that support SEM and focus ion beam (FIB) has the ability to do on a single platform. However, ion beam capabilities for electron microscopy can be prepared on custom-built systems. Few laboratories persuade ion beam setups such as France, UK, USA, and Japan. Minimal studies have been dedicated by *in-situ* TEM ion beam systems on nanomaterial study. Laser sources are incorporated with an electron microscope, and this can be utilized to generate heat and activate reactions inside the specimen. On the other hand, such a design is commercially not available yet. In a general system, the TEM column is modified to equip with the laser beam facilities. Typically, the laser first allows to triggering a reaction or employing definite stimuli within the specimen, while in second it is used to assure the emission of the electron source. Nowadays, an alternative and more cost-effective route has been developed by using inexpensive micro-fabricated light sources or optical fibers and attached with the electron microscopy specimen arm (http://www.nanofactory.com/news.asp?id=59&type=news).

5 Conclusion

In-situ transmission electron microscopy (TEM) has become a prominent tool for materials characterization. It provides an important fact on the structural dynamics of a nanomaterial during phase transformations and further ability to relate a material's properties and structure. *In-situ* microscopy is anticipated to continue to impact the wide range of fields of sciences and technology, allowing for a deeper understanding of nanoalloy materials dynamics and function as well as an in-depth examination of real-time conditions. These nanomaterials can theoretically exhibit novel properties and thus have immense technological implications. The comprehension of the stability and phase transformation of such particles is central to designing alloys for potential future applications.

Acknowledgements KT and KB would like to thank Advanced Imaging Centre (AIC) at IIT Kanpur and office of Dean R&D for providing extended microscopic facilities.

References

Banhart F (2008) In-situ electron microscopy at high resolution. World Scientific

Bhattacharya V, Chattopadhyay K (2007) Mater Sci Eng A 449:1003–1008

Bhattacharya V, Bhattacharya P, Chattopadhyay K (2002) In: Materials science forum. Trans Tech Publ. pp 427–432

Boyes E, Gai P (1997) Ultramicroscopy 67:219–232

Brinker CJ, Scherer GW (2013) In: Sol-gel science: the physics and chemistry of sol-gel processing. Academic Press (2013)
Butler E, Hale K (1981) North-Holland 9:239
Byrappa K, Adschiri T (2007) Prog Cryst Growth Charact Mater 53:117–166
Calvo F (2013) Nanoalloys: from fundamentals to emergent applications. Newnes
Calvo F (2015) Phys Chem Chem Phys 17:27922–27939
Chattopadhyay K (2005) Trans Indian Inst Met 58:1057–1067
Chattopadhyay K, Bhattacharya P (2003) Materials research: current scenario and future projections. vol 130
Chattopadhyay K, Bhattacharya V (2004) Embedded metal and alloy nanoparticles. In: Encyclopedia of nanoscience and nanotechnology. American Scientific Publishers, pp 217–232
Chattopadhyay K, Bhattacharya V (2009) J Indian Instit Sci 89
Chattopadhyay K, Goswami R (1997) Prog Mater Sci 42:287–300
Chen Q, Peng L-M (2011) Ultramicroscopy 111:948–954
Dehm G, Howe JM, Zweck J (2012) In-situ electron microscopy: applications in physics, chemistry and materials science. Wiley
Devi MM, Biswas K (2015) Mater Chem Phys 166:207–214
Devi MM, Tiwari K, Biswas K (2019) Metall and Mater Trans A 50:3959–3972
Fecht H, Perepezko J (1989) Metall Trans A 20:785–794
Fecht H, Zhang M, Chang Y, Perepezko J (1989) Metall Trans A 20:795–803
Ferrando R (2016) Structure and properties of nanoalloys. Elsevier
Ferrando R, Jellinek J, Johnston RL (2008) Chem Rev 108:845–910
Gai P, Boyes E (2010) J Phys: Conf Ser
Gai PL, Kourtakis K (1995) Science 267:661–663
Gai PL, Sharma R, Ross FM (2008) MRS Bull 33:107–114
Garcia Esparza AT (2011)
Grogan JM, Rotkina L, Bau HH (2011) Phys Rev E 83:061405
Han X, Zhang Z, Wang ZL (2007) NANO 2:249–271
He B, Zhang Y, Liu X, Chen L (2020) ChemCatChem
http://www.denssolutions.com/en/our-products/sample-heat-ing-systems
http://www.nanofactory.com/news.asp?id=59&type=news
http://www.protochips.com/products/aduro.html
https://hitachi-hta.com/products/electron-ion-and-probe-microscopy/transmission-electron-microscopes/h-9500-300kv-te
https://www.fei.com/products/transmission-electron-micro-scopes/titan/etem.aspx
https://www.gatan.com/products/tem-specimen-holders/heating-situ-holders
https://www.jeolusa.com/PRODUCTS/Transmission-Electron-Microscopes-TEM/Analytical-Data-Optimization/Practical-Remote-In-Situ-Microscopy-PRISM
Idrees Y (2013) Microstructural evolution in Zr and Zr alloy Excel under ion irradiation. McGill-Queen's University Press, Kingston
Jellinek J (2008) Faraday Discuss 138:11–35
Johnson E, Johansen A, Dahmen U, Gabrisch H, Hagege S (2000) Lawrence Berkeley National Lab., CA (United States)
E. Johnson, A. Johansen, L. Sarholt, U. Dahmen, in: Journal of Metastable and Nanocrystalline Materials, Trans Tech Publ, 2001, pp. 267–274.
Jones RW (1990) The Institute of Metals 1990:128
Khan PY, Biswas K (2015) J Nanosci Nanotechnol 15:309–316
Khan PY, Devi MM, Biswas K (2015) Metall and Mater Trans A 46:3365–3377
Krivanek OL, Chisholm MF, Nicolosi V, Pennycook TJ, Corbin GJ, Dellby N, Murfitt MF, Own CS, Szilagyi ZS, Oxley MP (2010) Nature 464:571–574
LaGrange T, Campbell GH, Reed B, Taheri M, Pesavento JB, Kim JS, Browning ND (2008) Ultramicroscopy 108:1441–1449
Massalski T (1992) Phase Diagrams. pp 206–210
Mei Q, Lu K (2007) Prog Mater Sci 52:1175–1262
Mølhave K, Gudnason SB, Pedersen AT, Clausen CH, Horsewell A, Bøggild P (2006) Nano Lett 6:1663–1668
Peng B, Locascio M, Zapol P, Li S, Mielke SL, Schatz GC, Espinosa HD (2008) Nat Nanotechnol 3:626–631
Ruska VE (1942) Kolloid-Zeitschrift 100:212–219
Siem* E, Johnson E (2005) Philosophical Magazine. 85:1273–1290
Sinclair R (2013) MRS Bull 38:1065
Suryanarayana C (1991) Materials Science and Technology
Suryanarayana C (2001) Prog Mater Sci 46:1–184
Tang D-M, Ren C-L, Wang M-S, Wei X, Kawamoto N, Liu C, Bando Y, Mitome M, Fukata N, Golberg D (2012) Nano Lett 12:1898–1904
Tiwari K, Biwas K, Palliwal M, Majumdar B, Fecht H-J (2020) J Alloy Compd 155160
Urban KW (2009) Nat Mater 8:260–262
Williamson M, Tromp R, Vereecken P, Hull R, Ross F (2003) Nat Mater 2:532–536
Zewail AH (2010) Science 328:187–193
Zewail AH, Thomas JM (2010) 4D electron microscopy: imaging in space and time. World Scientific
Zhu Y, Espinosa HD (2005) Proc Natl Acad Sci 102:14503–14508
Ziegler JF (2012) Ion implantation science and technology. Elsevier (2012)

Fostering Morphological Mutations to Metal Nucleobase Complexes

R. Kamal Saravanan, Ilesha Avasthi, Rajneesh Kumar Prajapati, and Sandeep Verma

1 Introduction

Nucleobases are critical component of DNA and RNA and are also been encountered as versatile molecules for crafting aesthetically pleasing metal coordinated supramolecular motifs, owing to nitrogen atoms predisposed for coordination and non-covalent interactions (Amo-Ochoa and Zamora 2014; Sivakova and Rowan 2005; Verma et al. 2010). In addition, their metal coordination ability could be tuned by functionalization with metal binding groups at suitable positions (Verma et al. 2010; Mohapatra and Pratibha 2017). These diverse coordination modes of modified purine derivatives has been exploited to create complex supramolecular architectures exhibiting remarkable applications in material science as well as in biology (Mohapatra and Pratibha 2017, 20112011). Moreover, nucleobases have also been invoked to form interesting self-assemble patterns on various surfaces such as HOPG, Mica, Si, and Au. (Saravanan et al. 2018). The ordered self-assembly pattern of nucleobases and their metal-coordinated frameworks on various substrates have critically been analyzed by using electron microscopy.

Scanning and transmission electron microscopes (SEM and TEM) are among the most versatile and powerful tools deployed to decipher the microstructure, morphological and elemental composition of panoply of materials ranging from metal nano-structures, carbon nanotubes, inorganic–organic hybrids to biological samples, bacteria, and viruses. In present article, we have demonstrated the extensive use of electron microscopy in characterization of AuNPs decorated modified purine-blended electrospun fibers for sensing applications and morphological study of metal–nucleobase coordination polymers.

R. Kamal Saravanan · I. Avasthi · S. Verma
Department of Chemistry, Indian Institute of Technology Kanpur, Kanpur, UP 208016, India

R. K. Prajapati (✉)
Center for Nanoscience and Soft Nanotechnology, Indian Institute of Technology Kanpur, Kanpur, UP 208016, India
e-mail: rajkp@iitk.ac.in

2 AuNPs Decorated Nucleobase-Blended Electrospun Nanofibers: SERS Sensor

Electrospun fibers obtained by electrospinning technique serve as a promising avenue toward the development of smart functional materials, owing to its high porosity, mechanical strength, and large surface-to-volume ratio (Xue et al. 2019; Peng et al. 2016). Recently, metal nanoparticles immobilized electrospun fibers have gained significant attention due to their potential applications in catalysis (Qiao et al. 2018), sensing (Su et al. 20142014) and tissue engineering (Yadid et al. 2019), to name a few. Moreover, AuNPs decorated electrospun fibers have also been successfully studied as surface enhanced Raman scattering (SERS) substrates for the sensing of various analytes (Chen et al. 2017). Morphology of electrospun fibers, as well as metal nanoparticles incorporated electrospun fibers, have been analyzed critically by electron microscopy techniques (Xue et al. 2019; Zhang and Yu 2014).

During our critical effort to fabricate metal nanoparticles decorated electrospun fibers, we have prepared electrospun nanofibrous mats with varying concentrations of 8-mercapto-9-propyladenine (L) and polyacrylonitrile (PAN) by blending L with PAN polymer (Saravanan et al. 2020). The morphology of as-obtained electrospun fibers were analyzed by field emission scanning electron microscopy (FESEM) leading to entangled, long and continuous fibers (Fig. 1). These fibrous mats were further incubated with citrate-capped AuNPs, and resulting nanocomposites were characterized by various electron microscopy techniques such as SEM and TEM, as well as Fourier-transform infrared (FTIR) spectroscopy and powder X-ray diffraction. Careful inspection by SEM revealed that concentration of AuNPs on electrospun fibers has been enhanced with

K. Biswas et al. (eds.), *Electron Microscopy in Science and Engineering*, IITK Directions 6,
https://doi.org/10.1007/978-981-16-5101-4_9

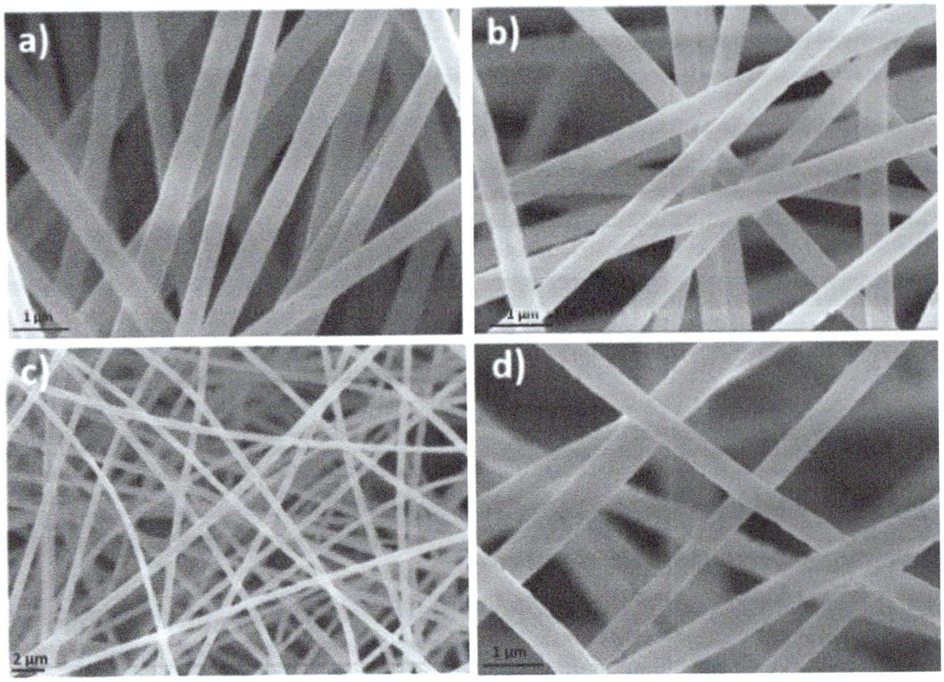

Fig. 1 SEM images of PAN/L electrospun nanofibers with various blend ratios a100/0 (P1); b 90.9/9.1 (P2); c 83.33/16.67 (P3); d 66.66/33.34 (P4) (% w/w). Reproduced with permission from Ref. (Saravanan et al. 2020) The Royal Society of Chemistry

increase in percentage of L (Fig. 2a–h), while Fig. 2i represents the HRTEM image of AuNPs/P4 nanocomposite (with 33% w/w of L) which indicates the presence of AuNPs on electrospun fibers.

Further, AuNPs decorated electrospun fibers nanocomposites were employed for SERS based detection of uric acid in aqueous solution, which is an important biomarker associated with several diseases. AuNPs/P_4 nanofibers composites (with 33% w/w of L) detected uric acid up to 10^{-7} M with the estimated average enhancement factor (AEF) for uric acid in SERS spectra to be 1.14×10^4 (640 cm^{-1} band) and 1.058×10^4 (882 cm^{-1} band). The limit of detection (LOD) was calculated by using regression method for 640 cm^{-1} peak and was found to be 1×10^{-7} M (Saravanan et al. 2020). The LOD achieved by our substrate was found to be lower than that of reported in literatures by various techniques.

3 Exfoliation of Cadmium–Purine Coordination Polymer

Layered frameworks when subjected to exfoliation result in 2D nanosheets through intercalation and isolation processes and can potentially be converted to 1D nanoscale structures.

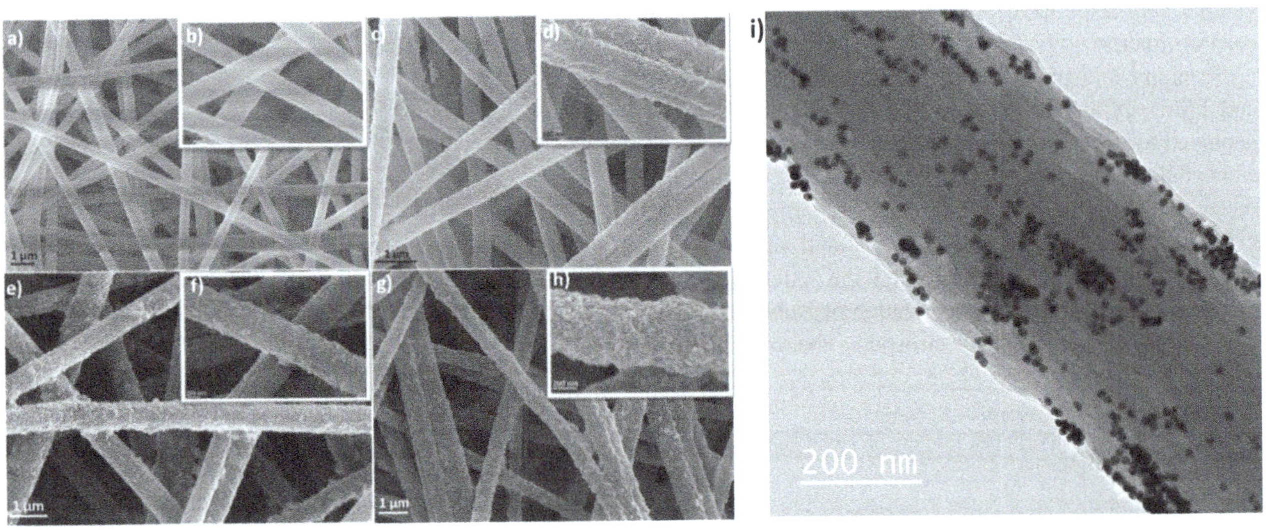

Fig. 2 FESEM images of AuNPs decorated PAN/L electrospun nanofibrous mats of P1 a, b; P2 c, d; P3 e, f and P4 g, h; and i HRTEM image of AuNPs/P4 composite. Reproduced with permission from Ref. (Saravanan et al. 2020) The Royal Society of Chemistry

These nanostructures inherit functional properties from their 3D bulk analogs. Herein, we have synthesized a derivative of adenine and subsequently its layered Cd(II)–purine coordination framework which was subjected to sonication-assisted liquid-phase exfoliation in ethanol or isopropanol to achieve 2D nanosheets (Avasthi et al. 2019). The same process of exfoliation when carried out in chloroform or THF resulted in 1D nanofibers. Further, a distinct conversion of nanosheets to nanofibers was also established at low temperatures. The characterization and analyses of the nanostructures and their conversion processes could successfully be achieved using scanning electron microscopy (SEM) and transmission electron microscopy (TEM) in addition to atomic force microscopy, energy dispersive X-ray (EDX), PXRD, and FTIR analyses.

Figure 3 depicts the SEM and TEM images of distinct nanosheets and long and continuous nanofibers obtained after exfoliation. Figure 4, however, highlights the conversion process of nanosheets to nanofibers in chloroform as recorded through SEM. Furthermore, these nanostructures

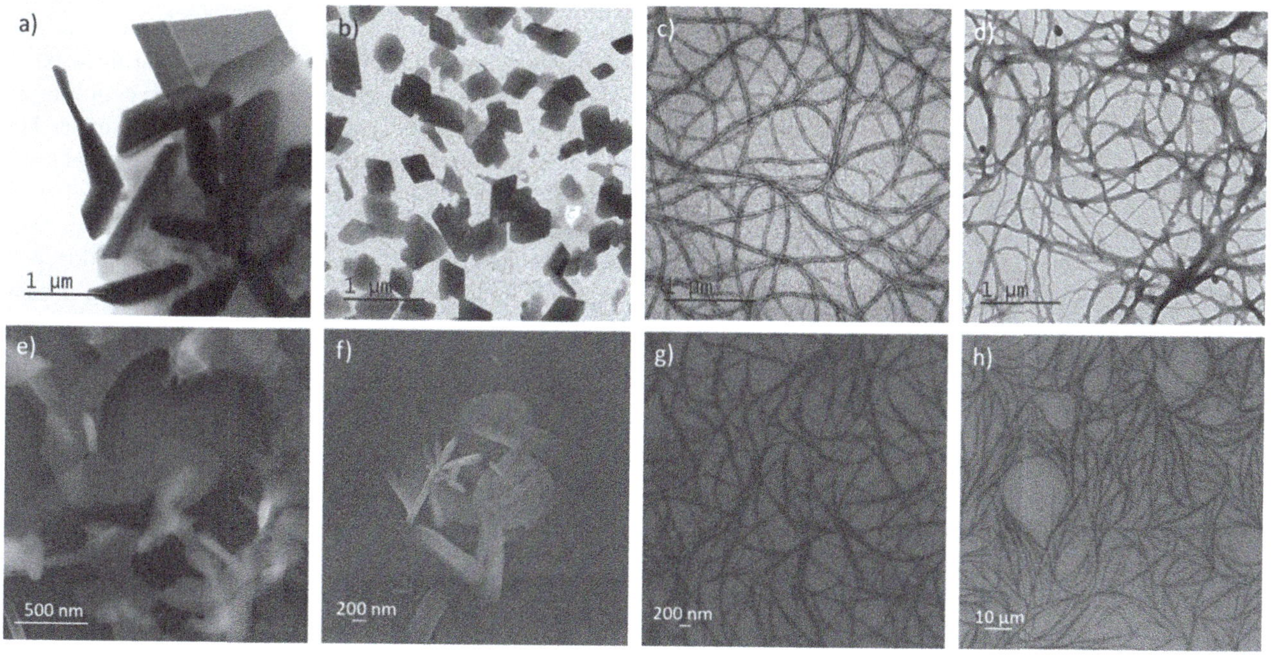

Fig. 3 TEM images of exfoliated Cd(II) complex in **a** isopropanol, **b** ethanol, **c** chloroform and **d** THF; SEM images of exfoliated Cd(II) complex in **e** isopropanol, **f** ethanol, **g** chloroform and **h** THF (where ethanol, isopropanol yield nanosheets and chloroform, THF yield nanofibers). Reproduced with permission from Ref. (Avasthi et al. 2019) © 2019 WILEY-VCH Verlag GmbH & Co. KGaA, Weinheim

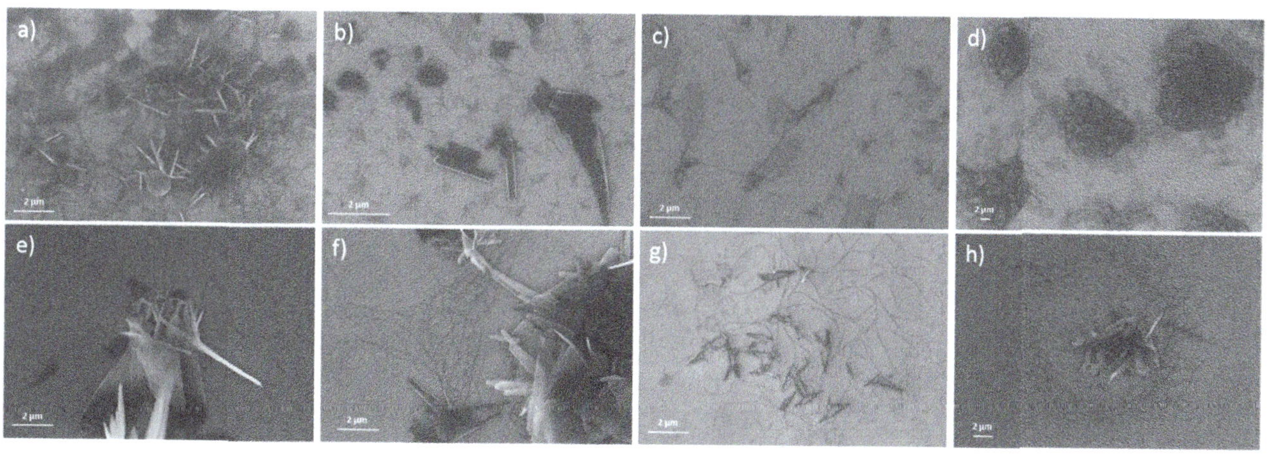

Fig. 4 Time-dependent SEM of Cd(II) complex exfoliated and incubated at 4 °C in chloroform at **a** 0-day, **b** 1-day, **c** 2-day, **d** 4-day and in THF at **e** 0-day, **f** 1-day, **g** 2-day, **h** 4-day demonstrating the transformation of nanosheets to nanofibers Reproduced with permission from Ref. (Avasthi et al. 2019) © 2019 WILEY–VCH Verlag GmbH & Co. KGaA, Weinheim

were probed for their elastic and capacitive properties using amplitude modulation-frequency modulation atomic force microscopy and Kelvin probe force microscopy, respectively, which revealed their potential applications in electronics and energy devices.

4 Copper–Purine Coordination Polymer: Thin Film Precursor

In another report, four N9 derivatives of 6-chloropurine were synthesized to subsequently achieve six Cu(II) complexes (Avasthi et al. 2017). These complexes were further established as thin film precursors to give copper(II) oxide thin films on quartz and Si(111) substrates by spin coating, first at room temperature in air and then CVD treatment at 650˚C. Thin films were prepared at this temperature under two conditions: (a) in air and (b) in inert atmosphere (under N_2) under standard pressure (760 Torr), on quartz and Si (111). The films were characterized using EDX, PXRD, and Raman spectroscopy followed by morphological study under SEM.

The films obtained on Si (111) surface under the two conditions has been shown in Fig. 5. The films were then subjected to electrical characterization using four-point probe method to calculate their sheet resistance indicating that rationally devised Cu(II) purine complexes could possibly find useful applications as a source/drain or gate of thin film transistor or as electrode in LEDs and solar cells (Wanjala et al. 2016) or in high-speed integrated circuits (Cale et al. 2000).

In conclusion, we have outlined the synthesis of modified purine blended electrospun fibers, which subsequently incubated by AuNPs and their morphology was investigated by using electron microscopy techniques. In addition to morphology of fibers, decoration of AuNPs on the surface of electrospun nanofibers was clearly revealed by SEM and TEM analysis as electron microscopes are versatile tool to analyze metal nanoparticles/electrospun fiber composites. Furthermore, As-fabricated AuNPs/electrospun fibers composites were demonstrated as potential substrate for SERS-based detection of uric acid with the detection limit of 10^{-7} M concentration. Detection of uric acid by such substrate might offer newer design paradigms for the sensors of biologically relevant molecules and biochemical pathways. Moreover, we have also exploited electron microscopy, for the characterization of nanostructures obtained as consequences of exfoliation of cadmium-purine coordination polymer, as well as to analyze the thin film made by copper–purine coordination polymer. The electron microscopy has not only allowed us to characterize the structures on the surface but also provided a deeper insight to establish their function at the nanoscale. These fundamental studies have assisted in establishing profound structure–property relationships which pave way for the development of useful functional molecular systems for various purposes. Such self-assembled novel nucleobase metal coordination polymers are envisaged to have potential applications in fabrication of smart functional materials.

References

Amo-Ochoa P, Zamora F (2014) Coordination polymers with nucleobases: from structural aspects to potential applications. Coord Chem Rev 276:34–58

Sivakova S, Rowan SJ (2005) Nucleobase as supramolecular motifs. Chem Soc Rev 34:9–21

Verma S, Mishra AK, Kumar J (2010) The many facets of adenine: coordination, crystal patterns, and catalysis. Acc Chem Res 43:79–91

Mohapatra B, Pratibha, Verma S (2017) Directed adenine functionalization for creating complex architectures for material and biological applications. Chem Comm 53:4748–4758

Imaz I, Rubio-Martínez M, An J, Solé-Font I, Rosi NL, Maspoch D (2011) Metal-biomolecule frameworks (MBioFs) ChemComm 47:7287–7302

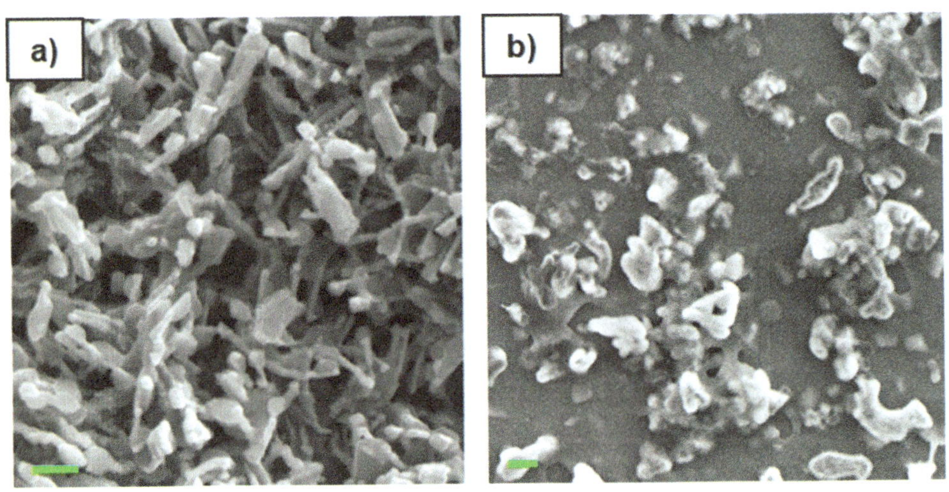

Fig. 5 SEM (Scale: 2 μm) for thin films in **a** air and **b** inert cond. (under std. pressure). Reproduced with permission from Ref. (Avasthi et al. 2017) The Royal Society of Chemistry

Saravanan RK, Avasthi I, Prajapati RK, Verma S (2018) Surface modification and pattern formation by nucleobases and their coordination complexes. RSC Adv 8:24541–24560

Xue J, Wu T, Dai Y, Xia Y (2019) Electrospinning and electrospun nanofibers: methods materials and applications. Chem Rev 119:5298–5415

Peng S, Jin G, Li L, Li K, Srinivasan M, Ramakrishna S, Chen J (2016) Multi-functional electrospun nanofibers for advances in tissue regeneration, energy conversion and storage, and water treatment. Chem Soc Rev 45:1225–1241

Qiao Z, Shen M, Xiao Y, Zhu M, Mignani S, Majoral J-P, Shi X (2018) Organic/inorganic nanohybrids formed using electrospun polymer nanofibers as nanoreactors. Coord Chem Rev 372:31–51

Su Z, Ding J, Wei G (2014) Electrospinning: a facile technique for fabricating polymeric nanofibers doped with carbon nanotubes and metallic nanoparticles for sensor applications. RSC Adv 4:52598–52610

Yadid M, Feiner R, Dvir T (2019) Gold nanoparticle-integrated scaffolds for tissue engineering and regenerative medicine. Nano Lett 19:2198–2206

Chen C, Tang Y, Vlahovic B, Yan F (2017) Electrospun polymer nanofibers decorated with noble metal nanoparticles for chemical sensing. Nanoscale Res Lett 12:451

Zhang C-L, Yu S-H (2014) Nanoparticles meet electrospinning: recent advances and future prospects. Chem Soc Rev 43:4423–4448

Saravanan RK, Naqvi TK, Patil S, Dwivedi PK, Verma S (2020) Purine-blended nanofiber woven flexible nanomats for SERS-based analyte detection. Chem Commun 56:5795–5798

Avasthi I, Kulkarni MM, Verma S (2019) Exfoliating a Cd II—purine framework: conversion of nanosheets-to-nanofibers and studies of elastic and capacitive properties. Chem A Eur J 25:6988–6995

Avasthi I, Khanna S, Tripathi SK, Verma S (2017) N9 substituent mediated structural tuning of copper-purine complexes: chelate effect and thin film studies. CrystEngComm 19:5202–5213

Wanjala KS, Njoroge WK, Ngaruiya JM (2016) Optical and electrical characterization of ZnS: Sn thin films for solar cell application. Am J Condens Matter Phys 6:1–6

Cale TS, Merchant TP, Borucki LJ, Labun AH (2000) Topography simulation for the virtual wafer fab. Thin Solid Films 365:152–175

Interplay of Stresses, Interfaces, and Nanoscale Effects: *TEM Investigations*

Anandh Subramaniam, R. M. Raghavendra, Ganesh Iyer, and Arun Kumar

1 Defects in Crystals

Defects are typically classified based on their dimensionality (http://home.iitk.ac.in/~anandh/E-book.htm) (Fig. 1). One inevitable defect in all real single crystals is the surface. In mechanics, the surface is sometimes referred to as the traction-free surface; albeit the fact that, in reality the under-coordination of the atoms at the surface lends to surface stress. Surface stress in metals is tensile in nature and leads to the compression of the crystal. Vacancies and dislocations are other common defects present in crystals. Dislocations, which are endowed with long range stress fields, can interact with the stress fields associated with other defects. The stresses under discussion are 'residual' in nature (Fig. 2). In typical polycrystalline materials, the effect of surface is limited, while the role played by grain boundaries (an internal interface) is prominent. The type and distribution of defects constitutes the defect structure in a material. Phases, defects and residual stresses and their distributions constitute a microstructure, which governs 'structure sensitive properties' (Fig. 3).

In nanoscale systems, two effects gain prominence: interactions due to the proximity of interfaces and the altered energetics of defects. Selected examples of the consequences of the same are (Schodek et al. 2009; Nalwa 2004): the destabilization of vacancies, a crystal becoming spontaneously dislocation free, and the alteration in the deformation mechanism. More such effects are highlighted in the current article.

In this article, the work of our group at IITK is kept primarily in view (Kumar et al. 2013a,2014; Rani et al. 2015,2017; Iyer et al. 2017), and the readers may refer to standard literature to gain a broader view of the subject matter. The focus of our group is on theoretical, computational, and experimental investigations of metastable microstructures, which include nanomaterials, coherent systems, internal interfaces, and crystalline defects. Three examples are considered to elucidate the interplay between stresses, interfaces, and geometry. These are: (i) the stabilization of a coherent state, (ii) an anomalous lattice expansion in spherical metals shells, and (iii) the alteration of the critical size for nucleation during a solid-to-solid diffusional phase transformation. The 'geometry' being referred to relates to features of the sample. We will come across interesting concepts, which include 'depth sensitive lattice fringe imaging,' 'liquid-like nucleation in nanoscale films,' and 'Poisson effect-driven anomalous lattice expansion in metal nanoshells.' These examples will serve to highlight the power of the use of transmission electron microscopy in conjunction with computational models. A range techniques associated with TEM/STEM (scanning transmission electron microscopy) have been used in the investigations, which include bright field imaging (BFI), high-resolution lattice fringe imaging (HRLFI), high-angle annular dark field imaging (HAADF), electron energy loss spectroscopy (EELS), and Moiré fringe contrast imaging. It will become amply clear to the reader that these studies provide insights into nanoscale phenomena which are practically inaccessible by other means.

Notes to the reader: The symbol r^* has been used for the critical radius in multiple contexts, each distinct from the other. The reader must be careful to distinguish these physically diverse scenarios. The meaning of the terms like domain, body, sample, crystal, and film has to be 'deciphered' keeping the context in view.

A. Subramaniam (✉) · R. M. Raghavendra
Materials Science and Engineering, Indian Institute of Technology, Kanpur, India
e-mail: anandh@iitk.ac.in

G. Iyer
Department of Mechanical Engineering, Institute of Infrastructure Technology Research and Management, Ahmedabad, Gujarat, India

A. Kumar
Department of Physics, J.C. Bose University of Science and Technology YMCA, Faridabad, Haryana, India

K. Biswas et al. (eds.), *Electron Microscopy in Science and Engineering*, IITK Directions 6,
https://doi.org/10.1007/978-981-16-5101-4_10

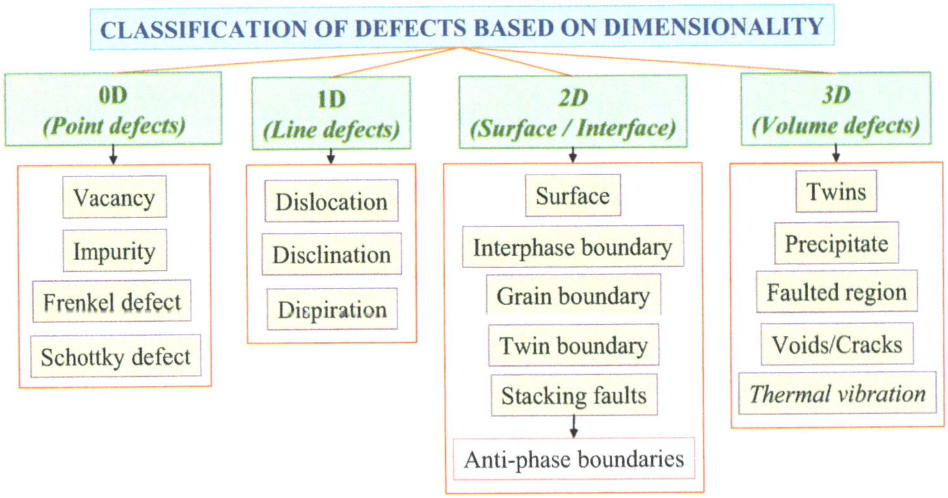

Fig. 1 Classification of defects in crystals based on dimensionality

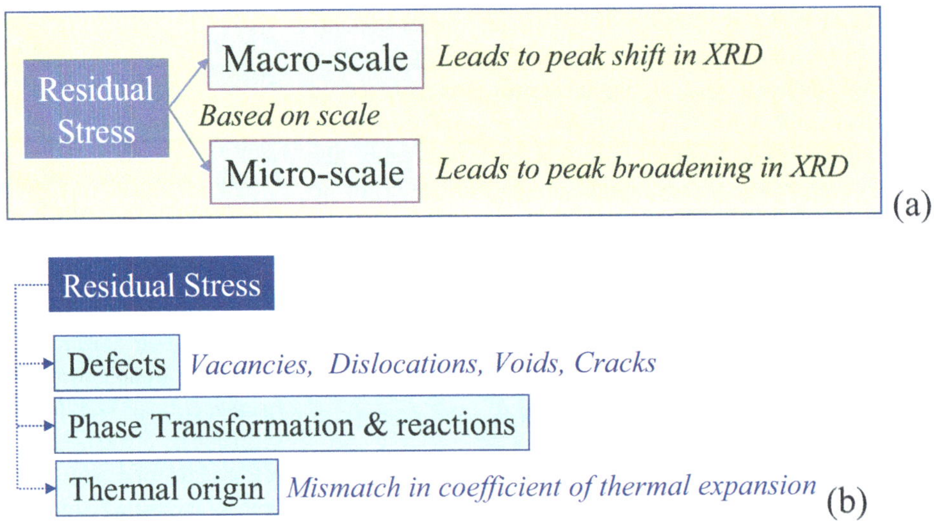

Fig. 2 **a** Classification based on scale and **b** origins of residual stresses in materials

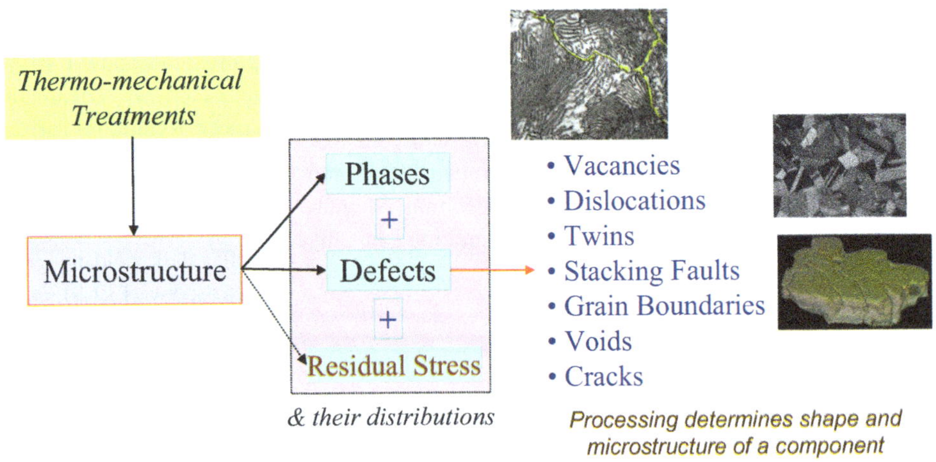

Fig. 3 'Functional' definition of microstructure. Thermo-mechanical treatments can be used to engineer the microstructure. The microstructure determines the 'structure sensitive properties'

2 The Interplay of Stresses, Interfaces, and Geometry

2.1 Dislocations in Finite Bodies

An illustrative system to comprehend the interplay of stresses, interfaces, and geometry is the study of dislocations in semi-infinite and nanoscale bodies. As alluded to before, the stresses being referred to in the current context are residual stresses. The stress fields of defects and the associated energetics are altered in finite bodies. In nanoscale systems, these effects are accentuated manyfold. An edge dislocation in a finite body can serve as a model example to illustrate the concepts involved. The stress fields of an edge dislocation in an infinite body (plot of σ_{xx} contours) is shown in Fig. 4a. If the body is semi-infinite, with the presence of a proximal free surface, the stress state is modified (Fig. 4b). As less volume of material is stressed, the energy of the dislocation is reduced, with respect to that in an infinite body. The energy of the system decreases with distance, and this results in an 'image force' (the gradient of the energy field is the force field). The image force is so termed, as the force of attraction toward the surface, can be computed using the construction of an 'image dislocation.' This force is a 'configurational force' and hence has to be seen in a different light as compared to that we typically exposed to.

As the dislocation is positioned within a few Burgers vectors from the surface, domain deformations and the interaction of the core of the dislocation with the surface

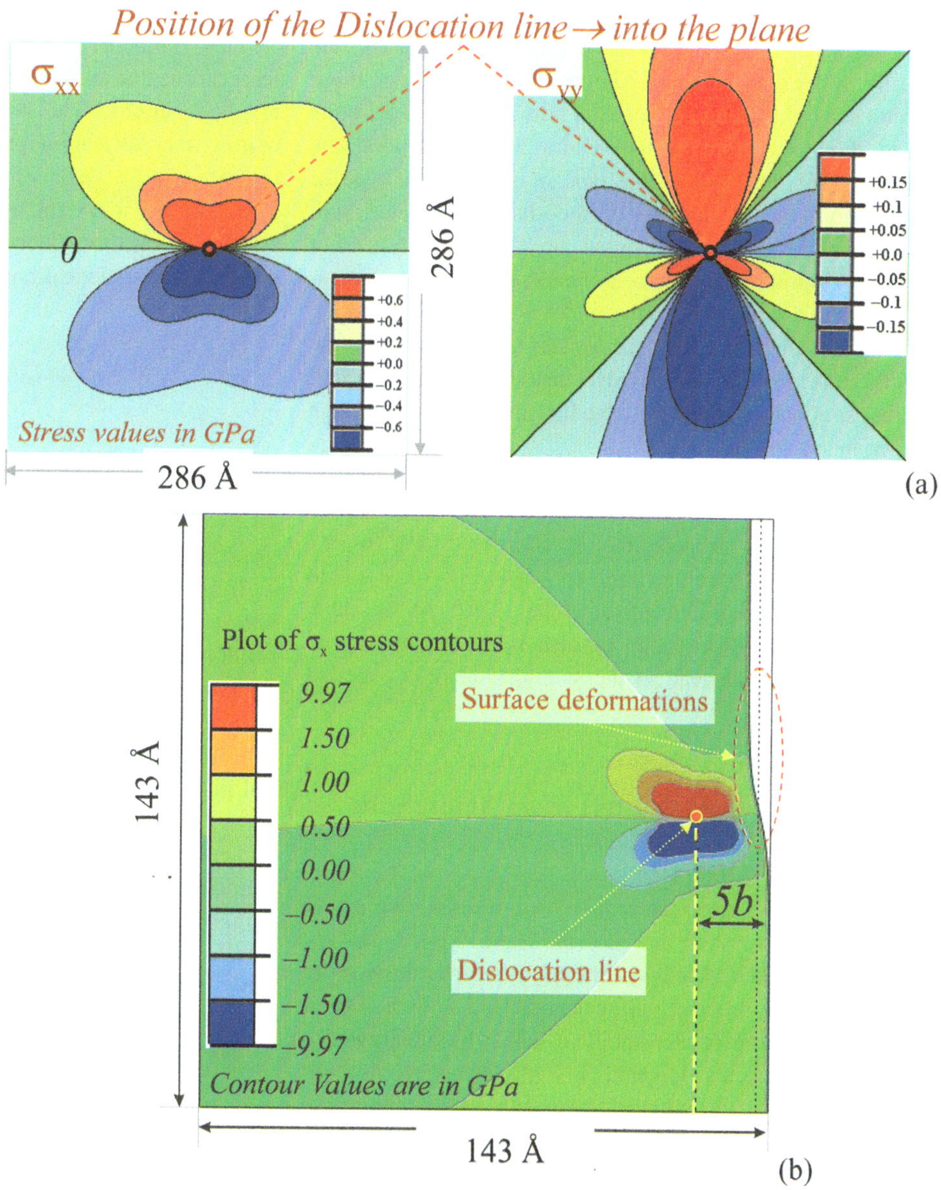

Fig. 4 **a** Edge dislocation in an infinite body. Note the left–right mirror symmetry and the top–bottom 'mirror-inversion' symmetry (which 'reflects' tensile stresses to compressive stresses). (b) In a semi-infinite body, with a proximal free-surface. The symmetries present in (a) are broken here

assume prominence. These effects further alter the energetics and forces involved. Eshelby showed in 1953 that a screw dislocation can be stabilized in a thin cylinder (Eshelby 1953). The corresponding scenario with regard to an edge dislocation was elucidated in 2012 by Kumar and Subramaniam (2012a) (the reader may refer to an article in directions for further details (Subramaniam and Kumar 2014)). In both these cases, the geometry of the body (thin cylinder or thin plate), its deformation under the stress fields of the dislocation, and concomitant reduction in the energy of the system results in the stabilization. Interestingly, in the case of the edge dislocation in a thin plate, the dislocation may exist in a state of neutral equilibrium (Kumar and Subramaniam 2011). For the case of two dislocations in a thin plate, we may observe the existence of 'metastable states of negative stiffness' along with 'unstable states of positive stiffness' (Kumar and Subramaniam 2013a).

This traction-free boundary condition existing at the free-surface is altered due to surface stresses. The stress state of the system is altered as shown in Fig. 5. Under these circumstances, an edge dislocation may experience a torque in addition to the force (Raghavendra 2018). In general, the 'geometry of the system' (the type of surface, the type of dislocation, the orientation of the dislocation, etc.) will determine the force and torque on the dislocation. For specific configurations, this can result an equilibrium position for the dislocation (Raghavendra 2018). It is interesting to note that after more than six decades a second origin of an equilibrium position for an edge dislocation has emerged! Perhaps, equally amazing is the fact that a monopole can experience a torque!

Image forces can result in regions near surfaces to become spontaneously dislocation free. This happens when the image force exceeds the Peierls force (PN force). Nanocrystals can become completely dislocation free due to this effect (Khanikar and Subramaniam 2010). As we show later, interfacial misfit loops are also subject to these considerations and can lead to the stabilization of a coherent precipitate.

2.2 Nucleation of Crystals in an Amorphous Matrix

In this and the next sub-section, we discuss two relate phenomena: nucleation and growth. There exists a propensity for an undercooled system to transform. First-order transformations proceed via nucleation and growth (David 2009). Nucleation occurs uphill in Gibbs free energy (G), while growth occurs downhill in 'G.' Nucleation involves the formation of the product phase of a certain minimum dimension, referred to as the critical radius (r^*). 'Embriyos' smaller than r^* revert to the parent phase, while 'super-critical' nuclei grow to facilitate the phase transformation.

Nucleation of crystals from an amorphous matrix serves as model system from both microscopic and mechanics point of view due to the following reasons (Pooja Rani and Raghavendra 2007).

1. It is easy to control the degree of transformation, as compared to that from a liquid.
2. Only the crystallite will give rise to lattice fringes in the HRLFI technique.
3. The matrix is isotropic and hence its elastic properties are captured by only two elastic moduli.
4. Homogeneous nucleation predominates.

It is to be noted that point (iv) is in stark contrast to nucleation in a typical crystalline solid, wherein, heterogeneous nucleation preferentially occurs at various defect sites.

The volume occupied by the nucleus (crystallite) is different from that of the glass, and hence, the transformation involves strains. The associated strain energy tends to oppose the nucleation process and with thus lead to an increase in the value of r^*, as compared to that for the nucleation of a crystal from a liquid. In the ambit of the classical nucleation theory (CNT), the process of nucleation occurs by a 'statistical random fluctuation' and the value of r^* is given by:

$$r^* = \frac{2\gamma}{(\Delta G_V - \Delta G_S)} \tag{1}$$

where, $\Delta G_S = \frac{E_{Strain}}{V}$ is the misfit strain energy per unit volume.

If the process of nucleation occurs close to a surface or in nanocrystals, the strain energy penalty is reduced, which results in a reduction in the value of r^*. Given that the thickness of a typical TEM sample is of the order of 10–50 nm, this naturally serves as nanoscale system. The details with respect to other geometries differ; however, the essential physics remains the same. The Cu-Zr-Al bulk metallic glass (BMG) serves as a model system for the study of nucleation due to the following reasons. (i) Glass can be formed by reasonably slow cooling. (ii) The diffusion is sluggish at room temperature, and hence, the occurrence of transformation during characterization (like TEM) is negligible. (iii) By working at a temperature in the 'nucleation dominant regime,' we can practically suppress growth.

The size of crystallites formed on devitrification can be determined by HRLFI. Other competing TEM techniques can also give us a rapid and accurate measure of the sizes, e.g., 'zero defocus' Fresnel contrast imaging (Bhattacharyya

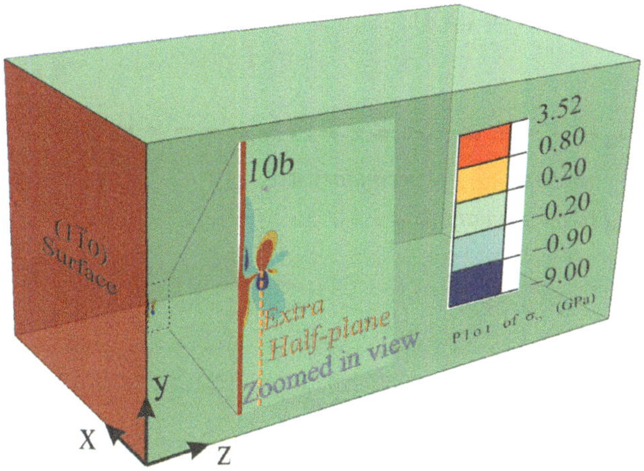

Fig. 5 Stress fields associated with an edge dislocation (plot of σ_{yy} contours) in a semi-infinite body, in the presence of surface stresses. The stress state is simulated using finite element method (FEM). The dimensions of the body are 500b × 500b × 1000b (b = 2.863 Å)

et al. 2006). The strain energy involved in the formation of the nucleus can be computed finite element method. A model for the same is shown in Fig. 6a. Figure 6b shows the state of stress (plot of σ_{yy} stress contours) in the presence of a nucleus (crystallite of $Cu_{10}Zr_7$).

The variation in the strain energy associated with a nucleus for two cases is shown in Fig. 7: (i) varying thickness of the amorphous film and (b) position of the crystal within the film (varying height). As expected, it is seen that the strain energy cost for nucleation decreases with a decreasing thickness of the amorphous film or as the nucleus is positioned closer to the surface. The computation of the r^* for homogeneous nucleation, via a plot of the change in the Gibbs free energy ($\Delta G_{homo}(r)$) with size of the nucleus (r), is shown as an inset to the figure. Three cases of nucleation of a crystals considered are: (i) from the liquid, (ii) at the center (t = 4 nm), and (iii) in a bulk matrix. As expected, the value of r^* increases with an increased cost of strain energy $r^*_{liquid} < r^*_{thin\,film} < r^*_{bulk}$.

Experimentally, the BMG sample can be made using suction casting. In the Cu-Zr-Al system, the composition of $(Cu_{64}Zr_{36})_{96}Al_4$ has good glass forming ability with a critical cooling rate of 40 K/s and critical diameter of 7 mm (Tanya Aycan Baser and Marcello Baricco 2008). Figure 8a shows the selected area diffraction (SAD) pattern showing the formation of amorphous structure. The corresponding real space image is shown in Fig. 8b (which displays the typical 'salt and pepper' contrast). Heat treatment of the BMG to induce nucleation was carried out in two kinds of samples: (i) bulk sample and (ii) nanoscale thin film (thinned down TEM samples). The crystallite/nuclei which first forms on annealing is $Cu_{10}Zr_7$ (Cmca, oC68, a = 12.68 Å, b = 9.31 Å, c = 9.35 Å (Alessandro Figini Albisetti 2012)).

As indicated before, the TEM specimen can be used as a nanoscale thin film. The thickness of the sample is an important parameter and can be determined using EELS. The EELS spectrum can be used to determine the local thickness of the sample (t) (Malis et al. 1988):

$$t = \lambda \ln\left(\frac{I_T}{I_0}\right) \tag{2}$$

where, I_0 and I_T are the areas under the zero loss peak and the entire spectrum and 'λ' is the inelastic mean free path. Using the standard values from literature, the local thickness of the sample can be determined (within about 20% accuracy). Figure 8c shows an EELS spectrum obtained using an in-column energy filter system in a Zeiss Libra 200FE instrument (a FEG gun instrument with a resolution of 0.9 Å, operating at 200 kV).

In the case of the bulk sample, the annealing was carried out first (200 °C for 4 h) followed by thinning to form a TEM sample. In the second case, the samples where thinned first followed by annealing (200 °C, 10 min). The choice of

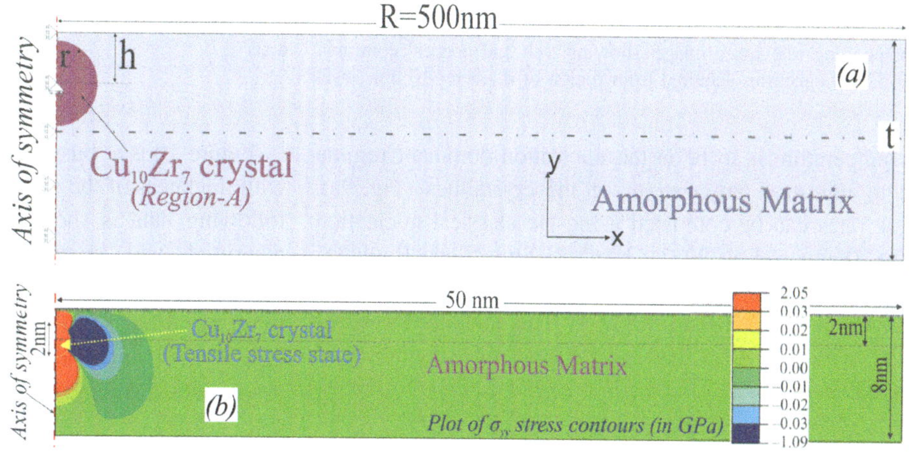

Fig. 6 **a** Finite element model used to compute the strain energy due to nucleation (of a crystal of radius 'r') in a thin film (of thickness 't'). Eigenstrains are imposed in region-A to simulate the stress state in the presence of a crystal. **b** Plot of σ_{yy} stress contours due to nucleation (r = 1 nm, h = 2 nm t = 8 nm)

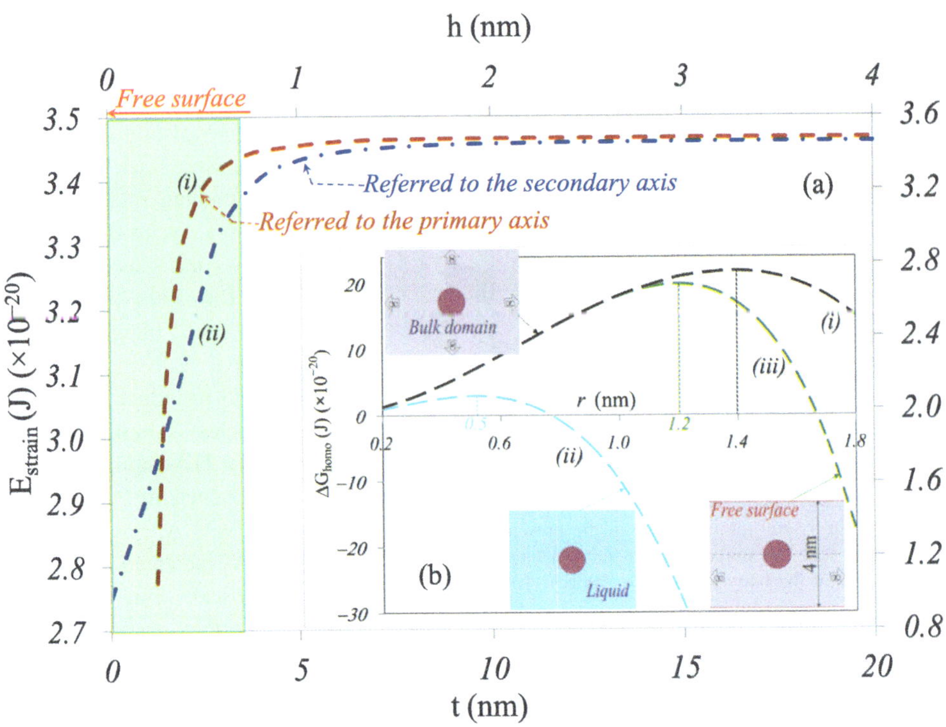

Fig. 7 Variation of strain energy (E_{strain}) with: **a** (i) 't' and (ii) 'h.' **b** Variation in ΔG_{homo} versus 'r' for nucleation in: (i) the bulk, (ii) the liquid, and (iii) the center of a film (t = 4 nm). Nanoscale effects predominate in the shaded region

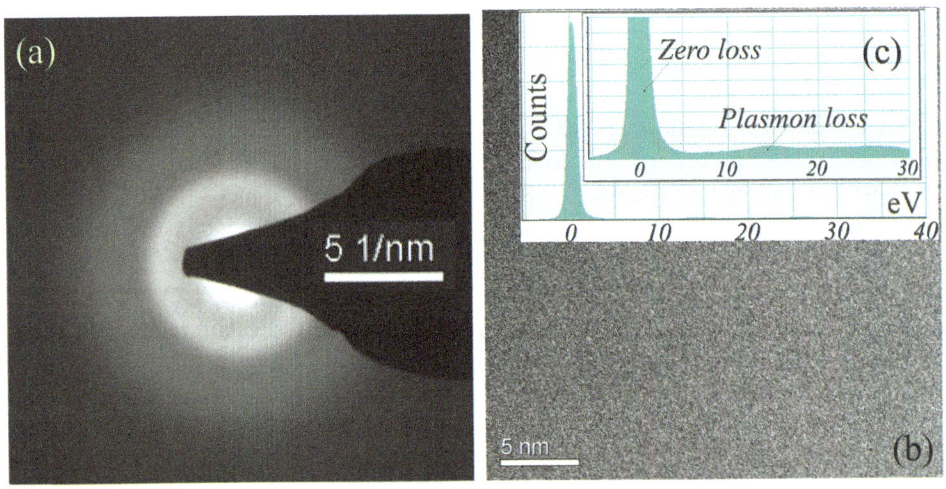

Fig. 8 **a** Diffuse rings in the SAD pattern showing the formation of an amorphous structure (suction cast $(Cu_{64}Zr_{36})_{96}Al_4$ alloy). **b** The corresponding real space image (showing 'salt and pepper' contrast). **c** An EELS spectrum acquired from region of diameter 10 nm (inset shows a region close to the zero loss peak). This spectrum can be used in the computation of the thickness of the specimen (as described in the text)

the temperature is to be in the nucleation-dominant regime and to minimize any growth of the crystallites (Fig. 9a). These rates can be computed using the classical nucleation theory (Kumar et al. 2013a; Karthika Suresh and Radhakrishnan and P. Kalaichelvi, 2016). The size of the nucleus can be determined by HRLFI (Fig. 9b). This technique is associated with an 'error bar' of at least one digital pixel (~0.032 nm).

Figure 10 is a 'busy plot' which shows the variation of r^* with thickness of the sample, along with other features. The following data is shown in the figure. (i) Experimentally measured and computed values of r^*_{bulk}, (ii) r^*_{liquid}, (iii) $r^*_{\text{thin film}}$ (computed and experimental), and (iv) $r^*(h)$ (with t = 8 nm). The experimentally determined value of r^*_{bulk} ~ 1.41 nm. Based on the data, we can make the following observations. (i) A very good match exists between

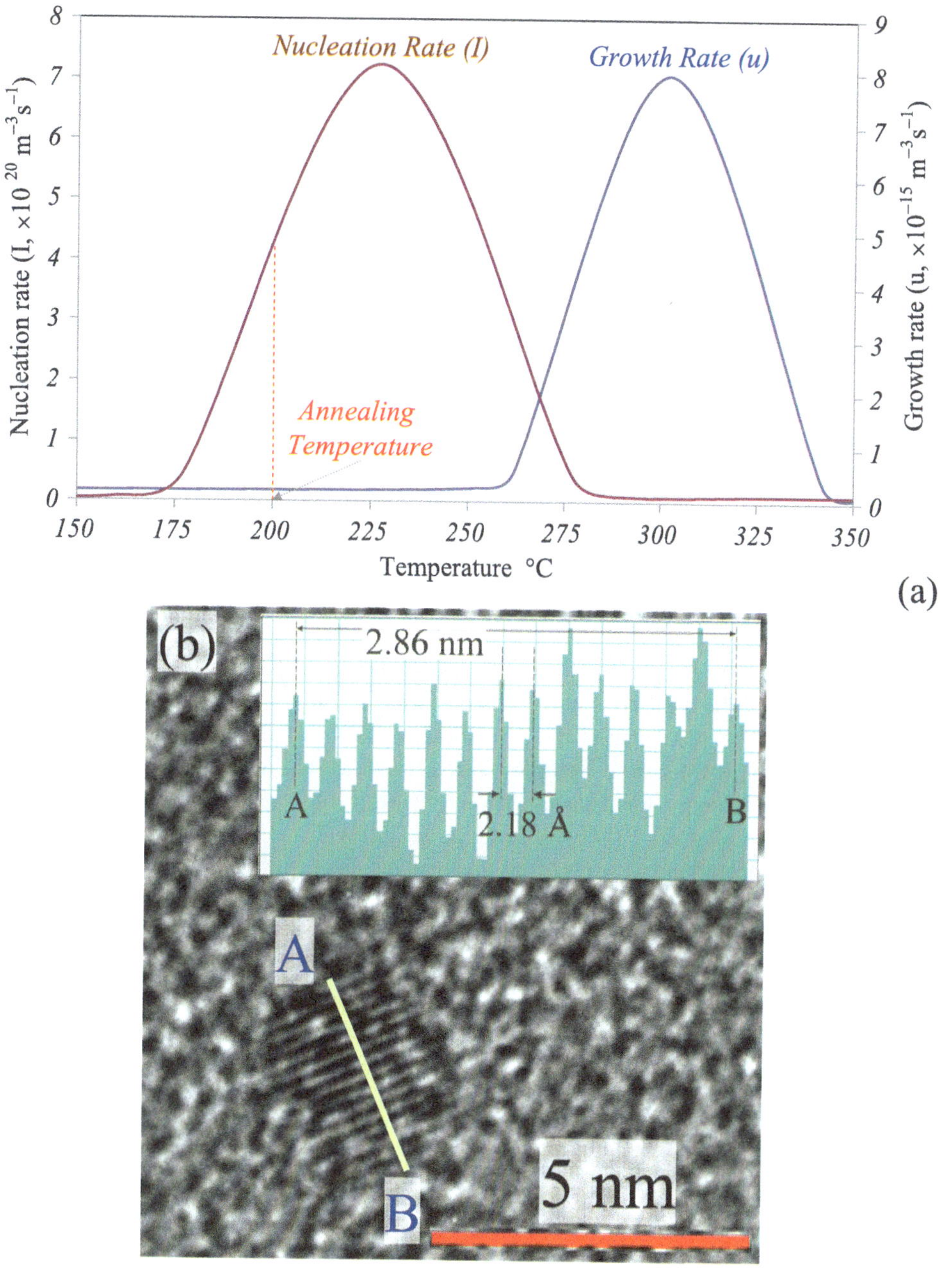

Fig. 9 **a** Plot of nucleation and growth rates for the crystallization of $Cu_{10}Zr_7$ crystal from the $(Cu_{64}Zr_{36})_{96}Al_4$ BMG. **b** HRLFI from a crystallite (d = 2.86 nm) embedded in an amorphous matrix. Inset shows a plot of the intensity across the line AB

the computed and experimental values of r^*_{bulk}. (ii) The decrease in the value of r^* for films with thickness less than ~ 9 nm is prominent. (iii) r^* decreases from the center toward the surface. This implies that a nucleation behavior approaches that from a liquid (i.e., $r^* \rightarrow r^*_{\text{liquid}}$) in case of nucleation in: (i) thin films and (ii) for positions of the crystal close to the surface.

A noteworthy feature is that 'bulk like' behavior is retrieved for films as thin as 12 nm. The variation of r^* with 'h' implies that we can perform '*depth (z) sensitive lattice fringe imaging*,' that is, determine the position (h) of the nuclei from lattice fringe images, This is interesting as lattice fringe images usually do not contain depth information related to the features observed.

2.3 Growth of Precipitates in Nanocrystals

In many systems, the precipitate is coherent with the matrix in the initial stages and progressively becomes semi-coherent and incoherent on growth. The terms 'coherent and 'semi-coherent' apply to interfaces, but are often used as adjectives to precipitates (as a whole). It is to be noted that precipitates can have some interfaces which are

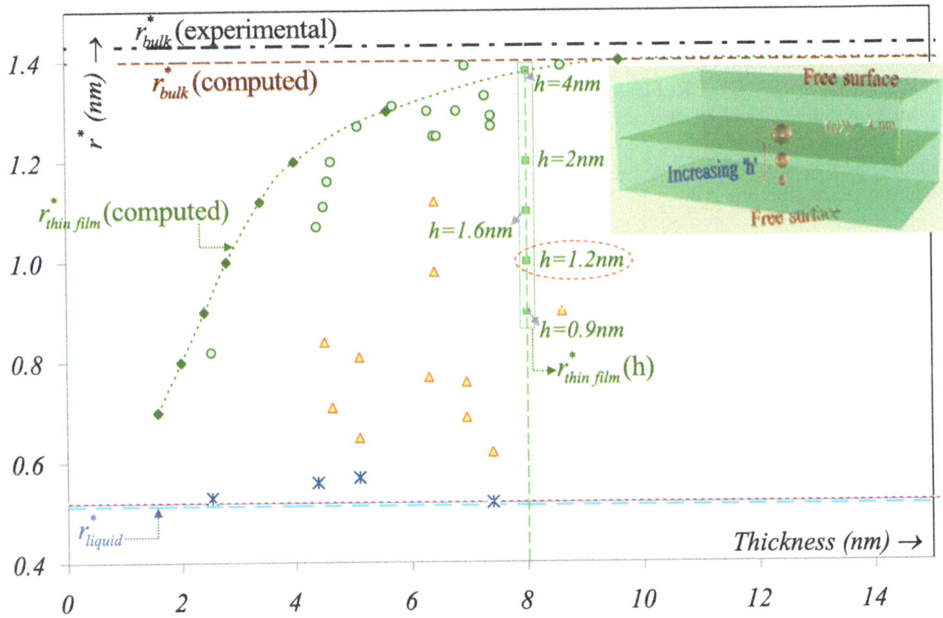

Fig. 10 Overlay of computed and experimental results. (i) The variation of r^*_{thinfilm} (computed) with 't.' (ii) r^*_{bulk} (computed and experimental) and r^*_{liquid}. (iii) Measurements using HRLFI. (iv) Variation of r^*_{computed} with 'h' (t = 8 nm, enclosed in a vertical box). Discrete point corresponds to measurements made using HRLFI. Inset to the figure shows a schematic of case (iv)

coherent with the matrix and others which are semi-coherent. The precipitation of γ-Fe (Fe-2 wt.% Cu) precipitate from a Cu-2wt.% Fe alloy has served as a model system for study for decades (Brown et al. 1968; Woolhouse and Ipohorski 1971; Watanabe et al. 2008). In this system, concomitant with the transitions of the interface character (Fig. 11), there occurs a shape transition and further a phase transformation of the metastable γ-Fe to the stable α form. Many systems, wherein precipitation occurs from a super-saturated solid solution, have been well studied in the context of precipitation hardening. The mechanism of the interaction of a dislocation with the precipitate switches from 'glide through the precipitate' (particle cutting) to Orowan bowing, as the interface character changes from coherent to incoherent (http://home.iitk.ac.in/~anandh/E-book.htm).

On solutionizing a Fe-2 wt.% Cu alloy and subsequently heat treating at lower temperatures (e.g., 550 °C), the metastable γ-Fe precipitate nucleates. The precipitate is endowed with a coherent interface to reduce the chemical interfacial energy (local), at the expense of strain energy ('long range'). The strain energy of a spherical precipitate of radius 'r_p' in an infinite isotropic matrix is given by Matthews (1979):

$$E^{\text{strain}}_{\text{ppt}} = \frac{8\,\pi\, r_p^3 f_m^2\, G_{\text{ppt}}}{3} \frac{(1+\nu_{\text{ppt}})}{(1-\nu_{\text{ppt}})} \quad (3)$$

where 'G' is the shear modulus, 'ν' is the Poisson's ratio, 'f_m' is the lattice misfit between precipitate and matrix. The subscript 'ppt' refers to the precipitate.

On growth beyond a critical size (r^*), the precipitate becomes semi-coherent via the formation of interfacial misfit

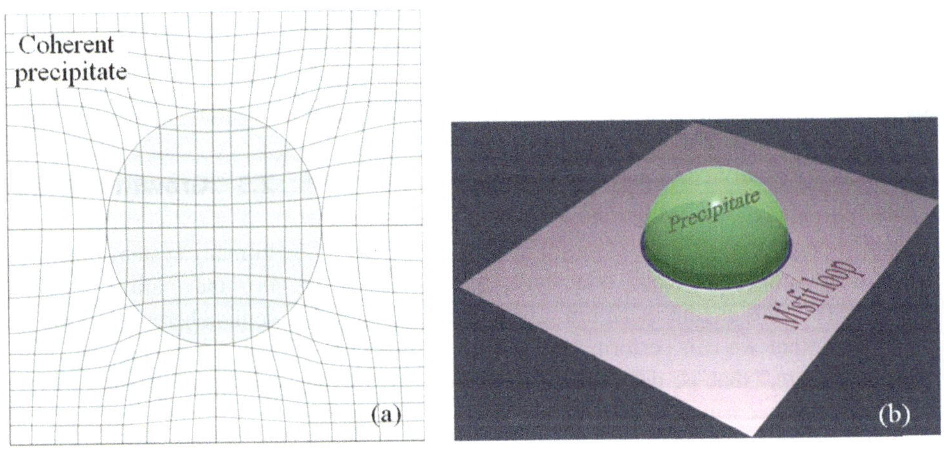

Fig. 11 Schematics showing the change in the character of the interface of a coherent precipitate on growth (e.g., in the γ-Fe precipitate in the Cu-2wt.% Fe alloy). **a** Coherent state with distortion of the atomic planes. **b** Semi-coherent with an interfacial misfit dislocation loop

dislocation loops (Matthews 1979). The energy (E_d) associated with circular a dislocation loop (of radius 'R') in an infinite body is given by Nabarro (1967):

$$E_d \approx \frac{Gb^2}{2(1-v)} R\left[\ln\left(\frac{8R}{\varepsilon}\right)+1\right] \quad (4)$$

where 'b' is the modulus of the Burgers vector and 'ε' is the 'core' cut-off radius (usually assumed to be in the range of 'b' to 5b). The 'core energy' has to be determined using atomistic models and is usually about 10% of the total energy of the system (Hirth and Lothe 1968; Bollmann 1970).

The critical size for the formation of the first loop along the 'equator' of the precipitate is (Woolhouse and Ipohorski 1971):

$$r* = r^*_{\text{bulk}} = \frac{b}{8\pi\,\omega(1-v)}\left[\ln\frac{8r*}{b} + \frac{3-2v}{4(1-v)} - 1\right] \quad (5)$$

where $\omega = [(1+\mathrm{v})f_m]/[3(1-\mathrm{v})]$ (Jesser 1969) is referred to as the strain parameter.

For the case of an interfacial misfit loop, the tensile and compressive fields lie in different materials. In finite bodies the stress state of the precipitate and the dislocation loop are altered with respect to that in an infinite body. If the precipitate is close to a free-surface, then domain deformations can lead to partial relaxation of the stress fields. In scenarios such as these, FEM has proved to be a powerful tool not only in determining the stress state of the body, but also in the computation of critical parameters related to the system (Kumar et al. 2014).

The discussions above, regarding the critical size for the formation of a misfit loop, were based on global energy considerations. An alternate view point is based on a local force balance (Kumar et al. 2013a). The local forces on the loop involve radial and circumferential/tangential forces, and off interface stability is a distinct possibility. It is interesting to note that a precipitate of a lower radius than the critical radius (i.e., $r_c < r^*$) can 'stabilize' an interfacial loop due to force balance on the loop. In this case, the line tension force tending to shrink the loop balances the coherency stresses trying to expand the loop. It is to be noted that at r_c it is not energetically favorable to form a loop. The value of r_c can be computed using:

$$r_c = \frac{b}{16\pi\,\omega\,(1-v)}\left[\ln\left(\frac{8r_c}{b}\right) + \frac{3-2v}{4(1-v)}\right] \quad (6)$$

Subsequent to the formation of a single interfacial misfit dislocation loop, two (Kumar et al. 2013b) and multiple loops can form, which progressively alleviate the coherency stresses and in the limiting case results in an incoherent interface. This scenario of coherent to semi-coherent transition in precipitates represents a 3D analog of that occurring in epitaxial films (Subramaniam 2004; 2003), wherein the edge component of the misfit dislocation is responsible for stress relief. Configurational forces on the dislocation have also been evaluated in these systems (Subramaniam and Ramakrishnan 2003), along with interesting effect arising from finite size domains (Arun Kumar and Kavitha and Anandh Subramaniam, 2012; Kumar and Subramaniam 2012b).

Figure 12 shows the FEM simulated stress state in the presence of precipitates of two different sizes. In (a), the precipitate is coherent, while in (b), it is semi-coherent. The

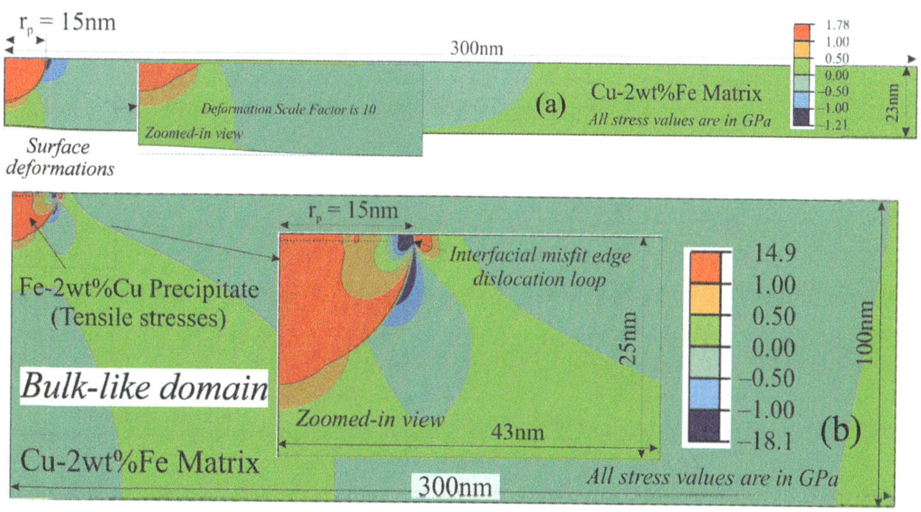

Fig. 12 Stress state (plot of σ_{yy} contours) due to coherent and semi-coherent precipitates. Symmetrical half of the film is shown in the figures. **a** Coherent precipitate in a nanoscale thin film (T = 46 nm). The inset shows a zoomed-in view, highlighting domain deformations arising due to the coherency stresses. **b** The state of stress in the presence of interfacial misfit edge dislocation loop in a 'thick' domain with T = 200 nm. The radius of the precipitate (r_p) is 10 nm

deformation of the domain due to the stress fields is to be noted in (a). The reversal in the state of stress (from tension to compression) due to the change in the character of the interface (in the vicinity of the dislocation) is to be noted.

Figure 13a, b shows methodology to determine the critical size (r^*). Figure 13a shows the plots of strain energy of the system as a function of the radius of the precipitate (r_p), with and without a misfit dislocation loop, in a 'bulk domain' (the thickness of the film (T) is 200 nm). Figure 13b shows the corresponding plot for a thin film (T = 46 nm). It is seen that at smaller sizes of the precipitate, the energy of the system increases on the introduction of a misfit loop. The

Fig. 13 Plot of strain energy of the system as a function of the radius of the precipitate (r_p), with and without a misfit dislocation loop: **a** bulk domain (T = 200 nm) and **b** nanoscale thin film (T = 46 nm). The intersection of the two curves gives the value of critical radius (r^*). (c) Variation in the critical radius (r^*) with the thickness of the film (T). Below a thickness of about 40 nm (= T^*), the coherent state is stabilized

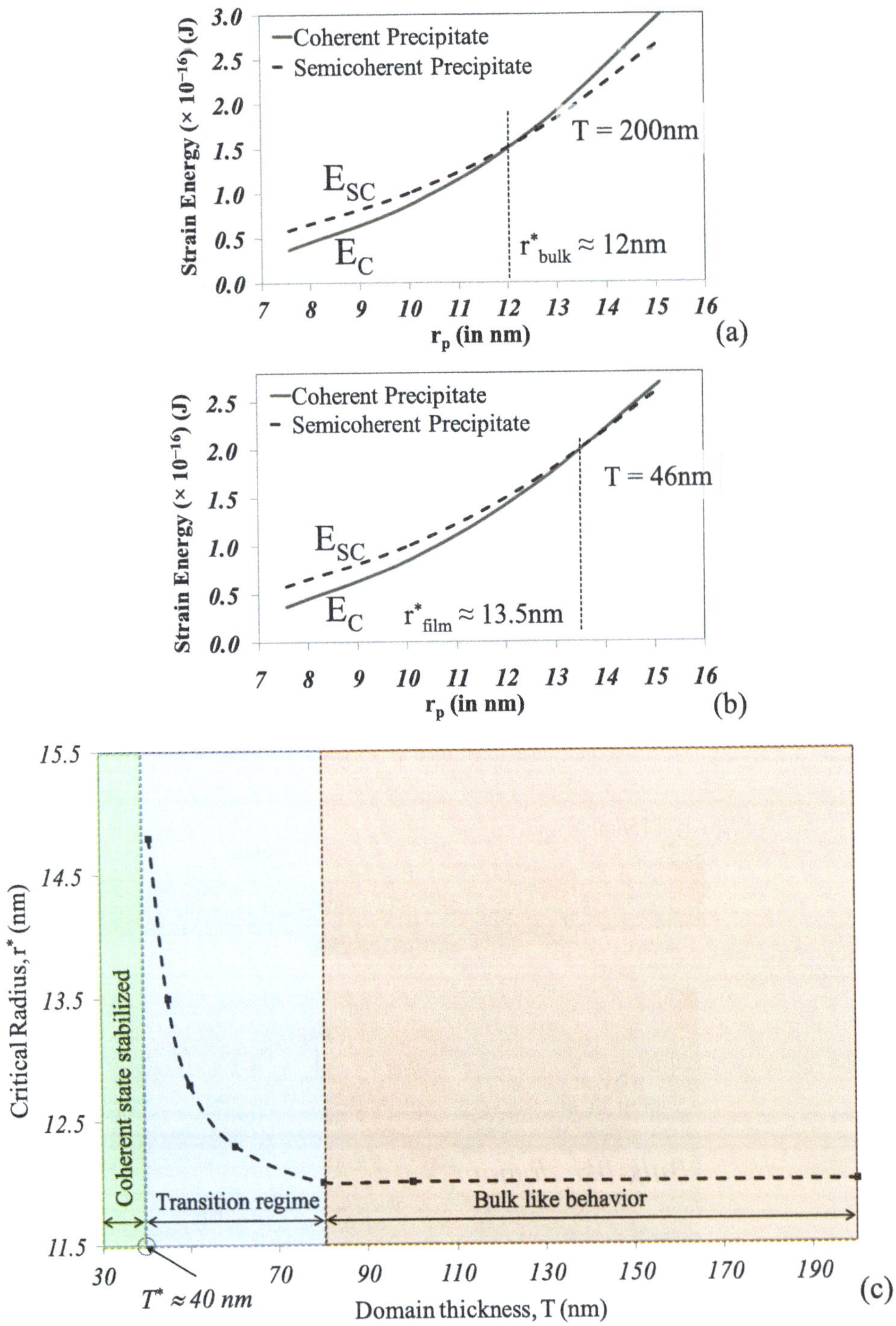

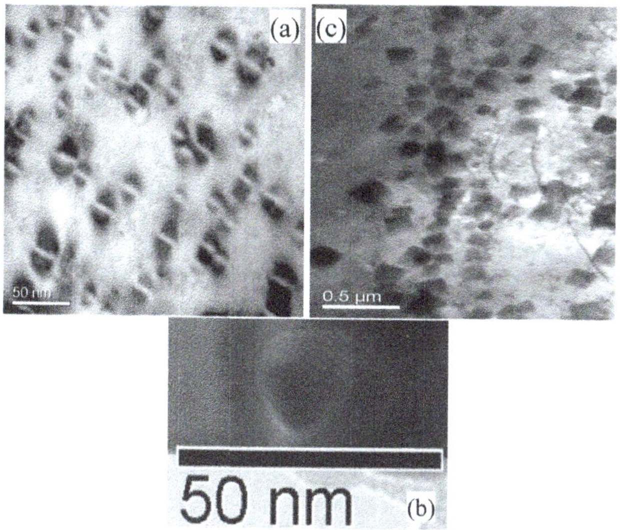

Fig. 14 TEM micrographs depicting the three stages during the growth of precipitates in a bulk sample. **a** A bright field image showing the coffee bean contrast associated with coherent precipitates (aged at 550 °C for 12 h). **b** Moiré fringe contrast arising due to an array of misfit dislocations at the interface of a semi-coherent precipitate (aged at 550 °C for 24 h). **c** Cuboidal incoherent precipitates, which lack strain field contrast (aged at 750 °C for 48 h). The value of the critical size r^* determined experimentally is about 11 nm

cross-over of the curves represents the critical size beyond which the semi-coherent state is energetically stabilized. As the thickness of the film is decreased, the strain energy due to a coherent precipitate reduces. Below a certain value of the thickness of the domain, the magnitude of r^* shows a sharp increase (Fig. 13c). It is seen from the figure that below a thickness of about 40 nm (labeled as T^*) the coherent state is stabilized.

In Fig. 14, we can see the different stages occurring during precipitate growth: (a) coherent precipitates (with strain field contrast), (b) semi-coherent precipitate (with moiré fringe contrast), and (c) incoherent precipitates. The typical 'coffee bean' contrast in the bright field image arises due to strain fields associated with the coherent precipitate (the crystal planes are locally bent to be at the Braggs' condition). An array of misfit loops decorates the interface in the semi-coherent precipitate and gives rise to the Moiré fringe contrast. This represents the partially relaxed state. On further growth, the precipitates lose their coherency and become cuboidal in shape.

In Fig. 15, precipitation has been carried out in a TEM sample (which is a thin film). The sizes of the coherent precipitates are to be noted. The deviation from the typical coffee bean contrast in the BFI is also to be noted. The heat treatment process has led to a variation in the thickness of the sample. This is best appreciated by creating a thickness map using scanning transmission electron microscopy (STEM) (Fig. 16). This local variations in thickness can play a role in the stabilization of coherent state (Rani et al. 2015).

In the picture presented above, certain interesting features have been omitted. Regarding precipitates in finite domains (like thin cylinders), the coherent state is stabilized in two different size regimes of the precipitate: one at small sizes and other at large sizes. In the intermediate size regime, the semi-coherent state is stable (Rani et al. 2017). This is reminiscent of the reentrant phase transition in condensed matter systems. This picture is true for cylinder diameters above a certain critical value. A phase diagram can be drawn, demarcating regions of stability of the coherent and semi-coherent states (Rani et al. 2017).

2.4 Surface Stress Actuated Lattice Expansion in Metal Nanoshells

We have already noted that surface stress can have profound effects in finite domains. Surface stress is tensile in metallic materials and can be compressive in polar surfaces. In nanocrystals, the compression induced by tensile surface stress can cause a reduction in the lattice parameter (Kumar and Subramaniam 2013b), and this fact has remained an unchallenged observation. In hollow metallic structures, the stress on the outer surface tends to compress the material, while that on the inner surface has the opposite effect. Hence, the resultant between the stress existing in the inner and outer surfaces determines the altered lattice parameter. Thus, hollow metal shells are an interesting class of structures, wherein there is interplay between geometry, stress, and scale. It is noteworthy that hollow spheres have been investigated in diverse contexts, which include anodes for batteries (Iyer et al. 2016), gas entrapment (Zheng et al. 2014; Shervani et al. 2017), and drug delivery (Subramaniam 2020).

Surface stress can be simulated by a two-scale methodology (Kumar and Subramaniam 2013b). The method was developed based on a concept proposed by Shuttleworth (Amstad and Reimhult 2012), wherein the atoms constituting a surface is brought into registry with the bulk by the introduction of biaxial eigenstrains. The parts to this computation are: (i) the determination of the lattice parameter of a layer (or bilayer) of atoms using density functional theory (DFT) and (ii) use of this value in a finite element model to compute the surface stress. The methodology allows us to study the effect of inner and outer surface stresses independently. This approach, albeit being approximate, can be

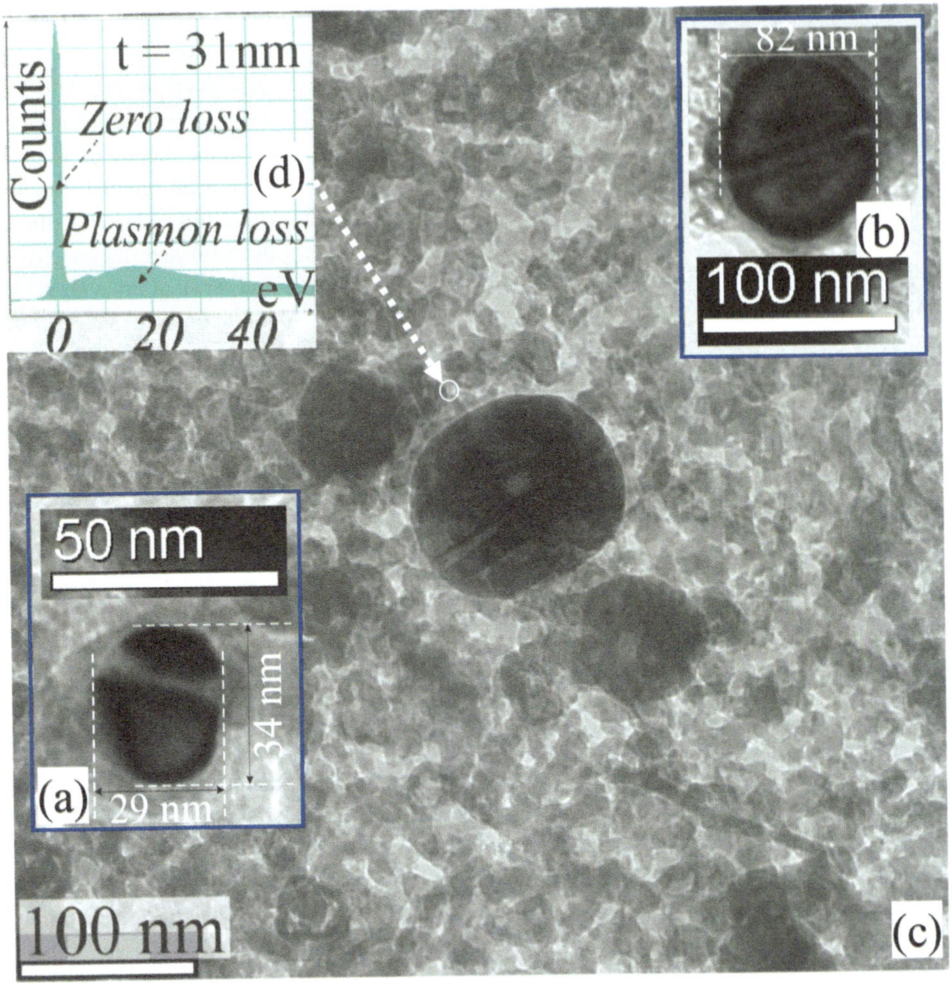

Fig. 15 TEM bright field images indicating the presence of coherent precipitates in thin film samples (**a–c**). The variation from the typical coffee bean contrast is to be noted. The sizes of the precipitate are considerably larger than r^*_{bulk}. **d** EELS spectrum is used to determine the local thickness

applied to lengthscales, wherein techniques like molecular dynamics prove to be time-consuming.

Let us consider a Ni nanoshell with an outer diameter (OD) of 80 nm and study the effect of varying shell thickness on the lattice parameter. By 'switching on' the outer and inner surface stress independently, we can study their effects on the lattice parameter, followed by a simulation, wherein the combined effect can be evaluated. The lattice parameter under consideration is along the radial direction (a_{radial}). Figure 17 shows the variation in lattice parameter with shell thickness. Three regimes can be identified in the plot: (i) thick shell (R1), (ii) thin shell (R2), and (iii) very thin shell (R3). In the thick shell regime (R1), the behavior is similar to that for a nanoparticle, wherein there is a reduction in a_{radial}. This occurs due to the domination of the outer surface stress (over the inner surface stress). In the case of thin shells (region R2), the reverse of the thick shell case is observed (i.e., the inner surface stress dominates over the outer one), and this leads to an increase in a_{radial}. This is an interesting result, as this is the first time that surface stress-mediated lattice expansion has been reported, in a metallic system. In both the regimes R1 and R2, the outer surface stress tends to compress the particle; which is but expected. The strange feature in the plot is R3, wherein the outer surface stress causes an expansion of the lattice. This implies that in R3 the lattice expansion is even more pronounced.

At the heart of this effect is the role of the Poisson's ratio (ν), and this can be evaluated by artificially varying the magnitude of 'ν' in the simulations (discrete points in Fig. 17). For values of 'ν' above the natural value for that for Ni (ν_{Ni} = 0.34), the effect is accentuated, while for lower values, the opposite is observed. For a value of $\nu < 0.2$, the anomalous behavior vanishes.

Experimentally, Ni hollow spheres are easy to synthesize, and hence, results obtained can be compared with the

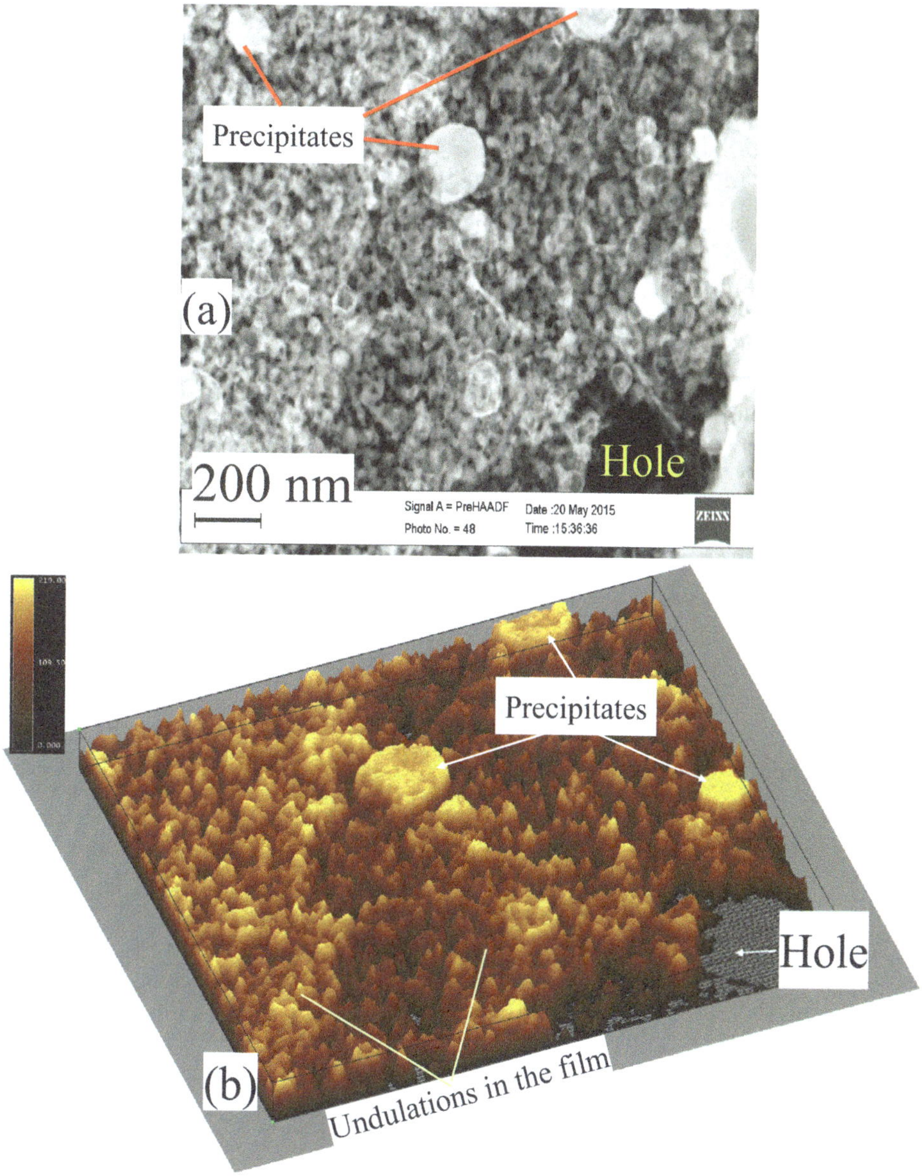

Fig. 16 **a** STEM map from a region with a coherent precipitate. **b** A thickness profile computed from STEM map. The local variations in the thickness are to be noted

computations. The effect of internal pressure on the lattice parameter of Ni hollow spheres has also been investigated (Shuttleworth 1950). The experimental confirmation of the aforementioned computational observations comes via TEM investigations (Fig. 18). Three sample HRLFI are shown in the figure, corresponding to the three regimes. It is difficult to obtain lattice fringes from thick shells, and hence, this has been replaced by a sample nanocrystal. The dimensions of the nanostructures and the corresponding a_{radial} values obtained are as follows. (1) Nanoparticle (D = 6 nm): $a_{\mathrm{radial}}^{\mathrm{exp}}$ = 3.46 Å, (2) thin walled MNS (OD = 150 nm, t = 25 nm): $a_{\mathrm{radial}}^{\mathrm{exp}}$ = 3.63 Å, And (iii) very thin walled MNS (OD = 100 nm, t = 10 nm): $a_{\mathrm{radial}}^{\mathrm{exp}}$ = 3.81 Å. It is seen that the experimental observations corroborate well with the computational results (Iyer et al. 2017).

A point to be noted is that obtaining HRLFI of 'ideal quality' is very difficult. This arises from multiple factors like: the stability of the particle under the electron beam and the difficulty in obtaining lattice fringes perpendicular to the radial direction. Needless to point out, multiple samples need to be studied to obtain repeatable results.

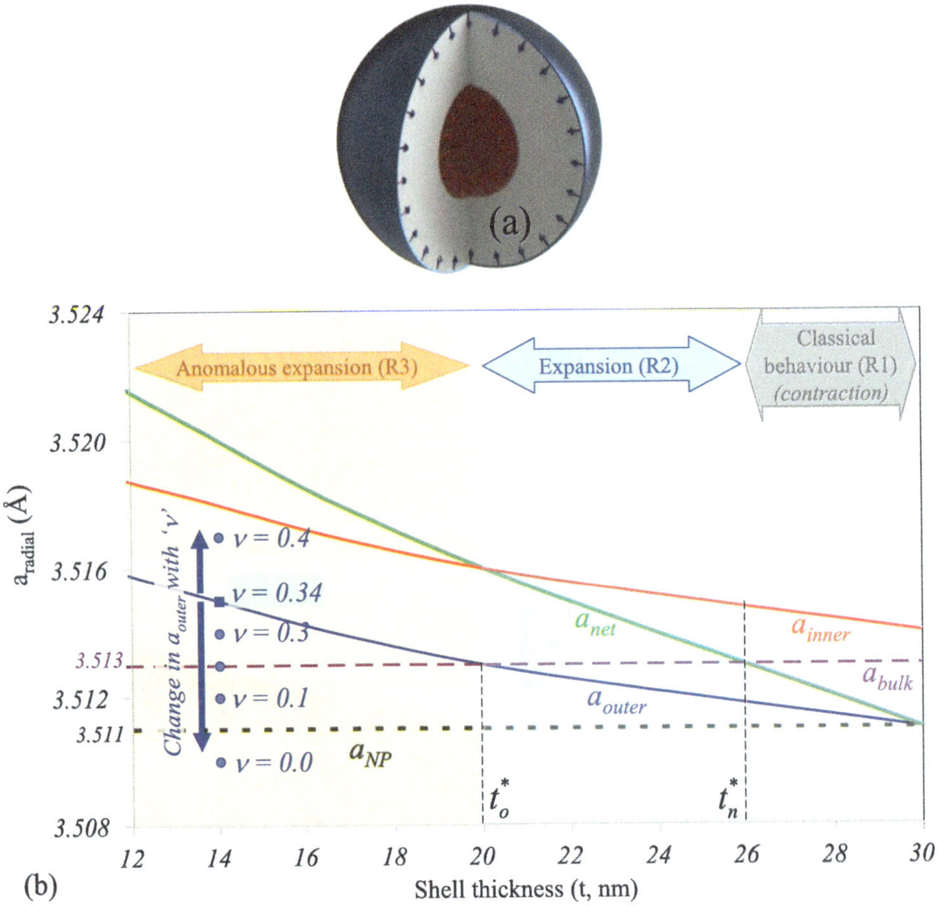

Fig. 17 **a** Schematic showing the effect of surface stresses existing on the outer and inner surfaces. **b** Variation in lattice parameter (a_{radial}) with shell thickness (Ni with OD = 80 nm). The effect of outer, inner, and combined surface stress on the lattice parameters is plotted as separate curves (labeled as a_{outer}, a_{inner}, and a_{net}). The effect of the value of Poisson's ratio on the lattice parameter (t = 14 nm, $\nu \in$ (0 to 0.5)) is overlaid on the figure. The horizontal lines correspond to the bulk lattice parameter (a_{bulk}^{Ni}) and that of a nanoparticle (a_{NP}). The nanoparticle has only outer surface stress acting on it

3 Musings

It is clear from the case studies considered that multiple tools are required to fully characterize the structures and to comprehend the physics involved. Multiple TEM techniques serve to reveal many facets of the sample and highlight the power of the tool.

If experimental techniques provide the 'body' of an investigation, then theories and computations endow it with a 'mind'. Hence, no investigation can be considered as complete without the synergistic role of experiments and computations. It is expected that better experimentation (along with the use of additional tools) and computations with higher accuracy can further unveil hitherto unanticipated secrets.

In one of the examples considered, it was noted that nanoscale effects are observed at relevant lengthscale of the order of few nanometers and 'bulk' behaviors was retrieved at a scale of greater than 12 nm. Specific systems have been considered to elucidate a specific effect (e.g., the Cu-Fe system was considered in the context of the stabilization of the coherent precipitate); however, it is expected that the observations have a much broader applicability.

4 Concluding Remarks

Transmission electron microscopy has proved to be a ubiquitous tool for the study of nanoscale structures and phenomena. Powerful computational tools have provided a firm conceptual footing to these investigations. Diverse techniques like high-resolution lattice fringe imaging, Fresnel contrast imaging and Moiré fringe imaging help unravel various facets related to the sample.

One can discover new effects and phenomena in nanocrystals, which have no 'bulk' counterparts. These include (i) the stabilization of the coherent precipitates, (ii) anomalous lattice expansion in hollow metallic shells, and (iii) 'liquid-like nucleation' in a solid-state diffusional transformation. Interestingly, surprises in this area are coming thick and fast and not surprisingly transmission electron microscopy is playing a major role in these discoveries.

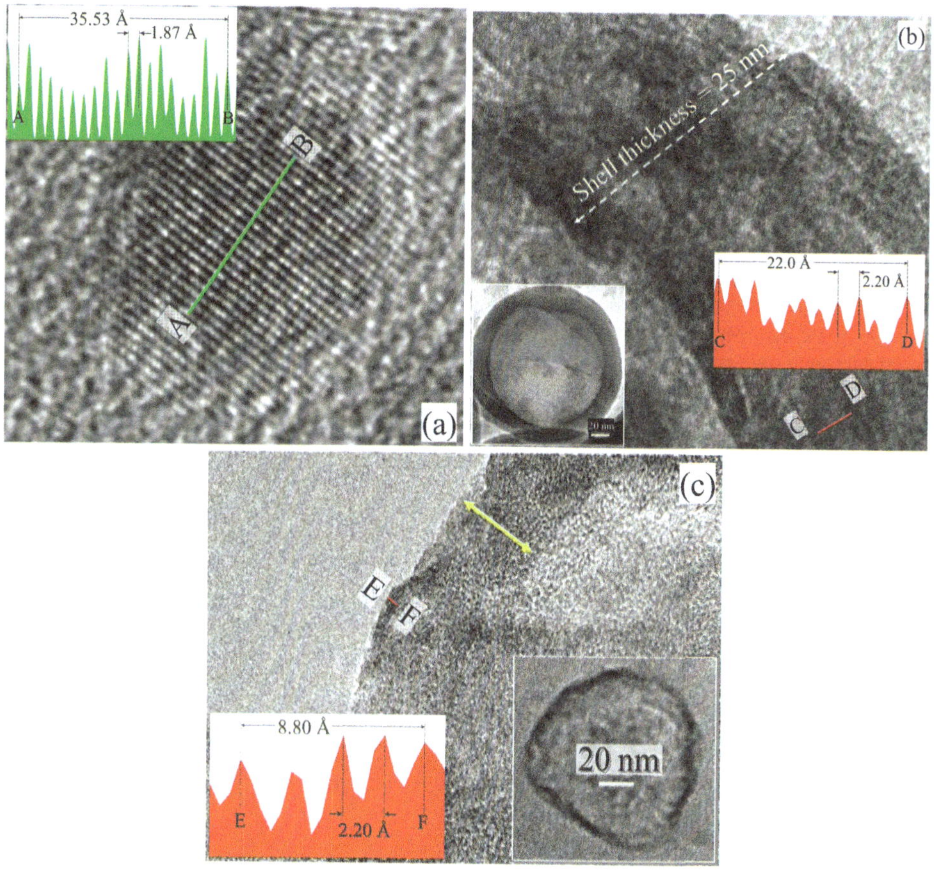

Fig. 18 HRLFI to determine the lattice parameter along the radial direction. **a** Nanoparticle (diameter = 6 nm). **b** A thin shell structure (OD = 150 nm, t = 25 nm). **c** A very thin shell structure (OD = 100 nm, t = 10 nm). The lattice spacing is measured using intensity patterns obtained across the lines in the HRLFI (AB, CD, and EF). Micrographs in the inset to (b) and (c) are bright field images from the hollow shells

The interconnectedness between stress, interfaces, and geometry may be considered ubiquitous, and it is expected that research with these facets in view will unveil amazing new phenomena and discoveries.

Acknowledgements The authors acknowledge the contributions of group members: Dr. Suboohi Sherwani and Dr. Pooja Rani for their contributions to the work, on which this article is based. Further we would like to acknowledge our collaborators and co-authors: Prof. Raj Pala, Dr. Raghvendra Tiwari, Dr. B. Vishwanadh, Prof. Somnath Bhattacharyya, Prof. Sri Sivakumar, Dr Gargi Mishra, Mr. Deb De, Prof. Kantesh Balani, Dr. Kawsar Ali, and Dr. Ashok Arya.

References

Albisetti AF, Biffi C, Tuissi A (2012) Synthesis and structural analysis of $Cu_{10}Zr_7$. J Alloys Compd 544:42

Amstad E, Reimhult E (2012) Nanoparticle actuated hollow drug delivery vehicles. Nanomed J 7:145

Kumar A, Kavitha KG, Subramaniam A (2012) Interfacial edge dislocation Interactions with free-surfaces in nanocrystals. J Nanosci Nanotechnol 11:1

Baser TA, Baricco M (2008) Glass forming ability of $(Cu_{50}Zr_{50})_{96}M_4$ (M=None, Al, Nb) bulk metallic glasses. Rev Adv Mater Sci 18:71

Bhattacharyya S, Subramaniam A, Koch CT, Ruhle M (2006) Aspects regarding measurement of thickness of Intergranular glassy films. J Microsc 221:46

Bollmann W (1970) Crystal Defects and Crystalline Interfaces. Springer-Verlag, Berlin

Brown LM, Woolhouse GR, Valdrè U (1968) Radiation-induced Coherency Loss in a Cu-Co Alloy. Philos Mag 17:781

David A (2009) Porter. Phase Transformations in Metals and Alloys, CRC Press, Boca Raton, Kenneth E. Esterling and Mohamed Y. Sharif

Eshelby JD (1953) Screw dislocations in thin rods. J Appl Phys 24:176

Gupta A, Shervani S, Amaladasse F, Sivakumar S, Balani K, Subramaniam A (2019) Enhanced reversible hydrogen storage in Nickel Nano hollow spheres. Int J Hydrog Energy 44:22032

Hirth JP, Lothe J (1968) Theory of Dislocations. McGraw-Hill, New York

Iyer G, De D, Kumar A, Pala R, Subramaniam A (2016) two scale simulation of surface stress in solids and its effects. Appl Surf Sci 371:343

Iyer G, Shervani S, Mishra G, De D, Kumar A, Sivakumar S, Balani K, Pala R, Subramaniam A (2017) Poisson effect driven anomalous lattice expansion in metal nanoshells. Appl Phys Lett 110:131603

Jesser WA (1969) On the theory of loss of coherency by spherical precipitates. Philos Mag 19:993

Suresh K, Radhakrishnan TK, Kalaichelvi P (2016) A review of classical and nonclassical nucleation theories. Cryst Growth Des 16:6663

Khanikar P, Subramaniam A (2010) Critical size for edge dislocation free-standing nanocrystals by finite element method. J Nano Res 10:93

Kumar A, Subramaniam A (2011) Materials analogue of zero stiffness structures. Philos Mag Lett 91:272

Kumar A, Subramaniam A (2012a) Stable edge dislocations in finite crystals. Philos Mag 92:2947

Kumar A, Subramaniam A (2012b) Finite substrate effects on critical thickness in epitaxial systems. J Adv Mater Res 585:39
Kumar A, Subramaniam A (2013a) Negative, zero and positive stiffness in extended Eshelby plates. Philos Mag Lett 93:703
Kumar A, Subramaniam A (2013b) Position dependant critical thickness in finite epitaxial systems. Appl Surf Sci 275:60
Kumar A, Kaur G, Subramaniam A (2013a) Critical sizes for coherent to semicoherent transformation in precipitates. Int J Mater Res 104:1171
Kumar A, Gautam M, Subramaniam A (2013b) On the Formation and Stability of Two Misfit Dislocations in the Cu-γFe System. J Mech Mater Struct 7:135
Kumar A, Gautam M, Subramaniam A (2014) Critical sizes for the stabilization of coherent precipitates. J Appl Phys 115:193509
Malis T, Cheng SC, Egerton RF (1988) EELS log-ratio technique for specimen thickness measurement in the TEM. J Electron Microsc Tech 8:193
Matthews JW (1979) In: FRN Nabarro (eds.), Dislocations in Solids. North-Holland Publishing Company, New York
Nabarro FRN (1967) Theory of crystal dislocations. Clarendon Press, Oxford, p 75
Nalwa, Singh H, Ed (2004) Encyclopedia of nanoscience and nanotechnology. American Scientific Publishers, Los Angeles, p 10
Rani P, Raghavendra RM, Subramaniam A (2020) On the variability of critical size for homogeneous nucleation in a solid-state diffusional transformation. arXiv:2007.02112
Raghavendra RM, Ganesh Iyer D, Kumar A, Subramaniam A (2018) Surface stress mediated image force and torque on an edge dislocation. Philos Mag 98:1731
Rani P, Kumar A, Vishwanadh B, Bhattacharyya S, Tewari R, Subramaniam A (2015) Stabilization of coherent precipitates in nanoscale thin films. Philos Mag 95:4130
Rani P, Kumar A, Vishwanadh B, Ali K, Arya A, Tewari R, Subramaniam A (2017) Liquid like nucleation in free-standing nanoscale films. Nanoscale (Communication) 9:12283
Schodek D, Ferreira P, Ashby M (2009) Nanomaterials, nanotechnologies and design: an introduction to engineers and architects. Butterworth-Heinemann
Shervani S, Mukherjee P, Gupta A, Mishra G, Illath K, Ajithkumar TG, Sivakumar S, Sen P, Balani K, Subramaniam A (2017) Multi-mode Hydrogen Storage in Nanocontainers. Int J Hydrog Energy 42:24256
Shuttleworth R (1950) The surface tension of solids. Proc Phys Soc A 63:444
Subramaniam A (2004) Critical thickness of equilibrium epitaxial thin films using finite element method. J Appl Phys 95:8472
Subramaniam A, Shervani S, Gupta A, Balani K (2020) Gases in nanocontainers, smart nanocontainers: micro and nano technologies. Elsevier p 499
Subramaniam A, Balani K, http://home.iitk.ac.in/~anandh/E-book.htm.
Subramaniam A, Ramakrishnan N (2003) Analysis of thin film growth using finite element method. Surf Coat Tech 167:249
Subramaniam A, Kumar A (2014) Edge dislocations in finite crystals: special effects and strange phenomena. Mech Solids Directions 14:88
Watanabe D, Watanabe C, Monzen R (2008) Effect of coherency on coarsening of second-phase precipitates in Cu-base alloys. J Mater Sci 43:3946
Woolhouse GR, Ipohorski M (1971) On the interaction between radiation damage and coherent precipitates. Proc R Soc A 324:415
Zheng G, Lee SW, Liang Z, Lee HW, Yan K, Yao H et al (2014) Interconnected hollow carbon nanospheres for stable lithium metal anodes, Nat Nanotechnol 9:618

Machine Write Up

JEOL 7100F FESEM: Advanced Center for Materials Science

JEOL 7100 field-emission scanning electron microscope (FESEM) was commissioned in service, in latter half of 2014. Ever since, this machine has been giving service to the entire IITK campus community, and beyond, day in and day out. It has run for over 4000 h for imaging and over 5000 h for EBSD. This state-of-the-art equipment is capable of resolving upto 3 nm at 15 kV. It is equipped with an ET detector (SE) and a retractable BSE detector. It has a Zr-O/W emitter. Some of the features of the equipment are.

Accelerating Voltage: 0.5 to 30 kV

Probe Current: 10^{-12} to 2 x 10^{-7} A

Tilt: -5°–70°

Rotation: 360°

Apart from these, it is equipped with some state of the art accessories which further enhance its characterization abilities.

EDS: Oxford Nano Analysis

EBSD: Oxford Nordlys detector

Stage: Gatan MT 2000E High temperature tensile stage (Tensile load: 5 KN; Temperature: RT to 500 °C)

Who can get time on this machine: Anyone from the country can make a request for time on this machine; however, researchers of IITK are given a preference.

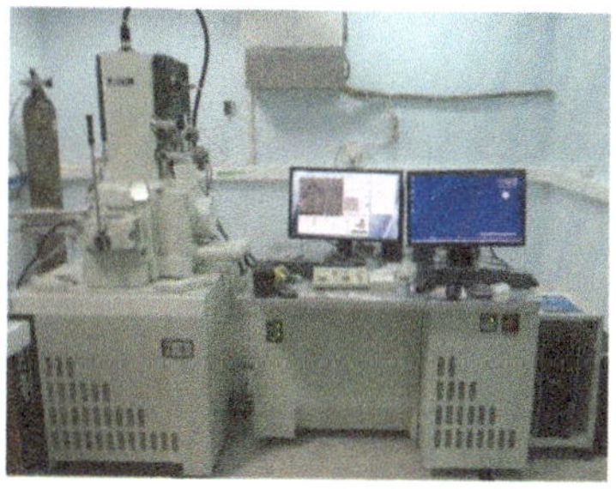

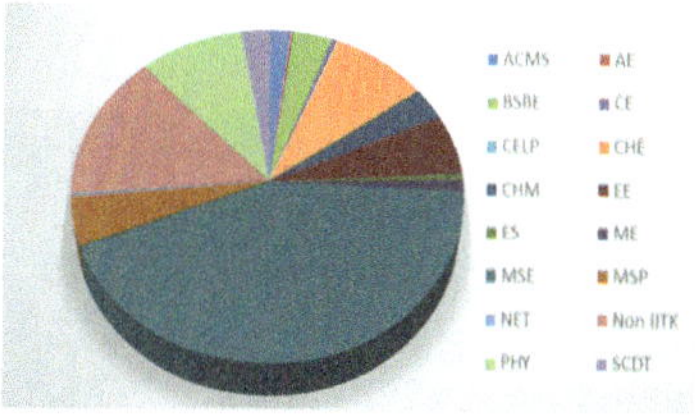

How to book: Researchers from IITK can book through the online booking system, the link to which is at ACMS website. Others can contact the concerned person. This facility would soon be available on I-STEM.

Contact		
Mr. M. Siva Kumar	**ACMS-112;**	**Email**: **rmuthu@iitk.ac.in**
P.I. Prof. Kantesh Balani	**Biomaterials lab**	**Email**: **kbalani@iitk.ac.in**

K. Biswas et al. (eds.), *Electron Microscopy in Science and Engineering*, IITK Directions 6,
https://doi.org/10.1007/978-981-16-5101-4

JEOL JSM 6010 LAW-SEM: Advanced Center for Materials Science

This is a compact SEM for the quick image analysis with high resolution and compositional information. The integral EDS detector can be used for micro-compositional analysis.

BSE Resolution: 5 mn at 20 kV

Magnification: 5–300000x

Accelerating voltage: 0.5 to 20 kV

Automatic SEM condition set-up based on sample type

Who can get time on this machine: Anyone from the country can make a request for time on this machine; however, researchers of IITK are given a preference.

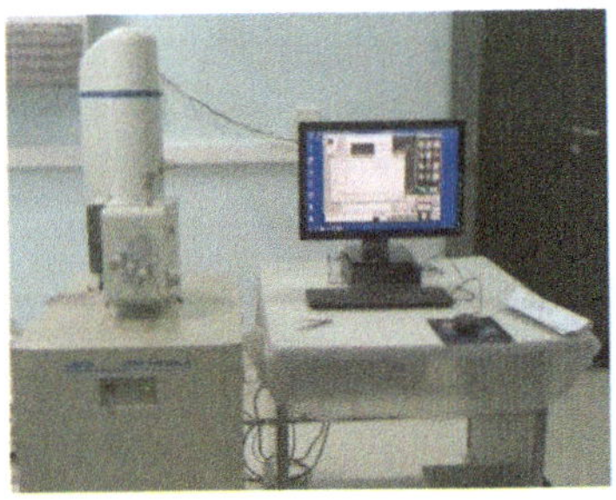

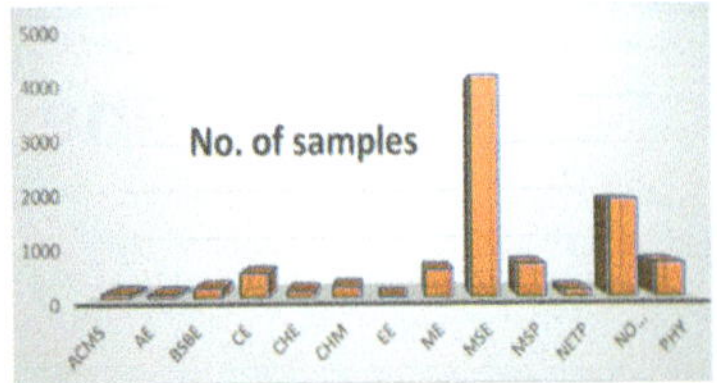

How to book: Researchers from IITK can book through the online booking system, the link to which is at ACMS website. Others can contact the concerned person. This facility would soon be available on I-STEM.

Contact		
Mr. M. Siva Kumar	**ACMS-112;**	**Email: rmuthu@iitk.ac.in**
P.I. Prof. Kantesh Balani	**Biomaterials lab**	**Email: kbalani@iitk.ac.in**

FEI QUANTA 200 W-SEM: Advanced Center for Materials Science

FEI Quanta 200 is a tungsten filament based scanning electron microscope (W-SEM). This equipment is more than 15 years old and still functioning as new. This equipment provides very high resolution SE and BSE images.

All types of materials ranging from metals to ceramic to powders to polymers, and even biological samples can be analysed in this machine. Some of the features of the equipment are:

SE Resolution: 2 nm at 20 kV

Accelerating Voltage: 0.5–30 k V

Magnification: 5–500,000X

Who can get time on this machine: Anyone from the country can make a request for time on this machine; however, researchers of IITK are given a preference.

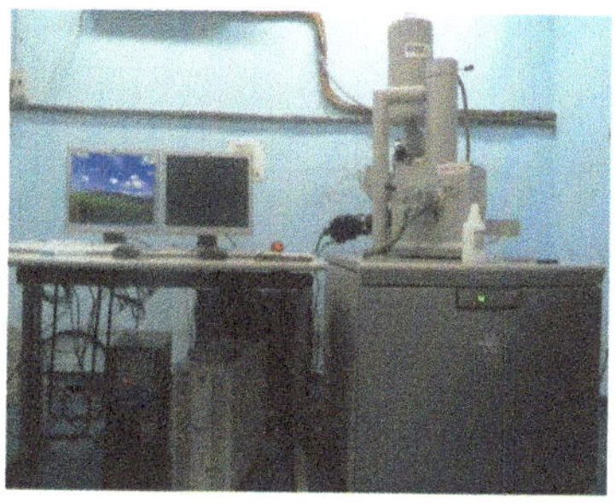

Contact		
Mr. M. Siva Kumar	**ACMS-112;**	**Email**: **rmuthu@iitk.ac.in**
P.I. Prof. Kantesh Balani	**Biomaterials lab**	**Email**: **kbalani@iitk.ac.in**

How to book: Researchers from IITK can book through the online booking system, the link to which is at ACMS website. Others can contact the concerned person. This facility would soon be available on I-STEM.

EVO 18 SEM: Biomedical Science and Bioengineering

EVO 18 SEM is an environmental scanning electron microscope (E-SEM) from Carl Zeiss, Germany. This equipment was installed in BSBE at 2011 and since then it has been operational continuously for 10 years now. The equipment is capable of imaging/analysing various types of samples, for example, metals, ceramics, and polymers, and hydrated samples, for example biological.

Filament: Tungsten

Secondary e-image resolution: 50 nm (Depends on sample)

E-SEM mode: The Variable pressure detector can analyze non-conducting and hydrated samples

BSE Detector: Available

EDX detector: Available

Tilt: 0°-60°

Rotation: 360° Degree

EHT: 200 V–30 kV **Magnification**: **50** ~ 100 K (Depends on sample)

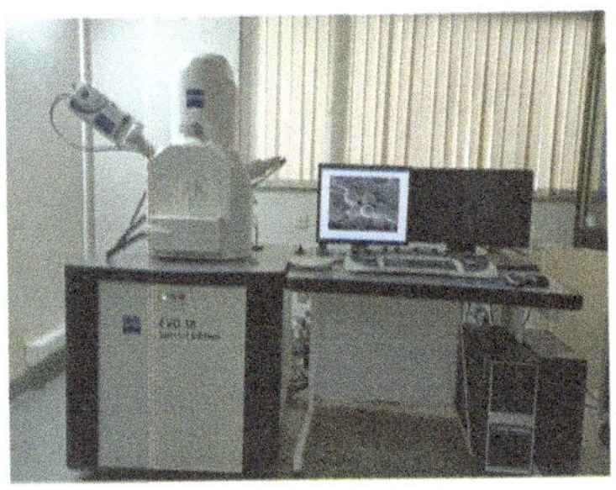

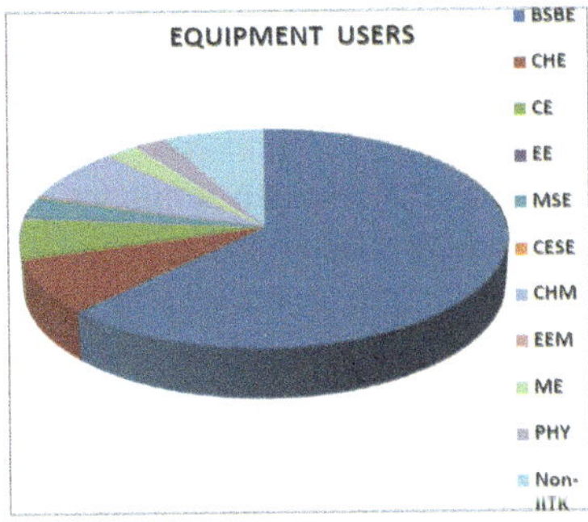

Who can get time on this machine: Anyone from the country can make a request for time on this machine; however, researchers of IITK are given a preference.

How to book: Researchers from IITK can book through an e-mail to the operator, for which the contact details are available at BSBE website.

Contact		
Mrs. Shraddha Singh	**BSBE T-111;**	**Email: ssinghs@iitk.ac.in**
P.I. Prof. D.S. Katti	**BSBE LN 16**	**Email: dsk@iitk.ac.in**

Field Emission Gun-Scanning Electron Microscope: Chemical Engineering

Post Graduate Research Laboratory (PGRL) is a user facility in the Department of Chemical Engineering at IIT Kanpur that provides sophisticated instruments and services for academic and industrial researchers to explore various research problems and address a variety of scientific and engineering challenges. In-house equipments at PGRL include a TESCAN high resolution Field Emission Gun-Scanning Electron Microscope (FESEM) MIRA[3] with STEM detector also by TESCAN and an EDS detector by OXFORD.

Salient Features of the Electron Microscope and the Detectors:

PGRL has a high brightness Schottky emitter field emission scanning electron microscope which offers multiple imaging modes for high-resolution imaging, wide field-of-view, or large depth-of-focus. The microscope can be operated at accelerating voltages from 1 to 30 kV. Imaging at very high resolution (1 nm at 30 keV and 2 nm at 1 keV) is possible with certain types of specimens. Its superb performance, particularly at low accelerating voltages (*i.e.*, 0.2–1 kV using Beam Deceleration Mode), makes it especially suitable for imaging the surface detail of polymeric, biological, and other low-density materials. In-lens (In-Beam Mode) secondary and back-scattered electron detectors enable very short working distances. Standard chamber secondary and back-scattered electron detectors are also available for larger working distances, and thus, larger fields of view.

Energy Dispersive Spectroscopy (EDS) Analysis provides elemental and chemical analysis of a sample inside the SEM with options of Point & ID and detailed elemental maps. The EDS detector at PGRL is LN_2 free type based on latest Silicon Drift Detector technology. It has a large SDD crystal size of 50 mm^2. The detectable element range is from Beryllium (Be) to Californium (Cf). The EDS system has following resolution Carbon (better than 56 eV), Fluorine (better than 65 eV) and Mangenese (better than 124 eV).

The TESCAN-STEM detector with simultaneous Bright Field (BF) and Dark Field (DF) imaging have a resolution of 0.8 nm at 30 kV. The detector consists of three semiconductor sensors for bright field and dark field imaging. Simultaneous acquisition has been provided for bright and dark field imaging and mixing of these two signals is also possible.

Contact

MR. Rajesh Singh	**PGRL-302**	**Email**: **rajeshsg@iitk.ac.in**
P.I. Dr. Debjani Banerjee	**PGRL-302**	**Email**: **debjani@iitk.ac.in**

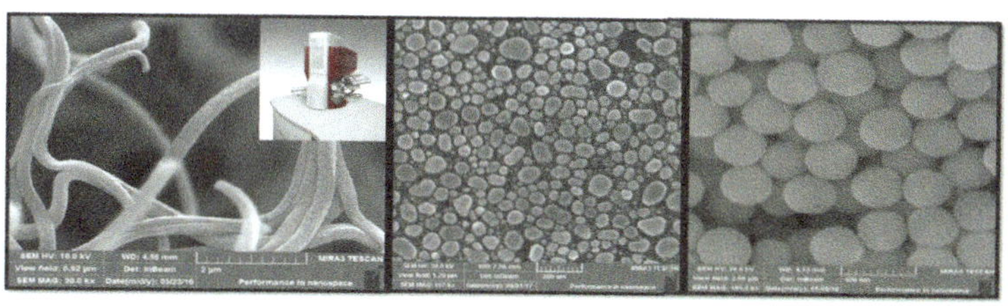

FEI Nova NanoSEM 450: Materials Science and Engineering

Nova NanoSEM 450 field-emission scanning electron microscope (FESEM) was commissioned in service, in the latter half of 2015. Ever since, this machine has been giving service not only to the entire IITK community but also to other academic institutes and industry all across the country. The primary features of the FESEM are as follows:

Resolution: 1.0 nm @ 15 kV Accelerating Voltage: 200 V–30 kV

Max Probe Current: 100 nA XY = 110 mm, Z = 25 mm, Tilt = +75 to −15°, 5 axis, motorized, eucentric stage Various Detectors:

In-lens SE detector (TLD-SE) Everhardt-Thornley SE Detector Low vacuum SE Detector (LVD) BSD in all modes

Continuous mixing of SE and BSE electrons

Integrated plasma cleaner. High and low vacuum operation. Apart from these, it is equipped with some state of the art accessories which further enhance its Characterization abilities.

TEAM-EDS Basic analysis system for SEM include OCTANE Plus. TEAM-EBSD Analysis system with Hikari XP

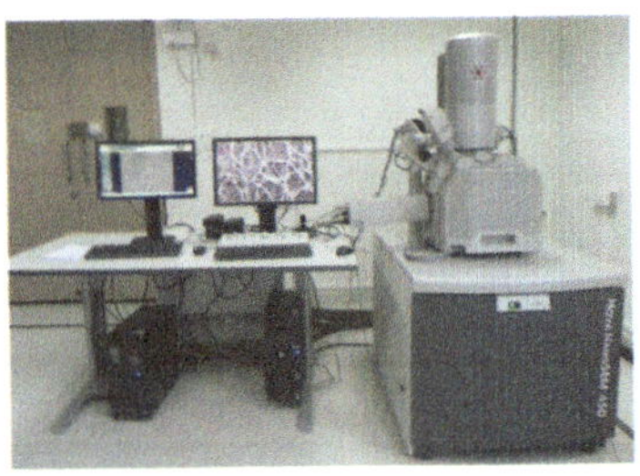

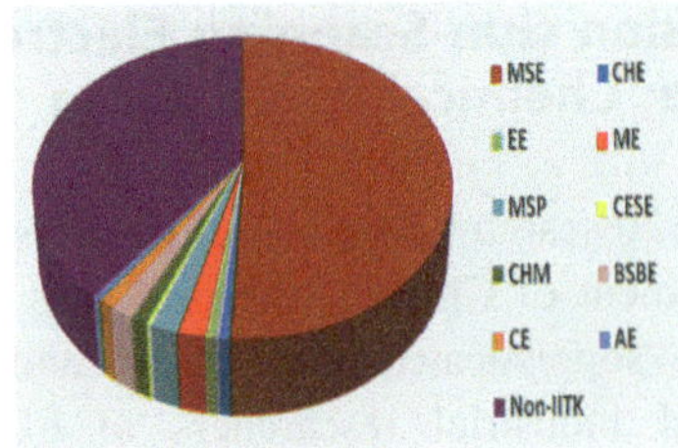

Who can get time on this machine: Anyone from the country can make a request for time on this machine; however, researchers of IITK are given a preference.

How to book: Researchers from IITK can book through the online booking system (Link: https://www.iitk.ac.in/mse/MSE-Facilities/SEM/) located in MSE website. Others can contact the concerned person mentioned below. This facility would soon be available on I-STEM.

Contact		
Ms. Samata Samal	**AIF-T101**	**Email**: **samata@iitk.ac.in**
P.I. Prof. Kantesh Balani	**Biomaterials Lab**	**Email**: **kbalani@iitk.ac.in**

CARL ZEISS EVO 50: Materials Science and Engineering

The CARL ZEISS EVO 50 has been in service since 2007. Ever since, this machine has been giving service not only to the entire IITK community but also to other academic institutes and industry all across the country. This SEM runs with Tungsten electron gun, which gives the highest current stability among all types of emitters.

Accelerating Voltage: 0.2–30 kV

Probe Current: 10^{-12} to 4.91 x 10^{-6}A

5-Axes Motorised Compucentric

Specimen Stage $X = 80$ mm

$Y = 80$ mm

$Z = 35$ mm

$T = 0°–90°$

$R = 360°$ (continuous)

Resolution: 3.0 nm @ 30 kV

Detectors: SE in HV-Everhart–Thornley BSD in all modes quadrant semiconductor diode

Apart from these, it is equipped with some state of the art accessories which further enhance its characterization abilities.

EDS: Oxford Nano Analysis

EBSD: Oxford Nordlys detector

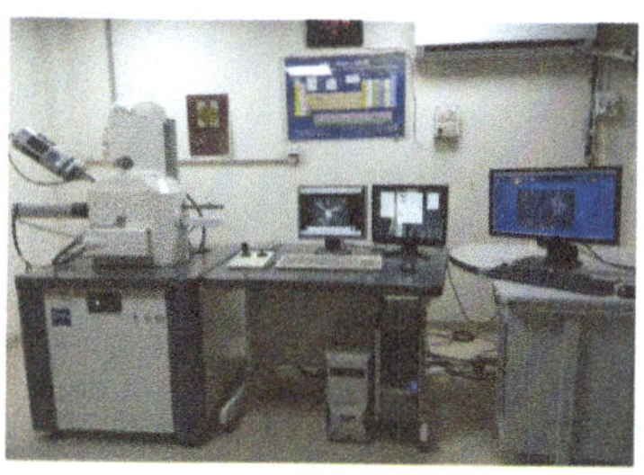

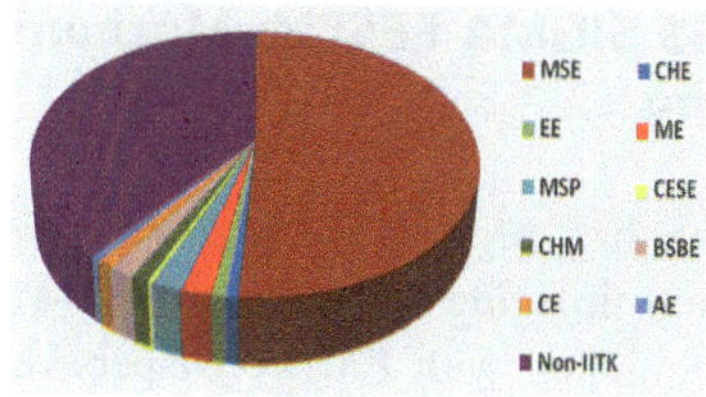

Who can get time on this machine: Anyone from the country can make a request for time on this machine; however, researchers of IITK are given a preference.

How to book: Researchers from IITK can book through the online booking system (Link: https://www.iitk.ac.in/mse/MSE-Facilities/SEM/) located in MSE website. Others can contact the concerned person mentioned below. This facility would soon be available on I-STEM.

Contact		
Ms. Samata Samal	**WL-103A**	**Email**: **samata@iitk.ac.in**
P.I. Prof. Kantesh Balani	**Biomaterials Lab**	**Email**: **kbalani@iitk.ac.in**

CARL ZEISS SIGMA FESEM: Mechanical Engineering

This machine has been in service since 2011. It has a high-resolution imaging capability with a resolution of 5 nm. It is equipped with Energy Dispersive Spectroscopy (EDS) from Oxford Instruments for identifying and quantifying elemental compositions and a retractable Backscatter Electron (BSE) Detector to effectively display the compositional differences in the specimen. This machine is fitted with Evacuator Plasma de-contaminator for clearer images with soft non-conducting materials. A sputter coater is available for gold coating. Apart from these, Gatan 300 N micro-tensile stage is also available.

Features: Acceleration Voltage: 0.1–30 kV

Stage: 5-axis motorised Cartesian, controlled through joysticks/software.

Tilt: −100 to 900

Rotation: 3600 continuous

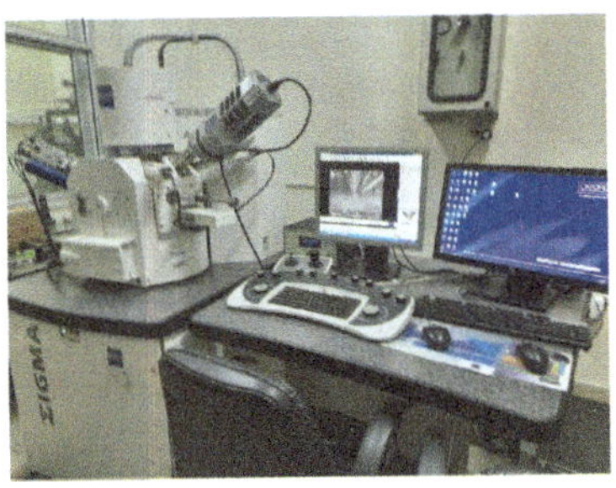

Booking: A slot can be booked by researchers from within or outside the institute. A slot request can be made through IITK Facility Management Portal. Slot request has to be made only 48 h before the commencement of the slot. Signed copy of the form has to be submitted to Mr. Anurag Goel (NL216).

Current Usage: The set-up is currently used by researchers from various academic departments of IIT Kanpur and the start-ups incubated at the SIIC IIT Kanpur.

Contact		
Ms. Mr. Anurag Goel	**NL-216**	**Email**: **agoel@iitk.ac.in**
P.I. Dr. Manjesh K. Singh	**Old IME Lab**	**Email**: **manjesh@iitk.ac.in**

Transmission Electron Microscope: Materials Science and Engineering

The Electron Microscope Facility (EM Facility) comprises a FEI Tecnai T20 Ultra Twin Transmission Electron Microscope. This microscope equipped with STEM detector, EDS detector, HAADF detector and Gatan digital imaging system. This microscope fitted with thermionic Gun compatible with W and LaB6, which operates at 200 kV. This analytical TEM provides nearly complete microstructural analysis such as imaging, micro-diffraction, nano-diffraction, CBED, lattice imaging, elemental analysis, STEM imaging, HAADF imaging for range of materials including metals, ceramics, semiconductors, thin films, polymers and biological materials. This machine attains a maximum resolution of 1.4 A° and the magnification extends up to 1 MX.

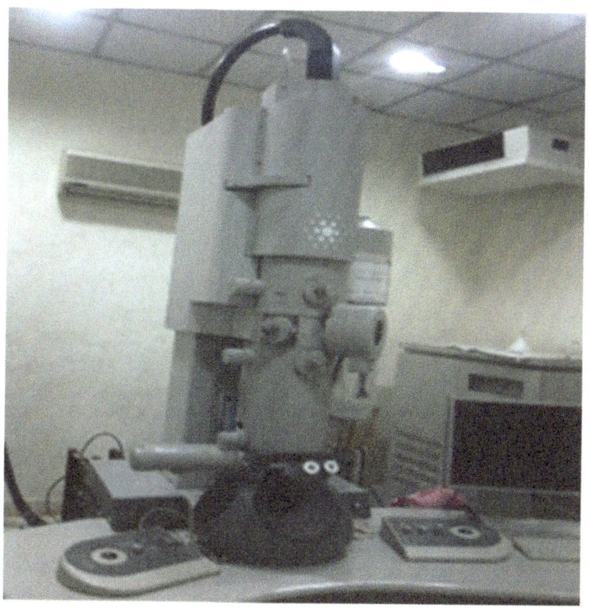

Contact		
Mr. Manohar Oraon	WL-207	Email: moraon@iitk.ac.in
P.I. Prof. Vivek Verma	FB-418	Email: vvivek@iitk.ac.in

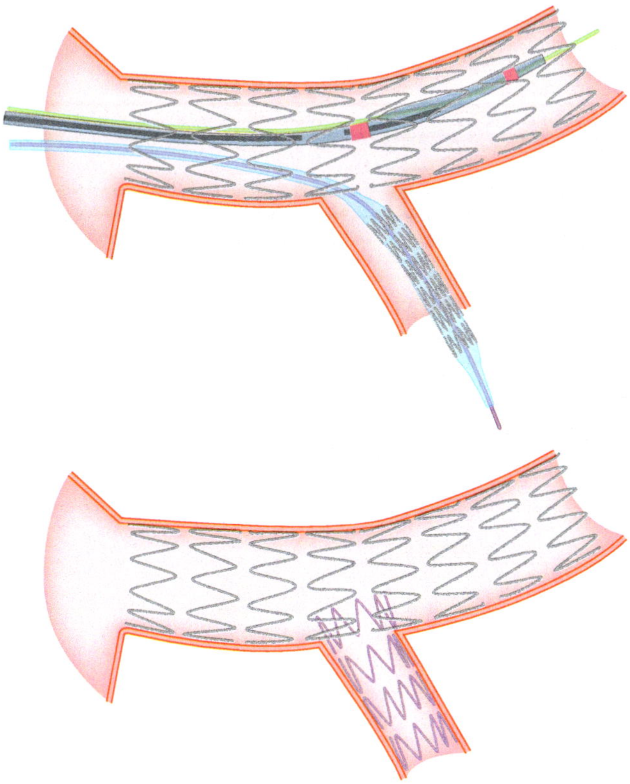

Fig. 4.25 T stenting. T stenting may be performed at the LM bifurcation if the SB (LCX) has a take-off angle of nearly 90 degrees and if the LCX has a small diameter

4.5 LM Trifurcation Stenting

Sometimes an additional artery arises at the bifurcation of the LM, forming a trifurcation. If this artery has a similar diameter to the LCX, it may be necessary to perform triple KBI and to implant stents in all three branches.

4.5.1 Stenting with (Triple) KBI

After stenting the LAD, you should perform KBI to achieve complete stent apposition and dilate the bifurcation to its normal diameter, as stated previously. As with bifurcation stenting, two-link stents should be implanted and the kissing balloons should be inflated at a relatively low pressure (8–10 atm) to avoid causing dissection/injury in non-stented segments of the SBs.

4.5.1.1 Lesion Preparation

You should follow the procedure recommended for bifurcation KBI. The individual branches should be adequately prepared to ensure that sufficient dilation can be achieved by low-pressure balloon inflation. The objectives of triple KBI are to reduce the risk of SB compromise by plaque shift or carina shift and to estimate the responsiveness of the distal LM bifurcation to low-pressure balloon angioplasty. When the LM bifurcation can be reliably expected to show low responsiveness, you should consider performing triple KBI with Lacrosse NSE balloons in order to optimize preparation of the trifurcation lesion.

4.5.1.2 Stent Placement

After implanting a stent in the LAD, you should perform POT and then triple KBI according to the following procedure (Fig. 4.26): (1) insert a new guidewire into the high lateral (HL) branch via the Crusade catheter; (2) perform KBI in the LAD and the HL branch; (3) insert a guidewire into the LCX via the Crusade catheter advanced along the HL guidewire; and (4) perform triple KBI. When wiring the SB, you should always pass the guidewire through the most distal cell at the carina.

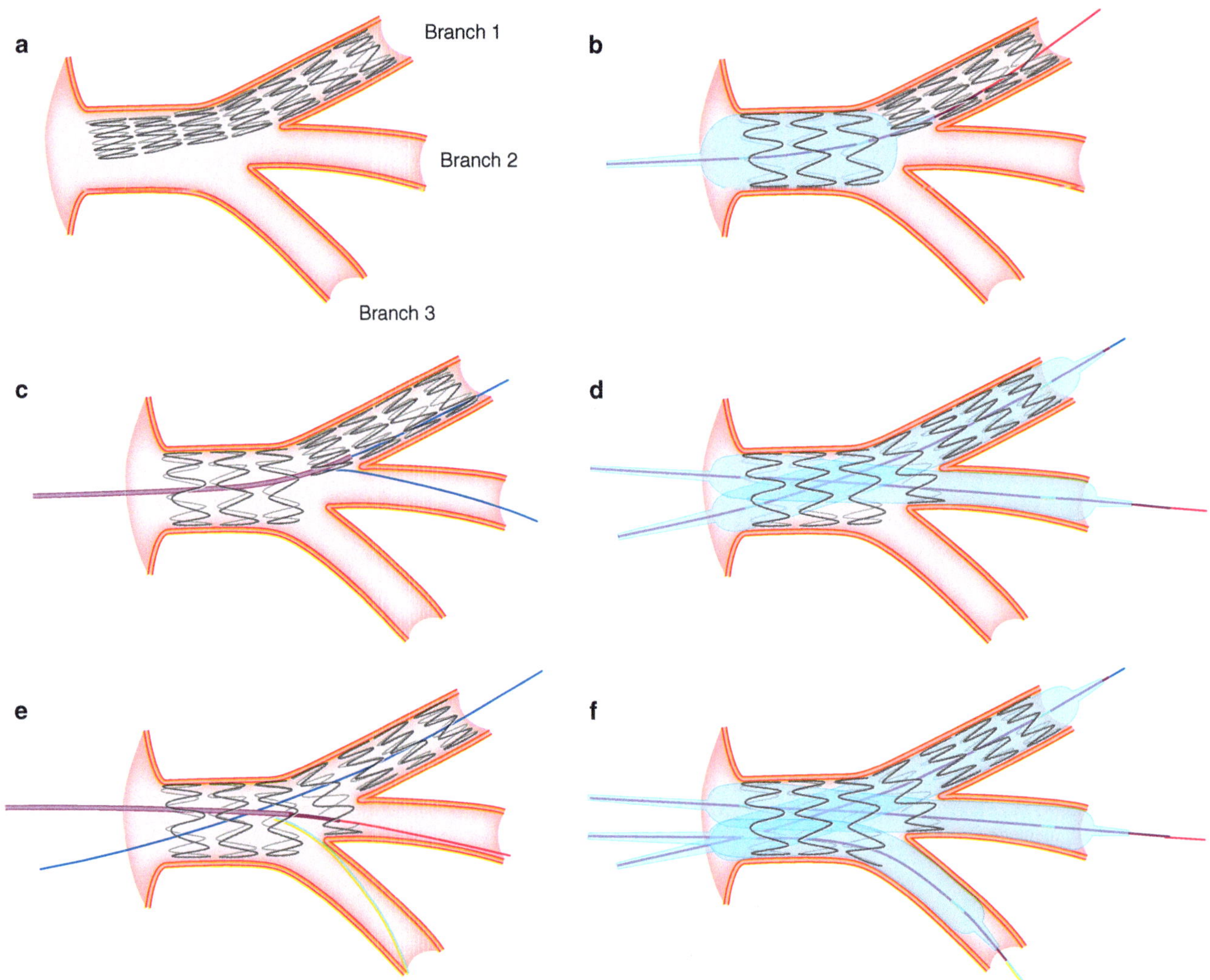

Fig. 4.26 Stent placement at the LM trifurcation. (**a**) Placing a stent in Branch 1. (**b**) POT. (**c**). Rewiring Branch 2 with the aid of the Crusade catheter. (**d**) Performing KBI in Branches 1 and 2. (**e**) Rewiring Branch 3 with the aid of the Crusade catheter advanced along the Branch 2 guidewire. (**f**) Performing triple KBI

4.5.2 Culotte Stenting at the LM Trifurcation

If lesions in the LAD and LCX are treated by culotte stenting, the HL branch will be compressed by both the LAD stent and the LCX stent, even if the culotte stenting is completed with triple KBI (Fig. 4.27). In other words, there will be dual carina shift toward the HL branch. If dual carina shift is considered to be approximately double that of a single carina, it is unlikely to be negligible, and persistent compression from dual carina shift may well increase the risk of restenosis at this branch.

Thus, a third stent needs to be implanted in the HL branch when treating LM trifurcation lesions because culotte stenting cannot prevent restenosis of the branch. An interventionalist who aims to recanalize all three branches at a trifurcation lesion should choose trifurcation stenting rather than culotte stenting. However, LM trifurcation stenting has been reported to achieve very poor mid-term outcomes with regard to patency of the HL branch.

The proximal HL largely overlaps the proximal LAD/LCX on CAG. If the HL branch is stented last, its ostium may not be covered sufficiently. Also, if triple KBI is only performed after stenting the HL branch following culotte stenting of the LAD/LCX, the guidewire inserted into the HL branch may bypass the culotte stents. On the other hand, if triple KBI is added to LAD stenting and to LCX stenting, trifurcation stenting will achieve full coverage of the three branches and ensure that all three stents obtain sufficient radial strength.

It is best to additionally perform triple KBI after HL stenting using the balloons maintained in the LAD and LCX. The stent in the HL branch should be positioned with its proximal edge protruding slightly into the LM lumen from the LAD-LCX carina (Fig. 4.28). IVUS can be used to confirm the position of the proximal edge of the stent.

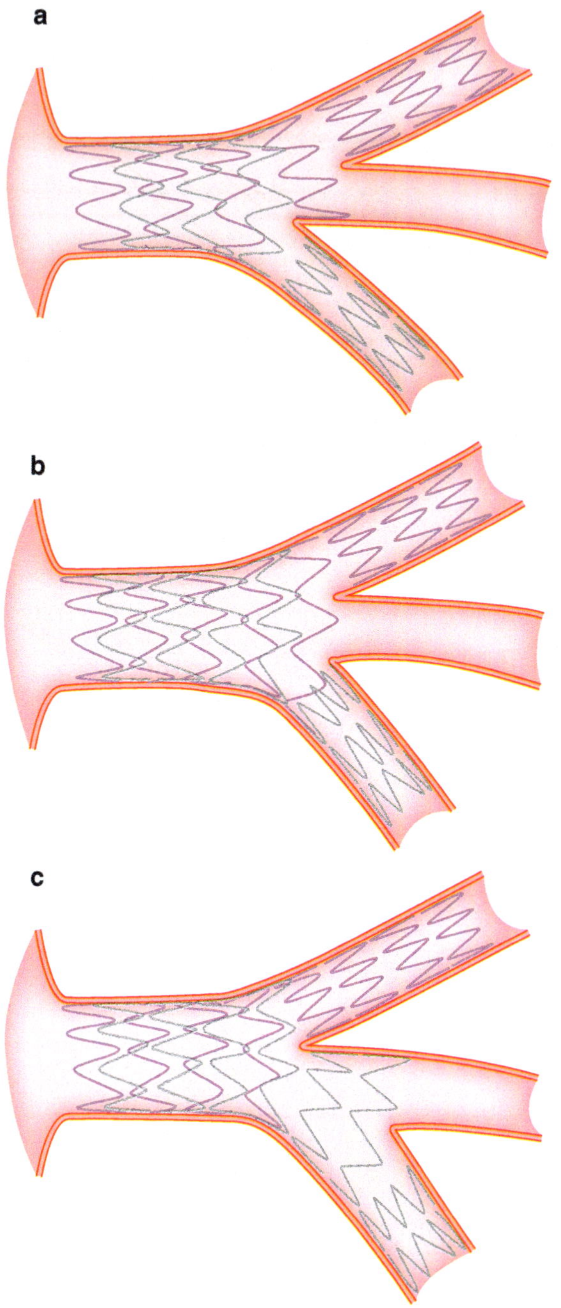

Fig. 4.27 Culotte stenting of various trifurcation lesions. (**a**) HL branch arising from the LAD ostium. (**b**) HL branch arising between the LAD and the LCX. (**c**) HL branch arising from the LCX ostium

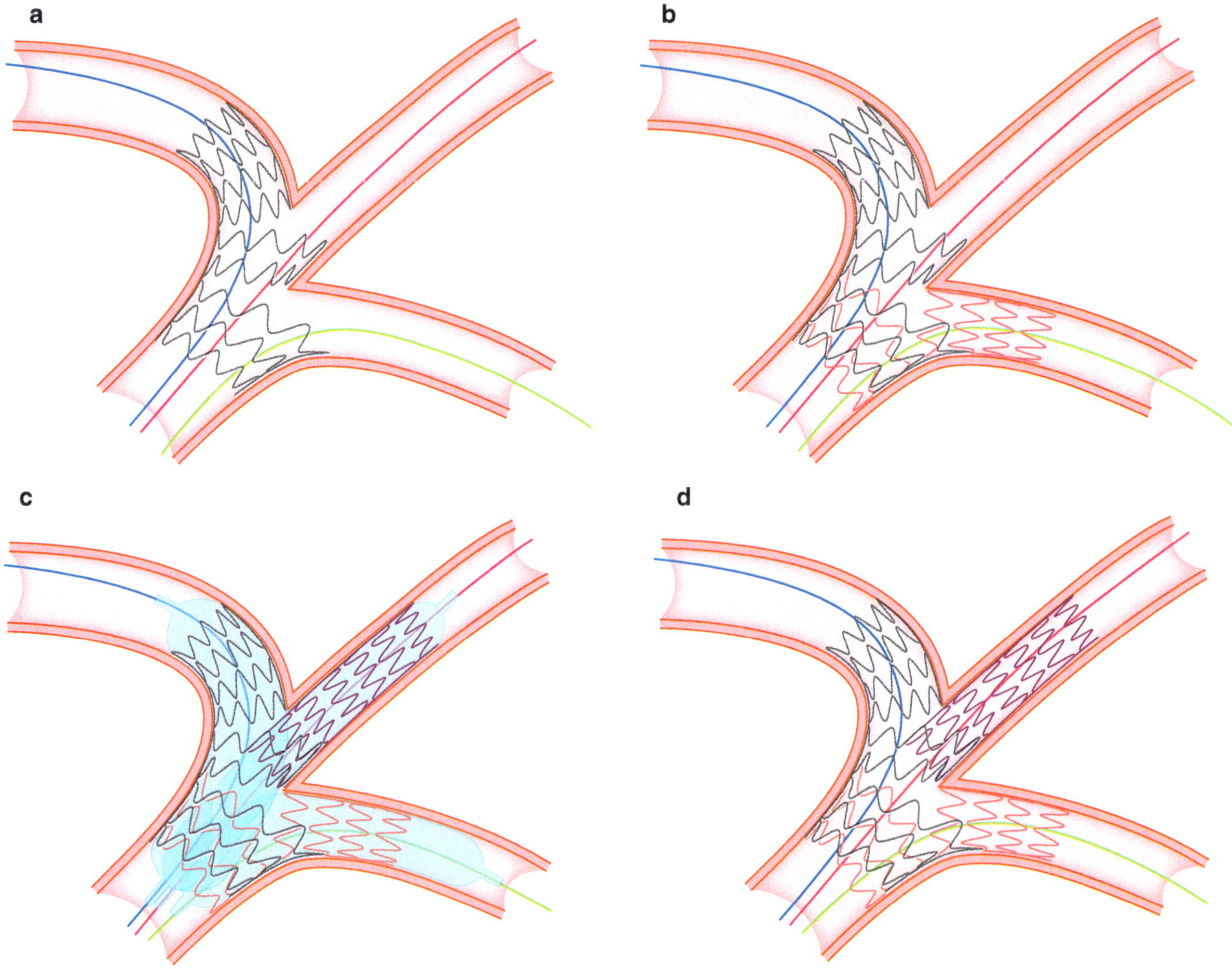

Fig. 4.28 Placement of the third stent in the HL branch (**c**, **d**) after culotte stenting of the LAD/LCX (**a**, **b**). With the balloons maintained in the LAD/LCX, HL stenting should be performed, followed by triple KBI

4.6 Case Study

This section provides an example of stenting an LM bifurcation lesion at my center.

To treat a true bifurcation lesion (Fig. 4.29), I introduced a Judkins left short-tip guiding catheter (Launcher SL4) into the LM.

I performed pre-PCI IVUS to estimate the sizes of the target vessels, as well as the characteristics and distribution of plaques. Attenuated plaque was found in the LAD, so I delivered a Filtrap catheter to protect the distal LAD and then predilated the LAD with a 3.0 mm balloon (Fig. 4.30a). After simultaneously inflating 3.0 mm and 3.5 mm kissing balloons in the LAD and LCX (Fig. 4.30b), I implanted a Nobori stent (3.5 × 24 mm) from the LM to the LAD and expanded it at a relatively low pressure (Fig. 4.30c). Subsequently, I performed POT by inflating a 5.0 mm balloon in the LM (Fig. 4.30d).

Then I manipulated a guidewire via a Crusade catheter to insert it into the SB (LCX). Angiography showed that the wire had failed to cross the stent through the most distal cell at the carina (Fig. 4.31a), so I performed SB rewiring (Fig. 4.31b).

After simultaneously inflating 3.0 mm and 3.5 mm kissing balloons in the LAD and LCX (Fig. 4.32), there was residual stenosis in the LCX. Therefore, I decided to switch to culotte stenting and implanted a Nobori 3.5-mm JV stent from the LM to the LCX with expansion at a relatively low pressure (Fig. 4.33a). I then performed POT by inflating a 5.0 mm balloon in the LM (Fig. 4.33b).

Next, wiring of the SB (LAD) was done via the Crusade catheter, and I confirmed by angiography that the wire crossed the stent through the most distal cell at the carina (Fig. 4.34a). After KBI (Fig. 4.34b), the bifurcation lesion was successfully recanalized (Fig. 4.34c).

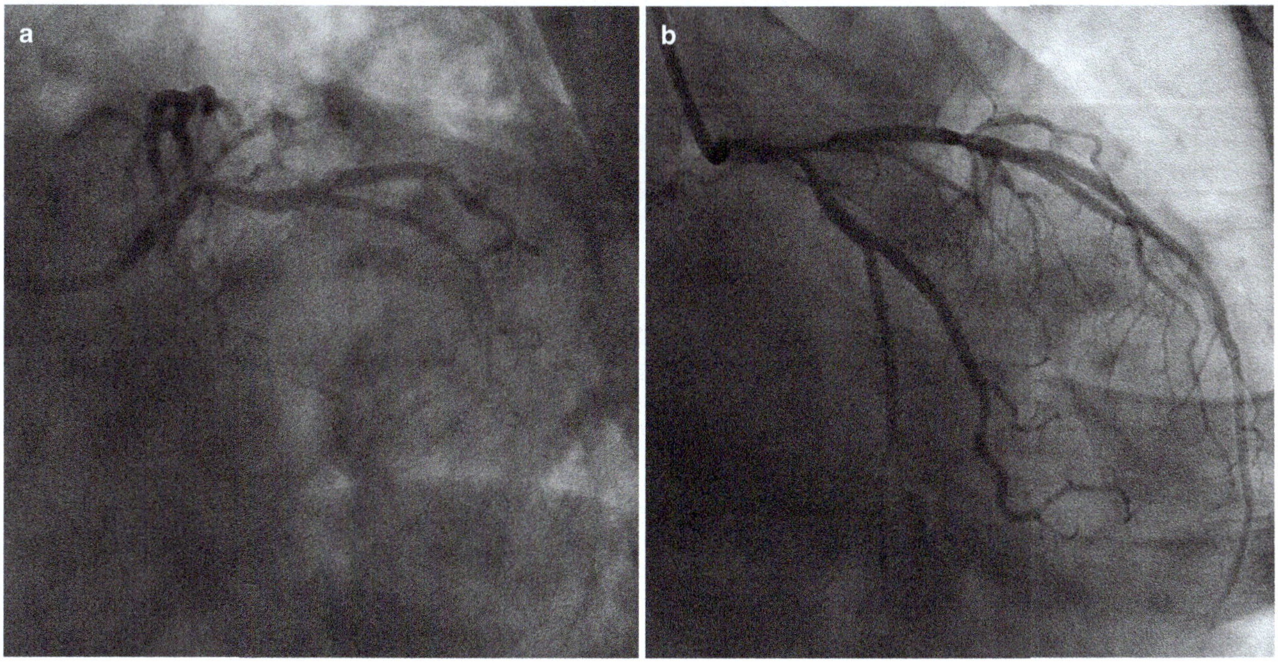

Fig. 4.29 True LM bifurcation lesion

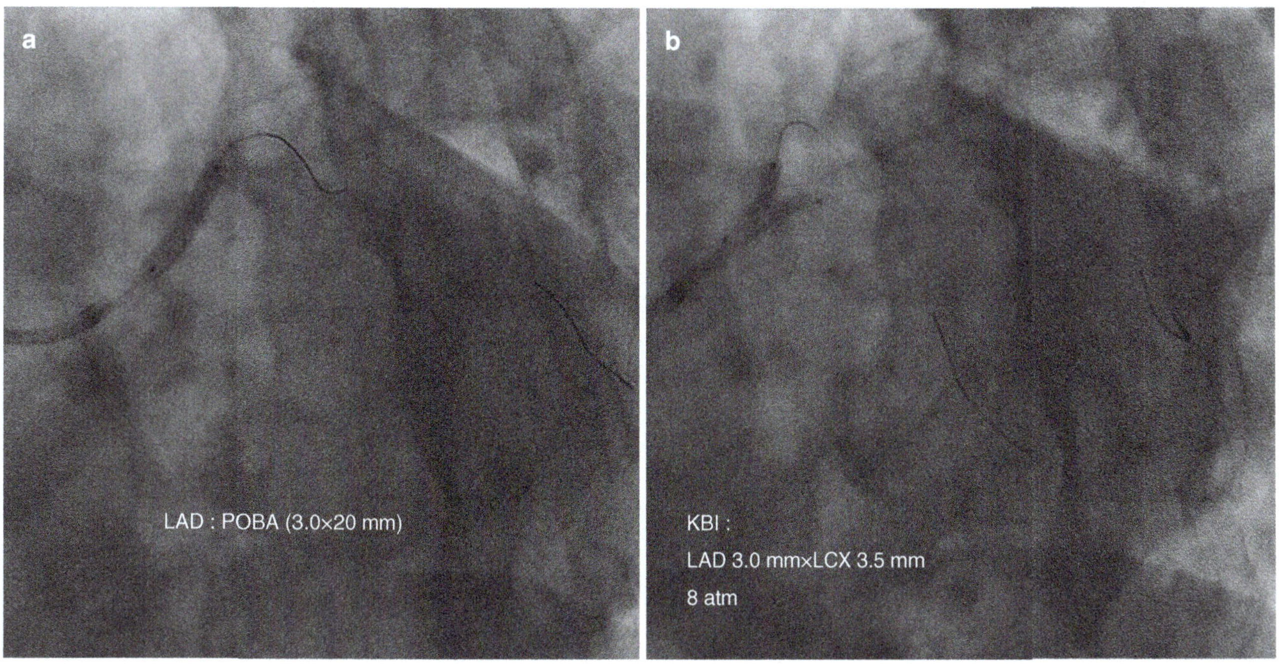

Fig. 4.30 KBI plus stenting of an LM bifurcation lesion. (**a**) POBA of the LAD was done using a 3.0-mm balloon. (**b**) KBI was performed with 3.0-mm and 3.5-mm balloons in the LAD and LCX, respectively. (**c**) A Nobori 3.5-mm stent was deployed in the LAD at a relatively low pressure. (**d**) POT was performed by inflating a 5.0-mm balloon in the LM

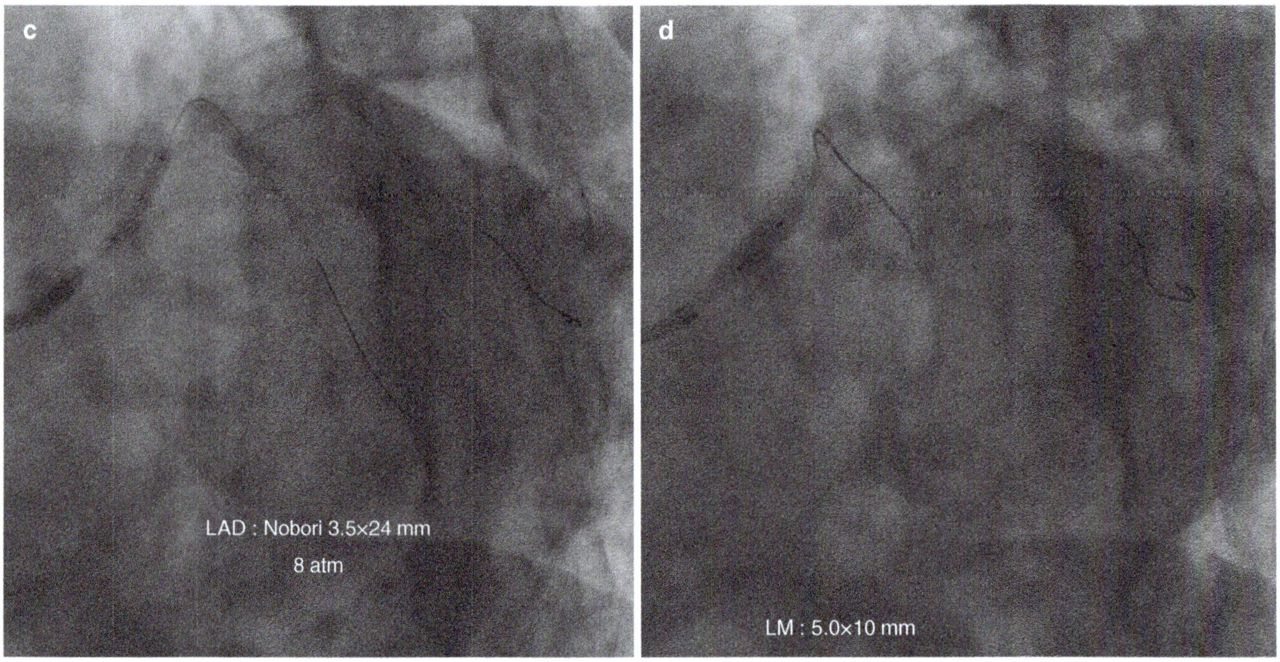

Fig. 4.30 (continued)

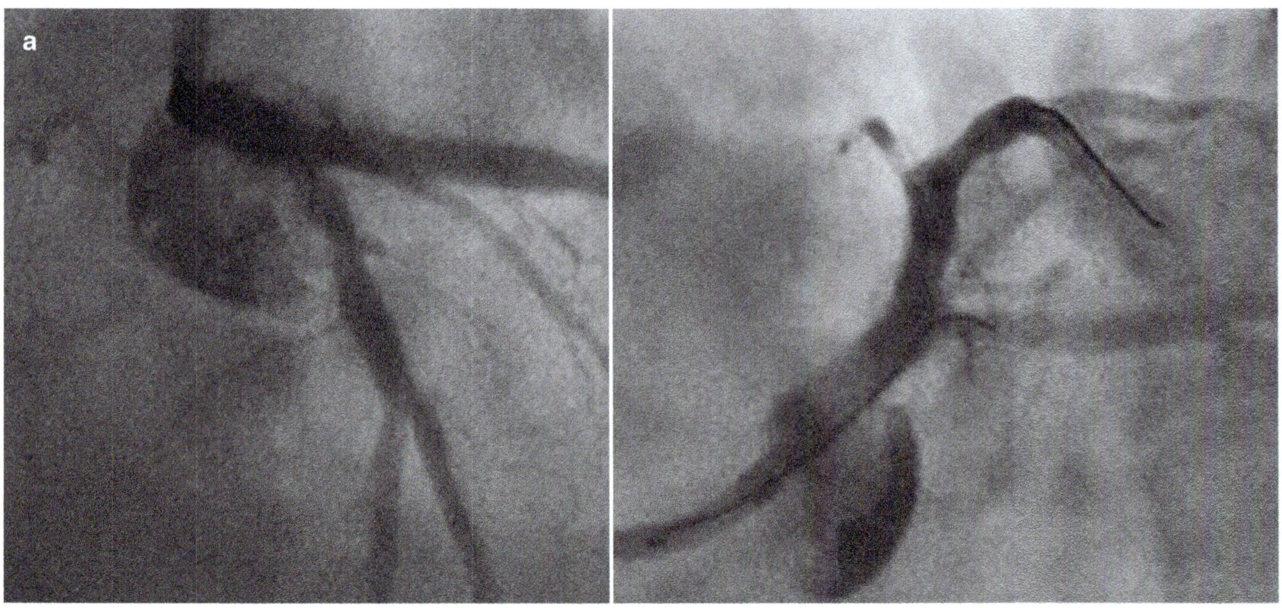

Fig. 4.31 SB (LCX) rewiring via a Crusade catheter. SB (LCX) rewiring was done under angiographic guidance. (**a**) The guidewire inserted into the SB has not crossed the stent through the cell nearest to the carina. (**b**) The SB guidewire now crosses the stent through the most distal cell at the carina

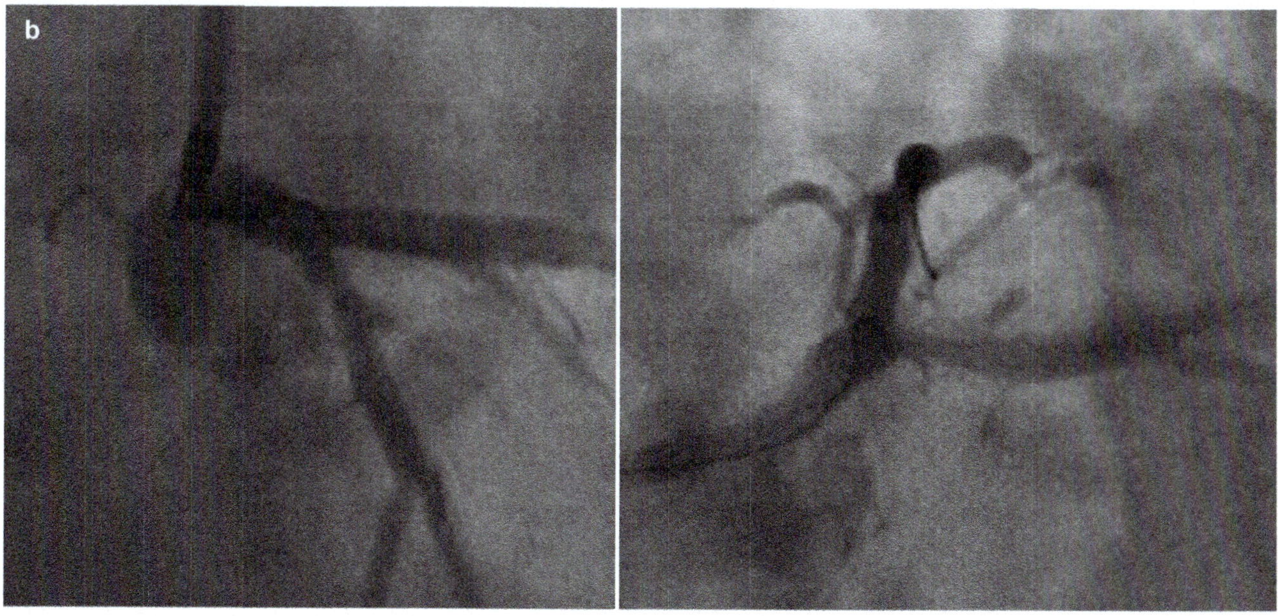

Fig. 4.31 (continued)

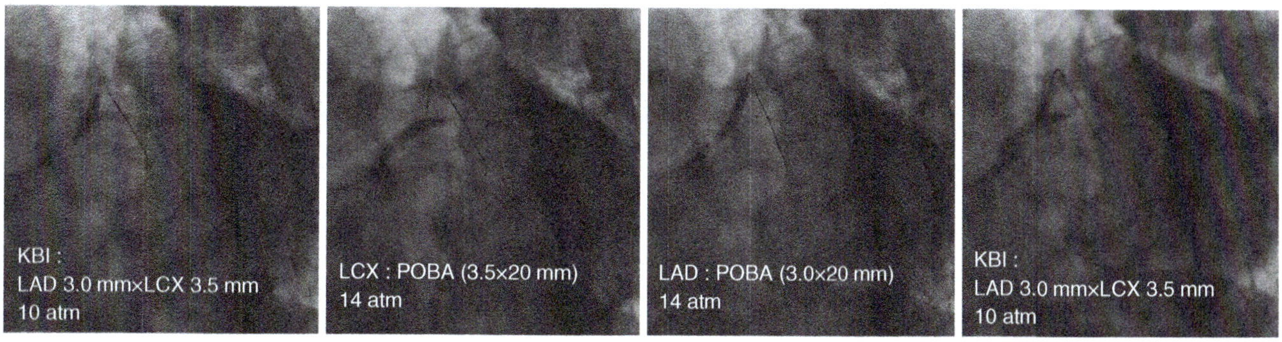

Fig. 4.32 Simultaneous balloon inflation in the LAD and LCX. A 3.0-mm balloon in the LAD and a 3.5-mm balloon in the LCX were inflated alternately at high pressure and then were inflated simultaneously (KBI)

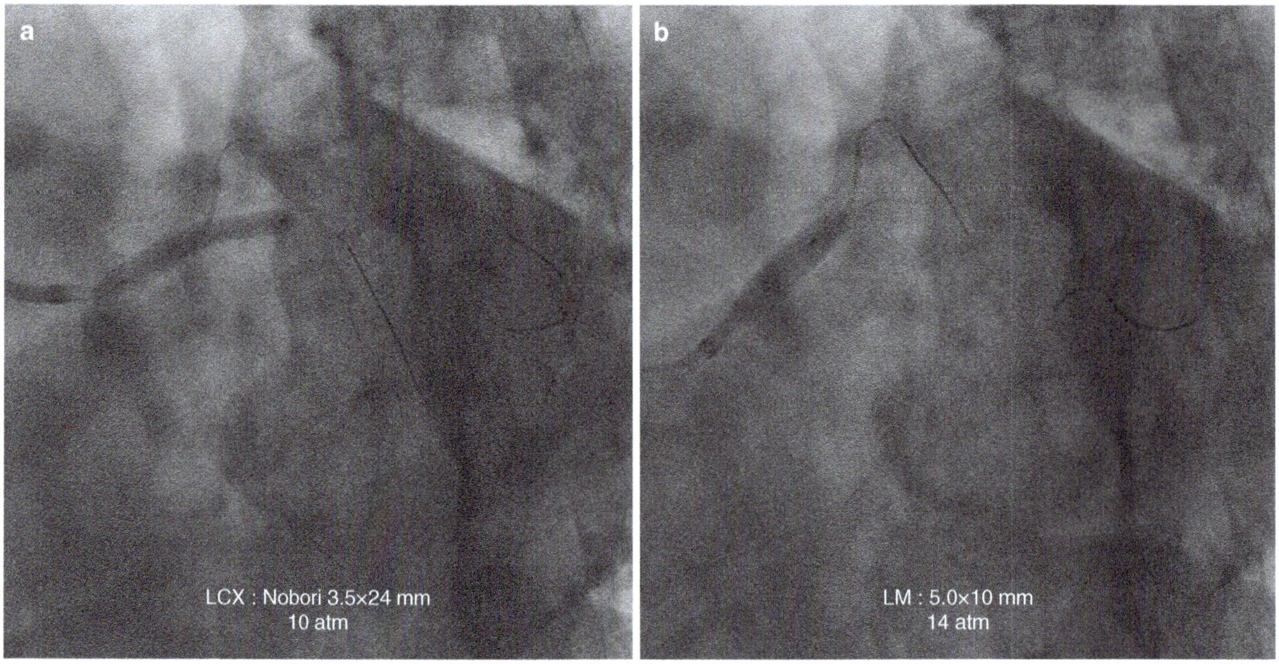

Fig. 4.33 Culotte stenting. After implanting a Nobori 3.5-mm stent in the LCX (**a**), POT was performed by inflating a 5.0-mm balloon in the LM (**b**)

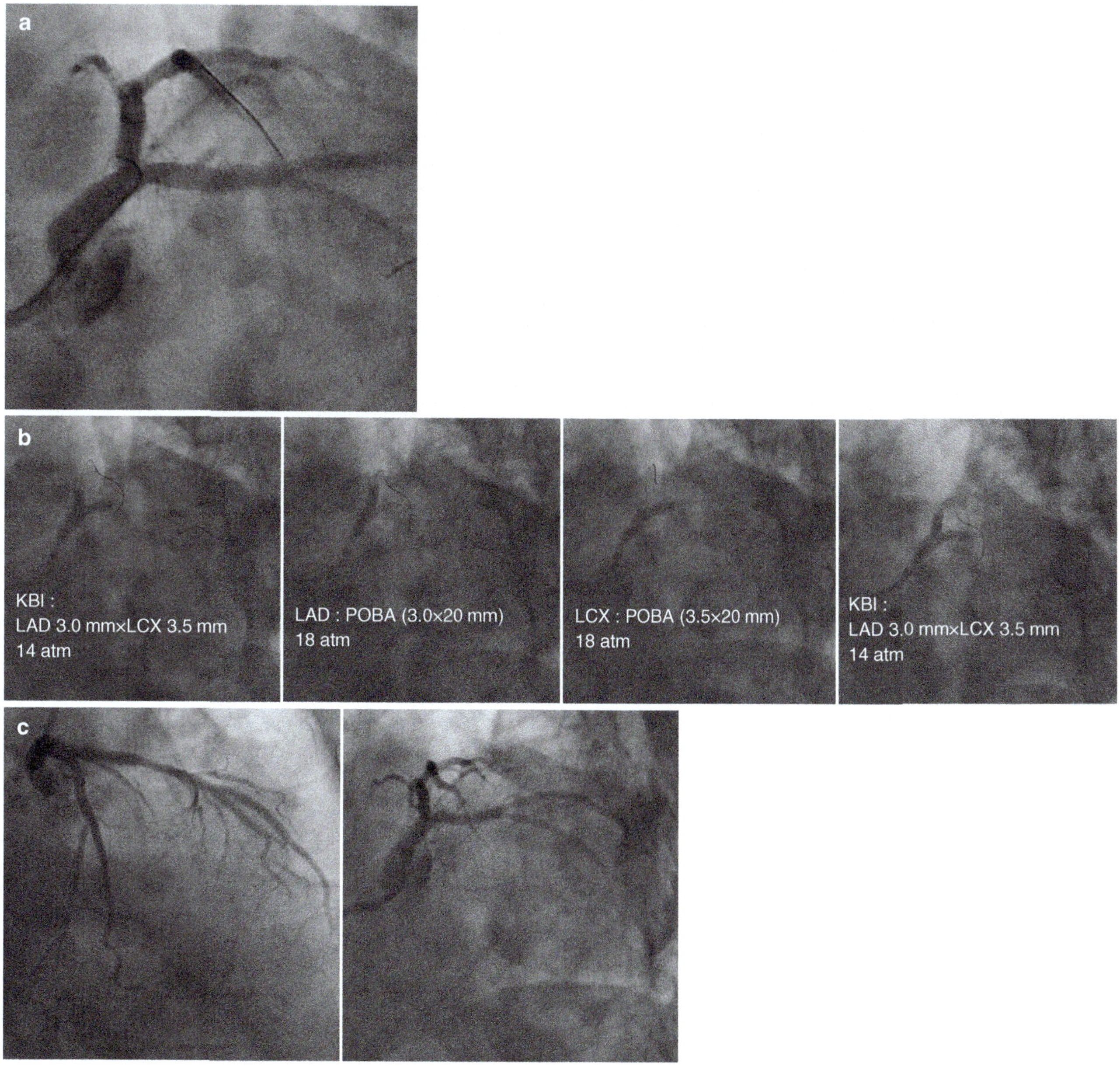

Fig. 4.34 KBI after culotte stenting. (**a**) Rewiring of the SB (LAD) was done via the Crusade catheter. (**b**) A 3.0-mm balloon in the LAD and a 3.5-mm balloon in the LCX were inflated alternately at high pressure, and then were inflated simultaneously (KBI). (**c**) Final angiography

5 Mitsudo's Non-pushing PCI Techniques

My 33 years of experience with PCI have taught me much, including the essential importance of non-pushing PCI techniques. Pushing devices forcibly may lead to injury in various ways because of stress on the target vessel. Although a device cannot be advanced at all without applying some force, the maximum tolerable force should be estimated (i.e., the force that can be applied to a device without causing damage/deformation), and force exceeding this threshold should never be applied. In addition, methods for advancing devices with minimum force should be determined. For example, it may be necessary to push hard on a device if it becomes blocked. Therefore, avoiding this situation is one of the ways to minimize the force required to advance a device.

5.1 When Is Pushing Allowed?

In general, I do not recommend forcibly pushing a device to advance it. However, there is one situation in which pushing is the only option and thus is permitted. This is when it proves difficult to advance a balloon or microcatheter across a lesion after successful wire crossing.

5.1.1 Microcatheter

It may be possible to cross a lesion, including one requiring rotablation, with a 0.014 inch guidewire, but not with a microcatheter. However, the microcatheter can often cross the lesion if the guidewire is exchanged for another that provides greater support.

During PCI for CTO, it is often necessary to rotate the microcatheter in addition to pushing it forward with minimal force in order to advance antegradely into a lesion, to retrogradely cross a collateral channel, or to deliver the catheter into a lesion requiring rotablation that has been crossed by a guidewire with microcatheter support.

Unlike the Tornus catheter, microcatheters must not be rotated excessively in the same direction because these catheters generally cannot tolerate the torque of excessive rotation. For example, the Caravel microcatheter only tolerates up to three clockwise or counterclockwise rotations. When more than three rotations are performed with the tip fixed, the shaft of this catheter tends to bulge and may become deformed. If this occurs after successfully tracking a channel, it may prevent withdrawal of the microcatheter. Therefore, you should never perform more than three clockwise or counterclockwise rotations of the Caravel microcatheter in succession. Of course, it is possible to perform three counterclockwise rotations initially and then repeat alternating cycles of six clockwise and six counterclockwise rotations. The Corsair microcatheter is better able to tolerate rotation, but it is safer to limit the number of successive clockwise or counterclockwise rotations to about ten with the Corsair and most other microcatheters.

5.1.2 Small-Diameter Balloon Catheter

If a microcatheter cannot be advanced, it should be exchanged for a small-diameter balloon catheter. Balloon catheters from 1.0 to 1.25 mm in diameter with good crossability are available. Monorail balloon catheters can only be pushed and can hardly be rotated. Therefore, you should use a balloon catheter that is suitable for the characteristics of the lesion.

Attempting to forcibly advance balloon that had become blocked will sometimes deform the balloon and enlarge its profile, preventing further advancement. Most of the recently developed balloon catheters have been modified to be more resistant to such deformation, but this problem has not been completely overcome. Therefore, bench testing should be performed to determine the force that can be applied before each balloon undergoes deformation.

A balloon with a stiffer tip is better for a hard and relatively linear lesion, since it can be advanced despite the

K. Mitsudo, *Non-Pushing PCI Techniques*, https://doi.org/10.1007/978-981-15-7043-8_5

hardness of the lesion. If the balloon has a soft tip, it will easily become deformed (Fig. 5.1), and you cannot advance a balloon with a deformed tip no matter how hard you push it. However, it may not be possible to advance a balloon with a stiff tip through a tortuous lesion because it is significantly biased toward the outer side of the vessel (Fig. 5.2b). On the other hand, such a lesion can often be crossed easily by a balloon with a soft tip that has little or no gap between its tip and the guidewire (Fig. 5.2c).

It is often difficult to advance a balloon through a hard and tortuous lesion. Therefore, it is usually better to exchange the guidewire for another with a stiff shaft that can provide greater support to straighten a tortuous vessel (Fig. 5.3) and then advance a balloon with a stiff tip. This can result in successful crossing of the lesion, but the balloon might be blocked by hard tissue within a long CTO. In this situation, dilating the entire proximal part of the occlusion with a small balloon will often facilitate easy advancement of the balloon catheter. Dilating the proximal part of the occlusion presumably reduces friction between the balloon and the occluded vessel, leading to better transmission of force, or changes the direction of the balloon at the point of blockade (Fig. 5.4).

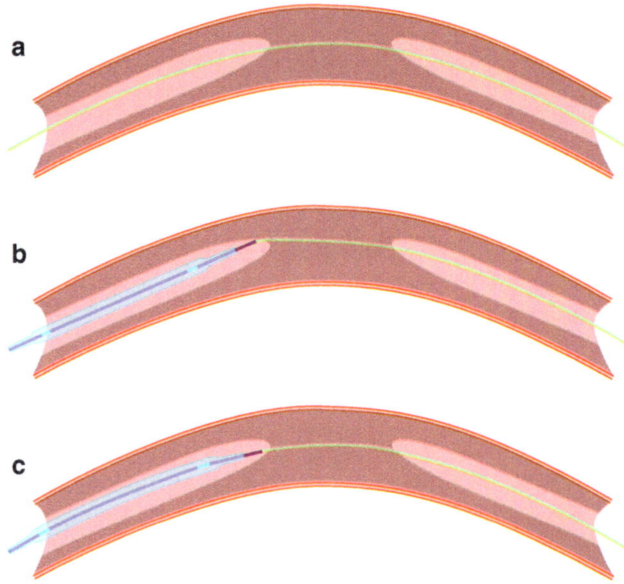

Fig. 5.2 Advancing a balloon through a hard and tortuous lesion (**a**). It can be difficult to advance a balloon with a stiffer tip because it is biased toward the outer side of the vessel (**b**). A balloon with a very small gap between its tip and the guidewire (providing better trackability) can often cross the lesion (**c**)

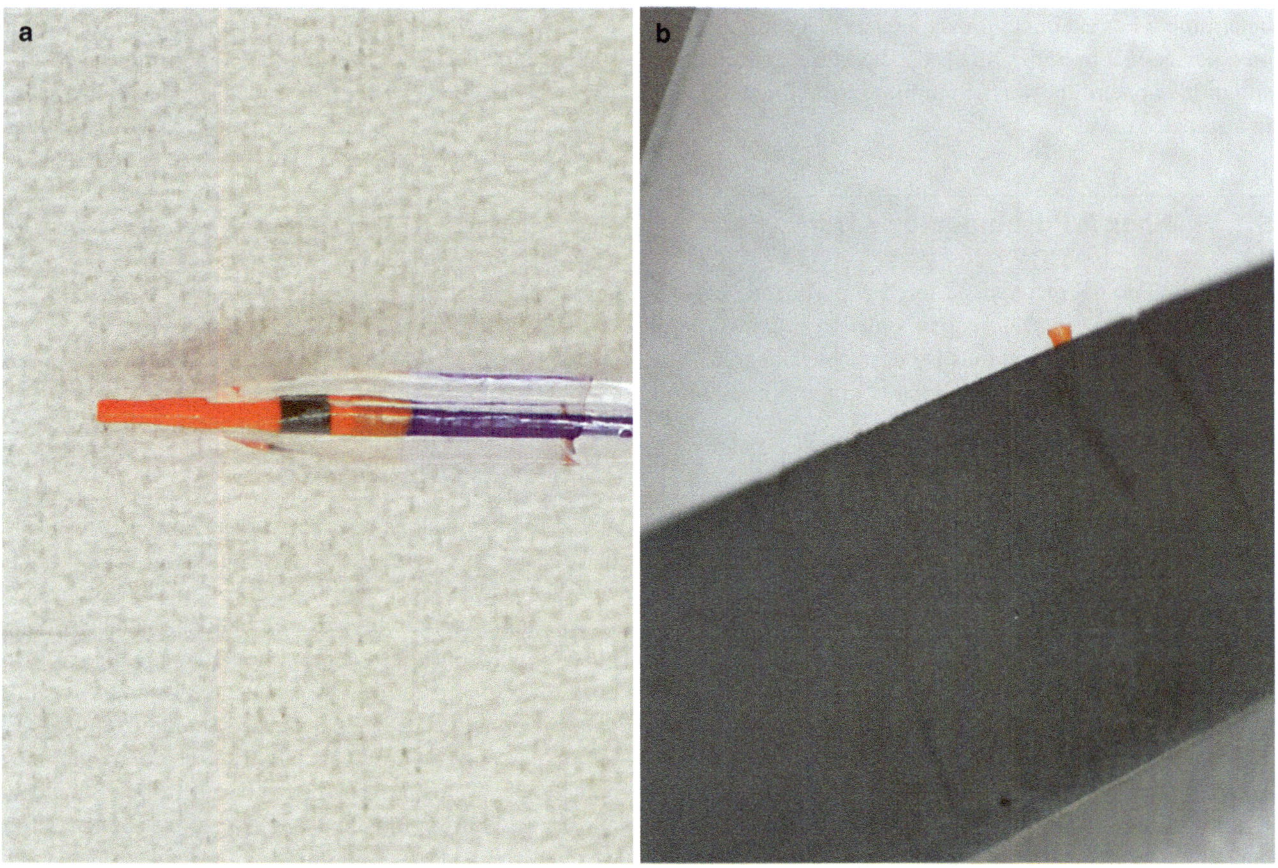

Fig. 5.1 Flaring of the balloon tip. If a balloon with a soft tip is pushed forcibly into a hard lesion, the tip may become deformed and flare out (**a**). If the tip becomes even slightly flared, it will be more difficult to advance the balloon through the lesion. Therefore, about 0.3 mm of the tip should be cut off (**b**) or the balloon should be exchanged for one with a stiffer tip

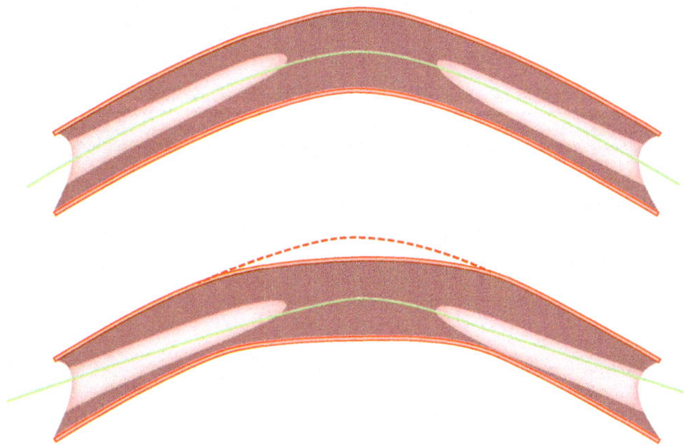

Fig. 5.3 Crossing a tortuous hard lesion. The guidewire should be exchanged for one with a stiffer shaft that provides greater support and straightens the tortuous lesion to facilitate crossing by the balloon

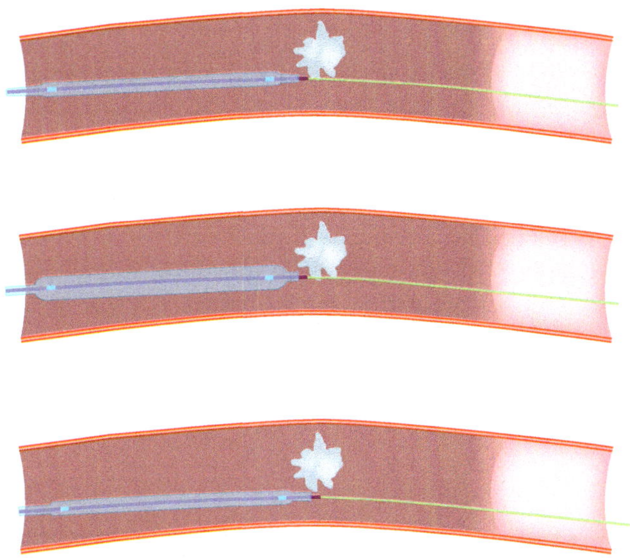

Fig. 5.4 Crossing a long hard lesion. If the proximal part of a long hard lesion is dilated, this will reduce friction between the balloon and the lesion and/or alter the direction of the balloon tip at the site of blockade to assist with crossing the lesion

5.1.3 Tornus Catheter

After failing to advance a balloon catheter across a lesion, a Tornus catheter should be tried. Three models of the Tornus catheter are available (2.1-Fr, 88 Flex, and Pro 2.1-Fr), all of which have a shaft composed of metal wires but are slightly different with respect to structure and characteristics (Fig. 5.5). I always choose the Tornus Pro if there is no particular contraindication.

The Tornus Pro has a 2.1-Fr shaft and its tip size is 0.025 inches. The Tornus 88 Flex is slightly larger, with a 2.6-Fr shaft and a tip size of 0.028 inches. If the entrance of the lesion is large enough to accommodate the 0.028 inch tip of the 88 Flex, its thicker shaft produces greater torque that promotes advancement. The Tornus Pro 2.1 Fr has the smallest tip (0.024 inches) and can be used for a tight stenosis that cannot be entered with the other Tornus models.

The Tornus cannot be advanced by rotation alone. To advance it into a tight stenosis, you have to simultaneously rotate the catheter and push it in quite strongly. In the RCA, even a deeply engaged guiding catheter may not provide sufficient support for the Tornus. Therefore, an anchoring balloon is often used in combination with the Tornus for RCA lesions.

There are several tips for manipulating the Tornus catheter. You should usually rotate a Tornus catheter counterclockwise in a stepwise fashion with the right hand while pushing it in with the left hand (Fig. 5.6). After one or two rotations, you should stop pushing with the left hand and return the right hand to its original position. You should then relax the left hand to release the Tornus and subsequently rotate it counterclockwise again. These processes are repeated until the catheter has received a total of 20 to 30 rotations. You should then completely relax the left hand to release the accumulated torque. The Tornus may advance spontaneously during torque release. Rotating it as much as possible at once, rather than repeatedly performing small rotations, will help the catheter to advance further.

After crossing has been achieved with the Tornus, most calcified lesions need debulking with a Rotablator, although some mildly calcified lesions may be treated by balloon angioplasty. To perform rotablation, the guidewire should be exchanged for a RotaWire after the Tornus has crossed the lesion. It is usually quite difficult to advance the RotaWire Extra Support guidewire through the Tornus catheter due to strong friction. This is particularly true if the lesion is long, hard, and tortuous (including CTOs), even if the measures described below are tried. It is easier to pass a RotaWire Floppy guidewire through the Tornus catheter.

You must never push a RotaWire forward strongly when advancing it through the Tornus catheter because the wire is likely to become kinked at the hub of the Tornus, making it impossible to advance further. Even if you manage to successfully pass a kinked RotaWire through the Tornus catheter, the kinking will make it difficult to deliver the RotaBurr and will affect debulking. To pass a RotaWire through the Tornus catheter, you should advance the wire carefully while rotating it. Do not use the attached clip for advancing the guidewire, but use a torquer to apply sufficient rotation to the wire. You should slide the torquer forward from the proximal edge of the RotaWire to near the hub of the Tornus. Advancing the RotaWire successfully may require many rotations, but you must never hurry or push it in forcibly. Instead, step-by-step advancement of the guidewire while rotating it provides the key to successful delivery through the Tornus catheter.

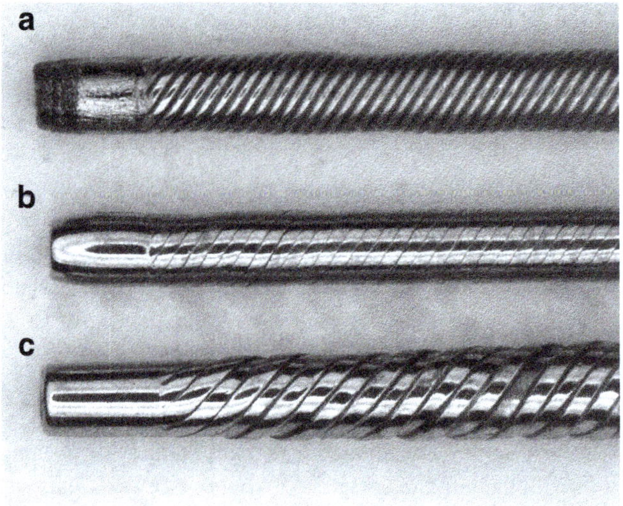

Fig. 5.5 The three Tornus models. (**a**) Tornus Pro. (**b**) Tornus. (**c**) Tornus 88 Flex

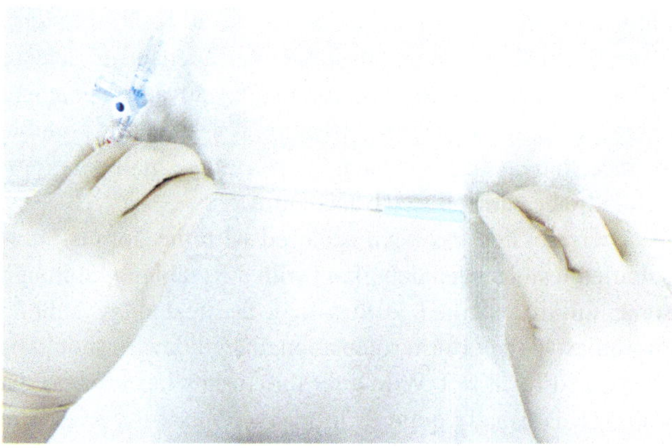

Fig. 5.6 Technique for advancing the Tornus. First, attach a torquer to the guidewire. Then rotate the Tornus catheter counterclockwise with the right hand while pushing it in with the left hand

5.1.4 Backup for the Guiding Catheter

As explained in Chap. 1, a guiding catheter should be selected that has a tip of the optimal size and curvature to maximize backup in the target coronary artery. That is, when the guiding catheter is engaged in the ostium of the target coronary artery, its tip should be parallel with the ostium and its shaft should be supported by the contralateral wall of the sinus of Valsalva so that it provides sufficient support when delivering devices.

If there is no guiding catheter with the optimal tip size/curvature and if greater back-up is needed, the following methods can be employed to enhance the back-up provided by any guiding catheter.

1. *Anchoring technique (see Chap. 1 [p. 14])*
2. *Deep engagement*

Deep engagement of the guiding catheter is an effective method of enhancing backup if the coronary artery ostium has a sufficiently large diameter and the vascular anatomy allows the catheter to be positioned coaxially in relation to the ostium (Fig. 5.7a). It is relatively easy to achieve deep engagement of a guiding catheter with a small diameter (e.g., 5-Fr) (Fig. 5.7b).

However, deep engagement of the guiding catheter is associated with a risk of coronary artery injury. Therefore, this method should only be used if the guiding catheter can easily be advanced by rotation alone without pushing it in.

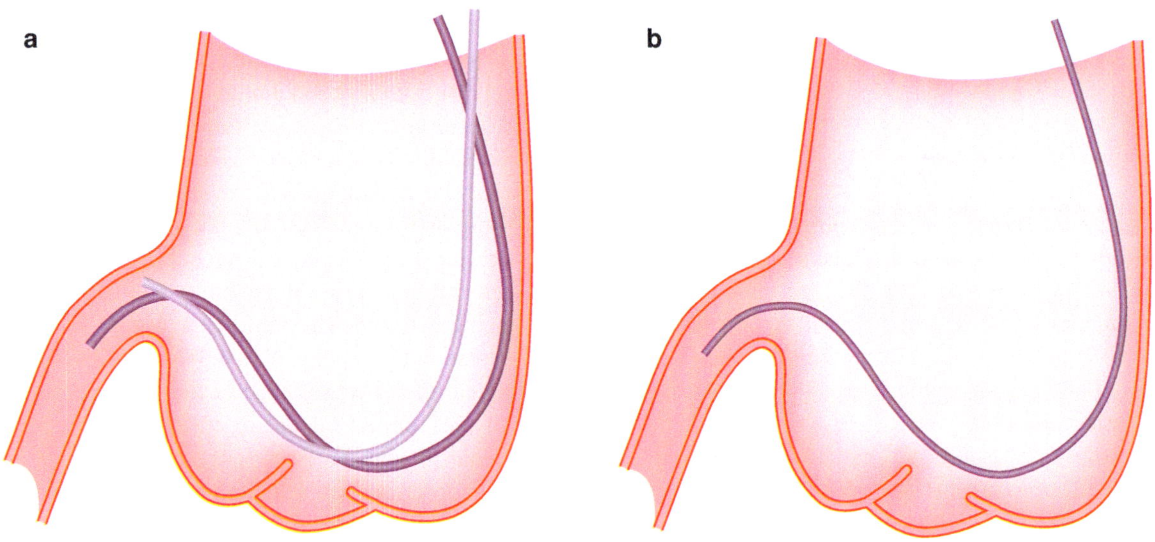

Fig. 5.7 Deep engagement of a guiding catheter. (**a**) To achieve deep engagement of an Amplatz guiding catheter in the RCA, the catheter should be pulled back slightly while rotating it clockwise so as that the tip is coaxial to the ostium. (**b**) It is easier to achieve deep engagement of a guiding catheter with a small diameter because its tip has a small radius of curvature

3. *Deep engagement with assistance from an over-the-wire child catheter or GuideLiner*

The child-in-mother technique can a useful supplementary method. However, the over-the-wire child catheter or Guideliner is not always suitable, and you may be unable to use either of them some circumstances. In that situation, you should exchange the current guiding catheter for another catheter with a tip designed to enhance backup. At many centers, it is difficult to always have access to all kinds of guiding catheters. Therefore, a guiding catheter can be heated and reshaped with an optimal curve or tip size or any additional three-dimensional changes that maximize backup (see Chap. 1 [Page 12]).

5.2 Guidewire

5.2.1 Fundamentals of Advancing a Guidewire

If the tip of a guidewire is deflected by an obstruction, excessive force must not be applied to advance it. If a guidewire becomes stuck in a severe stenosis or CTO and if the proximal part of the wire shows deflection, too much force must not be applied either. This is my absolute rule for guidewire manipulation. About 90% of procedural problems related to guidewires are attributable to using excessive force when attempting to advance the wire in various situations.

5.2.2 Guidewire Manipulation

A guidewire can be manipulated in four ways, which are pushing it forward, pulling it back, rotating it, and fixing its tip. These four manipulations should be combined appropriately to achieve the optimal wiring strategy for various purposes, such as (1) tracking a clearly visible channel, (2) exploring and tracking an accessible channel, and (3) crossing an occlusion.

Whatever wiring strategy is employed, it is of paramount importance to apply minimal force to the guidewire and to find a route that allows the wire to be advanced without pushing hard. If you cannot find a suitable route, the shape of the guidewire tip should be modified. If even a guidewire with a reshaped tip cannot be advanced, it should be exchanged for another wire that is appropriate for the circumstances, such as a guidewire with greater slipperiness, a guidewire with a tapered tip, a CTO crossing wire with a 0.014″ tip, or a CTO crossing wire with a tapered tip. Then you should search for a route along which the new guidewire can be advanced without pushing it hard by bypassing obstructions.

5.2.3 Rotating and Pushing a Guidewire

As explained in relation to PCI for CTO (see Chap. 1), a guidewire can be rotated in two ways, which are (1) fixed point rotation and (2) to-and-fro rotation.

To perform to-and-fro rotation of a guidewire, the entire (curved) tip is rotated around its axis (shaft) (Fig. 5.8). This method of rotation is often used to advance a guidewire to the entrance of a lesion or through the normal vessel lumen distal to a lesion. The wire is advanced while rapidly rotating it alternately clockwise and counterclockwise. Rotation of the tip is utilized to free the guidewire from irregularities of the vessel wall that have temporarily caught it and thus to minimize the force required to advance it.

If the guidewire becomes stuck while to-and-fro rotation is being performed, its tip stops rotating. If this happens, you should immediately stop advancing and rotating the guidewire, because forcible attempts to push the wire forward may cause intimal injury or deviation into the subintimal region. In this situation, you should pull the guidewire back slightly and then try to advance it again. If the guidewire is blocked by a hard lesion, the shaft should be rotated while keeping the tip fixed at the point of obstruction (fixed point rotation; Fig. 5.9), in order to cross the obstruction. This technique is typically used during SB wiring in bifurcation stenting when the guidewire targeting the SB becomes blocked by a stent strut. To assist the guidewire to bypass the obstruction, rotation of ≤90 degrees should be performed using the torquer without moving the tip of the wire. If the guidewire is advanced with even slightly stronger force than optimal during rotation, the tip will easily deviate from the obstruction. If the tip of the guidewire is deflected, you should pull it back slightly to straighten the tip. Combining this manipulation with fixed point rotation often helps to pass the obstruction.

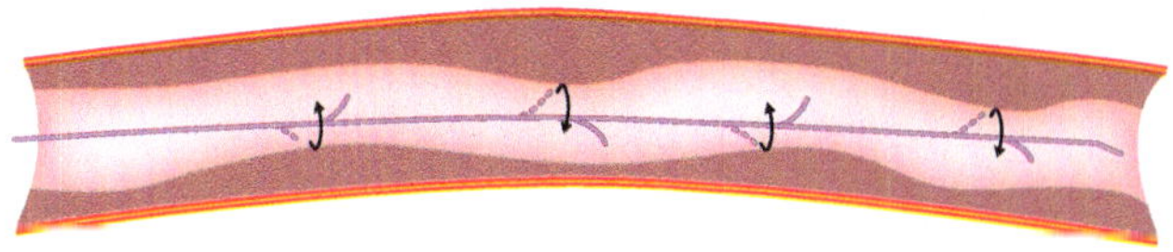

Fig. 5.8 To-and-fro rotation. A guidewire may be caught by irregularities of the vessel wall as it is pushed forward, leading to intimal injury if forcible attempts are made to continue advancing it. Performing to-and-fro rotation aims to free the guidewire from such irregularities by alternately rotating it clockwise and counterclockwise

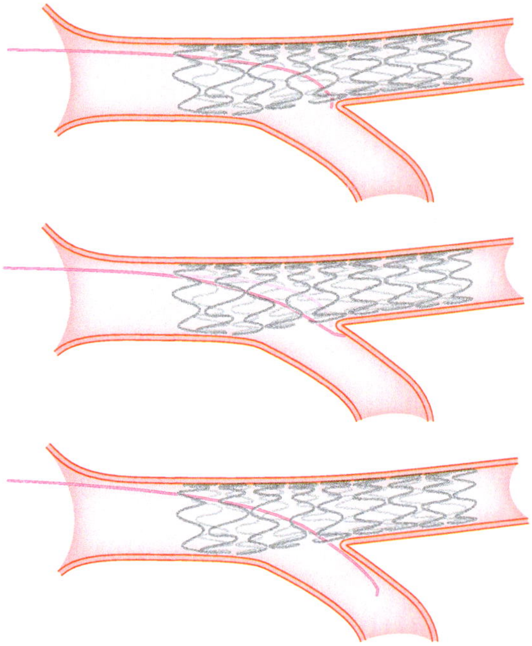

Fig. 5.9 Fixed point rotation. For wiring the SB during bifurcation stenting, the guidewire is advanced to the distal MB and then is pulled back with its tip oriented in the direction of the SB until the tip enters the branch. Applying fixed point rotation of ≲90 degrees to the guidewire at this stage will help to bypass obstruction by a stent strut so that it enters the SB. If the tip of the guidewire is deflected and does not enter the SB, the wire should be pulled back slightly to straighten the tip and fixed point rotation should be repeated to bypass the obstruction

5.2.4 Exploration with a Guidewire

If a channel across a CTO is thought to exist but it cannot be confirmed visually, you should try advancing a guidewire with a tapered soft tip in several directions to find a route along which the wire can go forward without deflection.

If the guidewire deviates into a subintimal space while you are attempting to cross a CTO and you can see an inflection point, the wire should be pulled back until it is just proximal to that point to bypass the obstruction that led to deviation.

While exploring to find a route to the SB at a bifurcation after reshaping the tip curve of a guidewire, slight rotation of the wire may be performed. However, such rotation only aims to orient the tip in the desired direction and should be considered as part of exploration.

5.2.5 Guidewire Selection and Supplementary Wiring Techniques (Crusade Microcatheter, Scoring Balloon [Lacrosse NSE Balloon] Angioplasty, Reverse Wire Technique, etc.)

It may be difficult to advance a guidewire through a very tortuous vessel, the SB of a tortuous vessel, a highly angulated SB, an SB distal to a coronary artery aneurysm, or an SB that is just distal to a stenosis. I have summarized the optimal guidewires and wiring strategies for these situations below.

1. Techniques for wiring a very tortuous vessel are described in detail in Chap. 1.7.8 (see p. 111). Although tortuous vessels with target lesions differ from the tortuous collateral channels used in retrograde PCI because of having a larger diameter and fewer bends, a similar approach to wiring is employed. That is, you should reshape a guidewire with a slippery soft tapered tip or non-tapered tip (polymer jacketed guidewire) to create a very acute (hairpin) tip curve and then should slowly advance the wire while applying nearly fixed point rotation (Fig. 5.10).
2. Wiring the SB at a bifurcation can be difficult in two situations. One is where the SB is located after a bend in the proximal MB (Fig. 5.11a). In this situation, you should follow the steps stated above when choosing and reshaping the guidewire for a tortuous vessel. Then you should twist the tip of the guidewire in the opposite direction to orient it toward the SB (Fig. 5.11b) and advance the wire slowly. This technique may require considerable experience with PCI. If another guidewire is advanced through the MB first, it will straighten the vessel and decrease the take-off angle of the SB, which may make it easier for the wire to enter the SB (Fig. 5.11c). A Crusade catheter can also be used to straighten a tortuous MB (Fig. 5.11d).

The other situation that makes wiring the SB difficult is if the branch arises with reverse angulation (Fig. 5.12). While you may follow the same advice for choosing and reshaping the guidewire given in (1) above, the wire will often fail to enter the SB. In this situation, the reverse wire technique can be very useful.

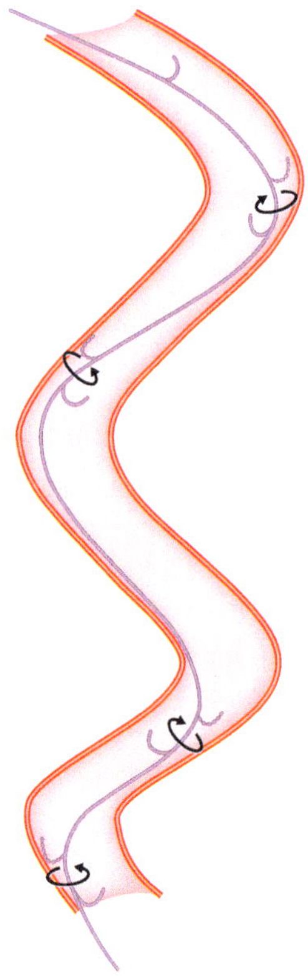

Fig. 5.10 Wiring a very tortuous vessel. To pass a guidewire through a vessel that is too tortuous to be crossed by a wire with a 0.014-inch tip, a slippery polymer jacketed guidewire should be reshaped to create a hairpin curve at the tip and then advanced while rotating it

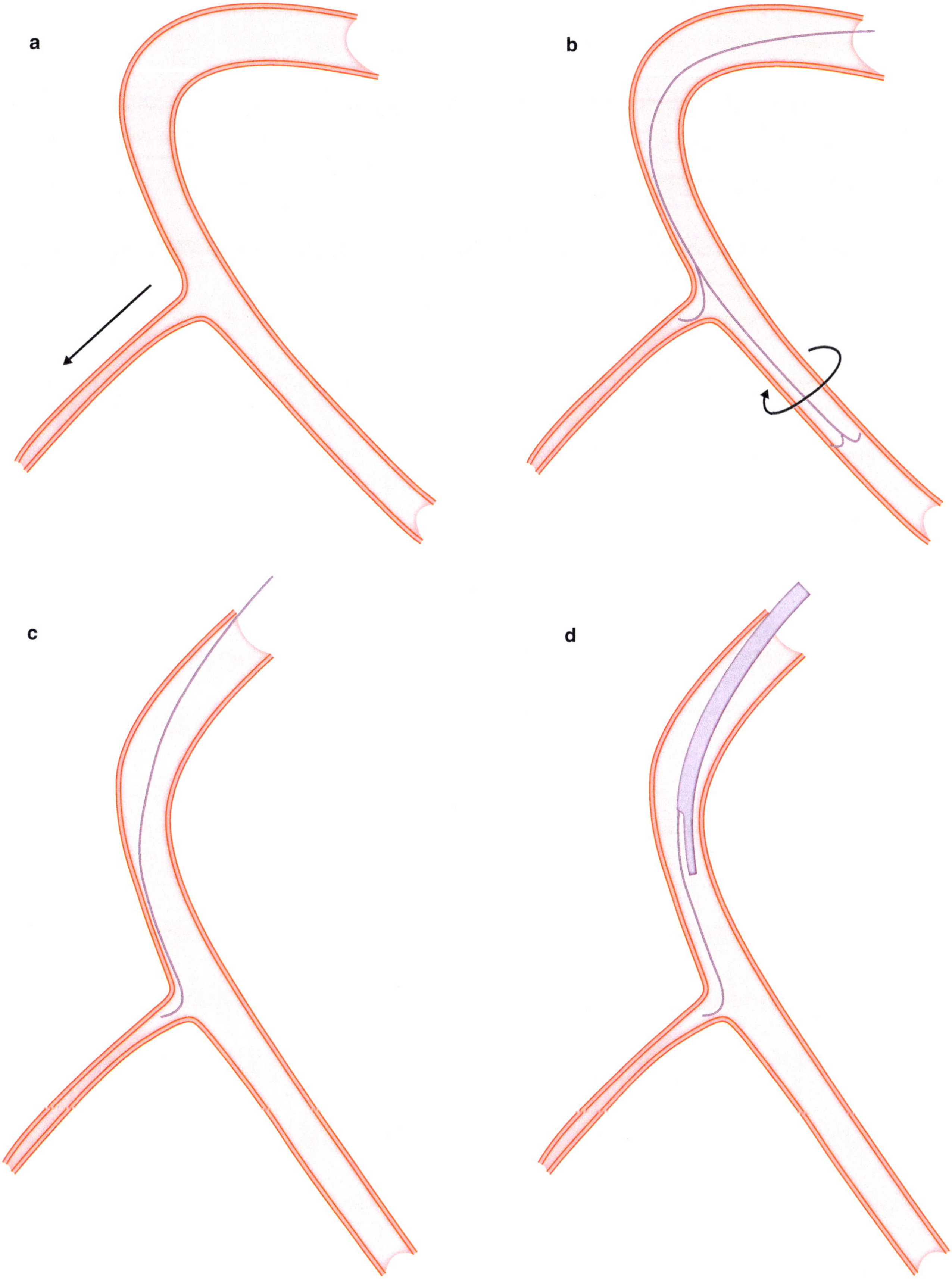

Fig. 5.11 Wiring a side branch (arrow in **a**). The guidewire is advanced into the distal MB and then slowly pulled back while orienting its tip toward the SB. To prevent the guidewire from slipping out of the ostium, the wire should be slowly advanced into the SB while applying rotation (**b**). Advancing another guidewire or a Crusade catheter into the MB may assist with isolation of the SB (**c**, **d**)

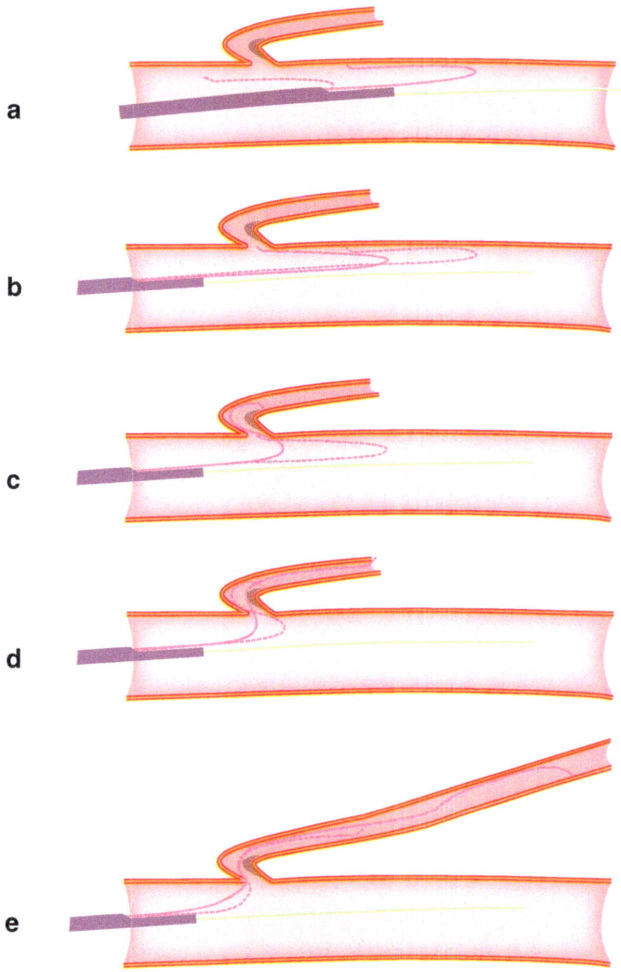

Fig. 5.12 Wiring a side branch with reverse angulation. The reverse wire technique is used for isolation of the branch

5.3 Balloon Angioplasty (POBA)

To pre-dilate a tight stenosis, it may sometimes be necessary to push a balloon catheter into the lesion, but this must not be done with too much force. Pushing a balloon catheter strongly into the lesion will deflect the proximal shaft of the catheter and apply stress to the vessel wall. Although the extent to which such catheter deflection contributes to dissection of the coronary artery proximal to the lesion or progression of stenosis is unclear, I have encountered progression of coronary stenosis that was possibly due to forcible advancement of a balloon catheter. Therefore, following the principle of "avoiding potential causes of adverse events whenever possible," measures should be taken to improve the crossability of a balloon catheter for pre-dilation, such as exchanging the balloon for one with a smaller diameter and inflating the new balloon.

5.3.1 Bifurcation Lesions

Entanglement of multiple guidewires in a bifurcation lesion may prevent delivery of a balloon catheter (Fig. 5.13). This is most commonly encountered when advancing a previously used balloon catheter to perform post-stenting KBI after rewiring an SB (Fig. 5.14). In such a situation, forcibly advancing the balloon catheter will dislocate the entangled guidewires and prevent guidewire crossing or even cause guidewire deformation. If it is difficult to advance a balloon catheter, you should always consider the possibility of guidewire entanglement.

If a Crusade catheter is used for SB rewiring, guidewire entanglement, if any, will be limited to several millimeters distal to the guidewire exit port of the catheter and entanglement is unlikely. Nonetheless, guidewire entanglement can occur even if SB rewiring is performed with a Crusade catheter, probably due to flexion or torsion of the guiding catheter. Two guidewires can become entangled even if their proximal topological relationship is always kept constant outside the body.

Therefore, interventionalists need to know countermeasures for guidewire entanglement. If entanglement of two guidewires prevents advancement of a balloon, the two guidewires should be kept in place and the balloon catheter should be withdrawn. You should then correct the torsion of the two guidewires by rotation in the correct direction (in practice, it can be hard to determine which direction this is) at the O-ring. Subsequently, re-advancing the balloon may resolve guidewire entanglement, although this is not always successful. Another method is to withdraw the guidewire from the distal MB into a balloon catheter that has been advanced to the site of entanglement and then readvance the guidewire for a short distance. This method can resolve guidewire entanglement and allow the balloon to pass into the stent (Fig. 5.14c, d).

In this setting, if the tip of the balloon is used to put slight pressure on the site of guidewire entanglement in the MB, withdrawal of the entangled guidewire into the balloon will not have much influence on the balloon's direction. If the guidewire is subsequently advanced a little from the tip of the balloon, the balloon will usually go forward smoothly into the MB. After withdrawal of the guidewire into the balloon, the balloon may sometimes become oriented toward the SB. If this happens, you should pull the balloon back a little and give its tip some freedom. Then you should readvance the balloon while avoiding guidewire advancement toward the SB or blocking of the wire by stent struts.

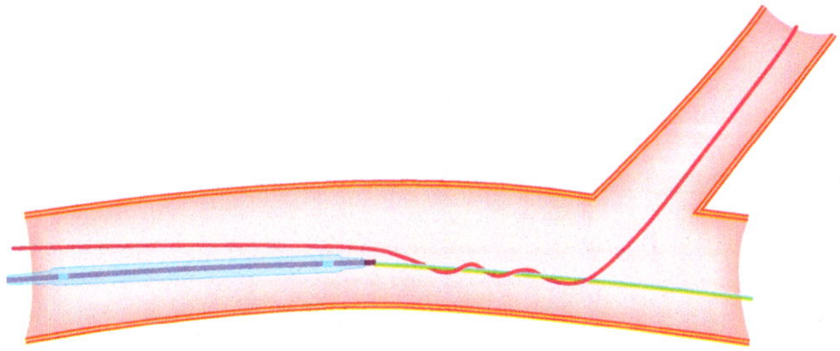

Fig. 5.13 Guidewire entanglement at a bifurcation lesion. Guidewire entanglement prevents delivery of a balloon

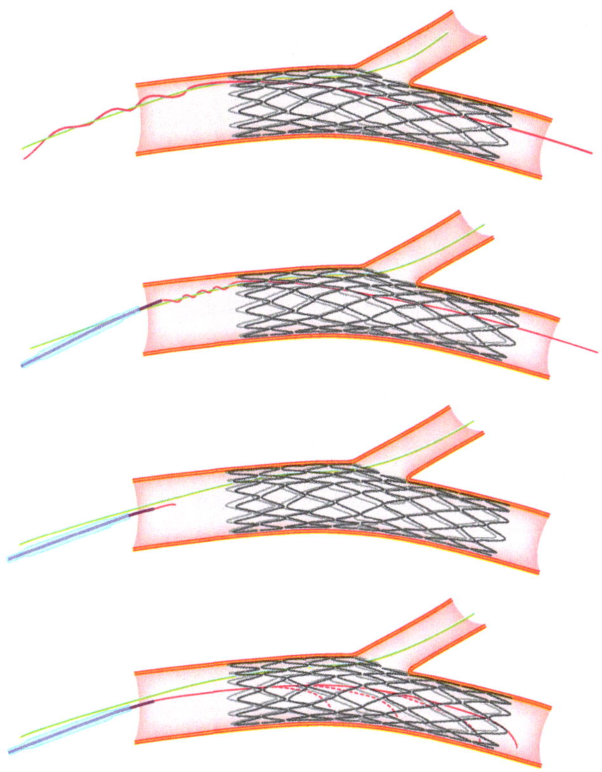

Fig. 5.14 Guidewire entanglement after SB wiring, precluding delivery of a previously used balloon to the MB

Although SB rewiring may be performed while avoiding guidewire entanglement, it is recommended to overcome entanglement by withdrawing the guidewire into a balloon that has been advanced to the site of entanglement in the MB and then advancing the balloon to the distal MB. This maneuver can resolve guidewire entanglement and permit smooth delivery of the balloon. As the tip of the balloon is oriented toward the MB, you can smoothly pass the balloon and the guidewire through a stent in the MB if the stent has been well apposed.

5.3.2 Balloon Size, Inflation Pressure, and Inflation Speed

It is often said that high-pressure balloon inflation causes dissection, but is this true? It is completely incorrect if dissection is taken to mean direct injury of an intact part of the vessel by the balloon (Fig. 5.15). The most common causes of dissection after balloon inflation are oversizing of the balloon and excessively rapid inflation.

Assume that a balloon is inflated in a straight vessel to exactly the luminal diameter so that the vessel wall comes into contact with the balloon but does not undergo expansion (Fig. 5.15b). Then balloon inflation will not injure the vessel regardless of the pressure employed. In this case, even if the balloon is inflated more rapidly, it will never injure the vessel. However, what will occur after inflation of a balloon with a larger size than the luminal diameter (Fig. 5.15c)? One can easily imagine that inflation could cause increasingly severe injury of the vessel as the balloon is inflated to a larger size and/or at a higher speed. In a curved vessel, vascular injury due to inflating an oversized balloon at excessive speed will predominantly occur at the edges of the balloon where the vessel wall undergoes greater excursion (Fig. 5.15d, e). In a curved vessel, high-pressure inflation of a balloon with low conformability can cause marked vessel wall excursion, and this increases the risk of dissection at the balloon edges. The risk of dissection also largely depends on the speed of balloon inflation after vessel wall excursion occurs at the balloon edges.

In general, insufficient preparation of the lesion (leading to suboptimal stent expansion) is associated with a high rate of restenosis and with an even higher rate of re-restenosis after repeat PCI for in-stent restenosis. You should remember that there are no satisfactory interventions for treating restenosis due to suboptimal stent expansion. Therefore, suboptimal expansion is an event that must be avoided. Because PCI is performed on this basis, it will often be necessary to increase the balloon inflation pressure to avoid suboptimal stent expansion. On the other hand, it is not always easy to predict the need for high-pressure balloon angioplasty. If a safe method of performing high-pressure balloon angioplasty is known, it should be employed routinely. I will explain my own method of high-pressure balloon angioplasty next.

To dilate a stenosis (Fig. 5.16a), a balloon (3.0-mm) that matches the luminal diameter of the vessel (3.05-mm) is selected and is inflated at its nominal pressure (6 atm). To remove an indentation in the balloon (Fig. 5.16b) and thus avoid insufficient lesion preparation, the pressure is increased to 18 atm (RBP plus 4 atm), achieving a final balloon diameter of about 3.3 mm (Fig. 5.16c). There is a risk

of dissection in the distal segment even if that segment has no plaque, and this risk is increased by more rapid balloon inflation.

In contrast, what will happen if a 2.75-mm balloon is selected with the intention of inflating it at a high pressure (18 atm) to a diameter of 3.05 mm? Although an indentation may remain after inflation at the nominal pressure (Fig. 5.16d), gradually escalating the pressure to 22 atm may remove the indentation and achieve a final balloon diameter of about 3.05 mm (Fig. 5.16e). This approach considerably reduces the risk of dissection in the distal segment.

The stenosis may sometimes be harder than expected. The approach I explained above aims to achieve optimal stent expansion by upfront high-pressure inflation of a slightly undersized balloon while ensuring the safety of high-pressure angioplasty by slowly escalating the inflation pressure. This reduces the risk of dissection associated with unplanned high-pressure inflation of a balloon to an oversized diameter.

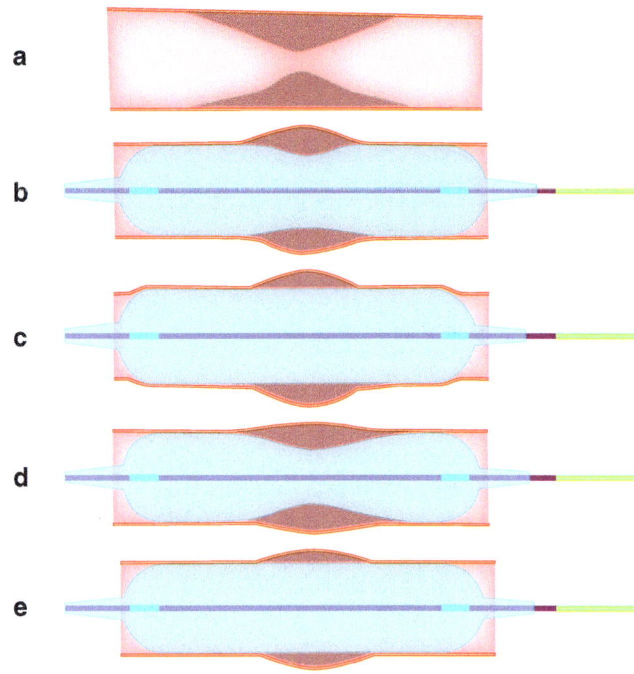

Fig. 5.16 My method of high-pressure balloon angioplasty. In a stenotic vessel (**a**), inflation of a balloon with a diameter matching the luminal diameter of an intact segment of the vessel at its nominal pressure results in insufficient preparation of the lesion (**b**). If this balloon is inflated at a higher pressure to achieve sufficient lesion preparation (and optimal stent expansion), the final balloon diameter will exceed the normal luminal diameter, possibly leading to dissection (**c**). An undersized balloon can be inflated at high pressure to a diameter matching the normal luminal diameter. If inflation to the nominal diameter results in insufficient lesion preparation (**d**), the undersized balloon can be inflated to an even higher pressure without exceeding the normal luminal diameter (**e**)

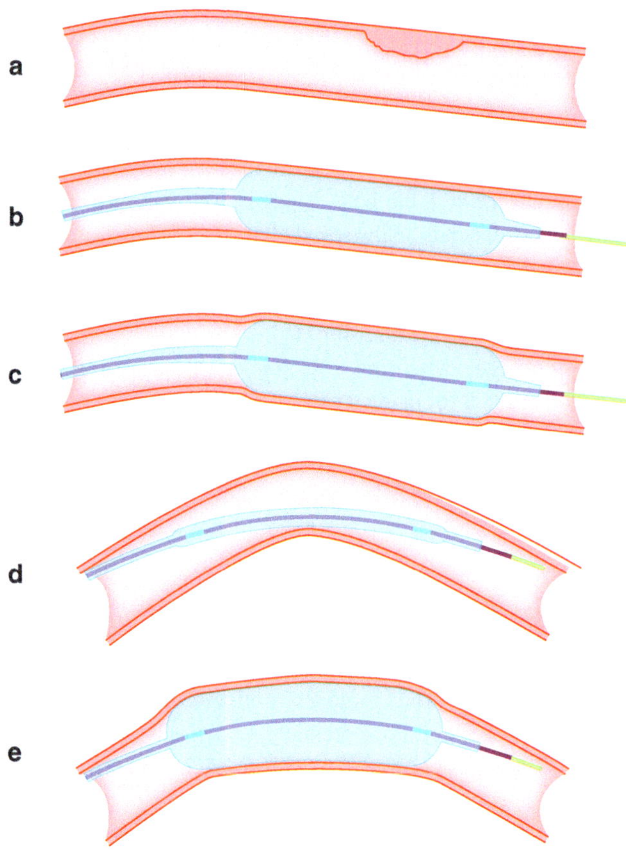

Fig. 5.15 Causes of dissection. If a balloon with a diameter matching the luminal diameter of an intact segment of a straight vessel is inflated across a lesion (**a**), the intact vessel wall will only just come into contact with the balloon and will not be injured (**b**). In contrast, the intact part of the vessel can be injured if the balloon has a larger diameter than the luminal diameter of the intact segment (**c**). In a curved vessel, even a balloon with a diameter matching the luminal diameter of the intact segment will apply greater stress on the vessel wall at its edges and can cause injury to the larger curvature of a bend (**d**, **e**)

5.3.3 Mechanisms of Dissection and Countermeasures

The previous subsection discussed the risk of dissection during angioplasty with a balloon when the distal marker is located in a segment distal to the lesion. However, dissection can also occur by other mechanisms during PCI, which means that precautions and countermeasures for dissection due to various mechanisms should be devised.

1. If the coronary artery distal to a lesion is vulnerable or contains plaque that is continuous from the stent landing zone, dissection is likely to occur at the distal edge of a stent/balloon. The risk of dissection is particularly high for the coronary segment distal to a CTO that has become vulnerable (due to lack of exposure to blood pressure) and also contains plaque.
2. It is well-known that balloon angioplasty can rupture stenotic plaque, causing controlled dissection, but local dissection may sometimes propagate distally during balloon angioplasty. To prevent this, the balloon should be inflated

slowly to minimize intima-media separation. Before performing POBA, you should identify hard lesions with a risk of propagating dissection and create longitudinal cracks in the lesion by rotablation or scoring balloon angioplasty. Dissection associated with longitudinal cracks is unlikely to propagate distally (Fig. 5.17a). In contrast, transverse dissection creates a blind end that is subject to stress from blood flow and thus is likely to propagate distally or even occlude the vessel (Fig. 5.17b).

3. A very high rate of dissection was reported after angioplasty with a previously available balloon. This balloon was found to have a very low slipperiness. In a vessel with irregular walls, parts of the balloon may have become adherent to the walls during inflation, after which further inflation of the balloon may have placed excessive stress on the vessel that led to dissection. Since all currently available balloons have improved slipperiness, dissection is unlikely to occur by this mechanism. However, the risk of dissection is increased by inflating the balloon too rapidly.

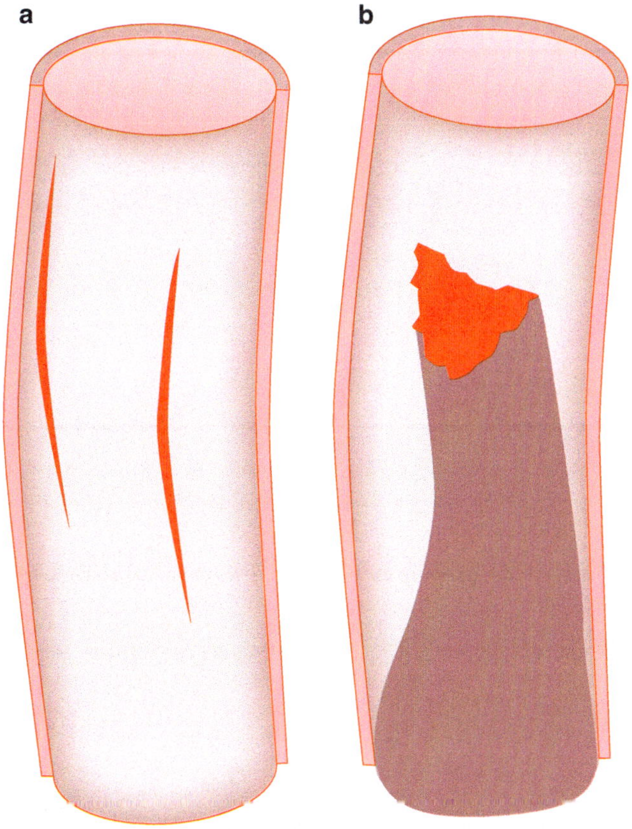

Fig. 5.17 Longitudinal versus transverse dissection. Unlike a longitudinal dissection (**a**), a transverse dissection (**b**) is subject to stress from blood flow that may enlarge the dissection or cause occlusion of the vessel

5.3.4 Scoring and Cutting Balloon Angioplasty

The balloons available for these procedures (Lacrosse NSE, ScoreFlex, and AngioSculpt) have distinct characteristics. Since creating longitudinal cracks permits the vessel wall to expand radially, I prefer to use scoring balloons that purely create longitudinal cracks. Specifically, I almost always use the Lacrosse NSE balloon because of its good crossability and the effectiveness of the pattern of cracks it creates.

The Lacrosse NSE balloon creeps forward and it can be advanced little by little without pushing forcibly. Even if a Lacrosse NSE balloon is stopped at the entrance of a stenosis, pre-dilating the lesion will allow it to creep forward if the scoring elements at the tip can be wedged in the lesion. If the tapered tip of this balloon distal to the distal marker can be inflated to the same shape as its proximal part, this indicates that the balloon will be able to creep forward again (Fig. 5.18a). Thus, this balloon has to be inflated until it is able to creep forward. If the balloon has been inflated sufficiently, it can usually be advanced little by little without pushing it forcibly. If the distal part is not inflated to the same shape as the proximal part (Fig. 5.18b), it is probable that the body of the balloon has not yet crossed the lesion.

If scoring angioplasty with a Lacrosse NSE balloon is not effective, cutting balloon angioplasty should be attempted. When cutting balloon angioplasty is performed, the cutting balloon must not be pushed forward either. Due to the risk of destroying the blade or bursting the balloon by injury due to the blade, performing rotablation or high-pressure balloon angioplasty should be considered prior to cutting balloon angioplasty.

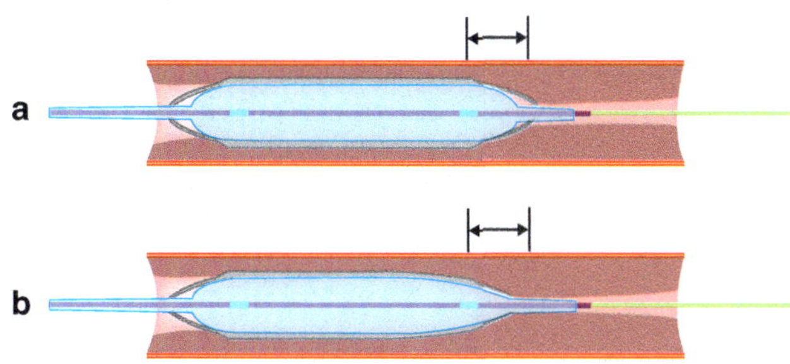

Fig. 5.18 Advancing a Lacrosse NSE balloon catheter. When the tapered part of a Lacrosse NSE balloon (indicated by the arrows) is fully inflated, the balloon can creep forward (**a**). Conversely, poor inflation of the tapered part indicates that it will be difficult for the balloon to cross the lesion (**b**)

5.4 Use of the Rotablator

At my center, rotablation is primarily indicated for debulking lesions with circumferential calcification or lesions that cannot be dilated sufficiently by balloon angioplasty (residual indentation of the balloon). Two rotablation guidewires are available, which are the RotaWire Extra-Support and RotaWire Floppy.

5.4.1 Tornus and RotaWire

Most of the lesions that need debulking with a Rotablator can only be crossed by the Tornus catheter. It is very difficult to pass a RotaWire Extra-Support through a Tornus catheter. Although this may sometimes be achieved in a straight vessel, it is usually impossible to advance a RotaWire Extra-Support through a Tornus catheter despite pushing and rotating it. However, a RotaWire Floppy can be advanced into a Tornus catheter by rotating it. To facilitate rotation and advancement, instead of attaching a clip to the guidewire (Fig. 5.19a), I attach a torquer (Fig. 5.19b). Attempts to forcibly push a RotaWire guidewire can easily result in kinking at the point of obstruction.

5.4.2 Debulking a Lesion at a Bend

If the lumen distal to a hard stenosis at a bend in a coronary artery is only slightly narrowed, the rotablation burr may become stuck immediately after crossing the lesion and be difficult to withdraw. This is likely to occur with the RotaWire Floppy, but is rare with the RotaWire Extra-Support. Therefore, the RotaWire Extra-Support should be used when debulking a severe stenosis located at a bend.

5.4.3 Reducing Guidewire Bias and Burr Bias

When a RotaWire, especially the RotaWire Extra-Support, passes through a bend in a vessel, the wire becomes biased toward the inner curvature of the bend (Fig. 5.20a). This inward guidewire bias may offset the outward bias of the burr. On the other hand, the burr shows bias toward the outer curvature that is opposite to the guidewire bias (Fig. 5.20b). If the guidewire passes through two bends in a vessel, the effect of crossing the first bend may bias the burr toward the inner curvature of the second bend.

The situation becomes complicated when the target vessel has two or more bends. As shown in Fig. 5.21a,

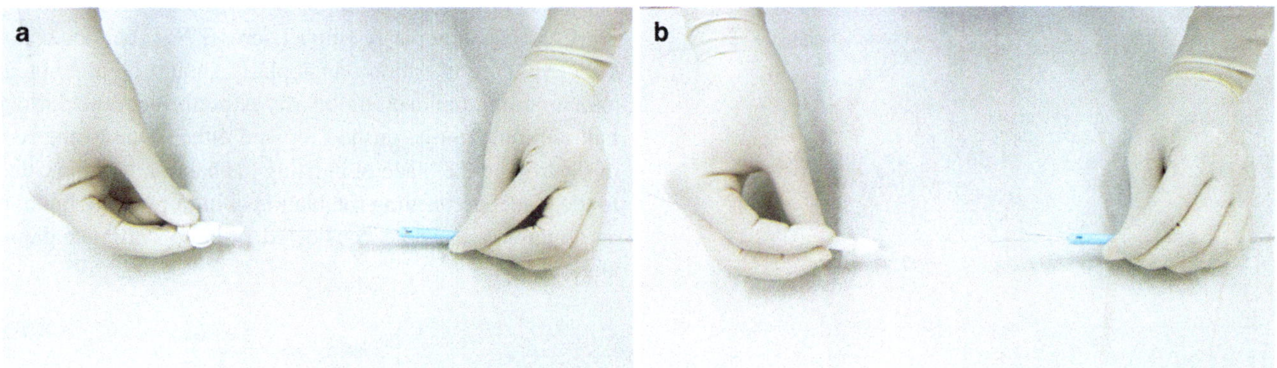

Fig. 5.19 Difficulty in advancing the RotaWire without rotation. (**a**) A clip can easily be attached to the RotaWire, but is of limited usefulness for rotating the wire. (**b**) A torquer can rotate the wire efficiently and help to advance it

the guidewire is biased toward the inner curvature of each bend. In contrast, the burr is biased toward the outer curvature of the first bend as a reaction to the guidewire bias, but this bias of the burr amplifies the guidewire bias at the second bend (Fig. 5.21b). If the guiding catheter is oriented so that guidewire bias at the first bend becomes equivalent to that at the second bend, the burr directs the guidewire bias toward the outer side, tending to eliminate the guidewire bias (Fig. 5.21c).

Performing rotablation with a biased burr will eventually result eccentric debulking of the lesion, and it will need to be entirely stented. It is sometimes difficult to deliver a stent to such a lesion, but it can be effective to use the child-in-mother technique to advance the stent part of the way.

a
b

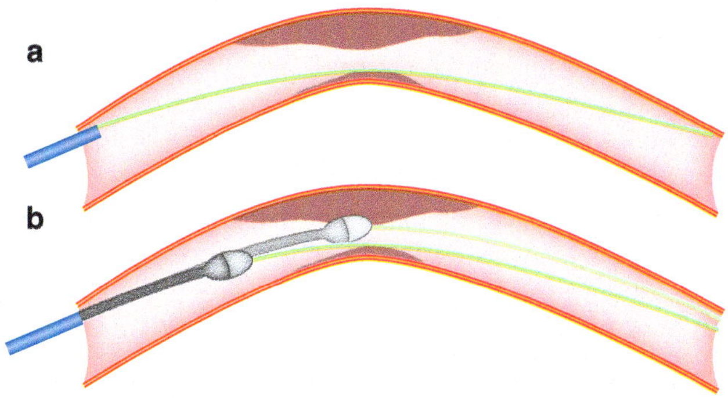

Fig. 5.20 Using the RotaWire Extra-Support when debulking a lesion at a bend. The guidewire is biased toward the inner curvature of the bend (**a**), while the burr passes along the outer curvature (**b**)

a
b
c

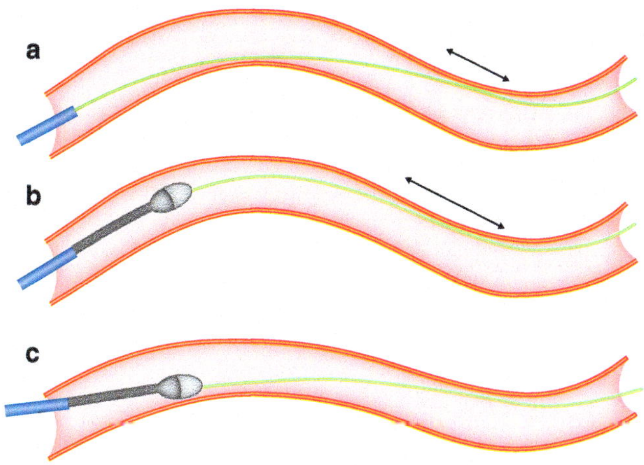

Fig. 5.21 Advancing the RotaWire across two bends. The burr is biased toward the outer curvature of the first bend, and this burr bias amplifies the guidewire bias toward the inner curvature of the second bend (**a**, **b**). Changing the orientation of the guiding catheter can reduce guidewire bias at the second bend (**c**)

5.4.4 Advancing a Burr

You can advance a rotablation burr into a stenosis by (1) lightly pressing the burr into the entrance of the lesion for several seconds or (2) repeatedly approaching the entrance with a pecking motion of the burr. I prefer to use the former method because the burr seems to follow the operator's intentions better, although there is no definite evidence to support this choice. You should advance the burr very slowly while running it at a constant rate of not less than 5000 rpm. In this context, I may add that you should not vibrate a balloon like a pecking motion when delivering it and must not vibrate a stent when delivering it.

5.5 ELCA

We assessed the benefit of ELCA in 116 patients undergoing PCI at my center during the period from 2001 to 2008. Among these 116 patients, 101 patients had CTO and 98 of them underwent 0.9-mm ELCA. ELCA was indicated for debulking of CTOs that could be crossed by a guidewire, but not by a balloon catheter.

After the introduction of retrograde PCI in October 2005, our use of ELCA declined dramatically and reached zero in 2008. A retrograde guidewire that has crossed a CTO can be introduced into the antegrade guiding catheter and trapped to create a guidewire loop, so that a retrograde microcatheter can almost always track the collateral channel and cross the CTO. If a retrograde microcatheter has crossed the CTO, an antegrade microcatheter or balloon catheter can also almost always cross the CTO. Thus, use of the 0.9-mm laser catheter for treating CTOs has been abandoned.

Since ELCA was recently approved for coverage by the national health insurance scheme in Japan, its benefit for the treatment of thrombotic occlusion has been reappraised. The importance of non-pushing PCI techniques should always be kept in mind when treating thrombotic occlusions. Since a thrombotic occlusion is soft, it can be readily crossed by advancing a laser catheter. However, you should always bear in mind that rapidly advancing a laser catheter is not a good idea. There is a risk of inadvertently pushing the catheter forward too vigorously.

A single laser energy pulse of up to 80 J only ablates 0.05 mm of tissue. At the maximum frequency of 80 pulses/sec, a laser catheter can only be advanced at a speed of 4.0 mm/s. Advancing the laser catheter more rapidly than 4.0 mm/s involves utilization of mechanical energy in addition to laser energy.

It may be considered reasonable to push the ELCA catheter to help it cross the CTO, but pushing will considerably reduce the ability to ablate soft tissue.

5.6 Stenting

5.6.1 General Precautions for Stenting

5.6.1.1 Lesion Preparation

The two objectives of preparing a lesion for stenting are (1) to facilitate smooth delivery of the stent to the target location without the need to apply force strong enough to deform the stent and (2) to dilate the lesion sufficiently to ensure optimal stent expansion.

To facilitate smooth stent delivery, it is most important to dilate the lumen of the lesion to a sufficient diameter for delivering the stent. In addition, lesion preparation should eliminate luminal irregularities. In particular, irregularities that create indentations visible in the short axis view on the larger curvature of a bend in the target vessel can interfere with advancement of a stent (Fig. 5.22a). In contrast, an irregularity that can only be seen in the long axis view will not block advancement of a stent (Fig. 5.22b).

How can a lesion be prepared sufficiently for optimal stent expansion? A stent can exert a maximum resistance of 3 kPa (3 atm) to prevent recoil of the surrounding vessel walls, which means that any stent can be deformed when compressed by vascular recoil with a force greater than 3 atm. It is well-known that a lesion should be pre-dilated until the balloon is fully inflated to eliminate all indentations. Thus, lesion preparation with balloon angioplasty (nominal pressure: 3 atm) is theoretically inadequate if any indentation remains in the balloon, although this has not been tested for economic reasons. To ensure optimal stent expansion, the vessel wall at the lesion needs to be made redundant (to reduce recoil).

Effective methods of adequately preparing a lesion for smooth stent delivery and optimal stent expansion include (1) debulking with a Rotablator, (2) scoring balloon angioplasty, (3) high-pressure balloon angioplasty, and (4) sufficient POBA.

POBA alone can prepare a stenotic lesion with soft fibrous plaque or lipid-rich plaque, while high-pressure balloon angioplasty may be required for a calcified lesion or a lesion with harder fibrous plaque. With a very hard lesion, scoring balloon angioplasty (e.g., Lacrosse NSE) can be performed to create cracks in the calcified or hard fibrous plaque, thereby reducing vascular recoil after balloon angioplasty. A calcified lesion that is too hard for scoring balloon angioplasty or that resists delivery of the scoring balloon should be debulked with a Rotablator.

1. The debulking devices available include ELCA and the Rotablator. Debulking with a Rotablator is most effective for preparing a calcified lesion for stent implantation. Rotablation can enlarge the lumen and also reduces the vascular burden of calcification and thus decreases rigidity of the vessel wall.
2. A lesion that seems difficult to dilate sufficiently by high-pressure balloon angioplasty even after debulking with a Rotablator should be scored with a Lacrosse NSE balloon. After performance of scoring balloon angioplasty, such a lesion will be easier to dilate by relatively low-pressure balloon angioplasty.
3. Adding high-pressure balloon angioplasty to scoring balloon angioplasty will fracture calcified plaque, thereby creating vessel wall redundancy and reducing recoil.

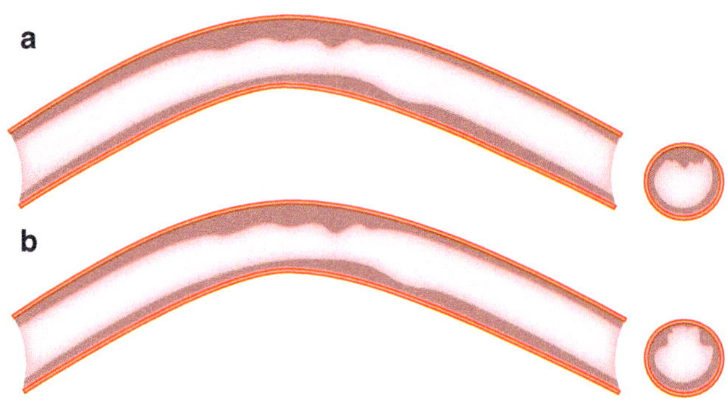

Fig. 5.22 Differences of luminal irregularities. Luminal irregularities on the larger curvature that appear to be similar in the long axis view may have a different distribution in the short axis view. Irregularities on the larger curvature that can also be seen in the short axis view may interfere with stent delivery (**a**), whereas irregularities only seen in the long axis view will not (**b**)

5.6.1.2 Difficulty with Stent Delivery: Predicting and Avoiding Problems

After apparently sufficient lesion preparation, it may still prove difficult to advance a stent during PCI. This is probably due to residual luminal irregularities after balloon angioplasty (Fig. 5.23a).

Difficulty delivering a naked stent can often be predicted by difficulty with delivering a balloon for lesion preparation. I use the child-in-mother technique (e.g., GuideLiner) if I encounter difficulty in advancing a balloon or if it becomes blocked after high-pressure balloon angioplasty.

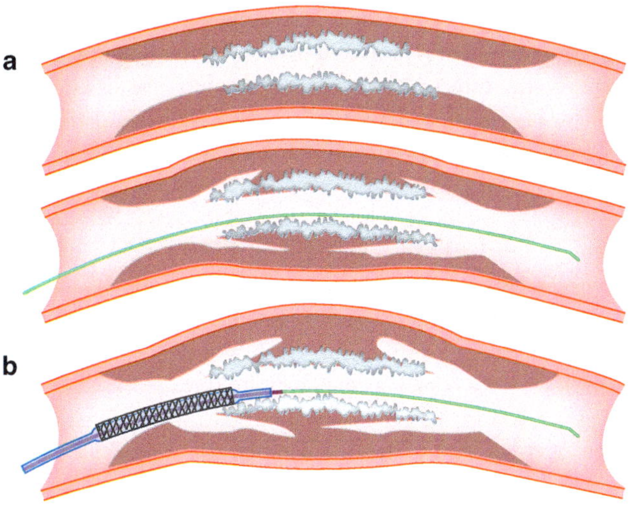

Fig. 5.23 Lesion at a bend with calcified plaque. (**a**) Sufficient dilatation of a lesion with calcified plaque can enlarge the lumen, but may cause dissection or indentation at the edge of the plaque that inhibits stent advancement. (**b**) Additional high-pressure balloon angioplasty may further enlarge the dissection or indentation at the edge of the calcified plaque, which may preclude stent delivery

5.6.1.3 Stent Delivery Strategy Based on the Pattern of Difficulty with Delivery

A stent that appears to be deliverable may become blocked and difficult to advance into the target lesion. If this happens, I choose the optimal stent delivering strategy according to the pattern of difficulty with delivery. I never push the stent hard or push it in while wiggling it. If it suddenly becomes impossible to advance a stent immediately after feeling that it was deflected, attempts to push the stent further are likely to deform it. It is safer and more reliable to advance the stent via a child catheter in order to bypass luminal irregularities.

If you notice that advancing a stent gradually becomes more difficult until it is completely impossible to move it further, you must not increase the force applied to the stent. In this situation, pushing hard on the stent will not help to advance it. Rather, some struts will be deformed at the edges or in the body of the stent, wherever friction is greater, eventually making the stent undeliverable to the landing zone. Instead, you should continue to apply the same force to stent delivery catheter as that which advanced it before, which will result in slight deflection of the shaft of the stent delivery catheter (Fig. 5.24a). If you then pull the catheter back slightly to eliminate the deflection and apply the same force again, the stent will advance a little (Fig. 5.24b).

This maneuver will achieve delivery of the stent into a short lesion, but may not prevent it from becoming stuck again in a long lesion. If the stent again stops advancing, it should be pulled back to eliminate deflection of the shaft and then pushed in again to advance it slightly. Such alternating pull-back and advancement of the stent will eventually achieve delivery. This is the safest and most reliable method, although it is time-consuming. However, if it becomes completely impossible to advance the stent after repeating this maneuver two or three times, the best option is to slowly withdraw the stent and switch to stenting via the child-in-mother technique.

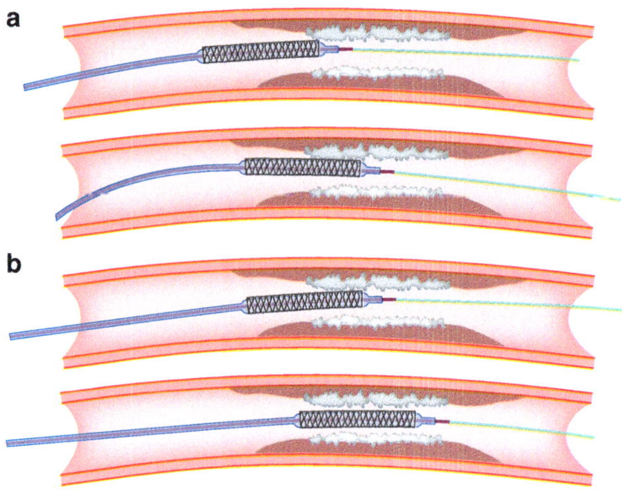

Fig. 5.24 When a stent is difficult to deliver. (**a**) To deliver a stent into a difficult lesion (e.g., a lesion with calcified plaque), it should be push in with slight force to deflect the shaft of the stent delivery catheter. (**b**) Then the catheter should be pulled back slightly to eliminate deflection of its shaft and slowly advanced again. This maneuver may help to bypass the obstruction and allow advancement of the stent. If the stent becomes obstructed again, this maneuver should be repeated. If several repetitions cannot achieve stent advancement, the stent should be withdrawn and then advanced via a child catheter. However, the stent should never be pushed in forcibly

5.6.1.4 Other Strategies

In recent years, the abovementioned strategy has been widely used to deliver a stent into a difficult lesion. In addition, the strategies discussed in previous chapters (e.g., the buddy wire technique, buddy balloon technique, slip-through technique, and trapping technique) are also effective. These techniques are worth trying if another guidewire has crossed a distal bifurcation lesion or an additional guidewire is available. However, a forcible attempt to advance an additional guidewire may fail or may cause deformation of a stent that has not been completely protected, so is questionable whether an additional guidewire should be inserted to facilitate stent delivery. The child-in-mother technique may be safer and more reliable for delivering a stent into a difficult lesion.

5.6.1.5 Stent Positioning

Before stably positioning a stent that has been delivered into a lesion, CAG should be performed to confirm that the distal edge of the stent has reached the target. If CAG takes too long, a stent that has reached the target will often move further before deployment and expansion. Even if it is expanded soon after performance of positioning CAG, the stent may advance further during expansion. After a stent has been advanced to the target, the stent delivery catheter should be pulled back slightly (so as to only straighten its shaft while not withdrawing the stent) before positioning CAG is performed. Whenever there is an interval between positioning CAG and stent deployment, positioning CAG (fluoroscopy) should be repeated immediately before inflating the SDB.

5.6.2 Using a Conformable Stent

5.6.2.1 What Is a Conformable Stent?

As is the case for bifurcation stenting, it is better to use a conformable stent for general coronary artery stenting. A conformable stent is preferred for the following four reasons: (1) less edge effect, (2) a low risk of fracture, (3) the ability to only apply bending stress to the vessel after fracture occurs at a link, and (4) less edge effect at the fractured stumps.

What makes a stent conformable? As shown in Fig. 5.25, less stress is produced when conformable stent is bent, so that it can be longitudinally expanded on the larger curvature and compressed on the smaller curvature. Thus, "conformability" of a stent is a synonym for "longitudinal deformability."

Particularly for bifurcation stenting, I prefer to use stents with fewer links (such as the Wiktor, GFX, S-6, S-7, Driver, S-stent, Nobori 3.5-mm, Element, and Integrity), as stated previously. I rarely use the Cordis and CrossFlex stents because the radio-opacity of the former is too high and the proximal part of the latter shows suboptimal expansion.

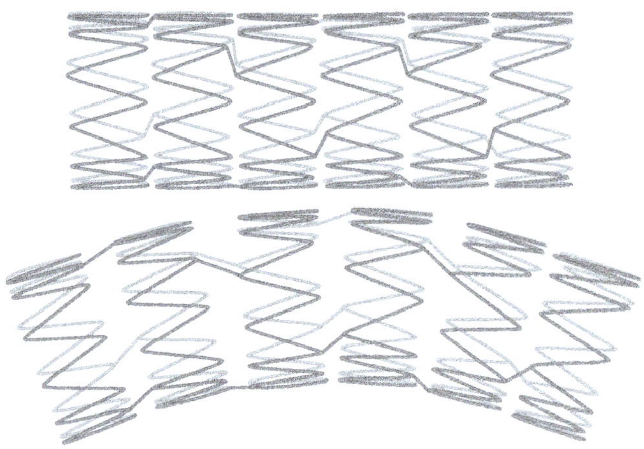

Fig. 5.25 Design of a conformable stent

5.6.2.2 Points to Consider

Based on the finding that stents with fewer links are more likely to undergo deformation, I have made efforts to develop techniques for successfully placing such stents without deforming them. I take great care to prevent deformation of stent struts by a balloon during its advancement into the SB of a bifurcation lesion or by the exit port of an IVUS catheter during withdrawal. I consider that the interventionalist is required to maintain the original shape of an implanted stent by using various techniques. However, stent deformation by other devices under the abovementioned circumstances is often localized and sometimes undetectable by CAG. Hence, stent deformity may often be overlooked during PCI.

The PROMUS Element is a two-link stent composed of eight short crowns, with struts linked by short oblique peak-to-valley interconnections and thus aligned in the identical phase. This configuration prevents overlap between adjacent struts and helps to achieve good conformability (longitudinal deformability) of the stent (Fig. 5.26).

Since I began to use the PROMUS Element stent, I have failed to prevent deformation several times despite taking great care during delivery, while its high conformability has deeply impressed me. Since I considered it my mission or raison d'etre to safely place this highly conformable stent without deforming it, I reviewed six cases of stent deformation among over 200 cases of coronary artery stenting to identify risk factors for stent deformation.

These six cases included the following: (1) a severely tapered lesion (Fig. 5.27), (2) a tapered lesion in a highly angulated vessel (Fig. 5.28), (3) an aorto-ostial lesion (Fig. 5.29), (4) a bifurcation lesion with a large-diameter proximal MB (Fig. 5.30), (5) a severely calcified lesion (Fig. 5.31), and (6) a lesion recanalized by stenting a false lumen (Fig. 5.32). In all of these lesions, a balloon for post-dilatation or SB dilatation had to be advanced into or across a stent with some struts that had not been apposed. The risk of stent deformation appears to be particularly high for lesions at a bend in the vessel or ostial lesions. Significant irregularity of the stent lumen (e.g., after deployment in a severely calcified lesion) or the balloon surface creates severe friction during balloon advancement, which can be another risk factor for stent deformation.

Such longitudinal deformation results in the struts being pushed together or pulled apart after stent deployment. Why is sufficient force to cause deformation applied to the stent? This primarily occurs because a stent strut or link has obstructed another device (Fig. 5.33). When additional force is applied to advance the device, the strut is very likely to undergo severe deformation. Accordingly, you should not attempt to push a device forward after hitting a stent strut and should take other measures that help to bypass the strut. In a tortuous vessel, in particular, even the tip of a balloon introduced to improve apposition of the proximal part of a stent is likely to hit a non-apposed strut (Fig. 5.34). In this situation, even slight application of force can cause severe deformation of the stent. To avoid such deformation, it is important to place the stent so that its struts will not be hit by other devices during the subsequent steps of PCI, such as delivery of the post-dilatation balloon.

I have encountered little stent deformation since I adopted several techniques (both old and new) to prevent collision of other devices with the struts and to eliminate these risk factors for deformation.

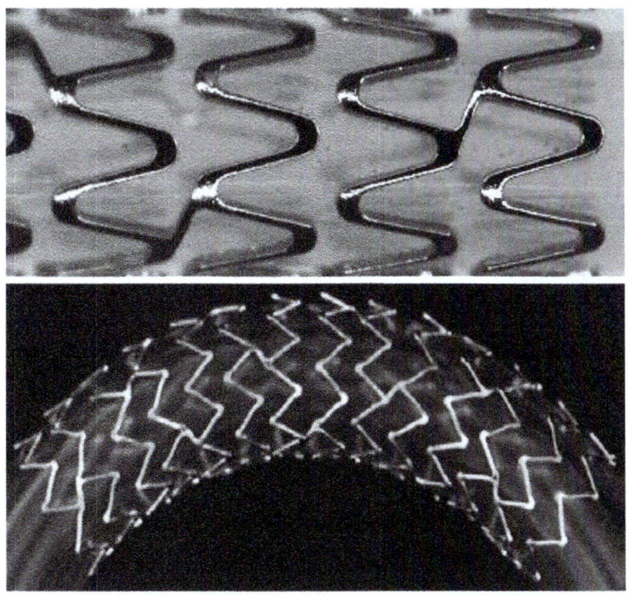

Fig. 5.26 PROMUS Element stent. At a bend in the vessel, the PROMUS Element stent applies less stress to the vessel wall as it can be longitudinally expanded on the outer curvature of the bend and compressed on the inner curvature

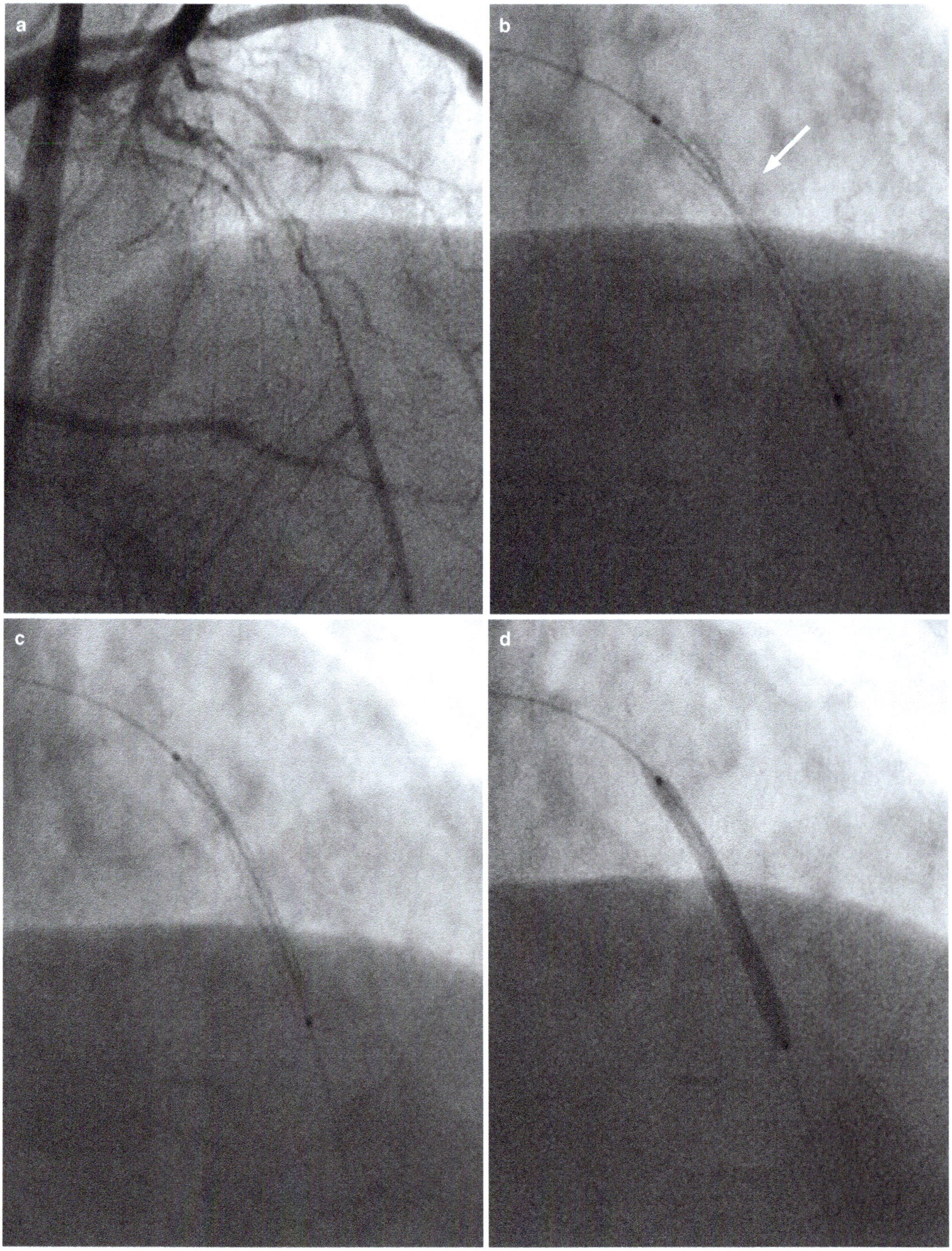

Fig. 5.27 Stenting an LAD lesion (**a**). Low-pressure inflation of the SDB to the target vessel diameter has not achieved optimal stent expansion at the point indicated by an arrow. When the stent delivery catheter was pulled back slightly, only the proximal marker moved and the distal marker did not, indicating that the stent has been shortened (**b**). Immediate withdrawal of the stent delivery catheter would establish deformation (shortening) of the stent and preclude delivery of a post-dilatation balloon. On the other hand, readvancing the stent delivery catheter resolved shortening of the stent due to its high conformability (**c**). Then the SDB was inflated slowly until all indentations were eliminated (**d**)

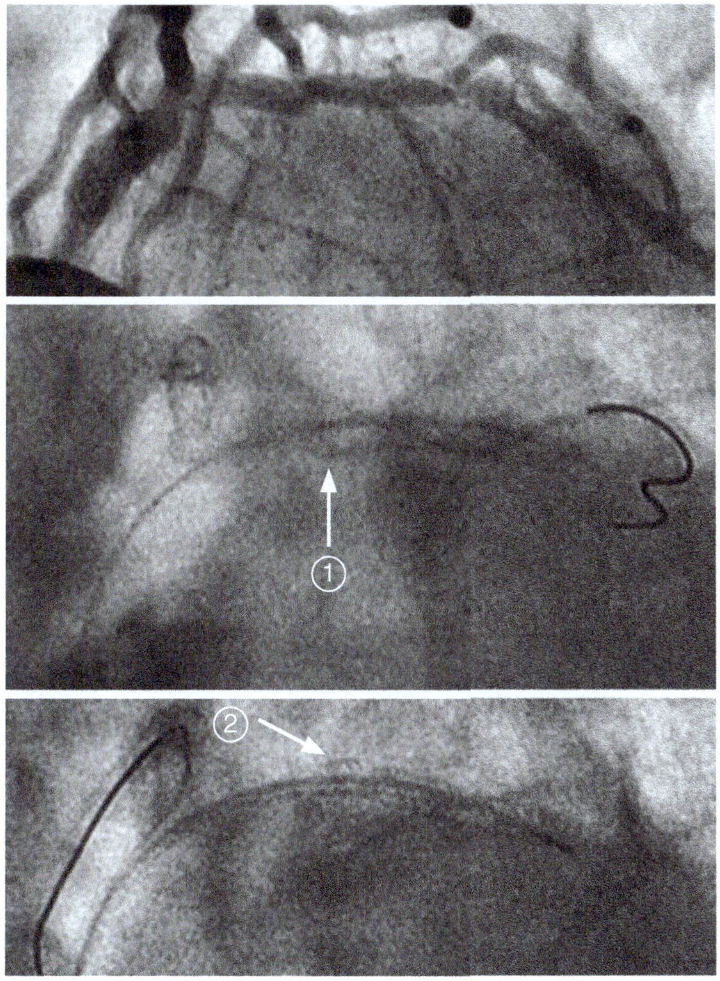

Fig. 5.28 LCX bifurcation lesion. After bifurcation stenting, an IVUS catheter was advanced into the stent and caused deformation of the stent edge on the larger curvature of the bend (arrow) due to proximal malapposition

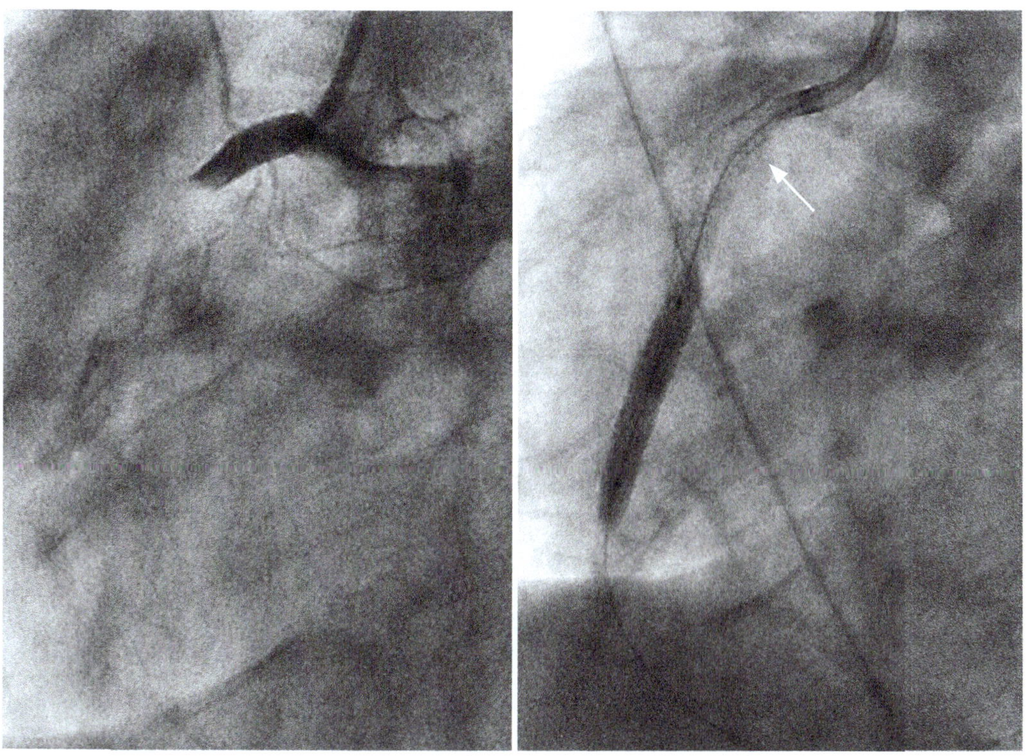

Fig. 5.29 Stenting an RCA lesion in a patient with acute coronary syndrome. Due to severe tortuosity of the RCA, the tip of a post-dilatation balloon contacted the stent as it was being advanced and caused shortening of the stent (arrow)

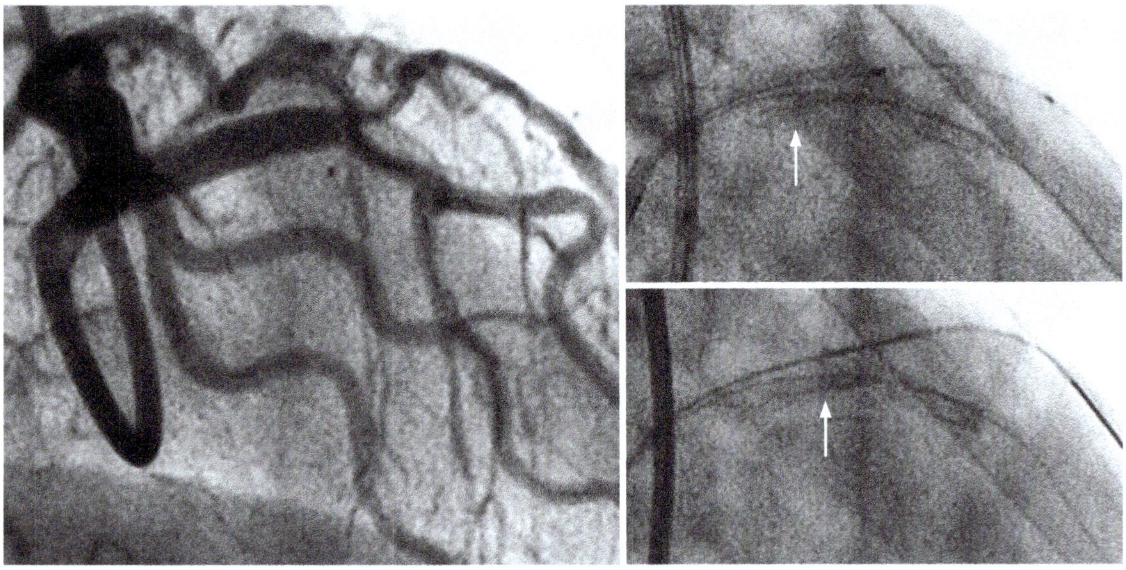

Fig. 5.30 LAD bifurcation lesion. Because the diameter of the proximal MB was much larger than that of the distal MB, POT was performed after stenting. When a balloon was advanced into the SB, it caused shortening of the proximal part of the stent (arrows), making it difficult to deliver a stent into the SB

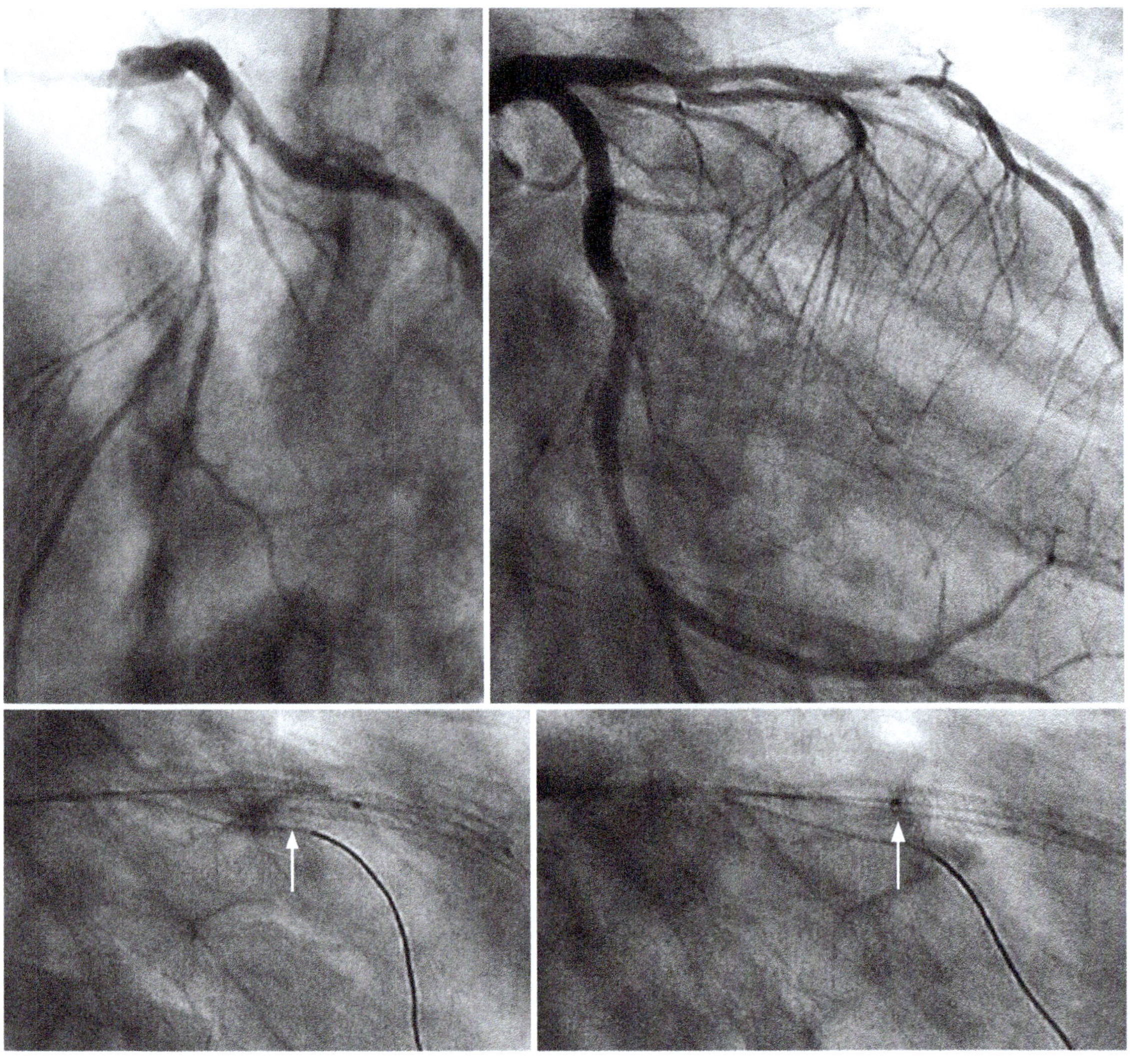

Fig. 5.31 Stenting a calcified LAD bifurcation lesion. After stenting, a balloon was advanced into the SB and caused shortening of the stent (arrows) due to malapposition

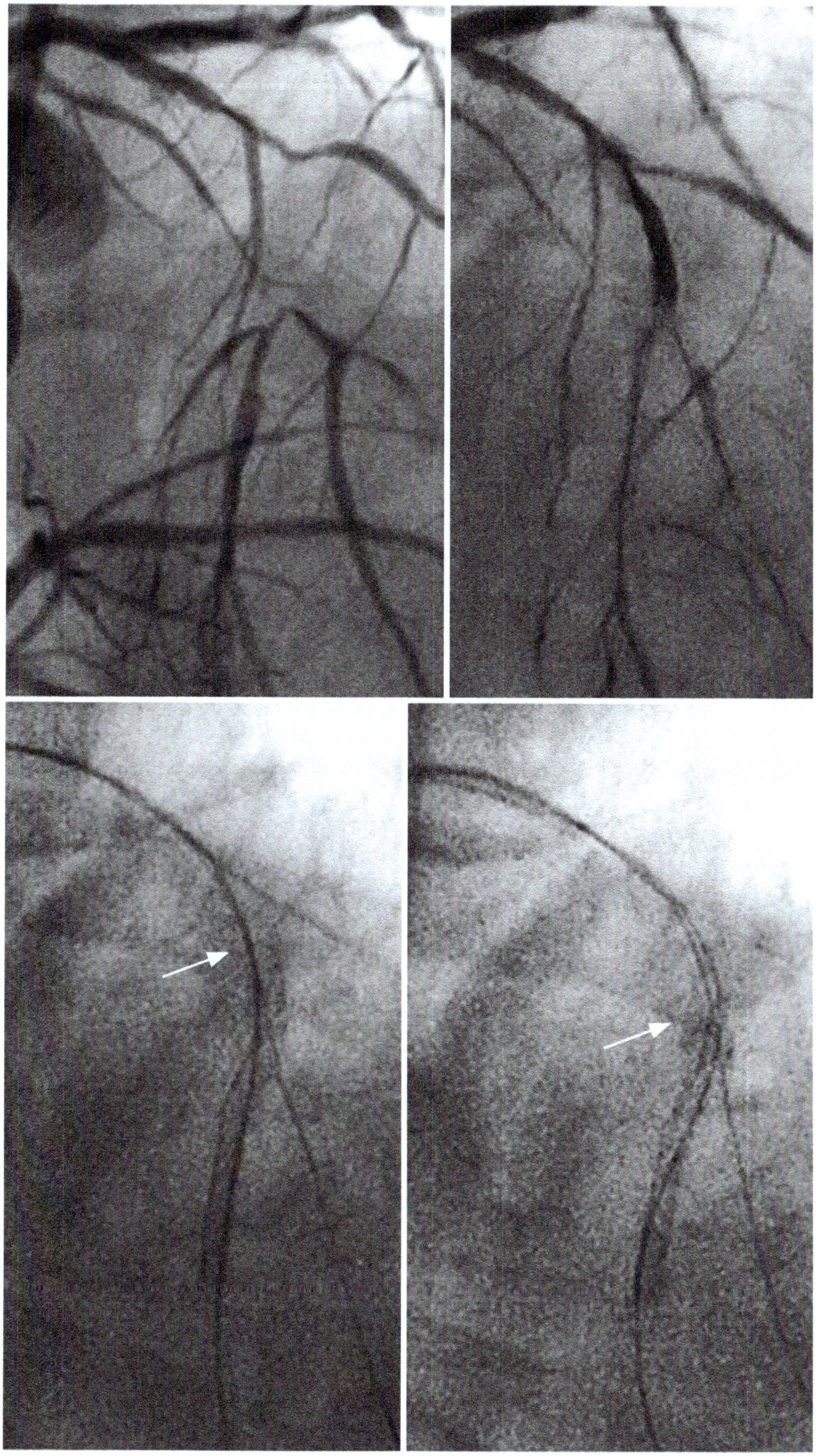

Fig. 5.32 CTO of the LAD successfully recanalized by reverse CART. After a guidewire had crossed the CTO through a false lumen, a stent was implanted in the false lumen. After stenting, a balloon was advanced into the SB and caused shortening of the stent (arrows) at the gap between lesion and stent. Planned SB stenting was abandoned because shortening of the stent (i.e., strut deformation) prevented delivery of a second stent to the SB

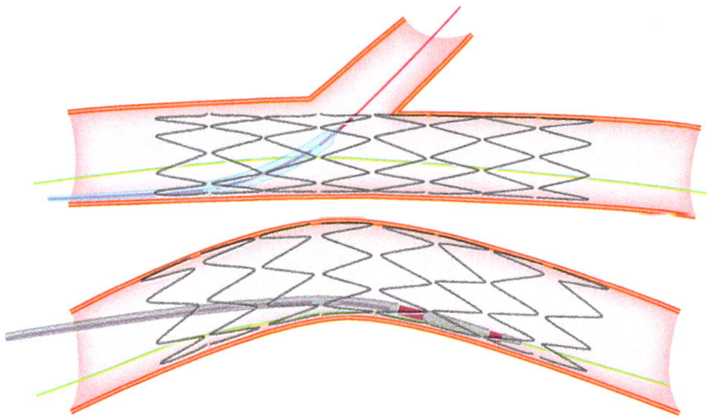

Fig. 5.33 Stent deformation by a balloon advanced into the SB or by an IVUS catheter during withdrawal after stenting. A stent may be deformed if a balloon is advanced forcibly or an IVUS catheter is withdrawn forcibly

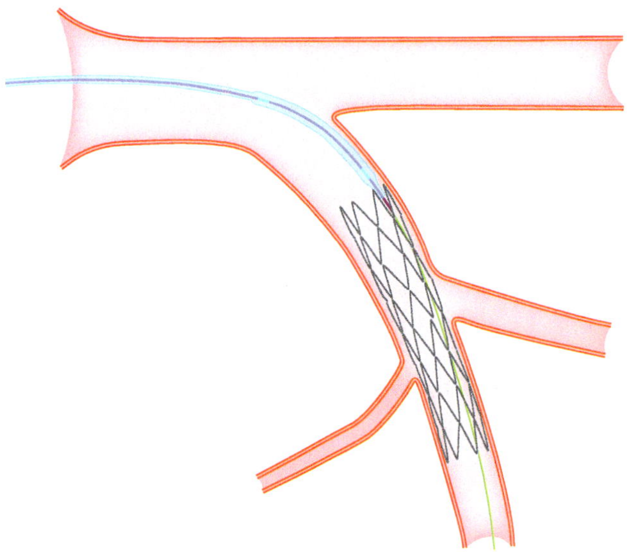

Fig. 5.34 Stent deformation by other devices at a curved bifurcation with a large-diameter proximal MB. A stent placed at such a bifurcation lesion is likely to show malapposition at its proximal part. When a balloon is introduced for POT, it may hit a strut and deform the stent

5.6.2.3 Practical Approach to Placing a Conformable Stent

The following strategies can be employed when placing a conformable stent:

1. In principle, use a guidewire that provides relatively strong support.
2. In a tapered vessel, place a stent with a size matching the diameter of the proximal segment of the vessel by inflating the SDB at a low pressure.
3. Prepare the lesion sufficiently to allow optimal stent expansion, even by low-pressure inflation of the SDB. Particularly if the distal segment of the vessel is calcified, debulking of the lesion should often be performed by scoring/cutting balloon angioplasty or rotablation.

For a bifurcation lesion, such as a distal LM bifurcation lesion:

4. Perform POT immediately after implanting a stent.
5. If difficulty is encountered when delivering a previously used balloon into a stent, withdraw the balloon into the guiding catheter and then rewrap it there by inflation at about 10 atm.
6. and 7. To deliver a balloon into the SB for post-stenting KBI, special techniques may be required.

1. Without using a guidewire that provides relatively strong support, it is impossible to alleviate bias of the stent/balloon toward the larger curvature of a bend in the target vessel (Fig. 5.35). For example, the Sion guidewire is not suitable for use when delivering a stent/balloon because it provides insufficient support. The Sion Blue Extra-Support wire, or another guidewire that provides equivalent support, is preferable.
2. The stent should be well apposed when it is initially placed. If there is malapposition of any strut, the stent can easily be deformed if the strut is hit by another device. At a large bend in the target vessel, a strut is likely to be hit by another device, even if the struts are all well apposed. In a tapered vessel, a stent with a diameter as close as possible to that of the proximal segment should employed. In a tapered vessel with a bend, a stent with a diameter that ensures optimal apposition in the proximal segment of the vessel should be used.

In a tapered vessel, there are two methods of placing a stent with a diameter matching that of the proximal segment. One method is to perform double stenting, while the other is carry out low-pressure implantation of a stent with a diameter matching the proximal segment, followed by distal and proximal post-dilatation. I generally employ the latter strategy. If the proximal vessel has a diameter of 3.5 mm, I choose to implant a 3.5-mm stent even if the distal vessel diameter is only 2.5 mm. If there is no plaque at the distal edge of the stent, there is little risk that low-pressure expansion of the stent (about 6 atm) will cause dissection.

If there is plaque at the distal edge of the stent and dissection unfortunately occurs at the stent edge, this can be overcome by implanting a short additional stent (about 8 mm long) with a diameter matching that of the distal vessel.

3. Lesion preparation: To achieve low-pressure stent expansion, it is necessary to sufficiently prepare (pre-dilate) the

lesion. Wherever stent expansion is suboptimal, a post-dilatation balloon or another device may become caught on a strut, possibly leading to deformation of the stent.

The diameter of the distal vessel (particularly the diameter of the distal MB at a bifurcation) may be much smaller than the diameter of the stent implanted in the proximal segment. An oversized stent will exert little expansionary force after implantation. Many stents exert a maximum force of only 2 to 3 kPa when expanded to their target diameter. If a stent is going to be expanded to a smaller diameter than the target, sufficient lesion preparation must theoretically be performed to allow sustained stent expansion with low-pressure balloon inflation (1.5–2.0 atm).

4. POT: In a bifurcation lesion, POT should only be performed to dilate the proximal MB to the final target diameter and thus improve apposition of the proximal struts. In a tapered non-bifurcation lesion, POT should also be performed before post-dilatation of the distal part of the stent if there is malapposition of the proximal struts.
5. Rewrapping: If a balloon is advanced into a stent for post-dilatation or KBI after being used for pre-dilatation and not rewrapped, considerable friction may be generated within the stent, and it can be impossible to move the balloon forward. If this happens, the balloon should be withdrawn into the guiding catheter and inflated at a relatively low pressure of about 10 atm, followed by rewrapping in a fine covering tube. After a balloon is rewrapped in this way, it can usually be delivered into a stent very easily.

   In the era of bulky balloons, the interventionalist had to withdraw a balloon completely and rewrap it outside the patient. To rewrap the balloon in those days, it was usually returned to its protective sheath and inflated at about 10 atm. The abovementioned rewrapping technique copies this old method of balloon rewrapping, but performs it inside the guiding catheter. Inflating and deflating a balloon in a smooth lumen with a relatively small diameter increases longitudinal folding of the balloon, which will then reduce friction during delivery of the balloon into a stent.
6. KBI or high-pressure MB dilatation: After wiring the SB through the MB stent and advancing a kissing balloon into the MB, you may sometimes encounter difficulty when advancing a kissing balloon into the SB across the MB stent. If the stent struts have been crossed by the tip of the balloon, but not by its shoulders, you may immediately perform KBI at a low pressure of about 6 atm. This will often facilitate advancement of the balloon into the SB. Even if performing KBI once fails to completely deliver the balloon into the SB, several cycles of balloon inflation/deflation can lead to gradual advancement of the SB balloon and eventually allow it to smoothly cross the stent into the SB. To avoid over-dilation of the proximal segment of the vessel, you must not allow the marker of the MB balloon to protrude beyond the proximal edge of the MB stent, and simultaneous inflation of the two kissing balloons should be confined within the stent.

   High-pressure inflation of the MB balloon alone can also be useful and is possible after withdrawal or sufficient advancement of the SB balloon.

   As is also the case in (7) below, you should never use the anchoring technique with the MB balloon delivered into the distal MB or any other balloon. This is because forcibly pushing a device that has been caught on a stent strut is very likely to cause deformation of the stent.
7. Checking and cutting off a damaged balloon tip, using a new balloon, or using the buddy wire/balloon techniques: If a balloon cannot be advanced toward the SB and if the site of obstruction appears to be distant from the balloon's distal marker, the tip of the balloon may be blocked by a stent strut.

Possible reasons for this are (1) the balloon tip has become frayed or (2) the angle between the tip of the balloon and the stent strut/vessel wall is too small or large.

As mentioned in (6) above, high-pressure inflation of the MB balloon alone, which is possible after withdrawal or sufficient advancement of the SB balloon, can be useful and is worth trying first. It may also be effective to withdraw the SB balloon into the guiding catheter or another site where it can be rotated freely and rotate it 180 degrees before readvancement. However, it is impossible to deliver a balloon into the SB across the struts of the MB stent if the tip has become frayed. Therefore, you should cut off the frayed tip of the balloon or exchange it for a new one.

If a balloon with an intact tip is difficult to deliver, you may advance a very small balloon past the obstruction and pre-dilate the stent cell.

Since the highly conformable PROMUS Element stent is prone to proximal deformation, the design was modified when developing the PROMUS Premier, which has four or five links in the three struts at its proximal edge. This modification has made the proximal 3 mm of the stent very rigid and thus increased the risk of fracture at the interface between the rigid and more flexible parts of the stent. Hence, the PROMUS series cannot escape one of the greatest defects of the first-generation DES. It is important for interventionalists to consider ways of making the best use of currently available conformable stents to achieve implantation without deformation and not to employ stents with a new design that may apparently make stenting easier, but is actually inferior.

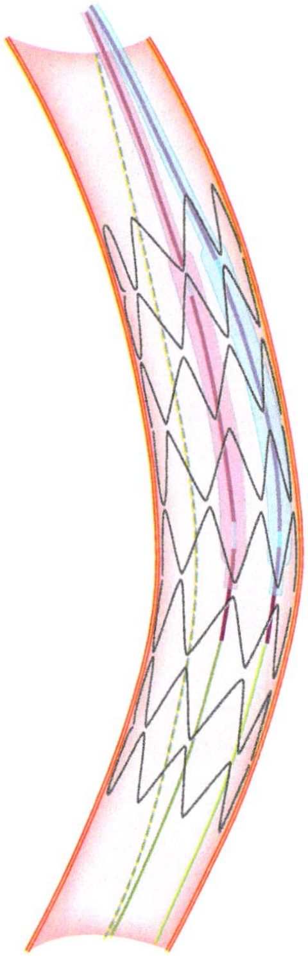

Fig. 5.35 Using a guidewire that provides strong backup. A guidewire or balloon catheter tends to track along the larger curvature of a bend in a vessel. Upfront use of a guidewire with strong backup may allow advancement of a balloon catheter along a different route. It can also be effective to first advance a balloon with good deliverability on an outwardly biased guidewire and then advance an optimally sized balloon along a guidewire with strong backup

5.6.3 Using a Child Catheter

After sufficient preparation of the lesion, you should repeatedly advance and pull back the balloon catheter. If you notice any difficulty in advancing or withdrawing the balloon catheter or a Crusade or IVUS catheter, you should consider using supplementary techniques for stent delivery.

The supplementary techniques for stent delivery include (1) the buddy wire technique (Fig. 5.36a), (2) the buddy balloon technique (Fig. 5.36b), (3) the slip-through technique (Fig. 5.36c, d), (4) the balloon trapping technique (Fig. 5.36e), and (5) the child-in-mother guide technique (Fig. 5.36f, g).

In recent years, use of a child catheter (the GuideLiner or equivalents such as Guidezilla and GuidePlus) has become widespread because a child catheter can be manipulated simply and reliably. However, the GuideLiner has a larger profile than a balloon or stent, and its tip becomes biased toward the greater curvature of a bend as it is advanced through a vessel, i.e., the same side where resistance to devices occurs. In other words, pushing a GuideLiner too vigorously may cause injury to the vessel (Fig. 5.37a). Advancing a balloon catheter first (Fig. 5.37b) or inflating a small-diameter (≤2 mm) balloon so that half of it protrudes from the Guideliner (Fig. 5.37c) may facilitate advancement of the catheter. However, it is safer to use a balloon inflated inside a pre-dilated distal segment or in an implanted stent as a coaxial anchor. Then the GuideLiner catheter can be advance reliably while slightly pulling back the anchoring balloon catheter (Fig. 5.37d).

When advancing a Guideliner across a proximally implanted stent into a distal segment, it is necessary to take great care to prevent stent deformation by the child catheter. A stent can readily be deformed if the tip of the GuideLiner even slightly comes into contact with a strut. Use of a coaxial anchoring balloon enables safer advancement of the GuideLiner.

When attempting to deliver a stent through a previously implanted stent, it may be impossible to advance the new stent from a GuideLiner catheter. If this happens, you should advance the GuideLiner and just keep it at the point of obstruction. With the support of this child catheter, you may then be able to advance the stent by applying gentle force. This method probably succeeds because the Guideliner fills the gap between the two stents (Fig. 5.38a) or because repositioning the guiding catheter corrects the bias of the catheter (Fig. 5.38b).

The sleeve of the GuideLiner can block advancement of a balloon/stent or may cause deformation of a stent. Usually, the tip of a balloon or stent comes into contact with the rim of the GuideLiner sleeve (Fig. 5.39a, b). To prevent this, the GuideLiner should be pushed in a little before advancing a device into it to ensure that the GuideLiner passes the tip of the guiding catheter and that the stent is advanced along the medial side of the sleeve (Fig. 5.39c).

The smallest catheter in the GuideLiner series is 5.5 Fr. If an even smaller child catheter is needed, a 4-Fr Heartrail Kiwami OTW catheter can be used.

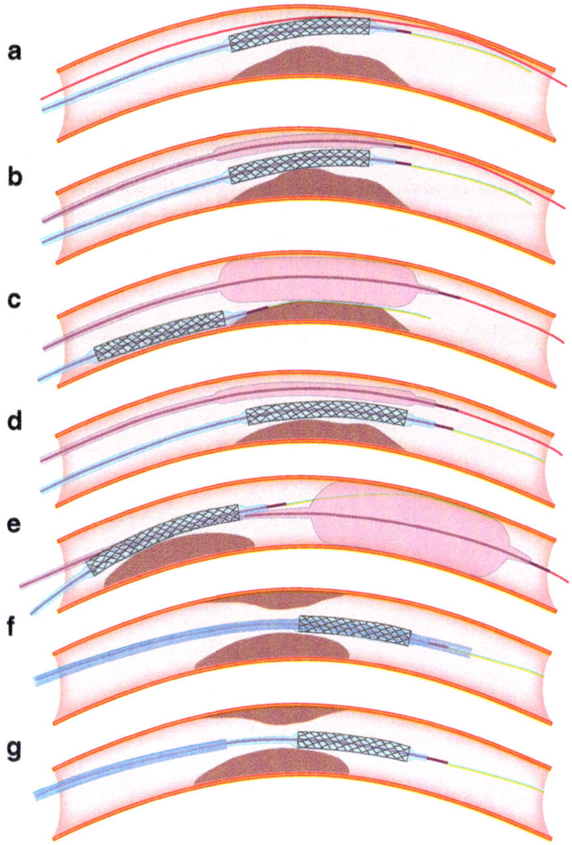

Fig. 5.36 Supplementary techniques for stent delivery. (**a**) Buddy wire techniques. (**b**) Buddy balloon technique. (**c**, **d**) Slip-through technique. (**e**) Balloon trapping technique. (**f**, **g**) Child-in-mother guide technique

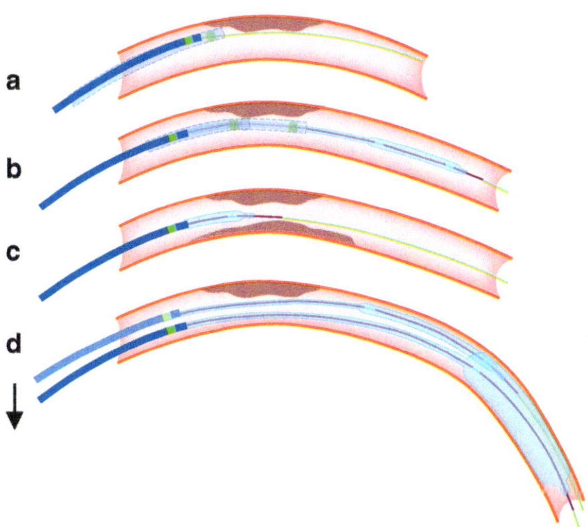

Fig. 5.37 Advancing a child catheter. (**a**) If there is a lesion on the larger curvature of a bend in the target vessel, attempts to forcibly advance a child catheter may injure the vessel, necessitating additional intervention. (**b**) Advancing a balloon first can reduce luminal irregularity and ensure smooth advancement of the child catheter. (**c**) Advancing and inflating a small-diameter ($\leq$2.0 mm) balloon first can facilitate advancement of the child catheter. (**d**) Inflating a balloon in the stent landing zone and then pulling the balloon catheter back slightly will change the orientation of the child catheter toward the smaller curvature of the bend, helping the catheter to advance beyond the lesion

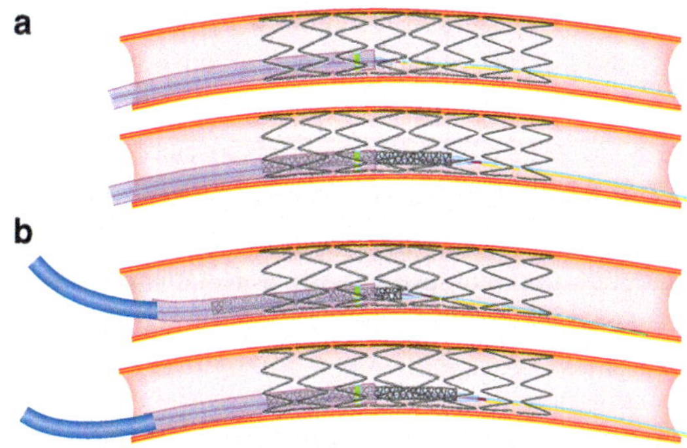

Fig. 5.38 Failure to advance a stent through a previously implanted stent. After advancing a child catheter to the point of obstruction, it can be easier to advance the other stent through the previously implanted stent, probably because the wall of the child catheter fills the gap between the two stents (**a**) or because repositioning the guiding catheter corrects the direction of the stent (**b**)

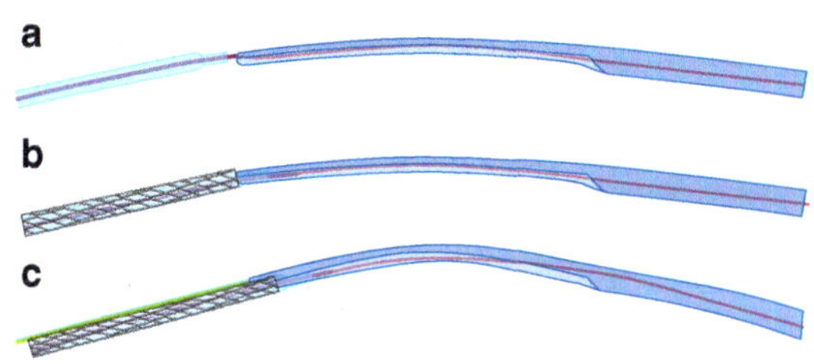

Fig. 5.39 Obstruction of a balloon/stent (**a**) or stent deformation (**b**) overcome by using a GuideLiner catheter. As it is advanced, the Guideliner catheter deviates outward in the guiding catheter and orients the device inward, thereby overcoming the obstruction (**c**)

5.7 IVUS

It is well-known that an IVUS catheter must not be forcibly pushed forward if it becomes difficult to advance. An IVUS catheter typically has a short OTW region and the shaft is not stiff. Accordingly, the shaft can easily be bent by pushing the catheter, leading to disconnection of the inner wiring.

If it becomes impossible to advance an IVUS catheter, you should suspect that its tip has been trapped by an irregularity on the larger curvature of the vessel wall. Therefore, you should pull the catheter back slightly and then immediately push it forward a little. Like a blocked stent or balloon catheter, this maneuver may allow the IVUS catheter to slip past the obstruction and advance again. If it becomes almost impossible to advance an IVUS catheter further after progressive escalation of difficulty in moving forward, it should be pulled back enough to eliminate deflection and then slowly advanced again. You should check whether the tip of the catheter can move forward even slightly, as is the case with a stent. If the tip moves forward a little, you should continue to push it with the same force until the shaft becomes deflected slightly in the proximal coronary artery. Then the maneuvers of pulling back and pushing forward are repeated.

If the hard transducer of the catheter becomes caught at a bend in the vessel, you should slide the core shaft back slightly

to increase the flexibility of the catheter tip and then follow the above procedure (Fig. 5.40a, b). After the catheter tip has passed the bend, you should slide the core shaft (i.e., transducer) forward again to restore the backup of the catheter (Fig. 5.40c).

If all of these attempts fail, it is necessary to enlarge the lumen by (1) balloon angioplasty (upfront or repeated) or (2) by debulking the lesion with a Rotablator. After failing to deliver the IVUS catheter although the lesion is sufficiently dilated or stented, supplementary techniques can be employed, such as (1) the buddy wire technique, (2) the buddy balloon technique, or (3) the trapping technique. I prefer to use a Guideliner to increase the backup of the IVUS catheter.

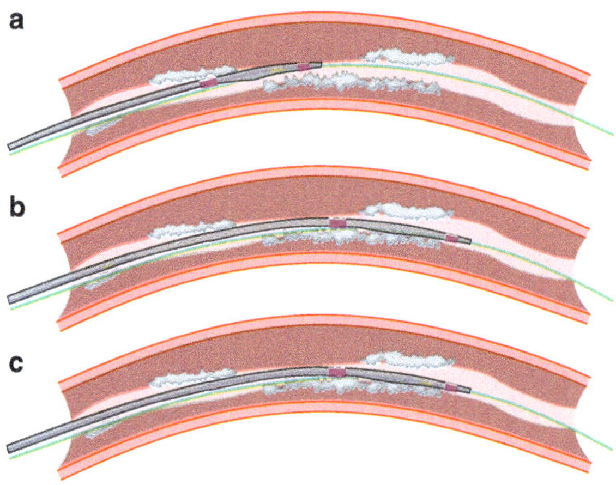

Fig. 5.40 Failure to deliver an IVUS catheter. (**a**, **b**) It can be difficult to deliver an IVUS catheter into a hard and tortuous lesion. If this problem is encountered, slide back the core shaft and then slowly advance the entire catheter. This will increase the flexibility and trackability of the catheter tip and may facilitate successful delivery of the catheter. (**c**) After the catheter tip has passed a bend in the vessel, slide the core shaft forward and then slowly advance the entire catheter

5.8 Anchoring Technique

The term "anchoring technique" covers several different concepts, which are reviewed here in relation to non-pushing PCI. "Anchoring" means taking measures to stabilize a guiding catheter or another device or to ensure smooth advancement by inflating and fixing a balloon in the artery lumen. In contrast, fixing a guidewire by inflating a balloon and then advancing a device along the fixed wire is referred to as "trapping."

Anchors can be non-coaxial or coaxial (Fig. 5.41). When a non-coaxial anchor is used, the device can only be advanced by pushing it forward (Fig. 5.41a). With a coaxial anchor, it is not always necessary to push the device forward, and it may be advanced almost spontaneously if the obstruction can be overcome by advancing a child catheter while pulling the anchor balloon back slightly (Fig. 5.41b).

I refer to inflating a balloon in a coronary artery or inside a guiding catheter for the purpose of fixing a parallel guidewire as "trapping." Trapping may be used to push forward a device or to avoid an obstruction and allow spontaneous advancement of the device (Fig. 5.41c, d).

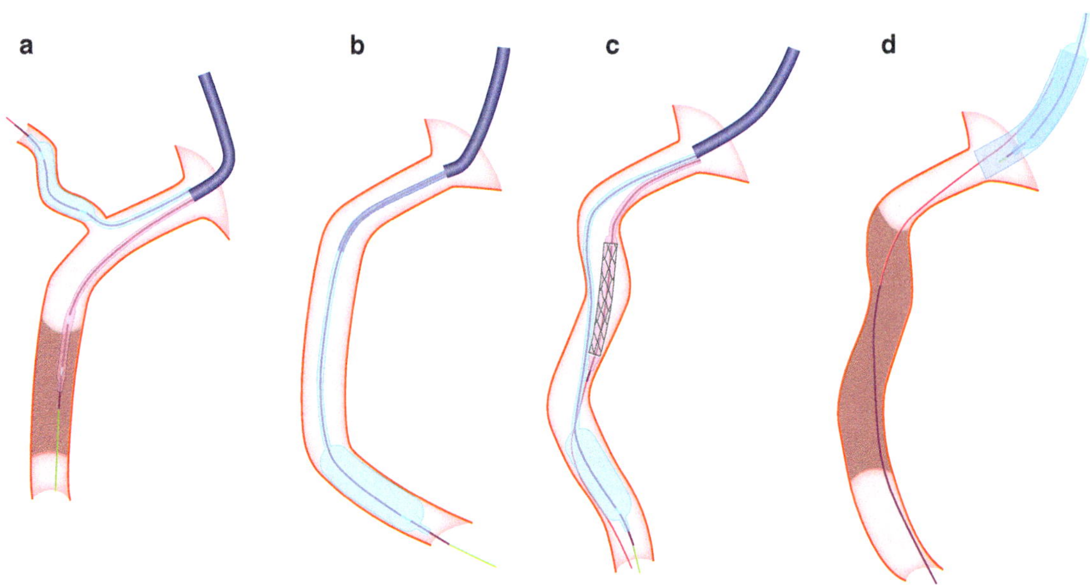

Fig. 5.41 Anchoring technique. (**a**) Inflation of a balloon in the SB to facilitate advancing a device. (**b**) Inflation of a balloon in the distal vessel to facilitate advancement of a child catheter. (**c**) Trapping with a balloon to avoid an obstruction and allow spontaneous advancement of a device. (**d**) Trapping a guidewire to facilitate advancement of a microcatheter

5.8.1 Anchoring technique

The original anchoring technique (Fig. 5.41a) employs inflation of a balloon in the SB to obtain strong backup for a guiding catheter when advancing a device into the MB. This technique is not required if the tip of the guiding catheter remains coaxial to the coronary artery ostium and if the shaft of the catheter can be brought into close contact with the contralateral wall of the aorta or aortic sinus or if the catheter can achieve the optimal power position.

Due to the vascular anatomy, it is sometimes impossible for any guiding catheter to achieve the optimal power position (Fig. 5.42). Under such circumstances, it is often very difficult to engage a guiding catheter in the target coronary artery ostium, and the catheter may become disengaged and slide out of the ostium during PCI. If an SB is available, you should advance a guidewire into the SB for anchoring along with engaging a guiding catheter at the coronary artery ostium. The anchoring technique is very useful to obtain strong backup for a device, as well as for stabilizing a guiding catheter.

The anchoring balloon should have a diameter one size (0.5 mm) larger than the lumen and a length of 15 mm, and it should be inflated at a low pressure of about 4 atm. Conversely, an undersized balloon inflated at high pressure often fails to be an effective anchor.

When using the anchoring technique to increase backup for a device, it is important to be focused on pushing the device carefully to advance it. As stated in Sect. 5.1 of this chapter (page 243), the anchoring technique is useful for advancing a balloon into a severe native stenosis. However, a device should never be advanced with the aid of an anchor when pushing is not allowed. For example, the anchoring technique is typically contraindicated when delivering a balloon into the SB after stenting of the MB.

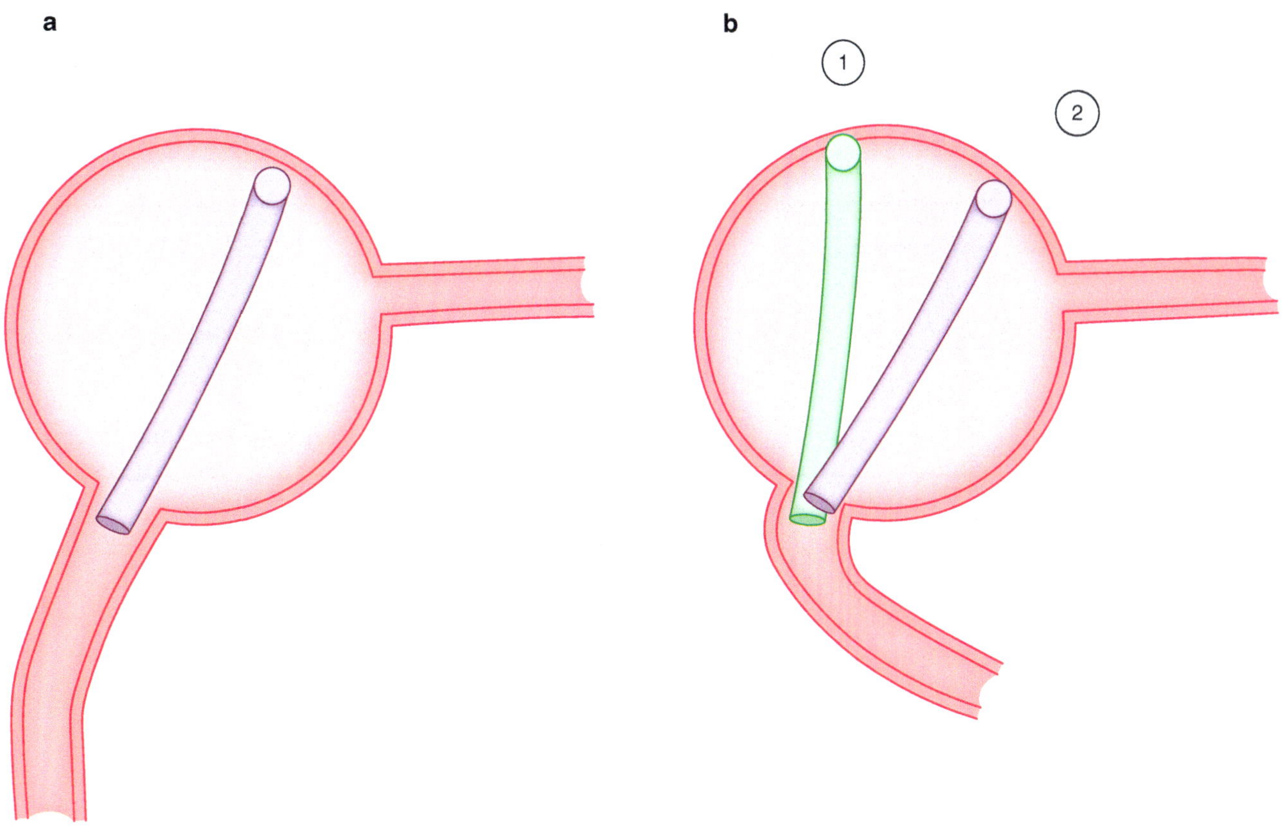

Fig. 5.42 Optimal power position. A guiding catheter achieves the optimal power position when the tip is coaxial with the coronary artery ostium and the shaft is brought into close contact with the contralateral wall of the aorta (**a**). If a coronary artery shows extreme angulation at the ostium (**b**), the guiding catheter cannot achieve the optimal power position. This is because keeping the tip of the catheter coaxial to the ostium decreases backup from the aortic wall (**1**), while ensuring sufficient backup from the aortic wall results in loss of coaxiality between the catheter tip and the ostium (**2**)

5.8.2 Coaxial Anchoring

Coaxial anchoring with an OTW or monorail balloon catheter is often used to advance a child catheter (Fig. 5.41b). If the guiding catheter has a small diameter, coaxial anchoring can be a very useful technique to assist stenting after deep engagement of the catheter. However, you should not use coaxial anchoring to push in a guiding catheter and instead should pull the shaft of the anchoring balloon back slightly to avoid the obstruction to catheter advancement. A balloon that has been used to pre-dilate the distal lumen is generally employed for coaxial anchoring. The distal end of the balloon should not be located beyond the distal edge of the stent. Sometimes, slightly pushing the anchoring balloon together with the child catheter for the last few millimeters cannot be avoided. If the child catheter still cannot be advanced, you should slightly push the tip of the child catheter into the site of obstruction and then gently insert a stent. The stent can often be delivered smoothly in this manner (Fig. 5.43).

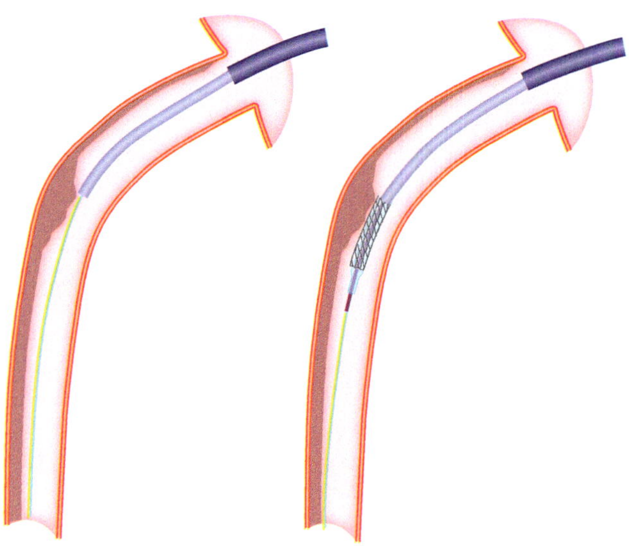

Fig. 5.43 Failure to advance a child catheter with coaxial anchoring. The child catheter should be advanced to the site of obstruction, after which it will fill the gap and facilitate delivery of a stent

5.8.3 Trapping

Trapping is a method of advancing a device by the same mechanism as coaxial anchoring. For trapping, a parallel guidewire is fixed and used to facilitate advancement of a device such as a stent (not a child catheter), which differentiates trapping from coaxial anchoring.

Usually, a trapping balloon has passed through the lumen and thus reduced the space available for advancing the device. If a retrogradely advanced balloon is used to trap a guidewire, the available space will become larger, permitting smoother advancement of the device.

A retrograde guidewire that has crossed a CTO is difficult to trap stably in the lumen proximal to the lesion. To advance a retrograde microcatheter, the retrograde guidewire often needs to be trapped very tightly. If it is not trapped, the retrograde guidewire may move back through the CTO into the distal coronary artery segment, necessitating another attempt to retrogradely cross the lesion.

After a retrograde guidewire has successfully crossed a CTO to reach the lumen proximal to the lesion, it should be introduced into the antegrade guiding catheter and trapped there, allowing a retrograde microcatheter to be reliably advanced across the CTO into the antegrade guiding catheter.

5.9 Guidewire Loop

A guidewire loop can be created by trapping, snaring, or externalization (Fig. 5.44). When snaring is used, the guidewire may escape from the snare, leading to the loss of the loop. It is safer to combine trapping with snaring (Fig. 5.44d). In most cases, a guidewire loop is created after a retrograde guidewire has crossed a CTO (see Chap. 1).

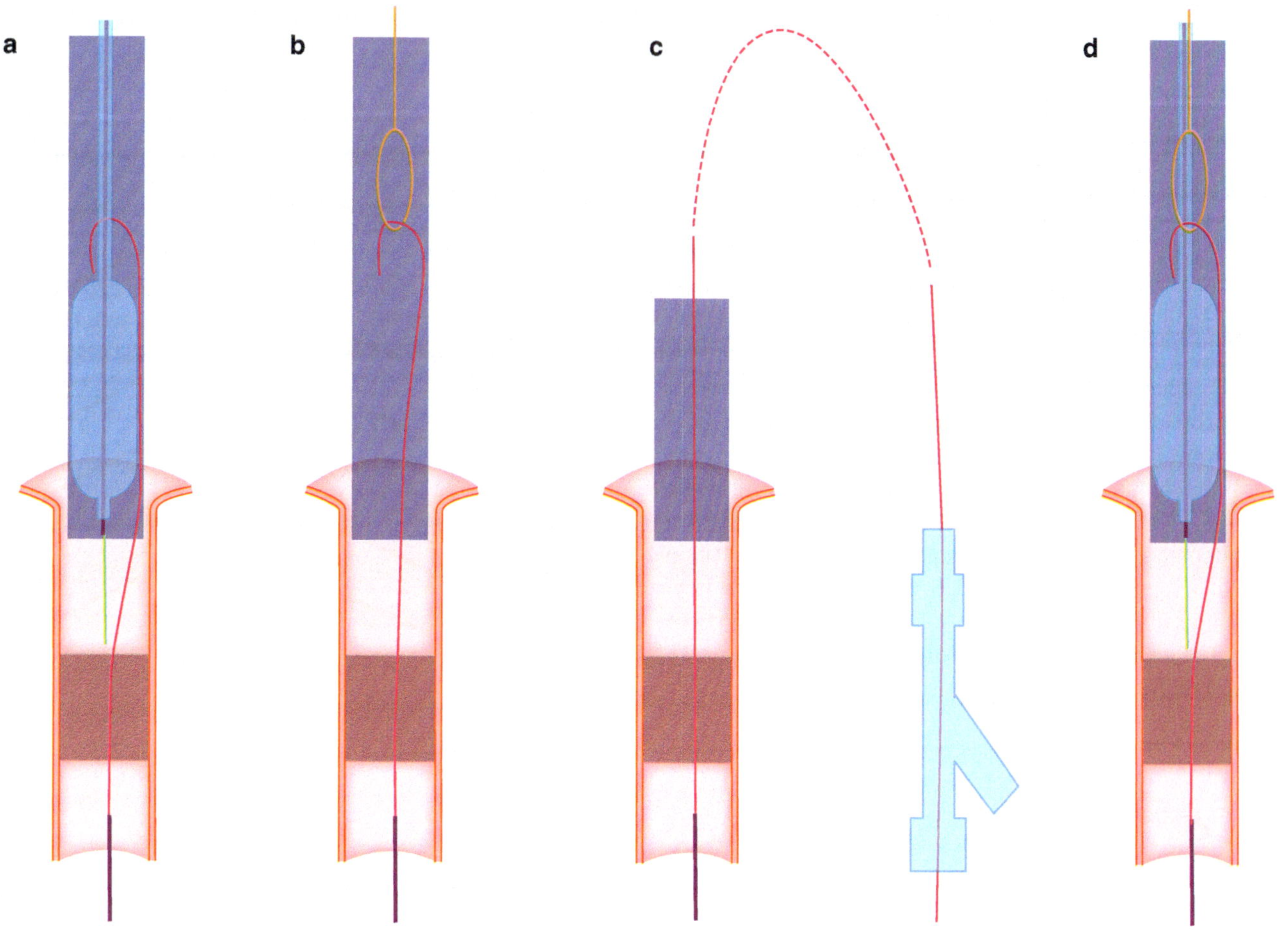

Fig. 5.44 Making a guidewire loop. (**a**) Trapping. (**b**) Snaring. (**c**) Externalization. (**d**) When snaring is employed, the guidewire may escape from the snare, so it is safer to combine trapping with snaring

5.10 Removing an IVUS Catheter

You should not forcibly push a wire/catheter/device to advance it. Likewise, you should not use excessive force to withdraw an IVUS catheter or another device if difficulty is encountered when withdrawing it.

5.10.1 If the IVUS Catheter Becomes Stuck during Withdrawal

After stent implantation, it is usual practice to employ IVUS to confirm stent apposition. After completing observation, the IVUS catheter can usually be withdrawn easily by slowly pulling it back after first sliding its imaging core forward to the limit. If the guidewire used with the IVUS catheter has a low tip load, it is better to push slightly on the guidewire while slowly withdrawing the IVUS catheter.

During withdrawal, the IVUS catheter may sometimes become stuck on the stent. In some cases, the catheter can still be withdrawn by exerting a slightly stronger force, but pulling harder on the catheter can also lead to it becoming tightly stuck. What happens when an IVUS catheter is caught during withdrawal? Is it reasonable to pull the catheter if there only seems to be a little difficulty in withdrawing it?

One way that an IVUS catheter can be caught during withdrawal is illustrated in Fig. 5.45. Advancement of a device or balloon may be blocked when the gap between the tip of the device and the guidewire or between the balloon tip and balloon membrane results in the tip being caught by irregularities on the larger curvature of a bend in the vessel (Fig. 5.45a). Conversely, a device may become stuck on irregularities on the smaller curvature of a bend during withdrawal (Fig. 5.45b).

During withdrawal of an IVUS catheter, it may be caught at the exit port (Fig. 5.46a). To stop the exit port from colliding with the vessel wall during withdrawal of the IVUS catheter, you should push the guidewire while pulling the catheter back, in order to direct the catheter toward the larger curvature at a bend in the vessel. It is important to confirm that the IVUS catheter has not been caught by irregularities of the vessel wall (Fig. 5.46b).

However, this can only be done when the guidewire has a soft tip. If this method fails to stop the exit port encountering the vessel wall, there are two other techniques to try. The first technique (used conventionally) is to remove the imaging core of the IVUS catheter and to introduce a guidewire with a stiff tip into its shaft. The stiff tip of the guidewire will straighten the IVUS catheter around its exit port and direct the catheter toward the larger curvature of a bend. This may shift the exit port away from the obstruction and facilitate withdrawal of the catheter (Fig. 5.46c). The second technique is to advance a balloon along the guidewire of the IVUS catheter as far as the exit port and thus create another gap to offset the gap at the exit port that is preventing smooth withdrawal of the catheter (Fig. 5.46d).

If the shaft of the IVUS catheter needs to be disassembled for removal of the imaging core, the second technique using a balloon is the only option. To permit delivery of a balloon catheter together with an IVUS catheter, a 7-Fr or larger guiding catheter is needed. This is one reason why I choose a 7-Fr guiding catheter for PCI of a bifurcation lesion, CTO, or severely calcified lesion.

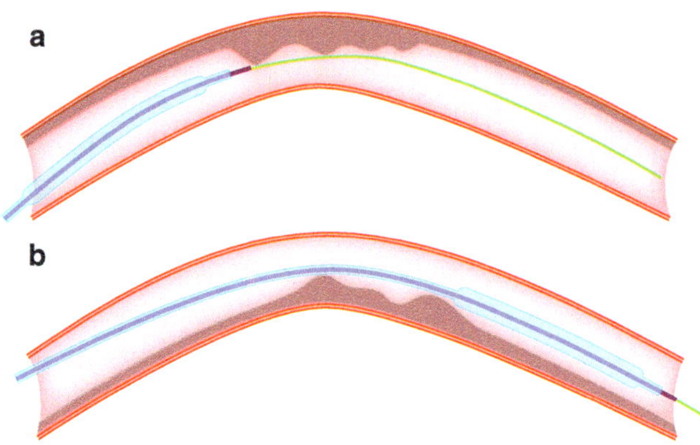

Fig. 5.45 Trapping of devices during advancement or withdrawal. During advancement, a device may be caught by irregularities on the larger curvature of a bend (**a**). During withdrawal, a device may be caught by irregularities on the smaller curvature of a bend (**b**)

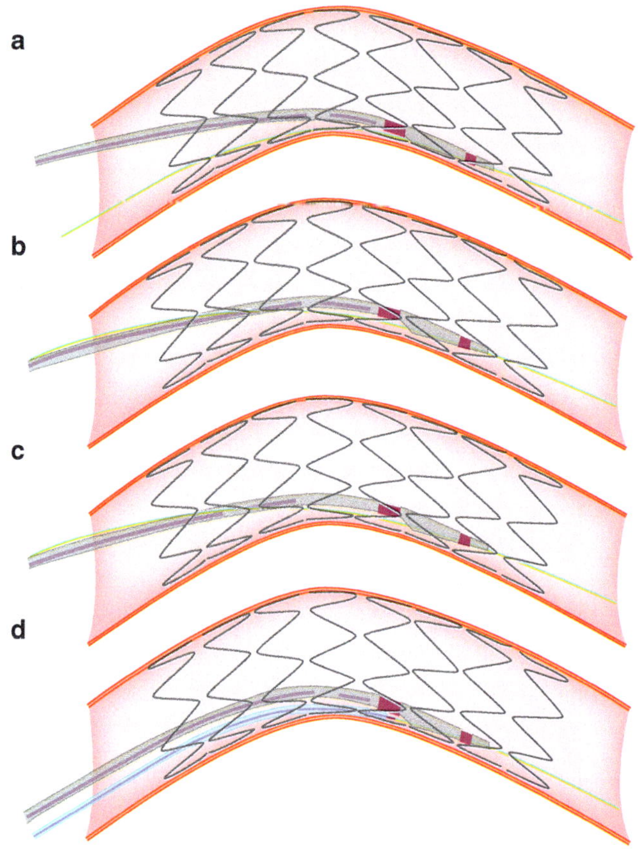

Fig. 5.46 Trapping of an IVUS catheter during withdrawal. (**a**) An IVUS catheter has a gap at its exit port, which may catch on a stent strut during withdrawal of the catheter. Forcible attempts to withdraw the catheter after it has become caught on a stent strut may lead to deformation of the stent. (**b**) Advancing a guidewire into the IVUS catheter may direct the catheter toward the larger curvature at a bend. (**c**) Sliding the imaging core back slightly and then advancing a guidewire into the IVUS catheter may straighten the catheter around the exit port and facilitate withdrawal. (**d**) Advancing a balloon along the guidewire to the exit port creates a large reverse gap, which will offset the gap at the exit port and facilitate withdrawal of the catheter

5.10.2 If the IVUS Catheter Is Caught, But Not Stuck

There might be little difficulty withdrawing an IVUS catheter through an implanted six-link stent (Cypher) or three-link stent (Xience).

However, you must pay attention if a device is even slightly caught by the strut of a two-link stent, because this may induce subtle stent deformation that cannot be identified by CAG and leads to subsequent in-stent thrombosis or restenosis. Of course, such stent deformation will not be found by IVUS if it occurs during withdrawal of the IVUS catheter. On the basis of favorable IVUS findings, many interventionalists might mistakenly regard such deformation as being unrelated to PCI. An IVUS catheter should be withdrawn slowly. If the catheter is even caught slightly during withdrawal, you should stop withdrawing it and use the abovementioned techniques to offset the gap before attempting to withdraw it again (Fig. 5.47).

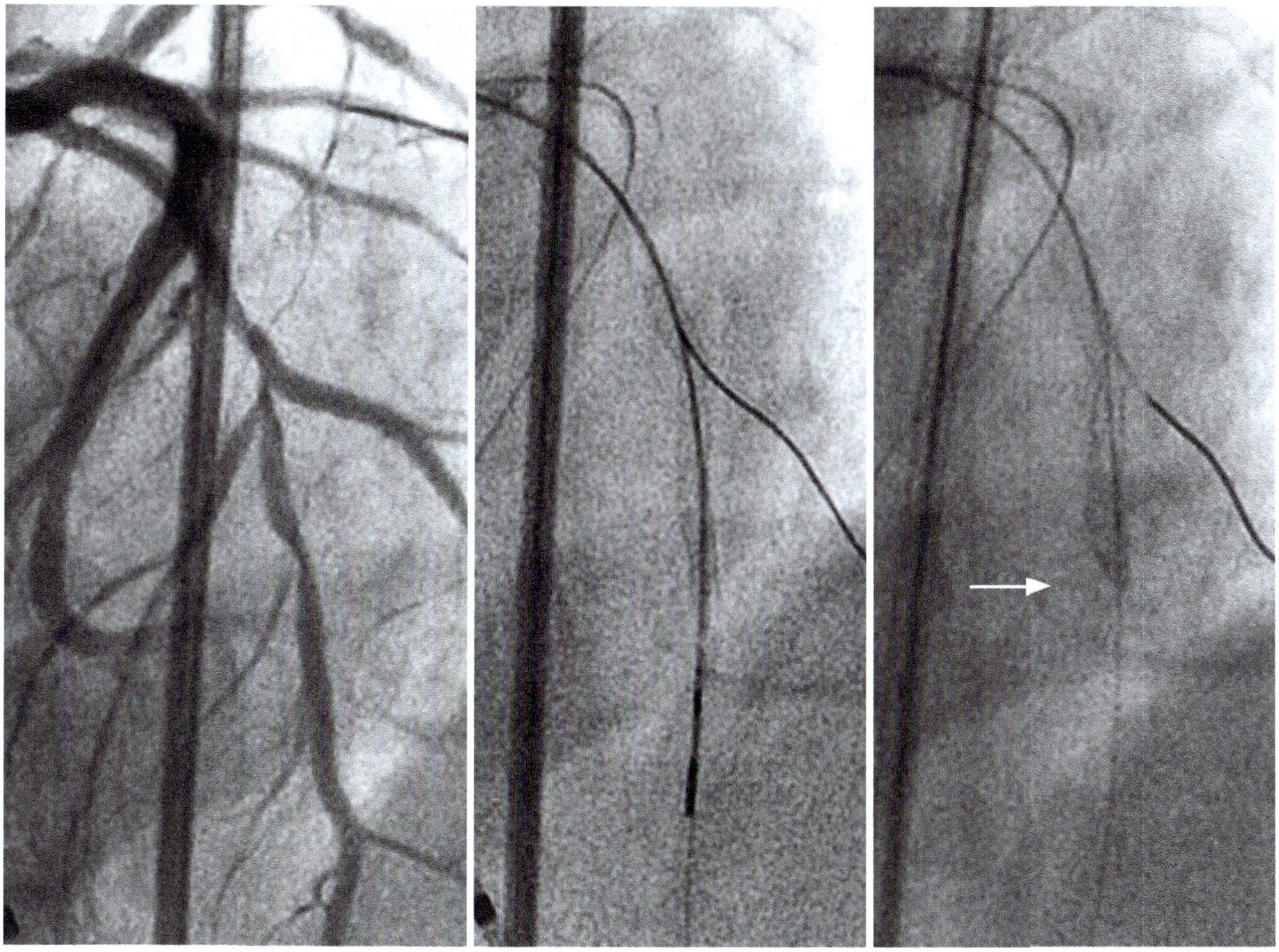

Fig. 5.47 IVUS after stenting of a LAD bifurcation lesion. The IVUS catheter was caught on the stent during withdrawal, causing stent deformation (arrow).

The manufacturer's authorised representative in the EU is Springer Nature Customer Service Centre GmbH, Europaplatz 3, 69115 Heidelberg, Germany. If you have any concerns regarding our products, please contact ProductSafety@springernature.com

Printed and bound by CPI Group (UK) Ltd, Croydon, CR0 4YY

30/09/2026

02225269-0003

The manufacturer's authorised representative in the EU is Springer Nature Customer Service Centre GmbH, Europaplatz 3, 69115 Heidelberg, Germany. If you have any concerns regarding our products, please contact ProductSafety@springernature.com

Printed and bound by CPI Group (UK) Ltd, Croydon, CR0 4YY
30/09/2026
02225271-0008

1 Mitsudo's PCI Techniques for CTO

1.1 Approach (Puncture Site)

There is still some controversy regarding the choice between the transradial (TR) and transfemoral (TF) approaches for intervention from the aspects of both preference and rationality. However, I do not think this is an essential matter. I select the TR approach whenever possible because it is less invasive irrespective of the PCI techniques I plan to use. I always choose the TF approach to perform antegrade PCI for CTO and PCI that can only be accomplished by stenting of a bifurcation lesion in female patients. I do this because a large-diameter guiding catheter is needed to achieve a "successful outcome" in every patient when performing these procedures, although recanalization of a CTO via the TR approach will be successful in many patients. The interventionalist's concept of a "successful outcome" may have a considerable influence on the choice between the two approaches. I select the approach and the size of the guiding catheter according to the rules described below.

1.1.1 Selection of the Approach

1.1.1.1 Guiding Catheter Size

The smallest-diameter guiding catheter that can be used is generally a good choice. I try to select a catheter with the smallest diameter that allows me to perform all of the PCI procedures that may be required for the target lesion (Table 1.1). Currently, a 7-Fr guiding catheter allows almost all procedures to be accomplished, apart from rotablation with a burr ≥2.15 mm in size. If a catheter with a larger diameter becomes necessary while you are performing PCI, you will need to replace both the catheter and the sheath with larger ones or you may even have to abandon the planned procedure. Conversely, you will never need to replace a larger catheter with a smaller one to accomplish the planned procedure.

A guiding catheter with a larger diameter does not always provide stronger backup. If there is plaque at the ostium, an 8-Fr guiding catheter is likely to damage the plaque, whereas a 7-Fr catheter may be passed through the ostium and engaged just beyond it, providing much stronger backup. If an 8-Fr guiding catheter is used in such circumstances, a catheter with side holes may be a good choice. Although a catheter with side holes can effectively prevent coronary ischemia, it cannot prevent ostial injury. In fact, using such a catheter may rather increase the risk of ostial injury because you cannot recognize that the tip has become wedged. This is why I question the selection of an 8-Fr guiding catheter with side holes for the purpose of obtaining stronger backup.

In contrast to an 8-Fr guiding catheter, a catheter with a smaller diameter (as small as possible) is less likely to cause ostial injury. When deeply seated, a smaller guiding catheter can often provide stronger local backup as it ensures coaxiality between devices and the target vessel.

However, performing PCI for CTO usually requires a combination of techniques, so one has to consider the optimal size of the guiding catheter to ensure success with all of the techniques that might be used. Antegrade PCI for CTO sometimes requires guidance by intravascular ultrasound (IVUS). If the guidewire exit port of the IVUS catheter is trapped by an implanted stent, a 7-Fr (or larger) guiding catheter is sometimes required to successfully remove the IVUS catheter together with the aid of a balloon without causing stent deformation (see Column 15 [page 174]). This is why I always use a 7-Fr guiding catheter from the start of PCI.

In female patients, I introduce a 7-Fr guiding catheter via the femoral artery rather than the radial artery because of its size. If a femoral artery is not available for catheterization, I choose the trans-brachial (TB) approach in female patients. When performing retrograde PCI, a 6-Fr guiding catheter may be sufficient, so the TR approach can be used even in female patients.

The TR and TB approaches should be avoided when performing PCI for occlusion of the left circumflex artery

K. Mitsudo, *Non-Pushing PCI Techniques*, https://doi.org/10.1007/978-981-15-7043-8_1

(LCX) because one of the two optimal orthogonal projections for viewing LCX lesions can be a projection from deep left anterior oblique (LAO) to the left outer (LO). In such projections, the brachium often overlaps the heart, which results in poor imaging conditions and prevents assessment of the anatomy of the target vessel.

Note that I always use the left radial artery for the TR approach. When choosing the TB approach, I always use the right brachial artery because a sheath introducer placed in the left brachial artery is too far from the interventionalist.

1.1.1.2 Fluoroscopic Angles for Biplane Cineangiography and Puncture Sites

As I will explain later, it is essential to view the target lesion in two orthogonal projections that provide the longest possible images of the longitudinal axis of the target vessel. I take care to exclude the arms and other interfering objects, particularly from lateral views.

In some cases, good images of the LCX (particularly its middle and distal segments) can only be obtained with the patient's arms raised above the head. Accordingly, the TR and TB approaches should be avoided when performing PCI for LCX lesions.

Sometimes, the biradial approach is employed in male patients, and the left radial/right brachial approach is used in female patients. However, these approaches are incompatible with the arm-raising posture and require the patient's left arm to be raised anteriorly, which severely limits the choice of fluoroscopic angles. Therefore, I only use these approaches in exceptional cases.

1.1.1.3 Influence of Severe Tortuosity and/or Stenosis

Both the TB and TR approaches should be avoided if diagnostic catheterization shows severe tortuosity of the innominate (brachiocephalic) artery, because such vascular anatomy may preclude these approaches. Conversely, the TF approach may occasionally require cannulation through more tortuous vessels that can make it difficult to manipulate the guiding catheter. In such cases, the TB or TR approach is a better choice.

Table 1.1 Optimum guiding catheter size

	Antegrade approach						Retrograde approach					
Target coronary artery	Male			Female			Male			Female		
	TF approach	TR approach	TB approach	TF approach	TR approach	TB approach	TF approach	TR approach	TB approach	TF approach	TR approach	TB approach
LMT	7	7	–	7	–	7	7(6)	7	–	7	(6)	7
LAD	7	7	–	7	–	7	7(6)	7	–	7	(6)	7
LCX	7	–	–	7	–	–	7(6)	–	–	7	–	–
RCA	7	7	–	7	–	7	7(6)	7	–	7	(6)	7

"(6)": a 6-Fr catheter can also be used
"—": this approach should be avoided whenever possible

1.2 Sheath

Whether I perform antegrade or retrograde PCI, I use a thick-walled, non-kinking sheath with a length of 40 or 45 cm for the TF approach. Although there are also long non-kinking sheaths that are flexible enough to easily follow a tortuous vessel, I do not use sheaths of this type (Fig. 1.1).

If a flexible sheath is introduced into a tortuous vessel, the guiding catheter must subsequently be advanced while straightening the sheath that has conformed to the tortuosities of the vessel, causing considerable friction between the sheath and catheter so that there is no benefit of previously introducing the sheath. If the guiding catheter is advanced further in an attempt to stabilize its tip, the tortuous region tends to become even more tortuous. This can result in failure to acquire backup and significantly impair manipulability of the guiding catheter (Fig. 1.1b).

On the other hand, a stiff, thick-walled, non-kinking sheath can pass through a tortuous vessel while somewhat straightening it and will remain almost straight itself. If a guiding catheter is advanced through such a straight sheath, there is less friction between the sheath and catheter. Thus, the catheter remains manipulable, and good backup can be acquired (Fig. 1.1c).

When using a stiff sheath, there is concern about the risks associated with vascular stress due to the "accordion" phenomenon. To reduce the risk of this phenomenon, I recommend repeated to-and-fro movement of the sheath, rather than simply continuing to push it forward until it advances smoothly. Specifically, I recommend pulling the sheath back and pushing it forward over a 2- to 3-cm distance after it has been advanced completely. This helps to stabilize the sheath within the vessel.

If a sheath cannot advance smoothly within a very tortuous vessel, do not advance it forcibly, but instead replace the guidewire with an extra stiff wire (Fig. 1.2). Alternatively, make a small curve at the top of the sheath (Fig. 1.3), and then push the sheath forward while rotating it. Using these methods, it is often possible to advance a sheath past the blockage in a vessel.

When performing TF interventions, including procedures for CTO, I always use a sheath with a length of 40 or 45 cm. I think that a long sheath has several advantages, while there are no disadvantages or inconveniences. One of the advantages of a long sheath is the small gaps between the guidewire, dilator, and sheath during advancement of the sheath (Fig. 1.4). Although I often use an inner sheath catheter to reduce the gap between the guidewire and the guiding catheter, using a long sheath makes the gaps between devices even smaller.

Therefore, there is a very low risk of injuring the vessel wall or scraping off plaque to cause embolism while a long sheath is being advanced. When exchanging a guiding catheter, the new catheter can be advanced smoothly beyond the abdominal aorta through a long sheath, and the inner sheath catheter protects the vessel wall while the catheter is advanced into the thoracic aorta.

Cholesterol embolization syndrome (blue toe syndrome) is an infrequent, but potentially fatal, complication of PCI. This complication became less frequent after I started to use an inner sheath catheter for PCI, and it is even less frequent since I started to use long sheaths.

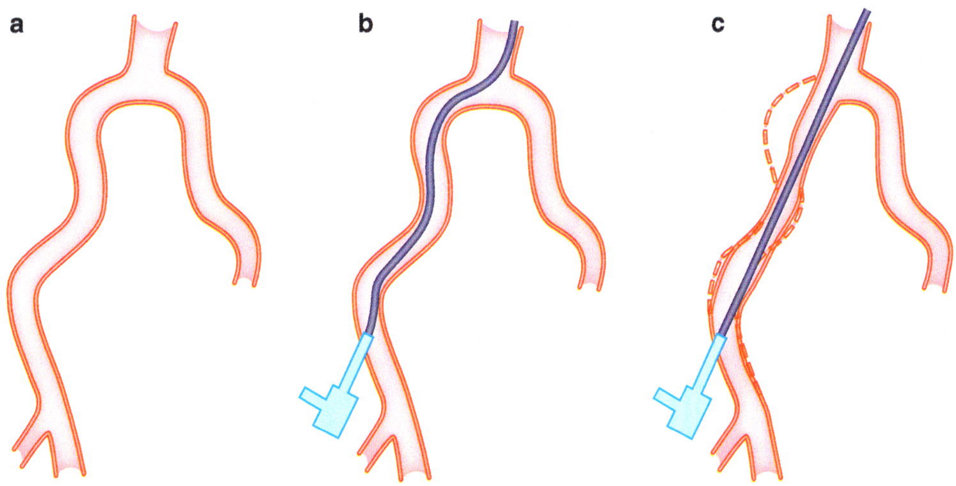

Fig. 1.1 Long non-kinking sheath. (**a**) Tortuous right iliofemoral artery. (**b**) A long, flexible, non-kinking sheath follows the tortuous vessel easily, but develops the same tortuosities as the vessel. To advance a guiding catheter, the sheath has to be straightened, which generates friction between catheter and sheath. (**c**) A stiff, thick-walled sheath passes through a tortuous vessel while straightening it somewhat and maintaining a linear shape. Therefore, there is less friction when a guiding catheter is advanced through the sheath. A sheath of this type is much more useful than the flexible sheath shown in *b*, both for advancing the guiding catheter and for obtaining sufficient backup

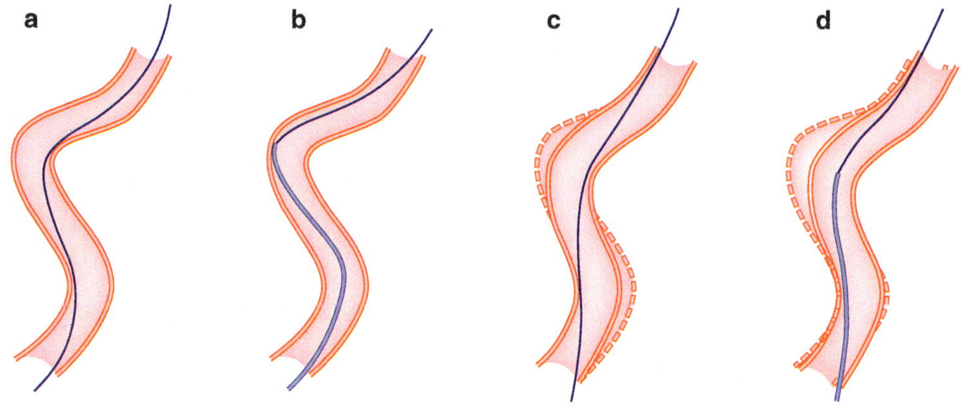

Fig. 1.2 Method of advancing a sheath through a very tortuous ilio-femoral artery—abdominal aorta. (**a**) When the guidewire in the sheath kit is advanced through a tortuous vessel, it passes along the inner curvature of each bend. (**b**) A stiff sheath cannot be advanced smoothly through such a vessel because its tip deviates in the outward direction at each curve, generating considerable friction with the vessel wall. (**c**) A guidewire with a stiff shaft can be used to straighten the tortuous vessel. (**d**) If a sheath is advanced along the stiff guidewire, outward deviation at the curves becomes smaller, and friction with the vessel wall is reduced. Thus, the sheath can often be advanced smoothly

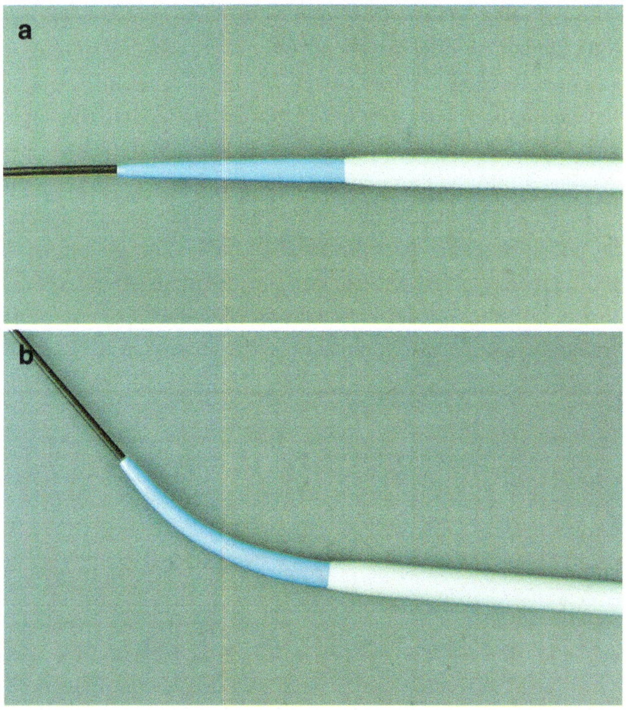

Fig. 1.3 Photograph of a sheath with a slightly bent tip. A sheath with a slightly bent tip can easily follow a tortuous vessel and can straighten the vessel after the tip has passed through it

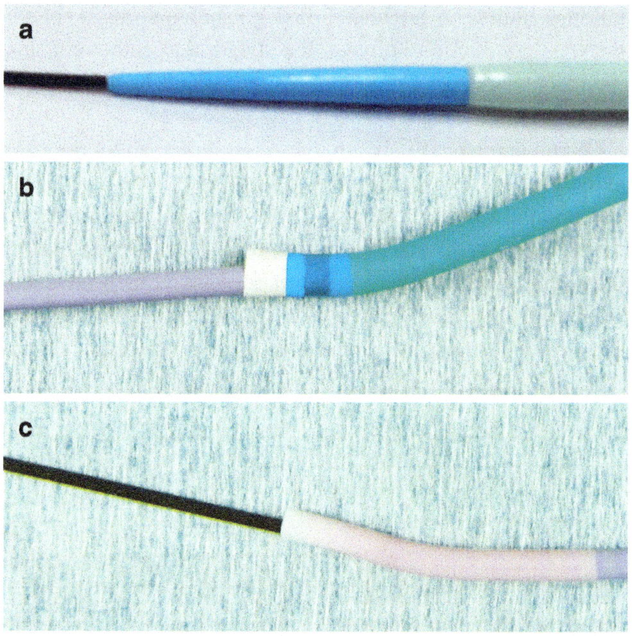

Fig. 1.4 Gaps between the sheath, dilator, and guidewire. The gaps shown in ***a*** are obviously smaller than those in ***b*** or ***c*** (gaps between a 7-Fr guiding catheter and a 5-Fr inner sheath catheter or between a 5-Fr diagnostic catheter and a guidewire, respectively)

1.3 Guiding Catheter

1.3.1 Selection of the Guiding Catheter

My method of selecting guiding catheters is very simple. For the left coronary artery (LCA), either the Launcher SL or EBU is my first choice, while the BriteTip AL or Launcher SAL is my first choice for the right coronary artery (RCA).

I have specified the manufacturers and model numbers of the guiding catheters above because I have good reasons for limiting my selection. Multiple manufacturers currently produce guiding catheters with identical model numbers, but the catheters of these different manufacturers show different levels of performance (even if they have the same model number), and many products fail to deliver the expected performance or rather cause problems for the operator.

1.3.1.1 Amplatz-Type Catheter for the RCA

I choose an Amplatz-type guiding catheter for PCI of the RCA, and not a Judkins-type catheter, for the reasons described below.

Since the Judkins guiding catheter only has a single curve, it permits more linear manipulation of the guidewire toward the RCA ostium compared with the Amplatz guiding catheter, which has two curves. However, this is not a decisive point. The Judkins catheter only provides weak backup, which is clearly noticeable when attempting to advance a balloon or another device over a guidewire that has been advanced through the guiding catheter. If the RCA ostium is oriented downward and not involved by a lesion, a deeply seated Judkins catheter can provide some backup. Alternatively, it should be pushed forward while being rotated clockwise to create an Amplatz-like shape. Adequate backup may be obtained if its shaft is pushed against the contralateral wall of the sinus of Valsalva. Anchoring the catheter is another way of obtaining better backup.

However, if you choose the Amplatz guiding catheter in this situation, you can obtain enough backup by engaging the guiding catheter in the RCA and keeping its shaft contralateral to the sinus of Valsalva. The greatest advantage of the Amplatz catheter is the ability to obtain backup from the entire sinus of Valsalva, including the contralateral wall and the aortic valve.

You may also use the Judkins catheter if there is a side branch available to anchor it. If there is no side branch, several problems will arise when performing PCI with the Judkins catheter, especially for occlusive ostial lesions. As shown in Fig. 1.5, the tip of the Judkins catheter may be blocked by the occlusion, and it may even be impossible to perform imaging of the target vessel. In the LAO view, the RCA ostium and the tip of the guiding catheter appear to be coaxial with each other, but it is difficult to achieve true coaxiality. If the target vessel has a large enough diameter from the ostium to a more peripheral site, coaxiality can be achieved by advancing the catheter tip a little further to that site. However, this is difficult with most ostial lesions. The right anterior oblique (RAO) and AP views will clearly show that the guiding catheter is not in a coaxial position, with the Judkins catheter tip generally being deviated rightward from the orientation of the RCA ostium. In this situation, it is impossible to advance the guidewire toward the entry point coaxially with the occluded vessel. Lack of coaxiality also reduces manipulability of the guidewire. When the guidewire is advanced forcibly, the guiding catheter may be pushed back or may become disengaged due to insufficient backup (Fig. 1.6). Antegrade PCI for CTO of the RCA ostium will never be successful with the Judkins catheter, except in some lucky cases such as when the occlusion is tapered.

If an Amplatz-type guiding catheter of an appropriate size is used, its tip can be disengaged and placed just beneath the RCA ostium (Fig. 1.7). Namely, it is possible to stably maintain the catheter tip coaxial with the RCA ostium and at the optimum distance. If a guidewire is advanced through a guiding catheter positioned in this way, it can be manipulated easily and is more likely to enter the true lumen at the site of occlusion.

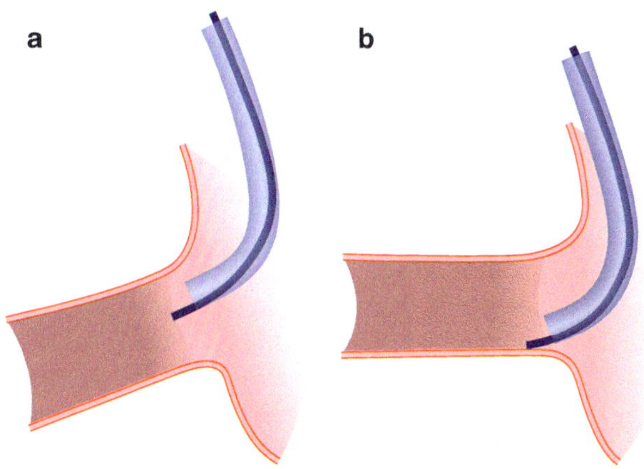

Fig. 1.5 Possible outcomes with the Judkins guiding catheter. If the tip of the catheter is located close to the entry point, as is usual when performing PCI for CTO of the RCA ostium, the penetration site and direction of the guidewire are dependent on the position and orientation of the catheter tip. A favorable outcome can be obtained if the tip of the catheter and the occluded vessel are completely coaxial with each other and if the catheter tip is oriented toward the desired entry point (**a**). However, the catheter tip is usually not coaxial with the occluded vessel, and its orientation is slightly deviated from the entry point (**b**)

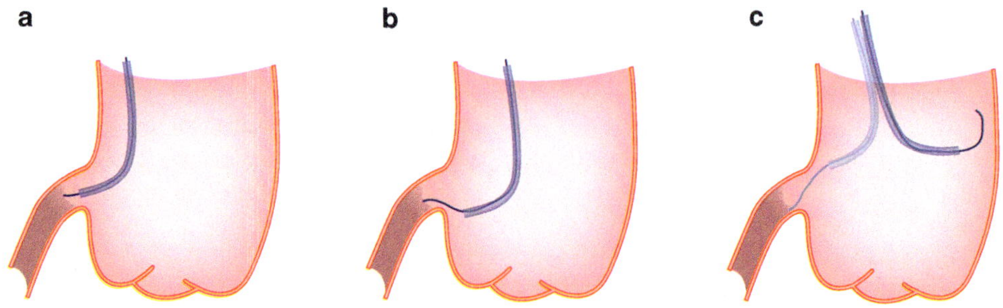

Fig. 1.6 Possible outcomes with the Judkins guiding catheter. If a Judkins right-type guiding catheter is used during PCI for CTO of the RCA ostium, the catheter may initially be coaxial with the occluded vessel (**a**). However, when a guidewire is advanced slightly through the guiding catheter (**b**), the catheter often becomes disengaged due to insufficient backup (**c**)

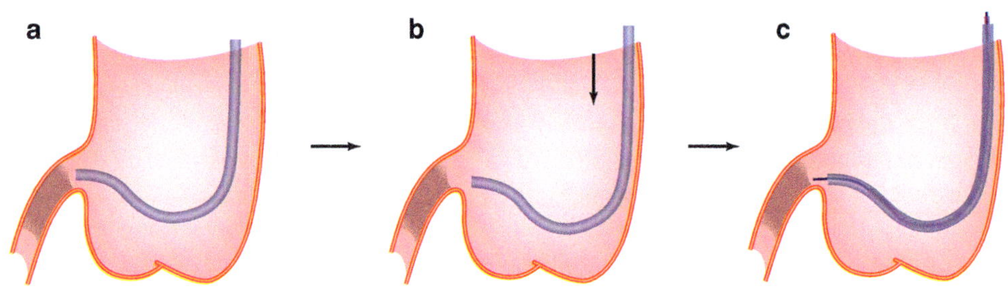

Fig. 1.7 Using an Amplatz left-type guiding catheter (AL) during PCI for CTO of the RCA ostium. If an Amplatz left-type guiding catheter is engaged, the pressure waveform will be damped, and tip injection will not provide sufficient information about the vascular anatomy and rather has the potential to injure the ostium. Engagement of this type of guiding catheter is risky because it makes both guidewire manipulation and angiography impossible (**a**). However, an AL-type guiding catheter with a specific shape can readily be disengaged when pushed slightly (**b**). A guidewire can be manipulated freely through the guiding catheter from a site slightly away from the entry point if the tip of the catheter is maintained just beneath the RCA ostium (**c**). With the guiding catheter in this position, the pressure waveform is also normalized and safe and high-quality angiography becomes possible

1.3.1.2 Tips When Using an Amplatz Left-Type Guiding Catheter for the RCA

Shape of the Catheter Tip

Guiding catheters that are made by different manufacturers, even those with an identical model number (e.g., "AL 1"), vary considerably regarding their performance and the shape of the curve at the tip. Figure 1.8 shows photographs of representative "AL 1" short-tipped guiding catheters made by three manufacturers (Group A). The tips have curves with different shapes. I use guiding catheters in Group A (e.g., BriteTip, Launcher, and Hyperion), which commonly have a "deep" second curve unlike those in Group B.

The advantages of having a deep second curve are illustrated in Fig. 1.9 (**a–c**). When a guiding catheter with a deep second curve is pushed forward, its tip spontaneously backs away from the RCA ostium while being maintained in a coaxial position to the ostium. When such a catheter is pulled back, its tip goes forward and enters the RCA. The former movement of the catheter tip (spontaneously backing away) makes it less likely that the RCA ostium will be injured and good backup is generated by pushing the shaft against the contralateral wall of the sinus of Valsalva. In contrast, a guiding catheter with a "shallow" second curve enters the RCA when pushed forward and disengages from the ostium when pulled back (Fig. 1.9 (**d–f**)). During both movements, the shaft of the catheter remains unstable ("floating") within the sinus of Valsalva, rather than generating good backup. Since such a catheter has to be pushed forward to play its role, it must have side holes. This inevitably increases the volume of contrast medium that is used as well as placing stress on the ostium, thereby increasing the risk of ostial injury.

Although I generally recommend using "AL 1" short-tipped guiding catheters for PCI of the RCA, I have always only employed the catheters in Group A for the above-mentioned reasons. Figures 1.10, 1.11, 1.12, and 1.13 (Figs. 1.10–1.13) show representative coronary angiograms (CAGs) of CTOs of the RCA that were treated by PCI using guiding catheters from Group A or Group B.

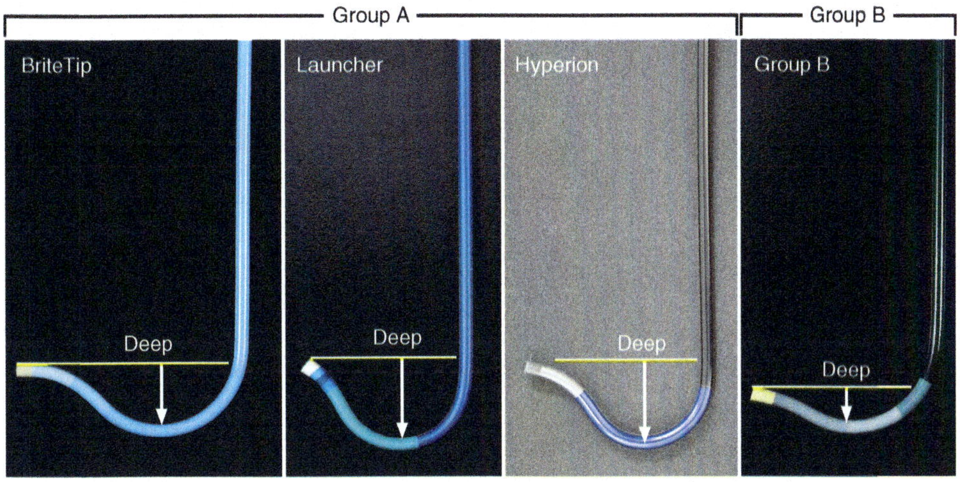

Fig. 1.8 Tip curves of short-tipped Amplatz left (AL 1 ST) guiding catheters produced by different manufacturers until 2015. Group A: BriteTip AL 1 ST, Launcher SAL 1, and Hyperion AL 1 ST. Group B: "AL 1 ST" guiding catheters produced by many manufacturers (Mach1 AL 1 ST is shown here). Group A guiding catheters are characterized by a greater distance between the tip and the bottom of the second curve (a "deep" second curve), while Group B catheters have a "shallow" second curve

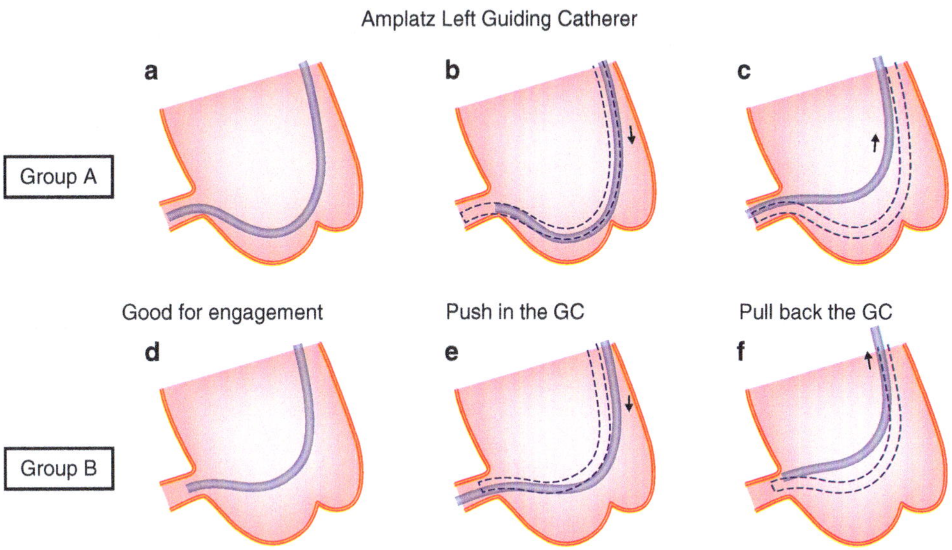

Fig. 1.9 Tip behavior of guiding catheters with different second curves. The upper row shows a guiding catheter from Group A. After initial engagement to the optimal depth (**a**), advancing the catheter results in it becoming less deeply engaged (**b**), while pulling back leads to deeper engagement (**c**). The lower row shows a guiding catheter from Group B. Initial optimal position (**d**). When the catheter is advanced, its tip tends to go deeper into the RCA (**e**). When the catheter is pulled back, its tip disengages from the ostium (**f**)

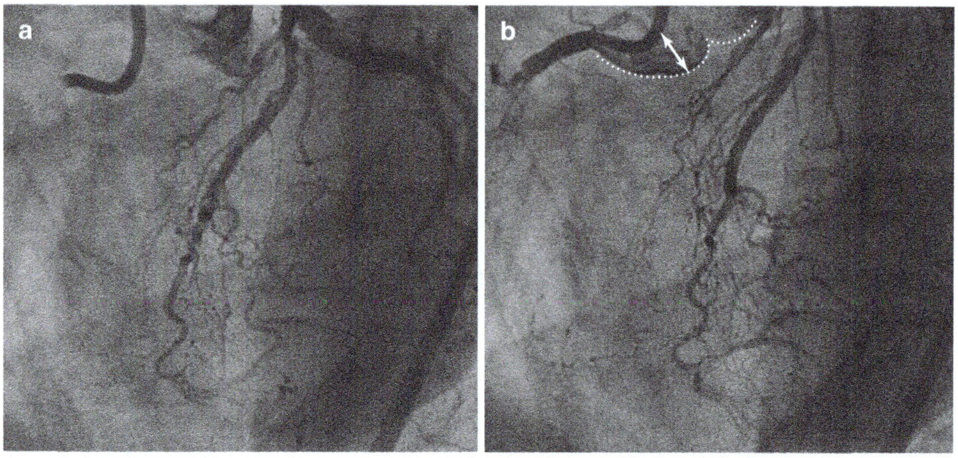

Fig. 1.10 PCI for CTO of the RCA using guiding catheters from Groups A and B: Initial use of a Group B catheter. PCI for CTO of the RCA was initiated with an AL 1 ST guiding catheter like a Group B type. (**a**) Because it had short first and second curves, the catheter could be easily manipulated within the sinus of Valsalva and was engaged in the RCA. Ease of achieving engagement is the greatest advantage of guiding catheters with such tip characteristics. (**b**) The tip of the catheter is coaxial with the RCA ostium and appears to be engaged well. However, the posterior side of the second curve of the catheter tip is floating within the sinus of Valsalva (arrows). The dotted curves indicate valve cusps

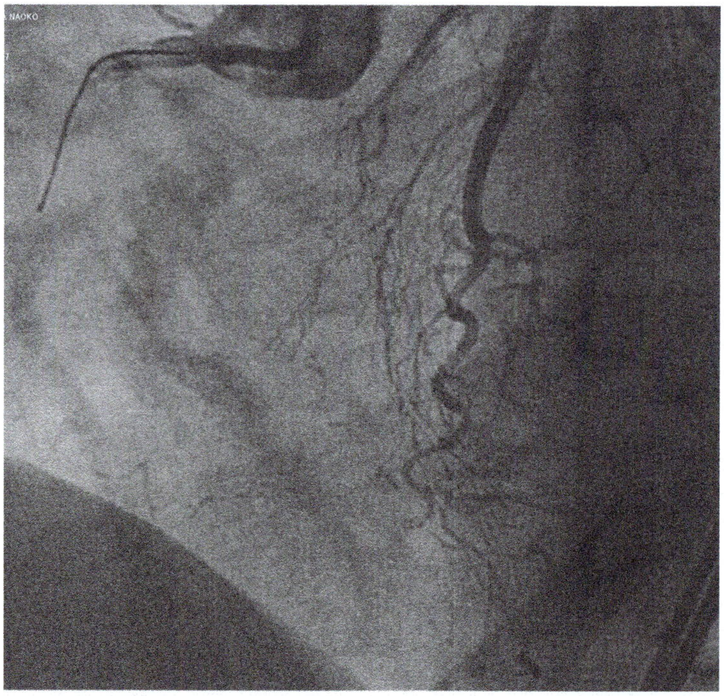

Fig. 1.11 PCI for CTO of the RCA using a Group B guiding catheter. When the guidewire is advanced toward the CTO, the guiding catheter is pushed back, and it can easily become disengaged because the posterior side of the catheter shaft is not supported by the contralateral wall of the sinus of Valsalva, as seen in the cusp images

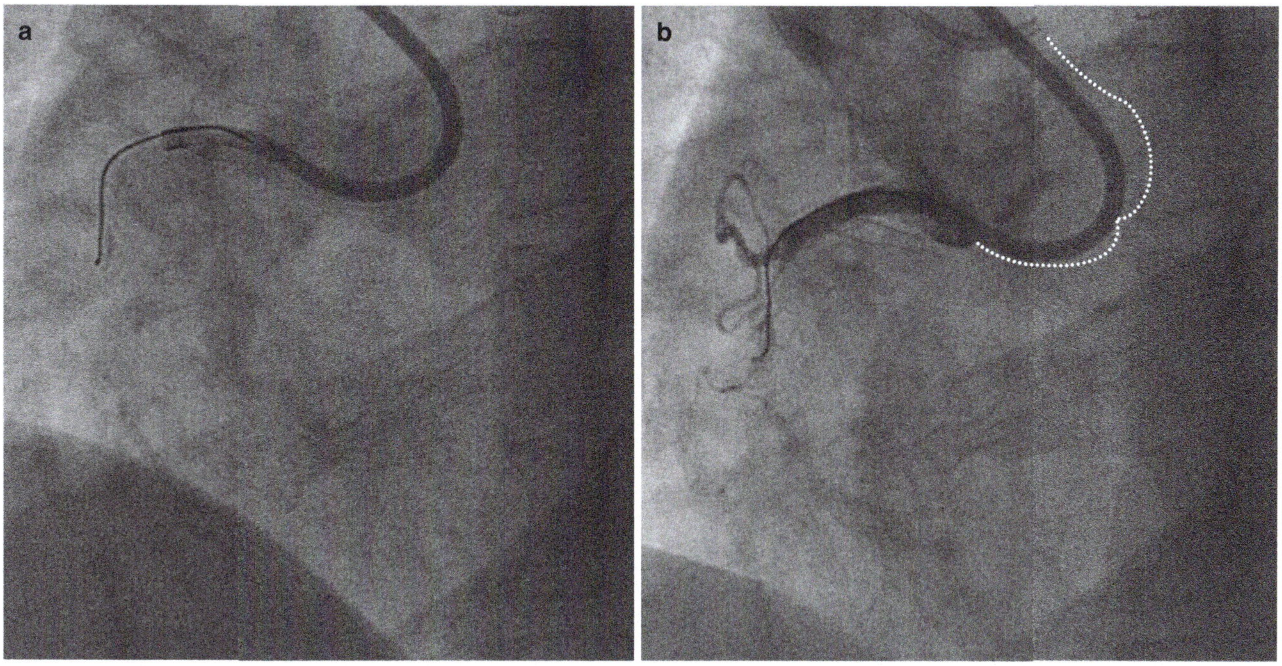

Fig. 1.12 PCI for CTO of the RCA after switching to a guiding catheter from Group A. (**a**) The tip of the guiding catheter has been engaged deeply, so the catheter will not be pushed back when a guidewire is manipulated. (**b**) CAG reveals that the catheter is coaxial with the RCA and its shaft is pressed against the contralateral wall of the sinus of Valsalva. Dotted curves show the cusps and the aortic wall

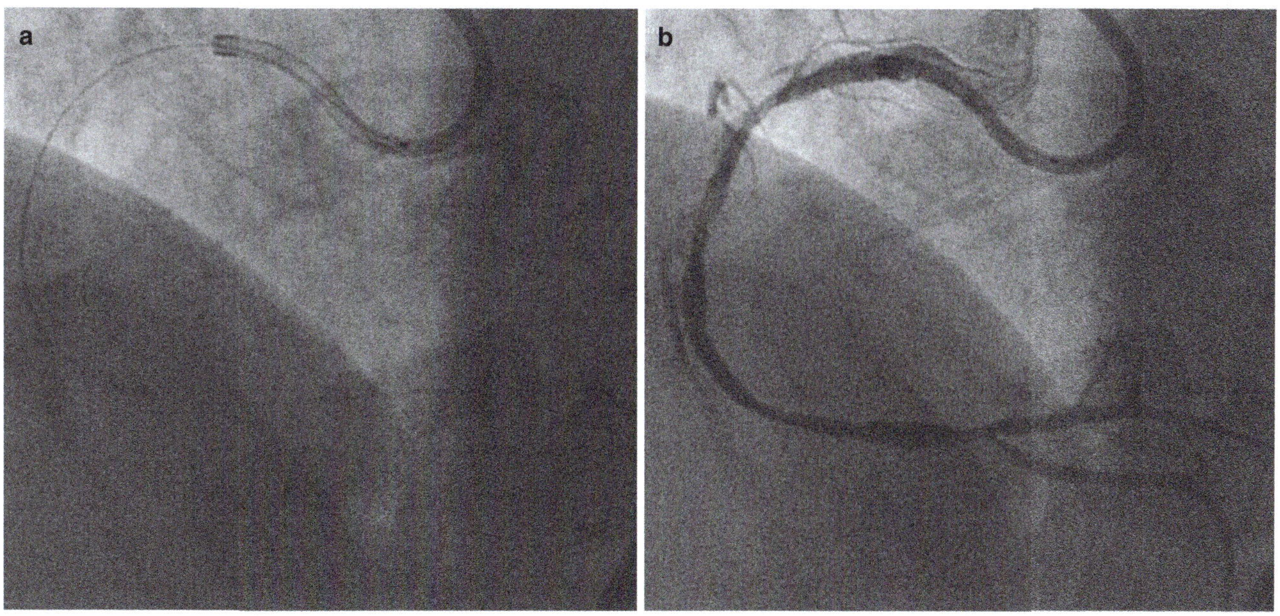

Fig. 1.13 Images of a Group A guiding catheter that has been optimally engaged by pushing (compare with deep engagement in Fig. 1.12). (**a**) Before injection, the pressure waveform and the position of the catheter tip indicate that the catheter is engaged optimally. (**b**) After injection

Size of the Catheter Tip Curve

The curve of the catheter tip is the optimum size if the distance between its tip and shaft is slightly shorter than the distance between the RCA ostium and the contralateral wall of the sinus of Valsalva (Fig. 1.14). Since contrast-enhanced CT makes it possible to measure the dimensions of the sinus of Valsalva, determining the catheter tip curve size based on measurement of the sinus is recommended at centers where contrast-enhanced coronary CT is routinely performed before PCI. The same method can be applied to determine the optimum size of the curve of a guiding catheter for the left coronary artery (LCA). Since I usually omit pre-PCI coronary CT, I initially try to engage a guiding catheter with an average-sized tip curve. If this initial attempt fails due to the wrong curve size, I then modify it. In principle, I choose a guiding catheter with a curve of such a size that the catheter becomes disengaged when it is advanced slightly.

My first choice is the BriteTip AL 1 ST for male patients and the Launcher SAL 1 for female patients. However, the size of the sinus of Valsalva varies among individuals, and some patients have an unexpectedly large sinus. At my center, BriteTip® catheters are available in sizes up to AL3.

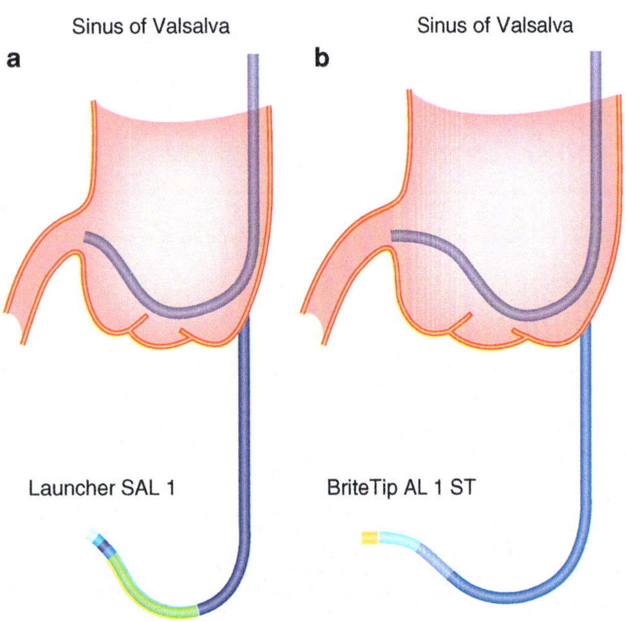

Fig. 1.14 Optimal size of the guiding catheter tip curve relative to the sinus of Valsalva. Ideally, the distance between the tip and the shaft of the guiding catheter is slightly shorter than the distance between the RCA ostium and the contralateral wall of the sinus of Valsalva. A female patient of short stature often has a small sinus of Valsalva (**a**), and the Launcher SAL 1 is generally optimal for such patients. A male patient of medium stature often has a medium-sized sinus of Valsalva (**b**), and the BriteTip AL 1 ST is usually optimal

Selecting a Guiding Catheter with or Without Side Holes and Management of a "Wedged" Waveform

In principle, I never use a guiding catheter with side holes for the RCA or the LCA. This is because the pressure waveform is not damped even if such a catheter becomes wedged, making it difficult to become aware of the increased risk of ostial injury, so that injury is more likely to occur. Let us consider the case where the catheter is not initially wedged, but subsequently the pressure waveform shows a "wedged" pattern when an Amplatz left-type guiding catheter is engaged. A good solution is to advance the guiding catheter by about 2 to 3 cm while monitoring the waveform without checking fluoroscopic images. This will usually result in slight disengagement of the catheter tip, and the wedged waveform will be normalized. If this maneuver fails, the guiding catheter should not simply be advanced further, but should be gently rotated counterclockwise and then slowly advanced under fluoroscopic guidance. This will lead to disengagement of the catheter with normalization of the pressure waveform.

If the guiding catheter has a relatively large tip curve compared with the size of the sinus of Valsalva, the pressure waveform may show a wedged pattern when the catheter is engaged, while the waveform often improves after exchanging the catheter for another catheter with a curve that is one size smaller. If a catheter with a smaller curve is not available, it will be necessary to (reluctantly) exchange it for one with side holes.

I create side holes in guiding catheters by using an 18-G injection needle to make two holes on the medial side of the second curve of the catheter. Each hole is created slowly and carefully by rotating the needle to-and-fro, rather than simply pushing it into the catheter (i.e., by gradually removing small particles of catheter material with the bezel of the needle). A hole created in this way remains patent for a long time. The second hole should be created in the same way by using a fresh needle. After creating the two holes, the tip of the catheter should be covered with the fingertips, and the catheter should be vigorously flushed with saline to completely remove all debris.

Pull Back to Advance the Tip and Push Forward to Disengage the Tip

As I mentioned before, you should pull a guiding catheter back slightly to advance the tip into the target coronary artery and should push an engaged catheter forward to disengage it. However, you may sometimes find that pushing a deeply engaged guiding catheter forward fails to move its tip toward the ostium.

If this happens, you should initially try to advance the guiding catheter slightly while gently rotating it counterclockwise. This maneuver may succeed in disengaging the catheter tip

without slipping it from the RCA ostium, although the catheter becomes slightly unstable. If this maneuver actually results in deeper engagement of the guiding catheter, you can pull the catheter back while gently rotating it counterclockwise until the tip just becomes disengaged. If the catheter is subsequently advanced slightly, the tip will often become stable again within the sinus of Valsalva, resulting in good engagement. If a guidewire has been advanced into the RCA from the guiding catheter, you should push it in slightly deeper and then advance the catheter. This maneuver will result in stable location of the catheter tip within the sinus of Valsalva.

Removing the Guiding Catheter from the RCA Ostium at the End of the Procedure

To remove a guiding catheter from the RCA at the end of the procedure, you should never simply pull the catheter back because removing it in this way is likely to cause ostial injury. As shown in Fig. 1.15, you should initially push the catheter further in while rotating it counterclockwise to disengage the tip. After the catheter tip has come out of the RCA ostium, you should slowly withdraw the entire catheter until the tip reaches the level of the aorta. If this method of disengaging the catheter fails, you can also slowly pull the catheter back while rotating it counterclockwise to disengage the tip. With the latter method, the tip of the catheter will go directly up to the level of the aorta, and you should then keep the tip at that level.

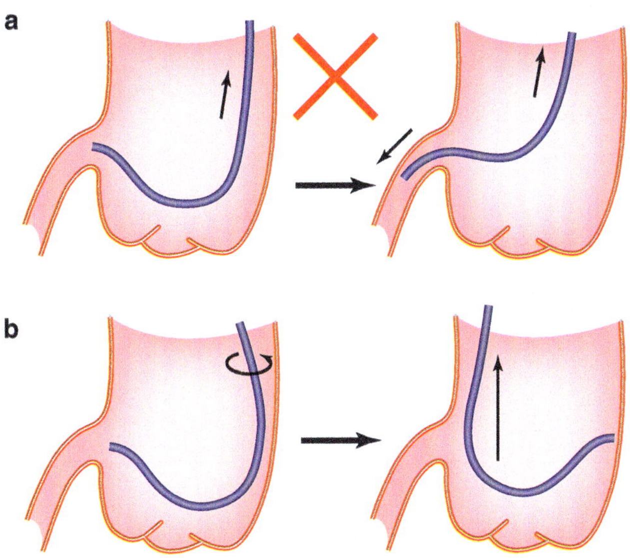

Fig. 1.15 Points to consider when removing a guiding catheter at the end of the procedure. You should never simply pull back on the catheter because removing a catheter in this way is likely to cause ostial injury (**a**). Instead, you should push the catheter in deeper while rotating it counterclockwise to disengage the tip. After the catheter tip has come out of the RCA ostium, you should slowly withdraw the entire catheter until the tip reaches the level of the aorta (**b**). If this method of disengagement fails, you should slowly pull the catheter back while rotating it anticlockwise to disengage the tip. With the latter method, the tip of the catheter will go directly up to the level of the aorta, and it should be maintained at that level

Removing the Guiding Catheter via the Femoral Artery

When removing a guiding catheter with its tip at the level of the aorta, you should utilize an inner sheath catheter and a guidewire to minimize stress on the aortic wall.

1.3.1.3 Short-Tipped Judkins Catheter or Extra Backup Catheter for the LCA

Among Judkins-type guiding catheters, I recommend using short-tipped catheters (preferably short-tipped catheters with a small first curve) for the LCA (Fig. 1.16). As early as 1985, Hartzler recommended the use of a short-tipped Judkins guiding catheter.

A short-tipped Judkins guiding catheter generates strong backup like an extra backup catheter, but has a tip that is oriented slightly in the medial direction, which makes it more likely to advance toward the LAD when pushed forward (Fig. 1.17). Even if there is plaque at the ostium of the left main trunk (LMT), it is easier to disengage a guiding catheter of this type while keeping it coaxial with the LMT. For these reasons, I choose a short-tipped Judkins-type guiding catheter when performing PCI for CTO of the LMT or LAD (Fig. 1.18).

On the other hand, a short-tipped Judkins catheter is inappropriate for PCI when the CTO is in the LCX because its tip is oriented slightly toward the LAD, i.e., contralateral to the LCX. The guidewire has to be redirected toward the LCX, so it becomes difficult to handle, and this guiding catheter only provides poor backup for the LCX. In contrast, an extra backup type of guiding catheter with an appropriate curve size will have the tip directed toward the LCX when it is engaged normally, and the tip will be directed further toward the LCX when it is pulled back slightly. Accordingly, I think that the extra backup guiding catheter is optimal when performing PCI for CTO of the LCX (Fig. 1.18).

To perform PCI for CTO of the LCA, I formerly used AL-type guiding catheters, but I rarely do so now. The main reason I no longer use AL-type catheters for LCA lesions is that this type of catheter is much more likely to cause coronary artery injury when it is removed from the LMT compared with the RCA. Over the years, techniques using Judkins or EBU guiding catheters without stressful engagement have become the mainstay of PCI for the LCA. These techniques include use of a guiding catheter with the tip shaped by heating to ensure coaxiality with the LMT, advancing the guiding catheter over a guidewire initially introduced into the target coronary artery (guidewire cannulation technique), and leaving the guidewire in place as a buddy wire (buddy wire technique).

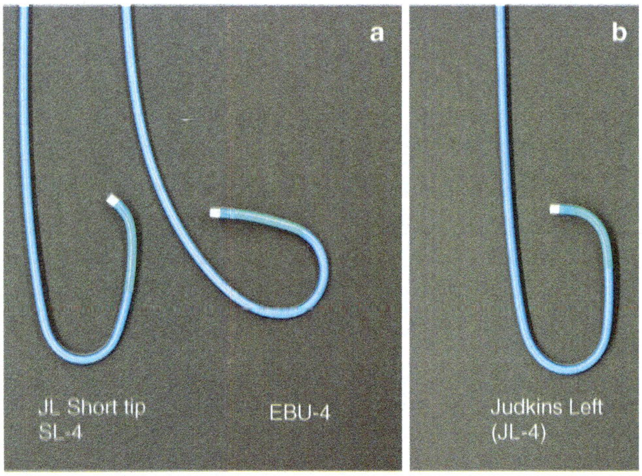

Fig. 1.16 Guiding catheters for the LCA. I only use the regular Judkins left (JL) guiding catheter (**b**) in exceptional circumstances. This type of guiding catheter has a first curve that is too long, so its tip is often oriented toward the roof of the LMT, potentially causing LMT injury and only providing poor backup. In contrast, the SL type of catheter with a short first curve (**a**) is rarely directed toward the roof of the LMT and is more likely to become coaxial with this segment of the LCA. The extra backup type of catheter is also more likely to become coaxial with the LMT and provide good backup

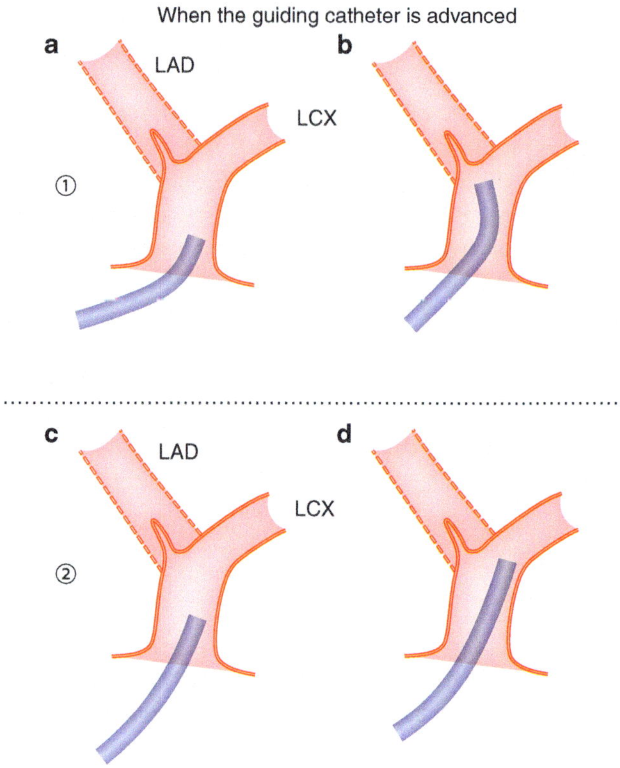

Fig. 1.17 Short-tipped (ST) Judkins left and extra backup guiding catheters for the LAD (especially the LAD ostium). (1) ST Judkins left catheter: If the tip is not engaged deeply, it may be difficult for the catheter to track the LAD (**a**). Even in such circumstances, the curve of the tip sends the catheter toward the LAD when the catheter is advanced (**b**) and makes subsequent manipulation of a guidewire easier. (2) Extra backup catheter: If it is difficult to direct the catheter toward the LAD (**c**), further advancement of the catheter may result in it entering the LCX (**d**) rather than the LAD

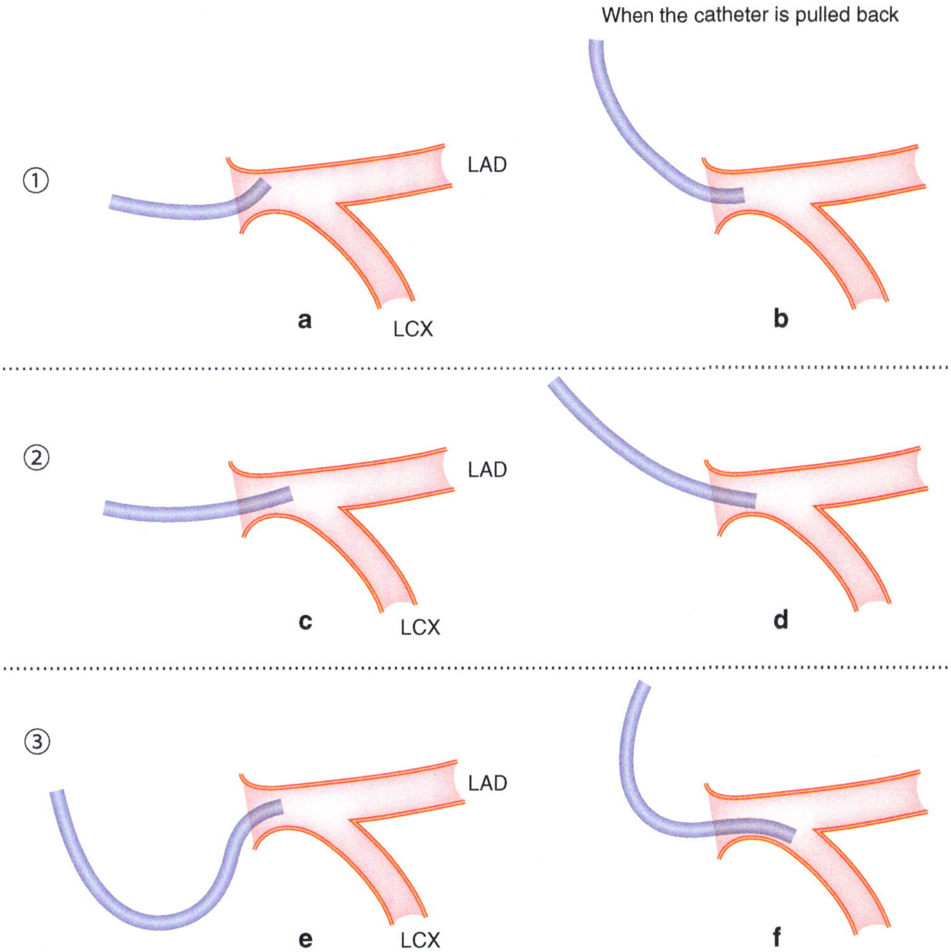

Fig. 1.18 Various guiding catheters for the LCX. (1) ST Judkins left catheter: This type of guiding catheter can sometimes be directed toward the LCX after it has been pulled back considerably. Once the catheter has been directed toward the LCX, its second curve becomes nearly parallel with the long axis of the aorta, which means that the catheter cannot provide strong backup while remaining coaxial with the LCX. (2) Extra backup catheter: A catheter of this type is easily directed toward the LCX when it is pulled back. Since its tip and shaft become nearly perpendicular to the long axis of the aorta, it is likely to provide good backup while remaining concentric with the LCX. (3) Amplatz left catheter: The tip of this type of catheter is likely to become coaxial with the LCX. However, in the position shown in *e*, this catheter cannot provide good coaxial backup with the LCX, and it has to be pulled back to gain coaxiality with the LCX. When this catheter is pulled back, control of its tip may be lost, leading to stress on the base of the LMT, or it may become deeply engaged or disengaged

1.3.1.4 Size of the Catheter Tip Curve

Interventionalists in the USA and Europe often use 3.5-cm extra backup guiding catheters to perform PCI for CTO of the LCA in male patients. For a Japanese male patient, I think a catheter of this size is too small, and I use a 4.0-cm guiding catheter. It is true that you can easily engage a 3.5-cm guiding catheter in the LCA, but it is hard to achieve the principal purpose of providing strong backup with a catheter of this size. For example, I usually select a 4.0-cm SL guiding catheter, which provides stronger backup than a 3.5-cm Launcher extra backup catheter. If a 4.0-cm extra backup guiding catheter is too large (though this only happens infrequently, as with the SL type), it should be changed to a 3.5-cm catheter. In principle, I choose a guiding catheter with a curve that is one size smaller for female patients. However, a guiding catheter of the size recommended for male patients may often be optimal for female patients, depending on the size of the aortic sinus of Valsalva.

You can successfully engage the guiding catheters listed in Table 1.2 in the LCA in 99% of patients, but will fail to achieve engagement in the remaining 1%. If failure occurs, I recommend inserting a copper wire into the tip of the guiding catheter for a distance of about 10 cm, reshaping the catheter tip and softening it by heating, and then immediately immersing the tip in cold water to maintain the new shape (Fig. 1.19). After removing the copper wire, you should engage the guiding catheter in the LCA ostium as soon as possible before the catheter undergoes further deformation due to overheating.

Table 1.2 Guiding catheters for CTOs in various coronary artery segments

			Male patients	Female patients
RCA	First choice		BriteTip AL 1 ST	Launcher SAL 1
	Variation		BriteTip AL 1–AL 3Launcher SAL 1	BriteTip AL 1–AL 3
	Rare		JR (shepherd crook), AR (downward orientation)	
LCA	LM, LAD	First choice	Launcher SL 4	Launcher SL 3.5
		Variation	Launcher SL 3.5, 4.5, 5.0	Launcher ST 4.0–5.0
	LCX	First choice	Launcher EBU 4.0	Launcher EBU 3.5
		Variation	Launcher EBU 4.5 Launcher EBU 3.5	Launcher EBU 4.0, 4.5
	Rare		AL	

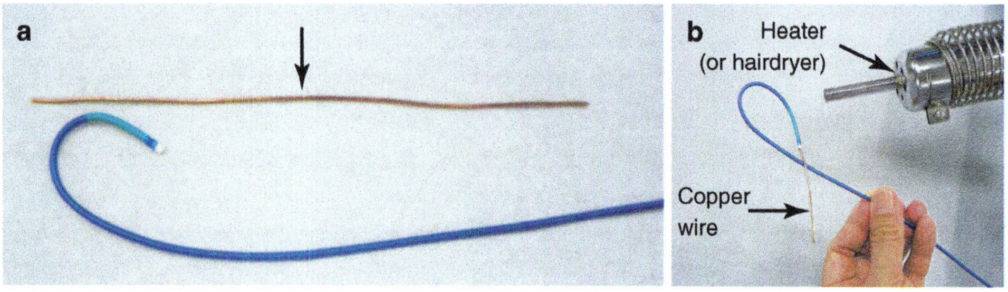

Fig. 1.19 Procedure for reshaping a guiding catheter (ST Judkins). (**a**) Cut a 15-cm-long piece of thick copper wire (desirably 0.8 to 1.0 mm in diameter), and sterilize it. (**b**) Insert the copper wire into the tip of the guiding catheter for a distance of about 10 cm, and curve the tip to obtain the desired shape. Evenly heat the tip with a heater (or a hairdryer) to soften it, and immediately immerse the tip in water to cool it, and ensure that it retains the new shape. After the catheter has been cooled, remove the copper wire, and promptly engage the guiding catheter in the target coronary artery

1.3.2 Anchoring Technique

When performing PCI for CTO of the RCA, AL-type guiding catheters of the appropriate size can provide good backup. However, it is sometimes necessary to continue PCI with a guiding catheter that has a curve which is too small for the sinus of Valsalva. This means that the guiding catheter cannot provide sufficient backup or ensure stable guidewire manipulation (Fig. 1.20a). In this situation, prompt use of the anchoring (anchor balloon) technique is recommended if a suitable side branch is available (Fig. 1.20b).

1.3.2.1 Size and Inflation Pressure of the Anchoring Balloon

The anchoring balloon should desirably be one size larger than the diameter of the side branch used for anchoring and should be short (10 to 15 mm). To perform anchoring, the balloon should be inflated at a low pressure such as 4 atm. If the side branch for anchoring is tapered, a long balloon will slip out when it is inflated. Even if the balloon is the optimal size, it will not have an anchoring effect or will slip out if it is inflated at a high pressure. If the side branch contains calcified plaque, a balloon that seems to be of the optimal size with reference to the branch diameter sometimes fails to have an anchoring effect when inflated at too high pressure.

1.3.2.2 If No Side Branch Is Available for Anchoring

If there is no side branch available for anchoring, the guiding catheter should be changed to a larger AL-type catheter to obtain sufficient backup from the contralateral wall of the sinus of Valsalva.

A side branch that is located too close to the target coronary artery ostium cannot be used for anchoring to increase backup. In fact, anchoring the catheter from such a side branch may rather decrease backup because the shaft of the anchoring balloon will not become coaxial with the coronary artery (Fig. 1.20b). However, even a side branch located close to the coronary artery ostium can be used for anchoring with another purpose in mind, i.e., to prevent the guiding catheter from slipping out of the ostium.

If the distance between the CTO and the coronary artery ostium is adequate to permit deep engagement of a guiding catheter, a child catheter such as the GuideLiner® can also be used to provide good backup.

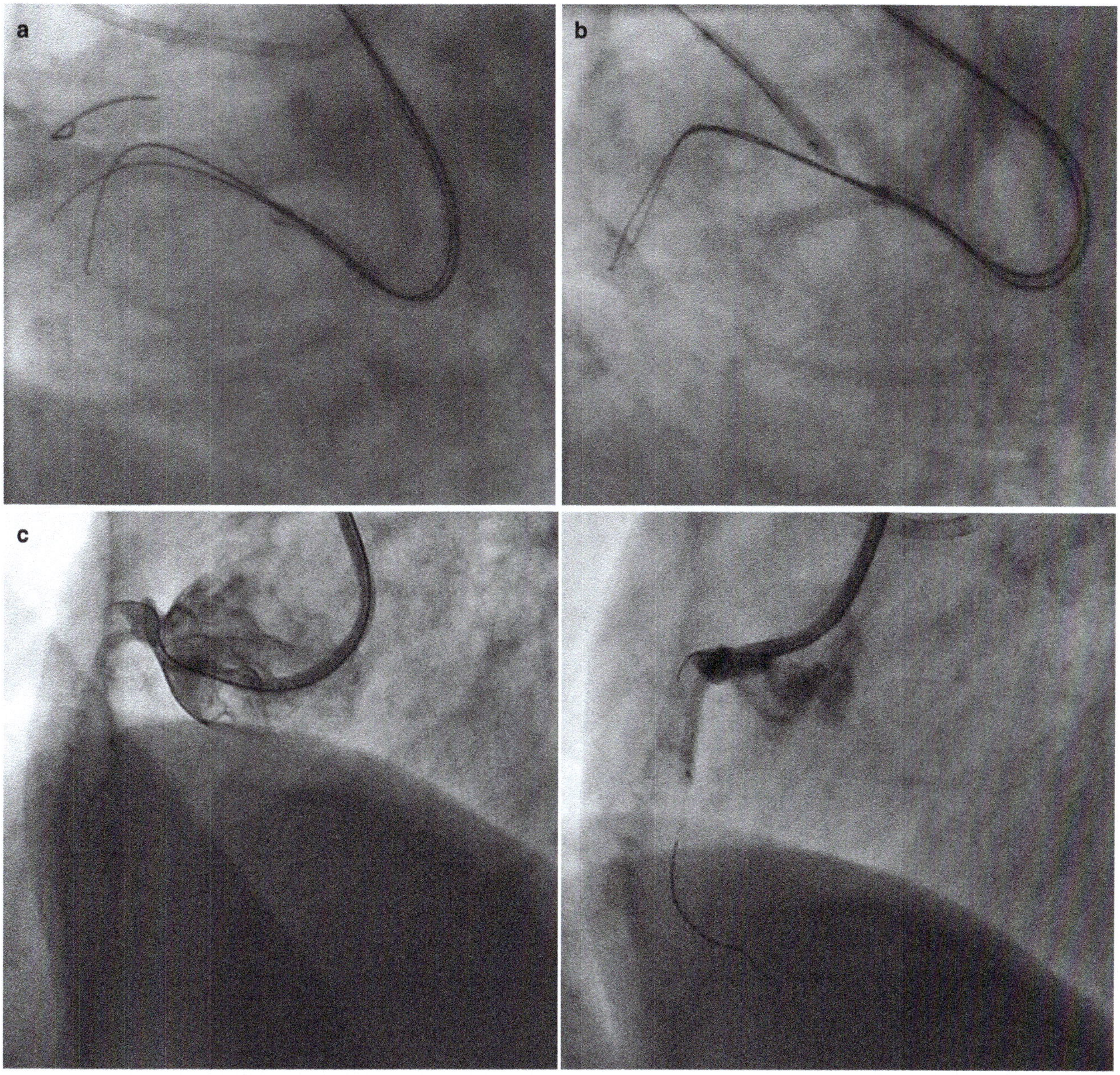

Fig. 1.20 Anchoring technique. (**a**) After starting PCI for a CTO of the RCA, loss of coaxiality between the guiding catheter and the RCA ostium occurred when the guidewire was advanced slightly. (**b**) Anchoring by using the conus branch maintained the guiding catheter coaxial to the RCA ostium and considerably improved guidewire manipulability. (**c**) Anchoring by using a side branch near the RCA ostium resulted in loss of coaxiality between the guiding catheter and the ostium. Exchanging the guiding catheter allowed coaxiality to be regained, but backup was somewhat impaired

Column 1 Guidewire Cannulation and Buddy Wire Techniques

If incomplete engagement of a guiding catheter results in laminar flow imaging of the target coronary artery (Fig. 1.21 a–d), it is difficult to obtain good images without taking additional measures. To achieve complete engagement of the guiding catheter for optimal imaging and backup in this situation, I sometimes introduce a guidewire first and advance the guiding catheter over the guidewire. When advancing the guiding catheter, I do not recommend forcibly rotating or pushing it forward. Instead, to-and-fro movement should be repeated in the appropriate direction while slightly rotating the catheter. If you still fail to achieve engagement of the guiding catheter, I recommend using another guidewire (plus a microcatheter) as a buddy wire. By this technique, you can advance the guiding catheter slightly while keeping it coaxial with the coronary artery ostium and can achieve engagement without generating much stress.

These techniques are also useful for engaging a guiding catheter with no side holes in a stenotic ostium so that it is slightly out of the wedged position.

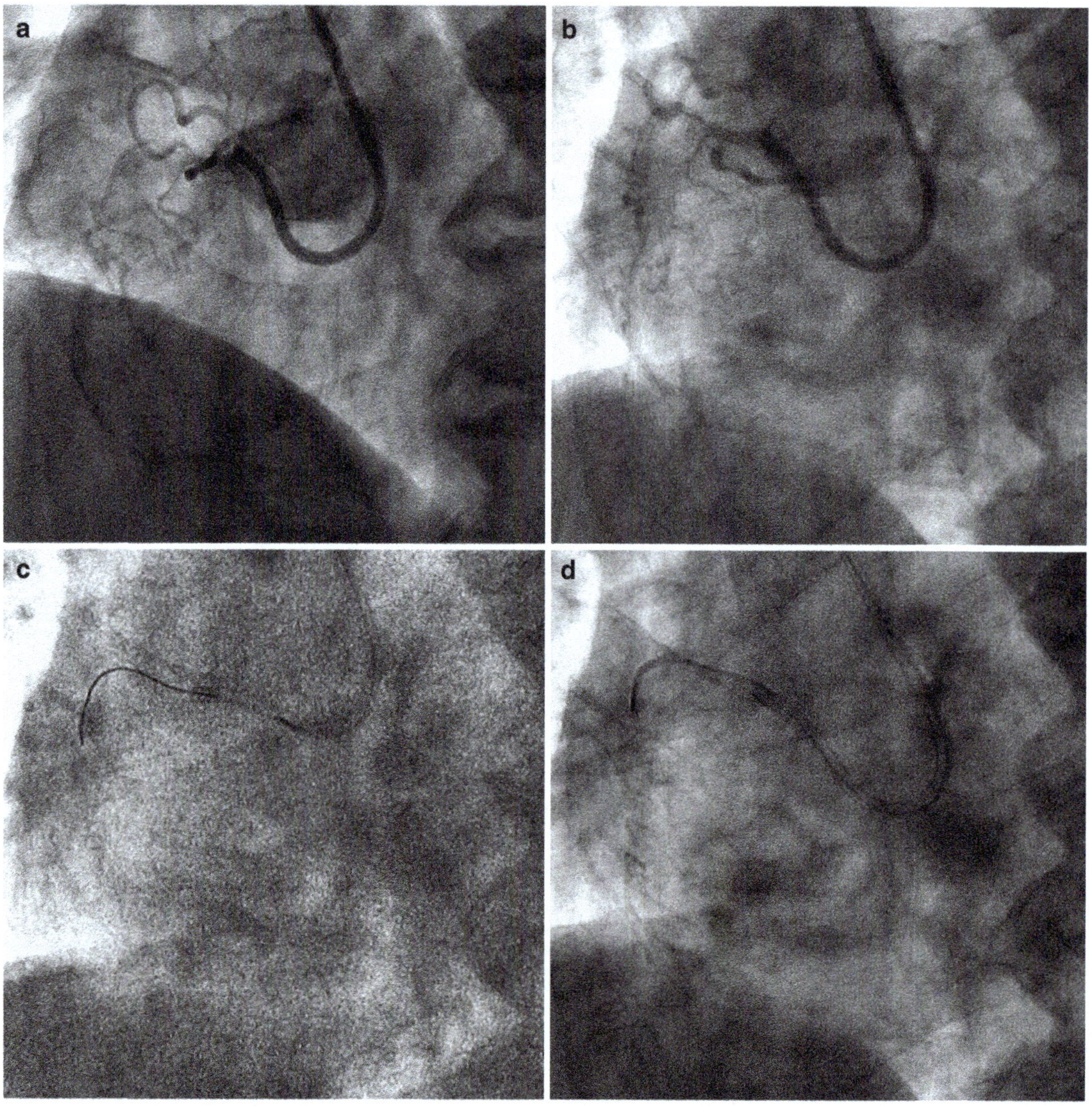

Fig. 1.21 (**a**, **b**) Incomplete engagement of a guiding catheter results in laminar flow imaging of the target coronary artery. (**c**, **d**) After introducing a guidewire, the guiding catheter could be engaged (**c**). In this case, deeper engagement of the guiding catheter to ensure enough backup would result in laminar flow imaging again. Therefore, a microcatheter was advanced, and tip injection was performed in order to assess the anatomy of the target vessel (**d**)

Column 2 Handling Coronary Arteries with Anomalous Origin

To engage a guiding catheter in a coronary artery with anomalous origin, you often must improvise when selecting the catheter and/or modify the engagement procedure.

[High take-off RCA]

Unlike a normal RCA, an RCA originating from the ascending aorta often arises in the left anterior position and runs downward. To achieve successful engagement in patients with such a "high take-off" RCA, you should choose an AL-type guiding catheter with a relatively large second curve and should direct its tip downward. One way to direct the tip downward is to seek the RCA ostium with the tip initially oriented down and to the left anteriorly (Fig. 1.22a). Another way is to pull up the catheter with its tip bent upward. When the tip is trapped by a dimple, upward movement should be continued slowly while keeping the tip at the dimple until the tip becomes oriented downward and coaxial with the RCA ostium. Then engagement of the catheter will be accomplished by slightly advancing the tip into the ostium (Fig. 1.22b).

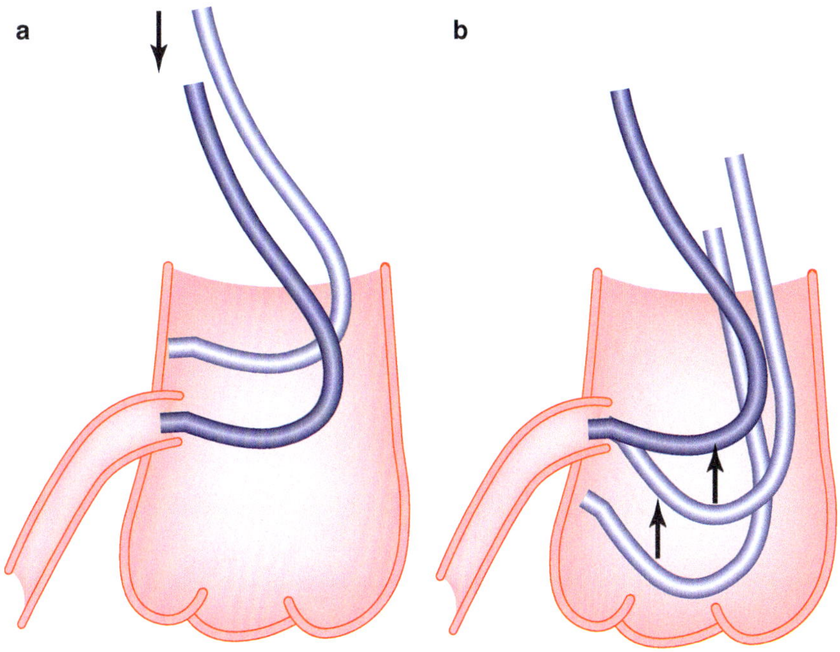

Fig. 1.22 High take-off RCA

[RCA originating from the left sinus of Valsalva]

To achieve engagement of a guiding catheter when the RCA originates from the left sinus of Valsalva requires complicated maneuvers. The RCA usually runs anteriorly to the right for a short distance from its ostium (normally located to the right and anterior to the aorta [sinus of Valsalva]) and then runs caudally. As is clearly seen on CT scans, if the tip of a guiding catheter is coaxial with the RCA ostium, the shaft of the catheter is almost perpendicular to the contralateral aortic wall (Fig. 1.23a). If the RCA originates from the left sinus of Valsalva, it runs anteriorly along the aorta from its origin. Therefore, if the RCA has such an anomalous origin, it is difficult to maintain the tip of a standard guiding catheter coaxial with the proximal part of the target vessel. Although a guiding catheter can be engaged in an anomalous RCA like this and the tip can be maintained coaxial to the ostium, engagement will not be deep enough to obtain good images or to provide strong backup (Fig. 1.23b).

An Amplatz left-type guiding catheter with a customized curved tip or a three-dimensional (3D) guiding catheter can be engaged at a relatively deep level and can provide enough backup for standard PCI, but it is often not sufficient for successfully crossing a CTO (Fig. 1.23c).

If a side branch is available for anchoring, the anchoring technique is most effective for helping to accomplish engagement of the guiding catheter. If there is no suitable side branch, using a child catheter such as the GuideLiner is somewhat effective (Fig. 1.23d).

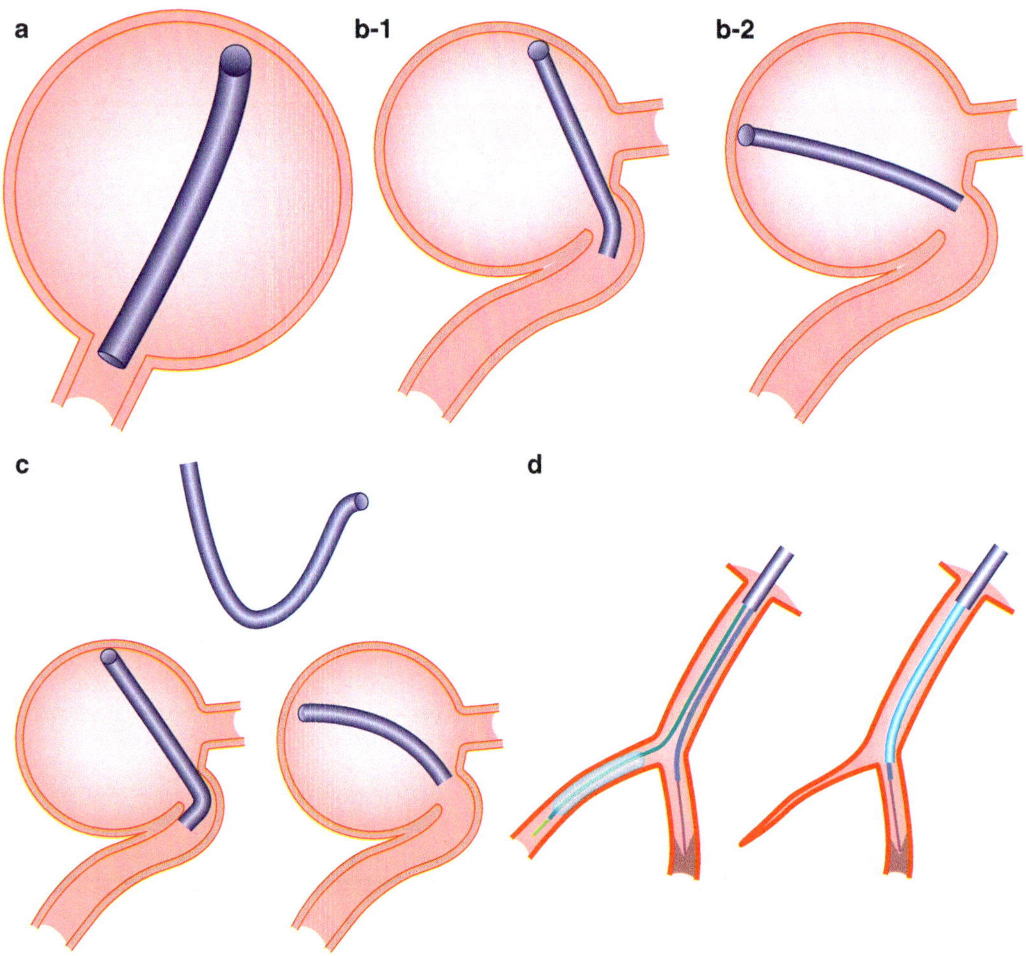

Fig. 1.23 RCA originating from the left sinus of Valsalva. (**a**) RCA with a normal origin. The shaft of the guiding catheter is perpendicular to the contralateral aortic wall, providing good backup. (**b**) RCA originating from the left sinus of Valsalva (1). A guiding catheter engaged in the ostium does not generate good backup (b-1), and engagement becomes less deep if the shaft is made perpendicular to the contralateral aortic wall (b-2). (**c**) RCA originating from the left sinus of Valsalva (2). A different guiding catheter may provide stronger backup, but this may still not be enough for treating a CTO. (**d**) The anchoring technique or use of a child catheter can be somewhat effective for helping to achieve adequate engagement of the guiding catheter

To treat an ostial CTO for which an antegrade guiding catheter cannot provide good backup, you should also consider crossing the lesion via the retrograde approach and forming a loop with an RG-3 to consolidate backup (Figs. 1.24 and 1.25).

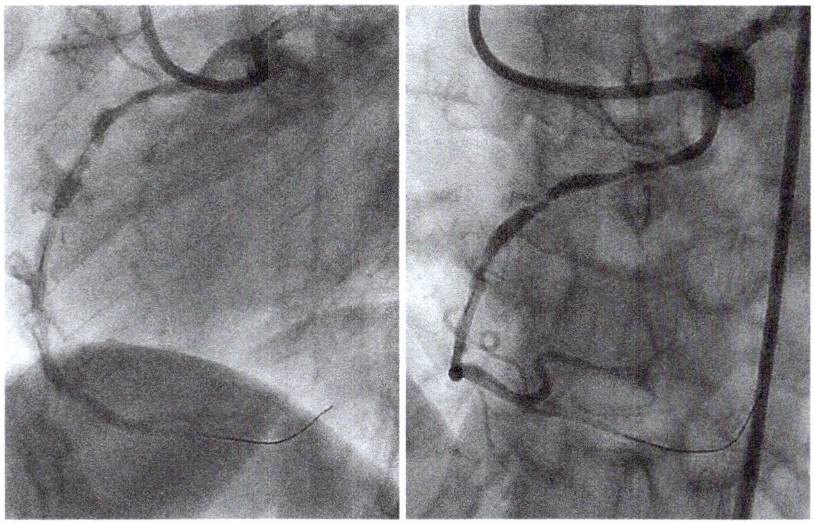

Fig. 1.24 RCA originating from the left sinus of Valsalva. Images obtained with an SL4. In the AP-CR view, the RCA changes direction just beyond the ostium. Therefore, it is difficult to engage a guiding catheter in the RCA and maintain it coaxial to the proximal part of the artery, resulting in poor backup

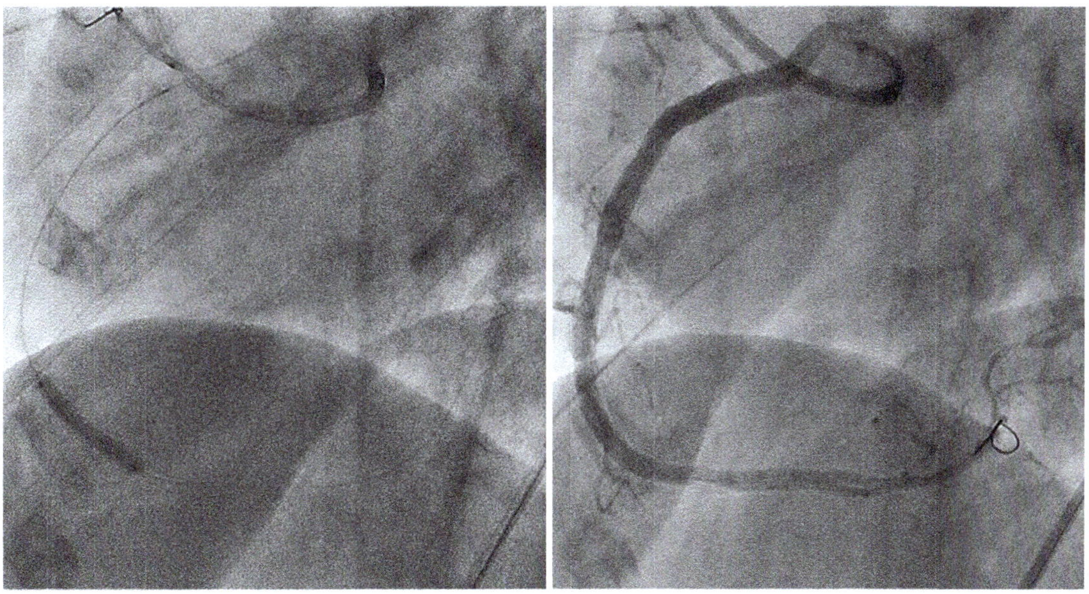

Fig. 1.25 Anchoring technique for balloon angioplasty and stenting combined with a GuideLiner for imaging

1.4 Anticoagulation Strategy

1.4.1 Administration of Heparin

Performing PCI for CTO requires prolonged manipulation of guidewires and other devices, which increases the risk of thrombosis. In particular, thrombosis occurring in a retrograde channel is often fatal and must be prevented. For complete thromboprophylaxis, it is necessary to ensure that a stable effect of heparin is sustained throughout the PCI procedure. Table 1.3 summarizes the recommended initial dose of heparin. At 5 minutes after administering the initial dose of heparin, you should measure the activated coagulation time (ACT). If the ACT indicates inadequate anticoagulation by heparin, you should administer an additional dose of heparin as indicated in Table 1.4. Measure the ACT every 30 minutes thereafter, and, depending on the results, administer an additional dose of heparin to keep the ACT at ≥300 seconds.

Blood for measurement of the ACT is often collected from the guiding catheter. When collecting blood for this purpose via the guiding catheter, you should take care to prevent contamination with even a small amount of contrast medium. If the ACT is ≥400 seconds after treatment with the standard dosage of heparin, this undoubtedly represents a measurement error arising from contamination of the blood sample by contrast medium during collection. If the ACT is around 300 seconds due to unrecognized contamination by contrast medium, the true ACT may be at a level associated with a significant risk of thrombosis. To completely exclude the risk of contamination by contrast medium, you should take care to optimize handling of the three-way stopcock during blood collection and pay attention to the dead space volume.

If the ACT is not prolonged at 5 minutes after the initial dose of heparin, administer a second dose, and repeat measurement of the ACT after another 5 minutes. If the ACT is still not prolonged, suspect heparin-induced thrombocytopenia/thrombosis (HIT/T), and switch heparin to argatroban. With this anticoagulation strategy using doses of heparin modified according to the ACT, no patient undergoing PCI for CTO at our center has developed thrombosis during intervention.

1.4.2 Blood Sample Collection for ACT Measurement

If venous access has been obtained with a sheath to provide blood samples for measurement of the ACT, blood collected via this route yields the most precise ACT values. If the sheath is the same size as the guiding catheter, it becomes difficult to collect blood from the side arm of the sheath. Using a sheath that is one size larger than the catheter makes it easier to collect blood and obtain precise ACT values. If there is no other route available, it becomes necessary to collect blood samples via the guiding catheter while taking appropriate precautions.

1.4.3 Precautions When Collecting Blood via the Guiding Catheter

If a blood sample is collected from the contrast injection port of a three-port manifold, much blood will need to be discarded first because of the large dead space. The volume of blood that needs to be discarded to prevent contamination with contrast medium is sometimes excessively large. At our center, we place a three-way stopcock near a Y-shaped connector and collect blood via the stopcock. When aspirating blood from the three-way stopcock to eliminate the dead space, the syringe should be kept horizontal or angled downward. Even if a large volume of blood is aspirated into a syringe angled upward, contrast medium always remains at the bottom of the three-way stopcock because of its high specific gravity. Take care to completely avoid contamination with contrast medium because this is essential for obtaining precise ACT values.

If the ACT is longer than 400 seconds or is prolonged without administration of additional doses of heparin, you should suspect that contamination with contrast medium has resulted in a falsely high ACT value and should repeat the test with a blood sample collected more carefully to exclude contamination.

If the ACT measured using blood contaminated with contrast medium is within the target range, the true ACT value will be below the range and will be at a level that is associated with a significant risk of thrombosis during PCI. It is important to always keep in mind the necessity of completely excluding contrast medium from blood samples collected through a guiding catheter for measurement of the ACT.

Table 1.3 Initial dose of heparin recommended for patients undergoing PCI

Characteristics	Initial dose of heparin
None of the characteristics listed below	Full (100%) = 10,000 U
Age > 75 years	About 80%
Body weight < 45 kg (females) or < 50 kg (males)	About 80%
On warfarin	About 80%

Table 1.4 Additional doses of heparin recommended for patients undergoing PCI based on ACT values

ACT value (sec)	Additional dose of heparin (U)		
	100%	80%	80% × 2 (64%)
120–170	5000	4000	3000
171–220	4000	3000	2000
221–270	3000	2000	2000
271–290	2000	1000	1000
290–300	1000	1000	500
300-	0		

1.5 Fluoroscopy and Imaging Strategies

1.5.1 Video Imaging Equipment and Fluoroscopy Angles

Selection of the correct video imaging equipment and fluoroscopy angles are among the most important considerations when performing PCI for CTO.

1.5.1.1 Is Biplane Imaging Essential?

I think that simultaneous biplane cineangiography of the heart is essential when PCI is performed for CTO, not only for diagnostic imaging but also for fluoroscopic guidance during guidewire manipulation.

In order to confirm the passage of a guidewire by monoplane cineangiography, images need to be obtained in different projections. Efforts have been made to reduce the frequency of imaging with monoplane cineangiography, such as obtaining an image while rotating the detector after locating the patient's heart precisely at the center of the two projections (isocenter). Despite such efforts, it is impossible to confirm passage of a guidewire until the wire has been advanced for a certain distance. Thus, more frequent imaging is needed with monoplane cineangiography to confirm the position of the guidewire after advancing the wire for a short distance.

Simultaneous biplane imaging allows the position and direction of the tip of a guidewire to be checked easily after advancing it for a short distance (Fig. 1.26). In practice, simultaneous biplane imaging is important for PCI because we manipulate guidewires and other devices while checking the fluoroscopy screen. I strongly recommend setting the biplane imaging equipment in the simultaneous mode since most biplane apparatus can be set this way.

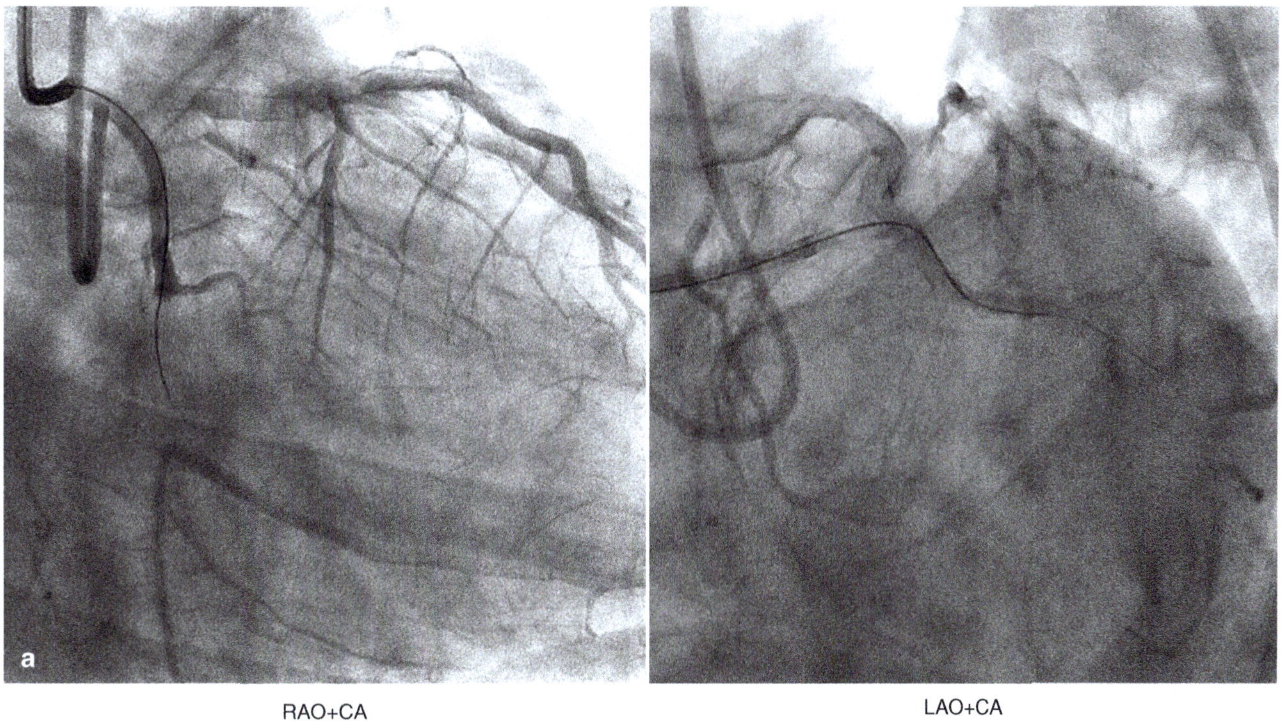

Fig. 1.26 Correcting the direction of the guidewire tip by simultaneous biplane cineangiography. (**a**) During PCI for a CTO in the middle segment of the LCX, simultaneous imaging in two orthogonal projections was employed to visually check whether the direction of the wire was correct or not. Although the guidewire appeared to be heading toward the exit point, simultaneous imaging showed that its tip was directed to the right in both the RAO + CA and LAO + CA views. (**b**) Based on this information, the direction of the guidewire tip was corrected leftward in both views, resulting in successful crossing of the CTO through the true lumen

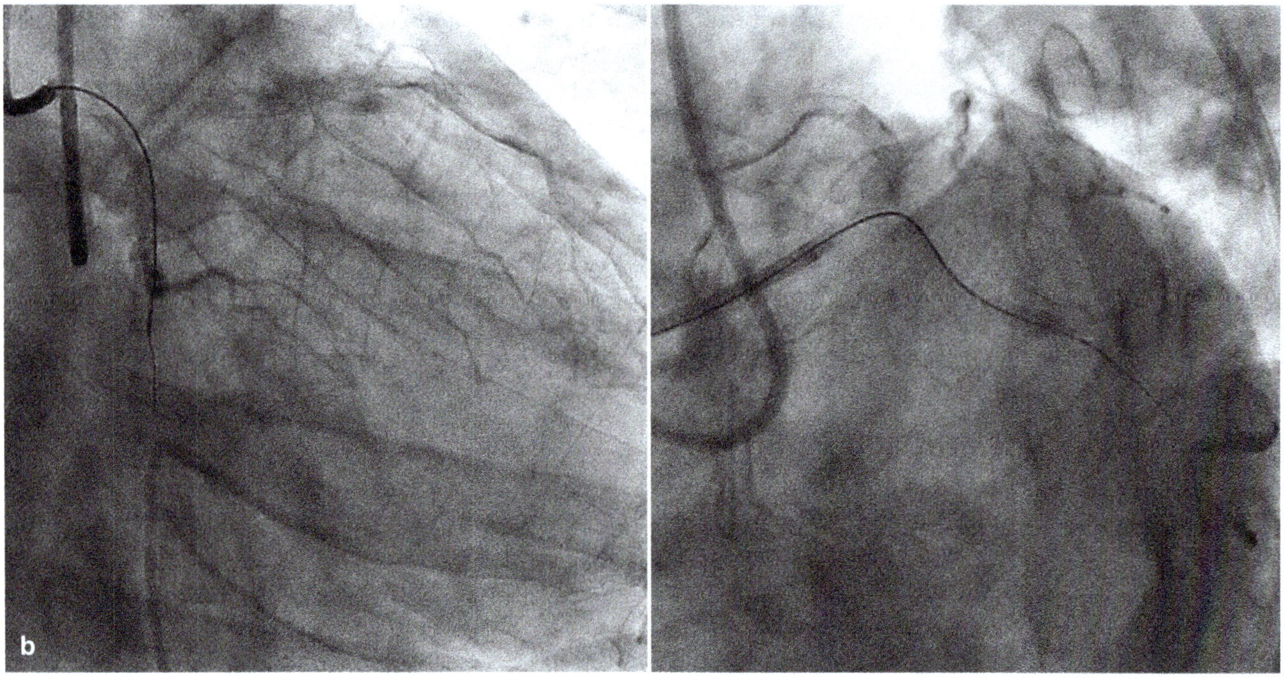

Fig. 1.26 (continued)

1.5.1.2 Direction of the Longitudinal Axis of the Target Vessel in the Region of Interest for Guidewire Advancement

The region of interest (ROI) is defined as the occluded region of the coronary artery from the point at the tip of the guidewire to a peripheral landmark or the site of a presumed bend (Fig. 1.27). When treating a long tortuous CTO such as the lesion shown in Fig. 1.28, the position of the ROI changes as the tip of the guidewire is advanced and the direction of the longitudinal axis of the target vessel in each ROI changes as well. In principle, two projections should be used to confirm that the guidewire tip is in the true lumen, and the two detector surfaces should desirably be set orthogonal to each other and parallel with the longitudinal axis of the target vessel when imaging. This is because obtaining two orthogonal projections minimizes the blind area (Fig. 1.29) and provides more accurate visual confirmation that the guidewire tip is in the true lumen (Fig. 1.30).

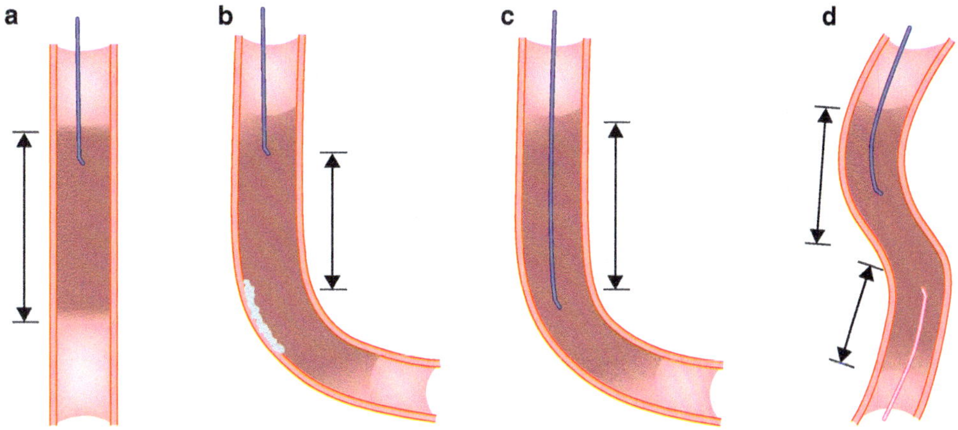

Fig. 1.27 ROIs (the ranges are indicated by arrows) during PCI for CTO. (**a**) If the lesion appears to be relatively straight from the entry point to the exit point on angiograms, the ROI is set from entry point to exit point. (**b**) If there is a landmark within the lesion, the ROI is set from the tip of the proximal guidewire to the landmark. (**c**) If there is a large bend in the lesion, the ROI is set from the entry point to the presumed bend. (**d**) Once the tip of the guidewire has reached the bend, a new ROI is set from the presumed bend to the next landmark, which might be the exit point (as in this case), a second bend, or any other feature

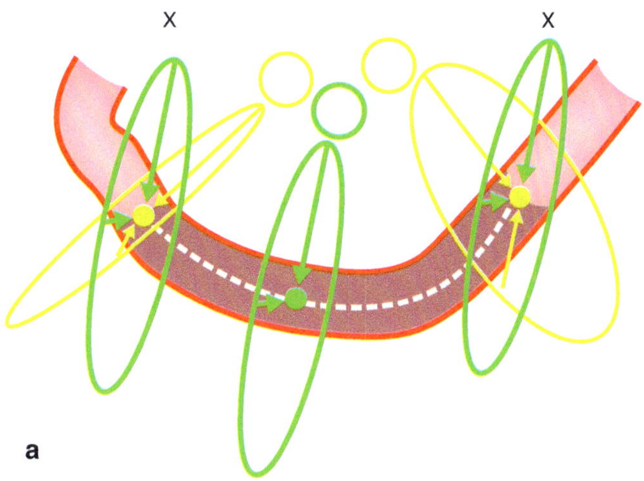

Fig. 1.28 Changes of the ROI while advancing the guidewire. (**a**) When treating a long tortuous CTO, the ROI will change as the guidewire is advanced. The detector surfaces should be set orthogonal to each other and parallel with the longitudinal axis of the target vessel inside the ROI. When treating a long CTO of the RCA extending from Segment #1 to the periphery of Segment #3, you would need to set four different ROIs as shown in this figure until the guidewire reaches the periphery. Appropriate projections for these ROIs are as follows: the AP + CR and LAO + CA projections for ROI 1 (from the ostium of the RCA to the bend in Segment #1); the RAO and LAO projections for ROI 2 (from the middle of Segment #1 to just proximal to the acute margin); the RAO (AP) + CA projection for ROI 3 (from the acute margin to the middle of Segment #3); and the AP + CR and LAO + CR projections (because of the bifurcation) for ROI 4 (from Segment #3 to the peripheral bifurcation of the RCA). (**b**) PCI was attempted for a CTO of the RCA that had occurred after coronary artery bypass grafting. Since the longitudinal axis of the proximal RCA was visualized well in the LAO + CA projection, the AP + CR projection was also chosen because it was orthogonal to the LAO + CA projection. (**c**) The longitudinal axis of the middle portion of the RCA was visualized well in the AP + CA projection, so the LAO + CR projection was also selected because it was orthogonal to the AP + CA projection. (**d**) Imaging of the peripheral RCA bifurcation should be able to clearly distinguish the two branches. Therefore, LAO + CR and AP + CR projections were chosen, although the detector surfaces partially overlapped

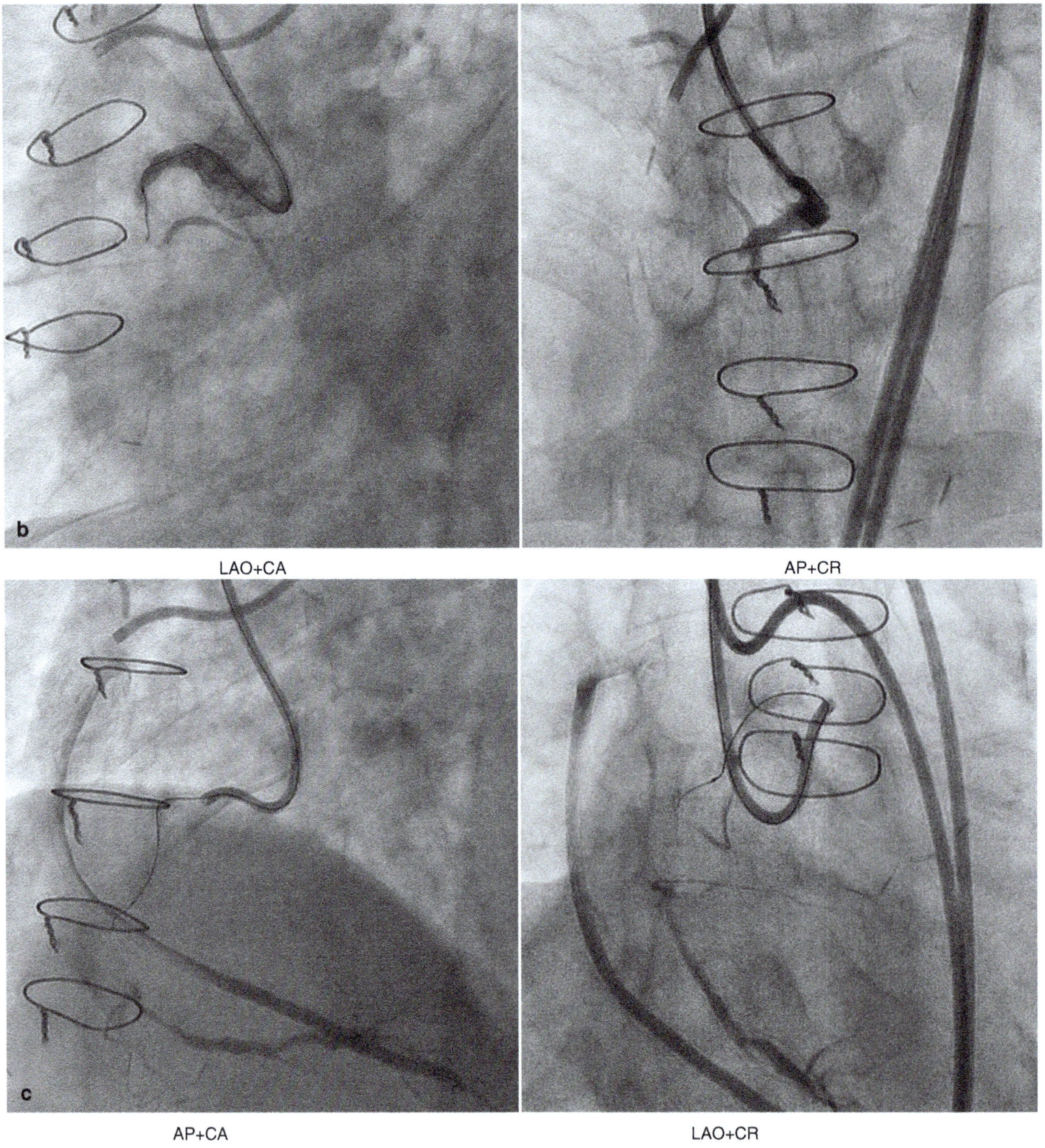

Fig. 1.28 (continued)

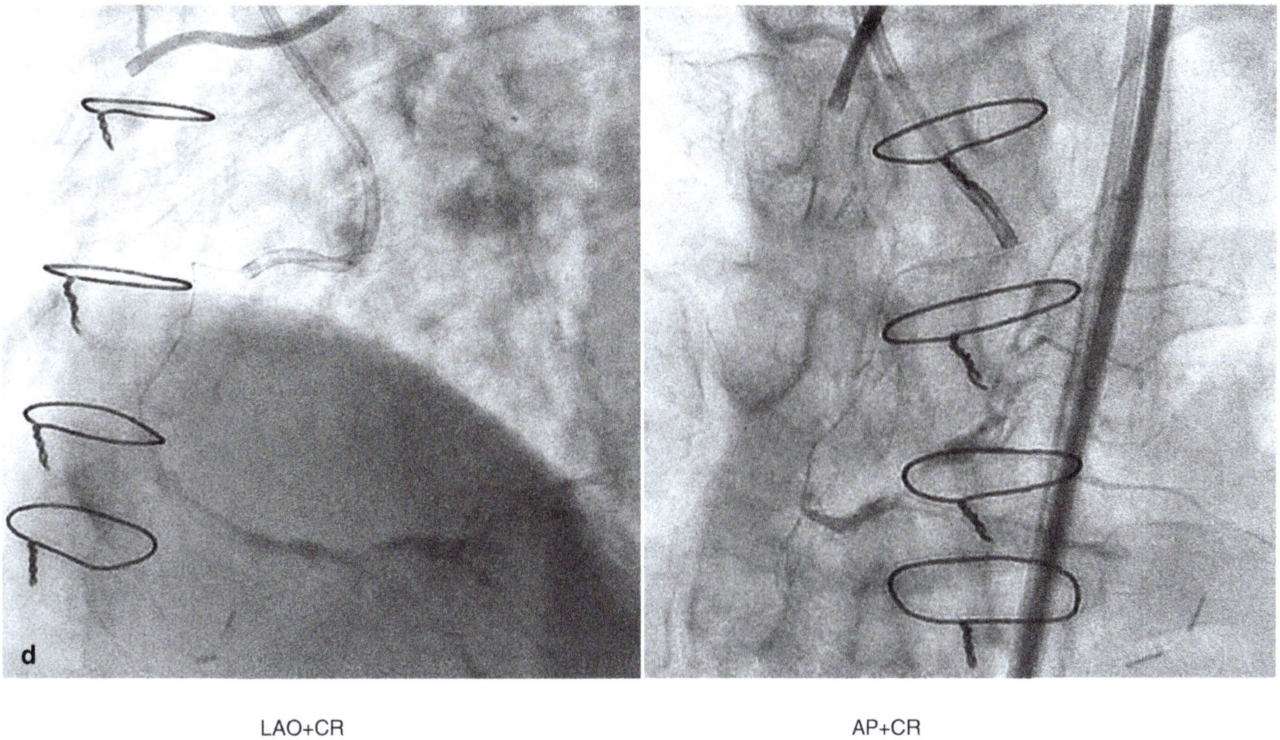

Fig. 1.28 (continued)

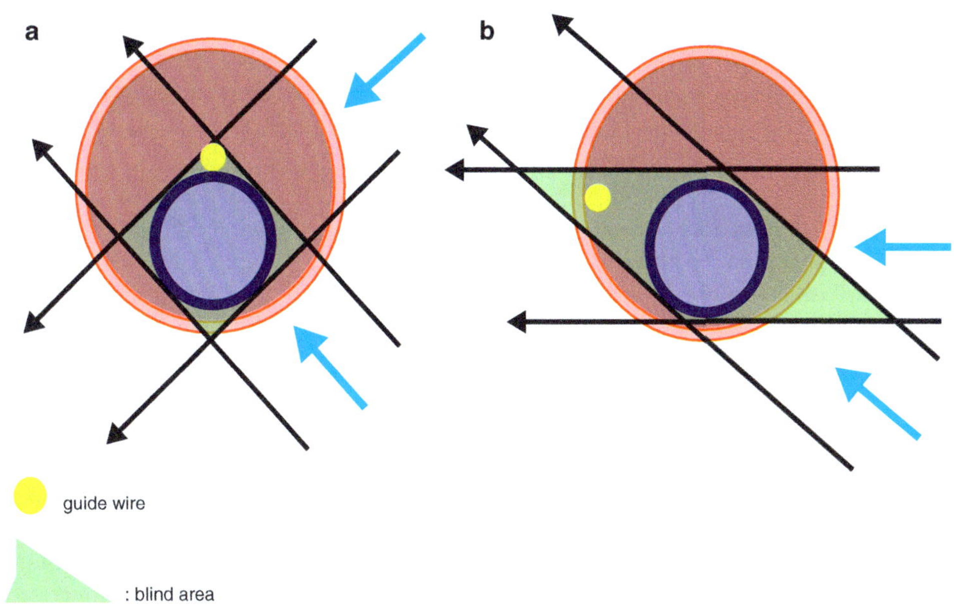

Fig. 1.29 Imaging in two orthogonal projections parallel with the longitudinal axis of the target vessel. (**a**) Even with imaging in two orthogonal projections, a guidewire in the blind spot (green in the figure) may be mistakenly thought to be in the true lumen, but the blind spot is extremely small. (**b**) Imaging in two non-orthogonal projections creates a larger blind area and is more likely to cause the interventionalist to think that a guidewire outside the true lumen is being advanced along the correct route

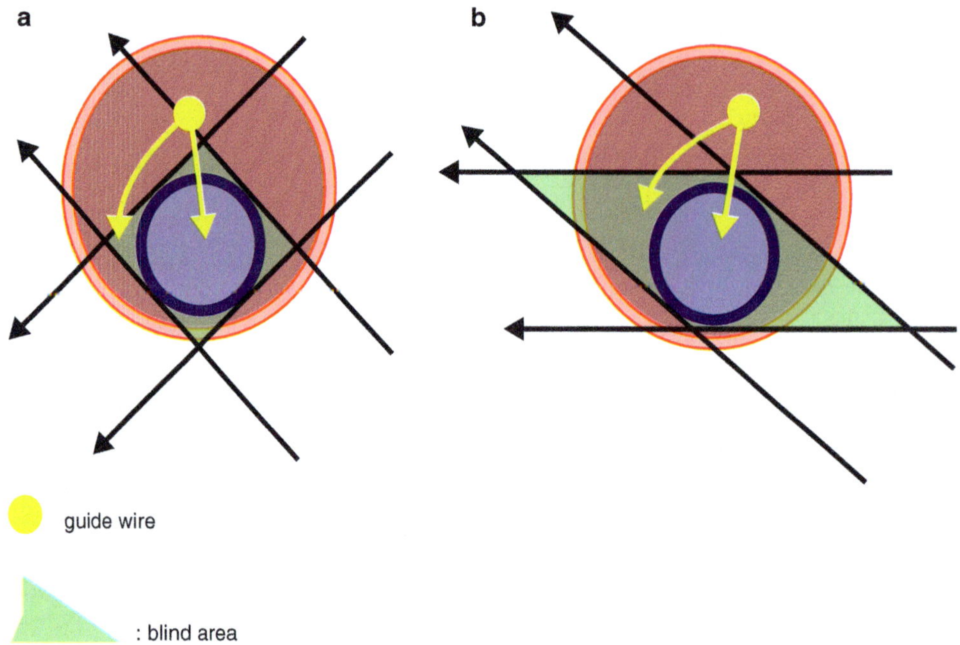

Fig. 1.30 Navigating the guidewire tip from a false lumen into the true lumen. (**a**) With imaging in orthogonal projections, there is less risk of erroneously navigating the guidewire while inside the blind area. (**b**) With imaging in non-orthogonal projections, the interventionalist is more likely to remain unaware of guidewire deviation and fail to navigate it into the true lumen

1.5.1.3 Selecting Two Orthogonal Projections

I will discuss the rationale for empirically selecting the optimal fluoroscopy angles and the angles parallel with the longitudinal axis of the target vessel, as well as how to choose the two orthogonal projections. In general, you should first choose a projection that appears to be orthogonal to the longitudinal axis of the target vessel in the ROI, i.e., the projection that gives the longest view of the vessel in the ROI (Fig. 1.31). If this projection is truly orthogonal to the longitudinal axis of the target vessel (providing the longest view of the longitudinal axis of the target vessel inside the ROI), then the vessel must be parallel with the detector surface. Based on this assumption, the angle of the second projection orthogonal to the longitudinal axis of the vessel in the ROI can be determined from the direction of the vessel on the detector surface.

If the vessel runs vertically on the first detector surface, the second detector surface should be set at a right angle in relation to the body axis, i.e., at 90 degrees in the RAO or LAO direction (Fig. 1.32). If the vessel runs horizontally on the first detector surface, the second detector surface should be angled in the cranial (CR) or caudal (CA) direction (Fig. 1.33). If the vessel runs to the upper right (at 45 degrees) on the first detector, the second detector surface should be rotated at 90 degrees to ensure identical angles from the LAO + CA or RAO + CR directions.

I would like to give some examples of determining the angles of detector surfaces that are parallel with the longitudinal axis of the target vessel. In practice, the longitudinal axis of the target vessel in the ROI is often not parallel with the first detector surface (Fig. 1.34a). In the above explanation of how to select the angle of the second detector surface, I assumed that the surface of the second detector was always parallel with the longitudinal axis of the vessel in the ROI (Fig. 1.34b). Rotation of the first detector surface at 90 degrees around the longitudinal axis of the target vessel on the second detector surface will make both detector surfaces parallel with the longitudinal axis of the vessel in the ROI (Fig. 1.34c).

Another practical example is shown in Fig. 1.35. Figure 1.35a presents the RAO + CA image that gives the longest view of the LCX. In this patient, the axis of the LAD ostium runs horizontally on this image (RAO + CA). When a 90-degree turn is made to LAO+ CA, the axis of the LAD ostium will be vertical, so LAO + CA will be the optimal angle (Fig. 1.35b).

Once the projection which gives the longest view of the longitudinal axis of the target vessel in the ROI has been determined, it is easy to select the second and third fluoroscopy angles. Therefore, it is important to know the standard projections that give the longest view of the longitudinal axis of each coronary artery segment in the ROI (Table 1.4). It should be noted that this table only shows standard projections, so it is most important to estimate the optimal projections from the diagnostic angiograms. One exception to these standard projections is treating a CTO at the bifurcation of a

large artery, when it is often important to consider whether the two projections can clearly distinguish multiple branches rather than focusing on orthogonality. Specifically, I choose the fluoroscopy angles for visualizing the LMT bifurcating into the LAD and LCX and the RCA bifurcating into the 4PD and 4AV as described below (Table 1.5).

As shown in Fig. 1.36a, the axis of the LAD ostium runs vertically in the LAO + CA projection. After the angle is rotated at 90 degrees toward the RAO, the axis of the LAD ostium runs horizontally on the image (Fig. 1.36b). Based on this information, the detector surface will be parallel with the longitudinal axis of the vessel in the RAO + CR projection (angled at 90 additional degrees in the CR direction). However, it is hard to clearly distinguish between the LAD and LCX in the RAO + CR projection, so I choose the two fluoroscopy angles shown in Fig. 1.36c and d when performing PCI for LAD/LCX bifurcation lesions.

When performing PCI for lesions from the middle part of Segment #3 of the RCA up to its bifurcation, I often choose the AP + CR and LAO + CR projections (Fig. 1.37). The two standard orthogonal projections that provide the longest view of the longitudinal axis of the vessel in Segment #3 of the RCA are the AP + CA (RAO + CA) and LL/LAO + CR projections (Table 1.5). However, the RCA bifurcation cannot be visualized clearly in these projections, so I always change the fluoroscopy angles as the guidewire approaches the bifurcation.

Although the fluoroscopy angles are basically determined as explained above, the patient's body or the other imaging equipment can sometimes preclude imaging in theoretically optimal orthogonal projections. If difficult imaging conditions prevent use of the optimal fluoroscopy angles for viewing the longitudinal axis of the vessel in the ROI, it becomes necessary to perform PCI while using angles that are quasi-orthogonal but achievable under the actual imaging conditions.

When obtaining a lateral view of the LAD, the patient's arms positioned along the body have little influence on image quality, while both of the patient's arms have to be raised above the head to obtain a good lateral view of the LCX. If the target lesion is located in the LCX and needs to be viewed laterally, you should therefore avoid using the TB or TR approaches.

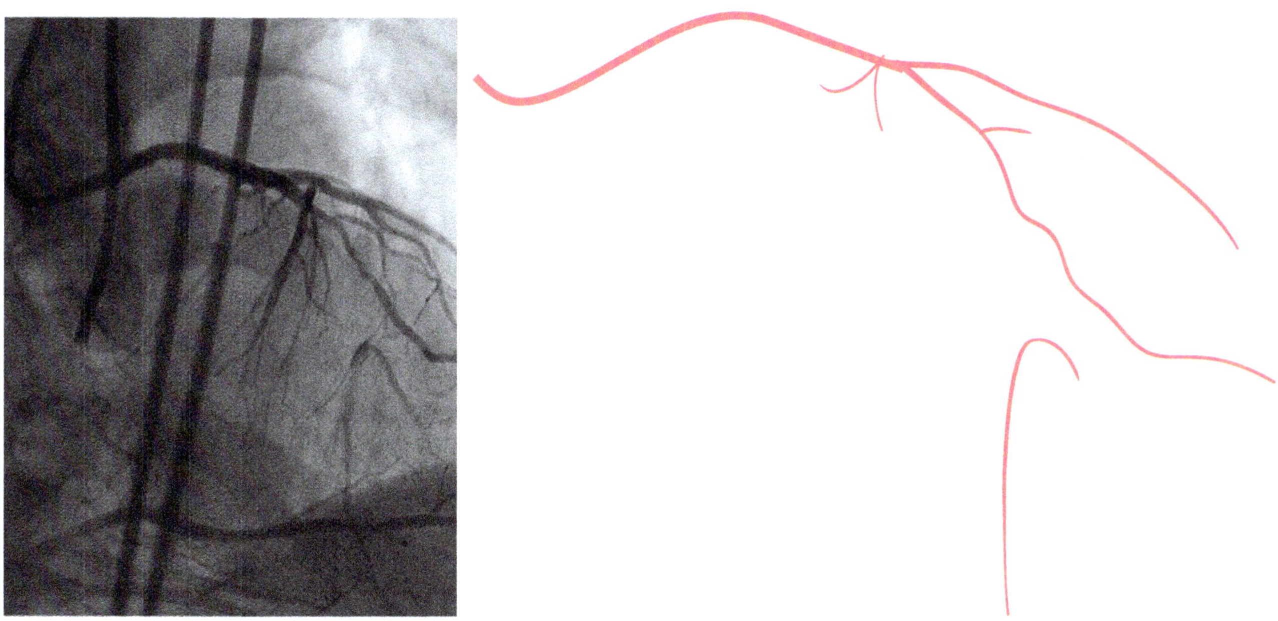

Fig. 1.31 Two orthogonal projections around the midportion of the LAD (1). The part of the LAD with the CTO runs vertically (from upper to lower) on the detector surface in the AP + CR projection. If the LAD is parallel with the detector surface, rotating the detector at 90 degrees in relation to the body axis will provide orthogonal views of the vessel. The longitudinal axis of the target vessel should run vertically on the detector surface in the new projection

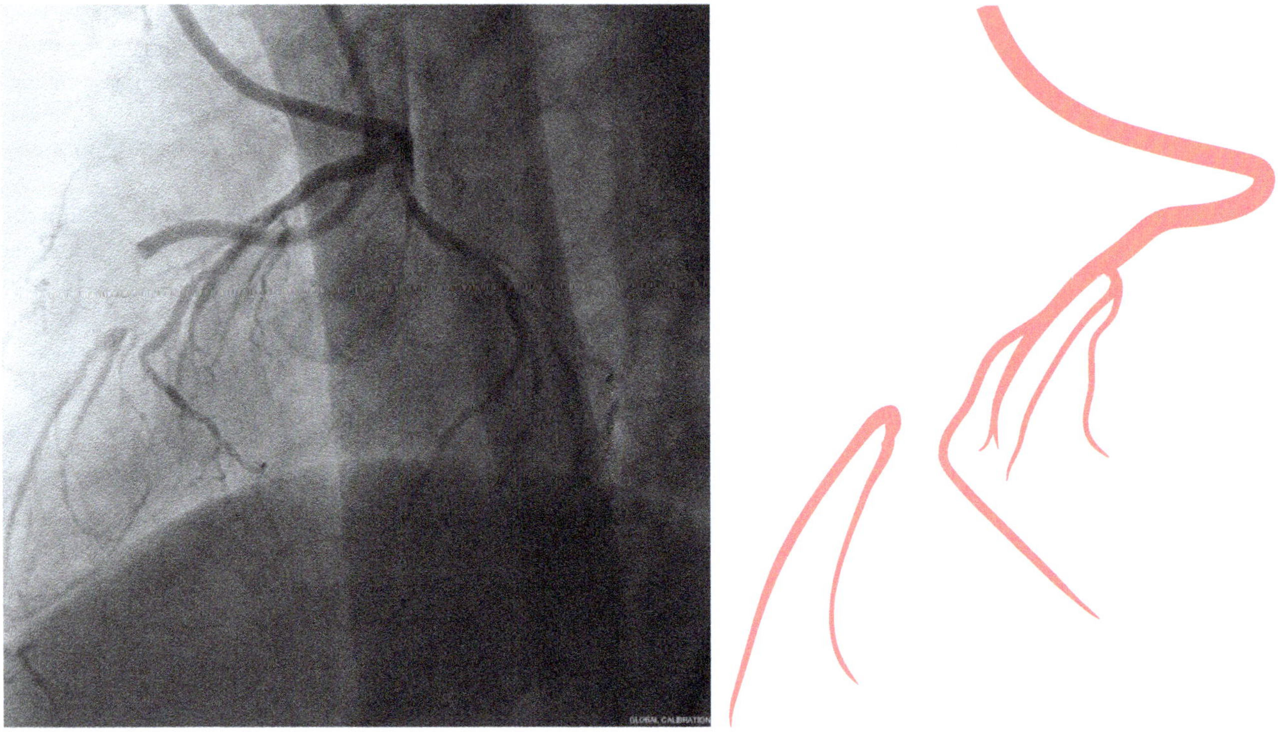

Fig. 1.32 Two orthogonal projections around the midportion of the LAD (2). After rotation of the second detector by 90 degrees (LL + CR), the target vessel does not run vertically, but instead runs rightward on the cranial side and leftward on the ventral side. Therefore, the first detector should optimally be set in the AP + larger angled CR projection

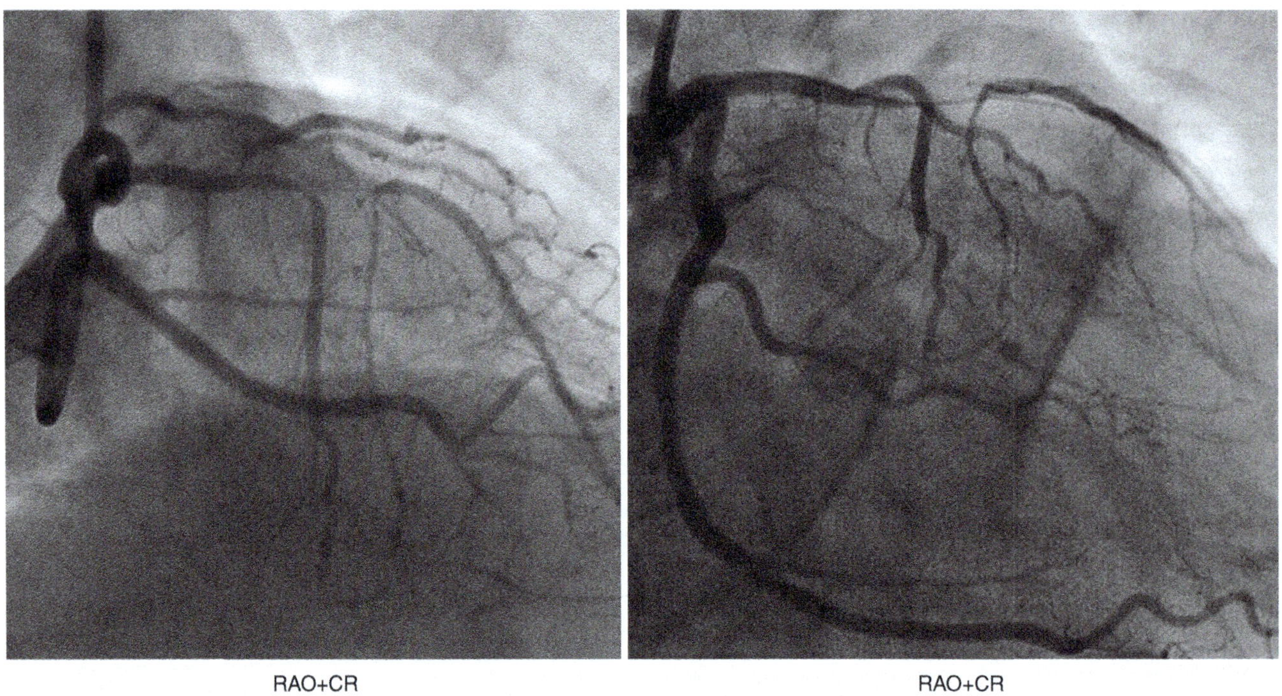

Fig. 1.33 Selecting two orthogonal projections (RAO + CR and RAO + CA). In the RAO + CR projection, the target vessel with the CTO is almost horizontal. After the projection is rotated by nearly 90 degrees toward the CA, the target vessel is still horizontal. This indicates that the vessel is being viewed in two projections that are orthogonal to its longitudinal axis and that the LAD of this patient runs to the left and anteriorly from its origin while remaining perpendicular to the body axis

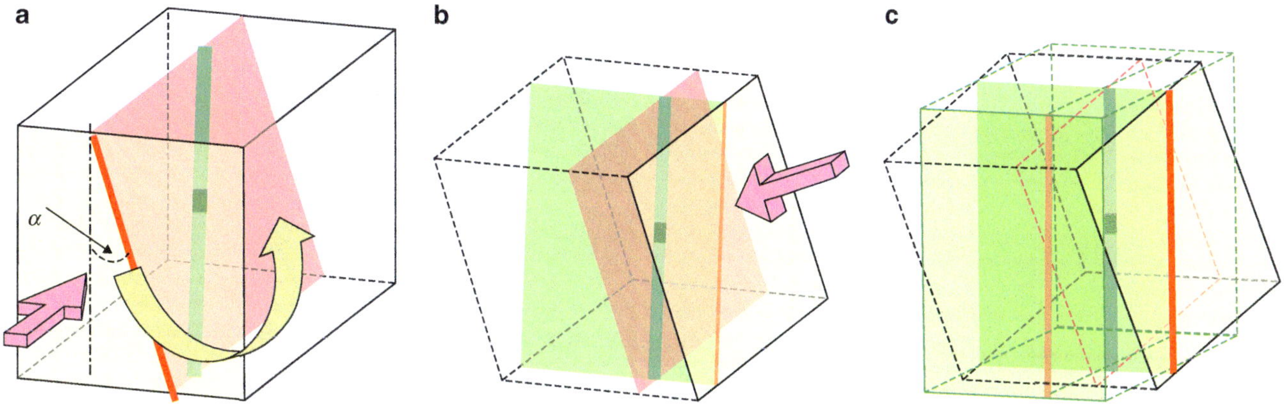

Fig. 1.34 Viewing the longitudinal axis of the target vessel on the detector. (**a**) The green line depicts the axis of the ROI (dark green line). It is assumed that the axis will appear as the red line when projected on the anterior detector surface. The detector surface is not always parallel with the longitudinal axis of the target vessel in the ROI. To make the surface parallel with the axis of the vessel, the detector should be rotated 90 degrees around the axis viewed on its surface. For example, assuming that the angle α between the axis of the target vessel and the vertical axis of the detector surface is 30 degrees, as shown here, the detector should be rotated toward the LAO projection at an angle of about 30 degrees in the CR direction or should be rotated toward the RAO projection at an angle of about 60 degrees in the CA direction to make it parallel with the vessel. (**b**) This is the result of rotating the detector from the position shown in *a* at 90 degrees toward the LAO projection and at an angle of 30 degrees in the CR direction. Since the detector surface is parallel to the longitudinal axis of the target vessel in the ROI, the longest view of the vessel is obtained in the projection perpendicular to a plane encompassing the axis. In biplane cineangiography, the other projection is normally the AP projection (shown in *a*). When using biplane imaging equipment, it is usual to search for the optimal position of the lateral detector while keeping one detector in the AP projection. As orthogonality of the two planes can be checked visually, it is easier to set the position of the lateral detector in this way. (**c**) To make the surface of other detector parallel with the longitudinal axis of the target vessel, the detector should be rotated at 90 degrees again in the direction perpendicular to the longitudinal axis of the plane shown in *b*. The new detector position provides a view of the target vessel in a projection orthogonal to a plane encompassing its longitudinal axis, thus giving the longest view of the vessel. With biplane imaging equipment, fine adjustments to the orientation of the AP detector can be made in this way to achieve imaging in two orthogonal projections

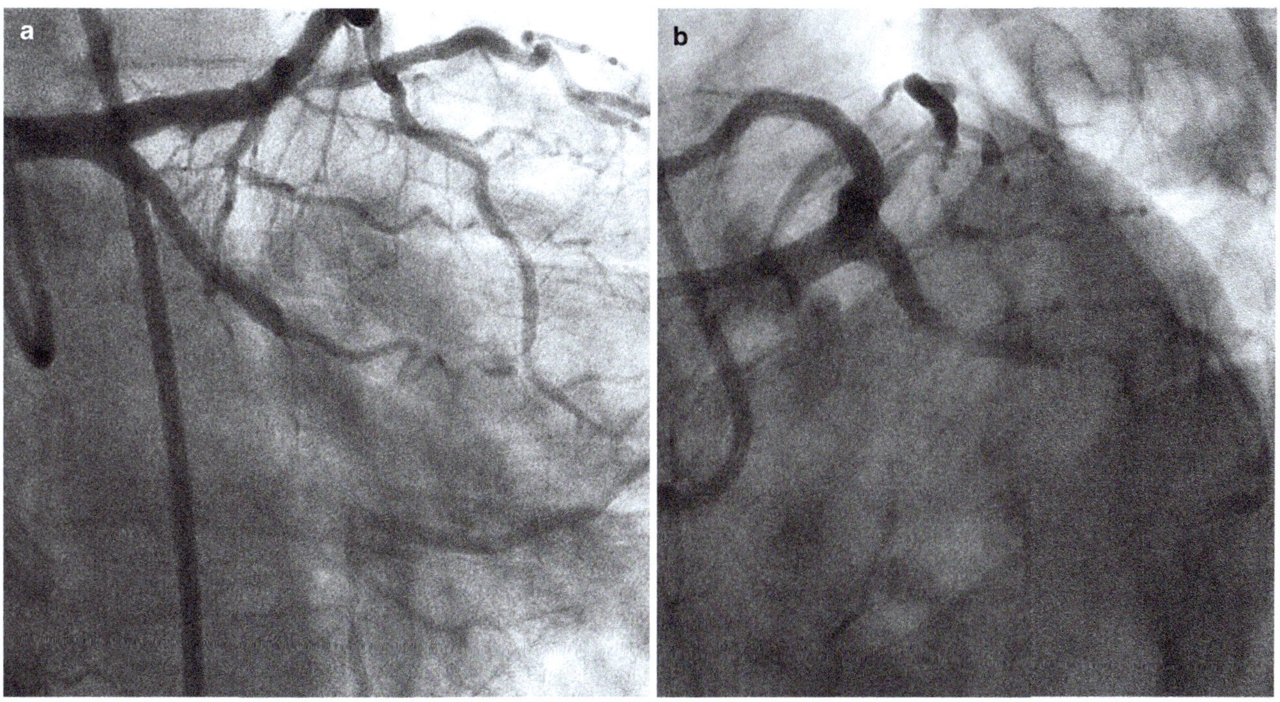

Fig. 1.35 Optimal projections for viewing LCX lesions. (**a**) In this patient, the longest view of the LCX encompassing the CTO is obtained in the RAO + CA projection, and the LAD runs horizontally in this projection. (**b**) After the detector is rotated 90 degrees (LAO + CA), the LAD runs vertically, and the LCX lesion is viewed at an angle of 90 degrees. Performing fluoroscopy in two optimal projections allows accurate detection of guidewire deviations

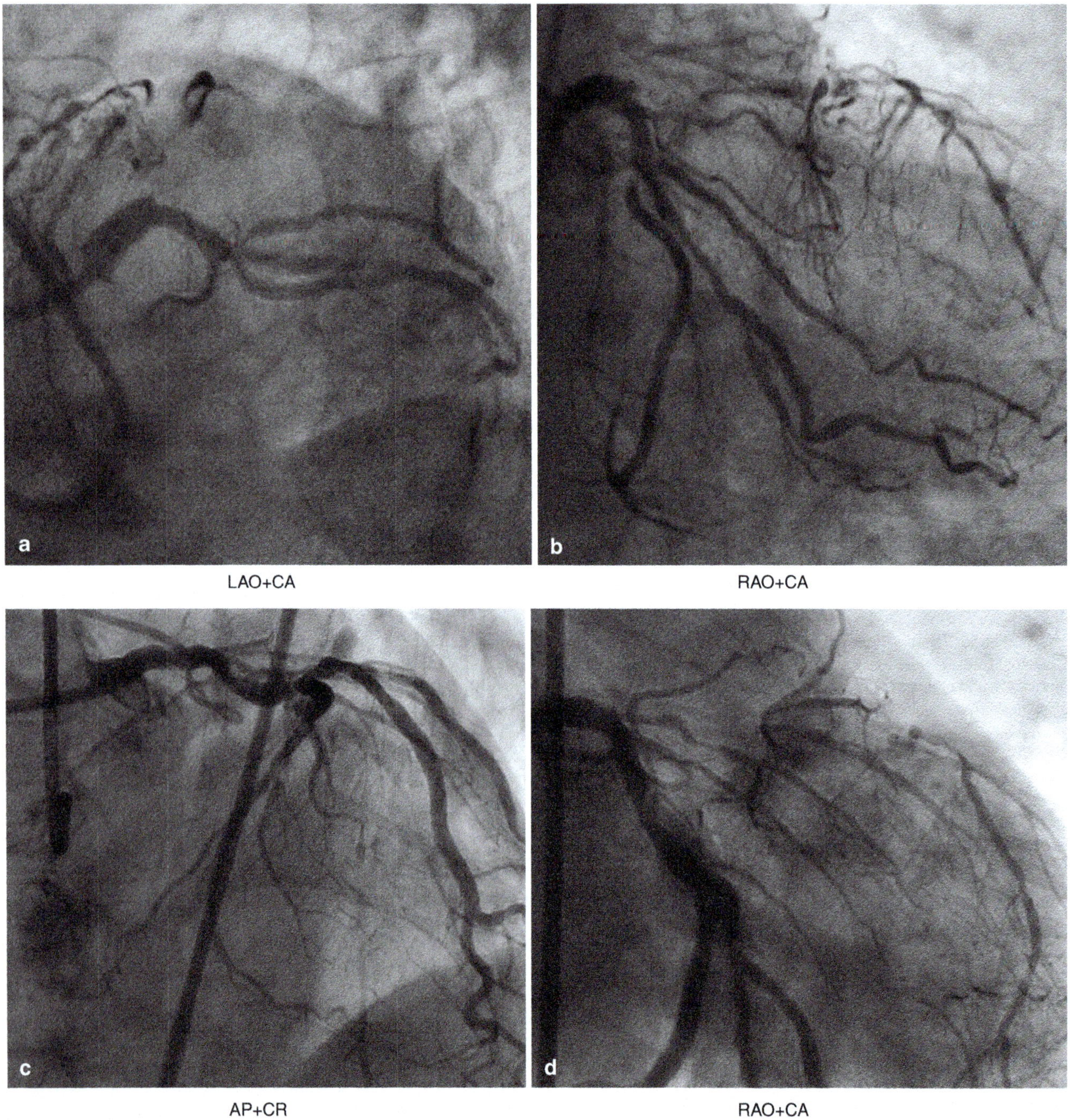

Fig. 1.36 Fluoroscopy of the LAD ostium. (**a**, **b**) In the LAO + CA projection (**a**), the LAD runs upward vertically from the ostium to Segment #6, remaining almost perpendicular to the detector surface. In the RAO + CA projection (**b**) (after rotating the detector 90 degrees toward the RAO projection), the target vessel runs horizontally. Rotating the detector 90 degrees in the CR direction alone (no change to the RAO) will obtain a projection perpendicular to the longitudinal axis of the target vessel in the ROI. However, it is difficult to clearly distinguish between the LAD and LCX in the RAO + CR projection. Therefore, you should use this projection (**a** & **b**) while advancing a guidewire through the LAD ostium. After the ROI moves to Segment #6 of the LAD, the LAO + CA projection provides a markedly shortened view of the target vessel. Accordingly, after the guidewire has entered the LAD, you should move the AP detector to the RAO + CR projection. However, none of the available biplane imaging equipment can provide simultaneous images in two RAO planes each angled in the CA and CR directions. (**c**, **d**) In this situation, a good solution is to rotate the AP detector in the AP + CR direction. Since many biplane imagers do not allow the two detectors to be set at angles that are too tight, you need to determine the optimal fluoroscopy angles compatible with the equipment being used

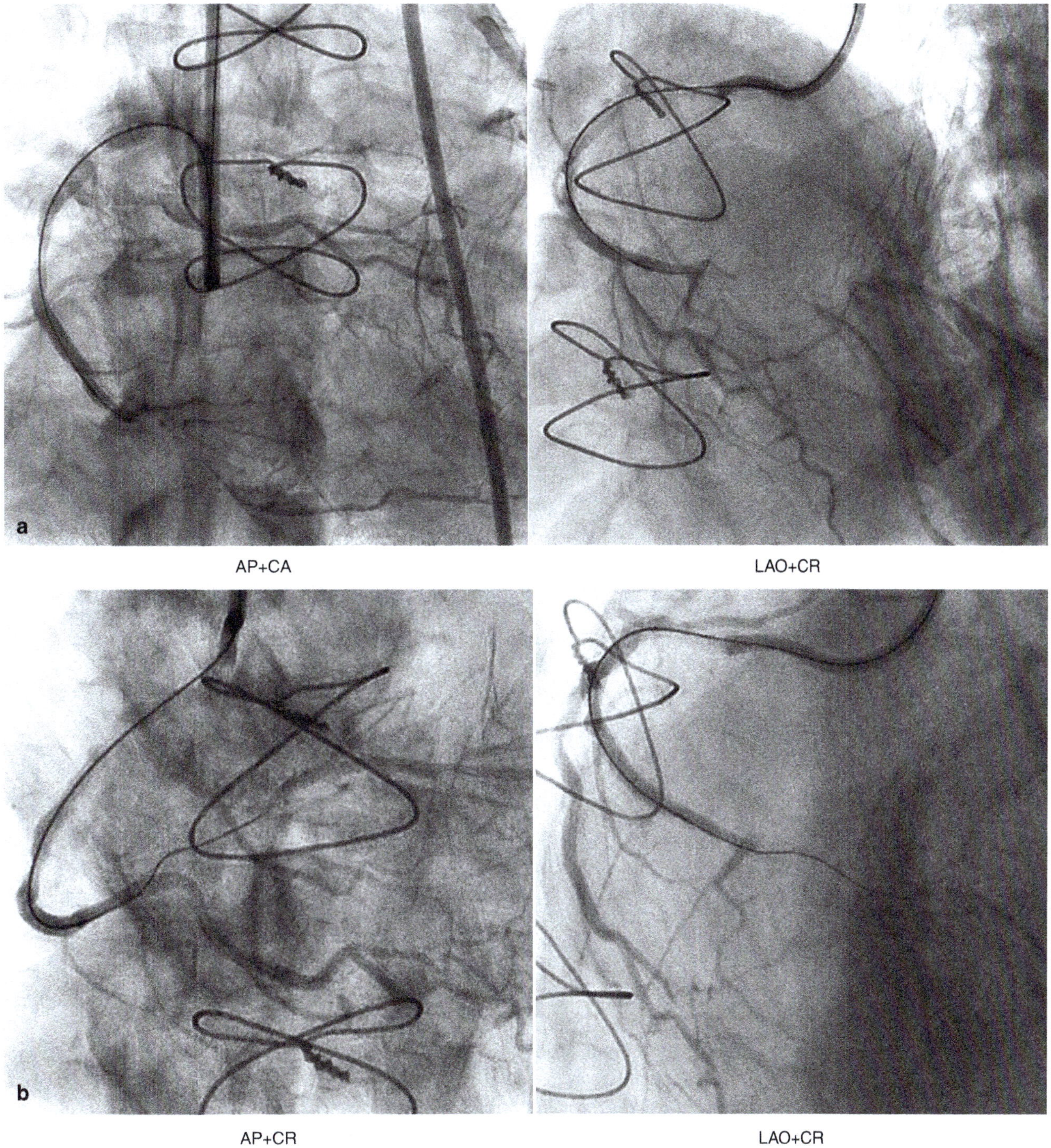

Fig. 1.37 Fluoroscopy of the RCA bifurcation. (**a**) The two optimal projections orthogonal to the longitudinal axis of the distal part of Segment #3 of the RCA are often the AP (RAO) + CA and LAO + CR projections. However, it is hard to distinguish #4PD from #4AV in the AP (RAO) + CA projection. (**b**) To view the distal bifurcation of the RCA, I use the AP + CR and LAO + CR projections that allow the two branches to be clearly distinguished, although there is partial overlap of the two detector surfaces

Table 1.5 Fluoroscopy projections providing the longest view of the longitudinal axis of the target vessel in the ROI

RCA			LCA		
ROI	Projection		ROI	Projection	
	Posteroanterior	Lateral		Posteroanterior	Lateral
RCA ostium	AP + CR	LAO + CA	LMT ostium	AP + CR	(LAO) + CA
RCA (#1-#2)	RAO	LAO	LMT to the bifurcation	RAO + CR	LAO + CA
RCA (#2-#3)	AP + CA(RAO + CA)	LAO + CR	LAD (#6-#7)	AP(RAO) + CA	LAO + CA
RCA (#3-#4)	AP + CR	LAO + CR	LAD (#7-#8)	AP + CR	LL + CR
				RAO + CA	AP + CR
			LAD (#11-#13)	AP(RAO) + CA	LAO + CA

Column 3 Fluoroscopy Angle and Detector Surface

In this textbook, I use the fluoroscopy angle and the detector surface to explain the optimal imaging strategy. The fluoroscopy angle means the angle of the projection, which can be precisely expressed as RAO, LAO, CR, CA, (and AP, LL), or combinations supplemented with the respective angles. The longest view of a vessel is obtained when it is viewed in the direction orthogonal to its longitudinal axis, and there will be no shortening in this projection. By combining this projection with a second projection obtained by rotating the detector 90 degrees around the vessel axis, two orthogonal projections of the target vessel are obtained.

At that time (or moment), the detector surface is perpendicular to the fluoroscopic axis and parallel with the longitudinal axis of the target vessel. It is very difficult to manually calculate a second angle that is at 90 degrees from the first angle and to express this as a fluoroscopy angle relative the first angle and the direction of the vessel axis. While computerized calculation is easy, it requires data about the direction of the target vessel on the image to be input. As I have described in detail in the text, it is not so difficult to rotate the other detector around the axis of the target vessel in the ROI projected on the surface of the first detector to obtain the second projection. Whether the second detector has been positioned correctly at 90 degrees can be checked by observing if the surfaces of the two detectors are orthogonal to each other. While this method cannot ensure complete orthogonality of the two detector surfaces, I think that achieving approximately orthogonal projections is sufficient.

1.5.1.4 Isocenter

During all PCI procedures, including those for CTO, you should always perform "isocentric" coronary cineangiography, i.e., imaging with the patient's heart positioned exactly at the center of rotation of the arms of the imager (Fig. 1.38). All of the fluoroscopy equipment introduced recently has been designed to position the focus of the X-ray tube and the center of the detector surface on a line that passes through the center of rotation, so positioning the patient's heart at the center ensures isocentric imaging.

To position the patient's heart at the center of rotation, you should rotate the arms laterally and adjust the height of the examination table so that the patient's heart is at the center of the detector surface while checking the image. Once adjusted, the examination table height must not be changed when the arms are rotated. This ensures that the patient's heart always remains at the center of the detector surface. Basically, you do not need to obtain test images or adjust the examination table height to optimize the position of the patient's heart even after changing the direction of projection, so this method of isocentric imaging saves time and also reduces radiation exposure for the patient.

Isocentric imaging is even more useful when performing biplane cineangiography of the coronary arteries. Many biplane imagers are equipped with isocentric posteroanterior and lateral arms, while some allow adjustment of the height of the lateral arm, a function that is apparently useful but removes isocentricity. However, once the lateral arm has been adjusted, it can be troublesome to reposition the patient's heart at the center of both detectors after changing the fluoroscopy angles. This procedure takes time and increases radiation exposure for the patient, so it is better not to cancel the isocentricity of the arms, even when using an imager with such a feature.

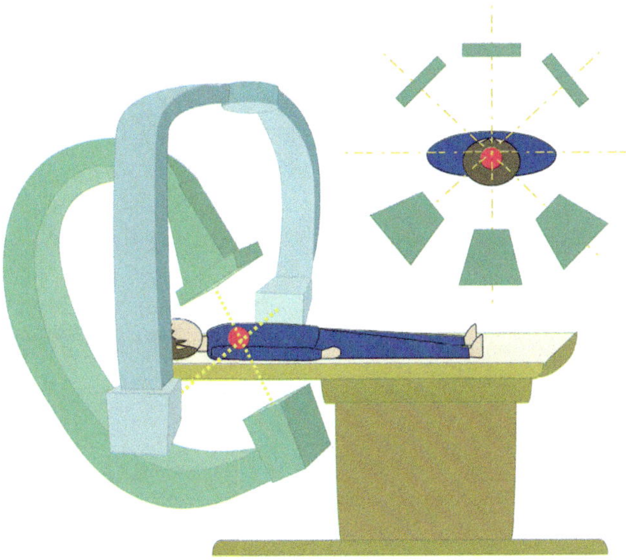

Fig. 1.38 Setting the isocentric position. Once the height of the imaging table has been adjusted to position the patient's heart at the center of rotation of both arms of the imager, there is no need to adjust the table height further when the projection is changed

1.5.2 Bilateral Angiography and Collateral Flow Angiography (Contralateral Imaging, etc.)

Some interventionalists still perform PCI for CTO without contralateral imaging, but I think that contralateral imaging is basically an essential part of PCI for CTO. When PCI is done for native coronary artery CTO, contralateral imaging is only unnecessary if angiography can visualize the true lumen of the target coronary artery distal to the occlusion via an ipsilateral collateral vessel (Fig. 1.39).

When you have a manual sensation that the guidewire has entered the true lumen of the vessel distal to the occlusion, the tip of the guidewire can actually be located (1) in the true lumen distal to the occlusion, (2) in a very soft subintimal space distal to the occlusion, (3) in a small side branch, or (4) outside the vessel wall but within the pericardium. In this situation, contralateral imaging is essential to visually confirm the exact position of the tip of the guidewire and to navigate the guidewire (if it has deviated) into the true lumen with reference to an appropriate landmark.

If contralateral imaging for diagnosis of in-stent occlusion visualizes the target coronary artery distal to the occlusion, including part of the stented region (Fig. 1.40), there is no need to repeat contralateral imaging during PCI. However, contralateral imaging will be required during PCI if the occlusion extends to the distal end of the stent (Fig. 1.41), because the guidewire may slip into the subintimal space after passing through the stent in this situation.

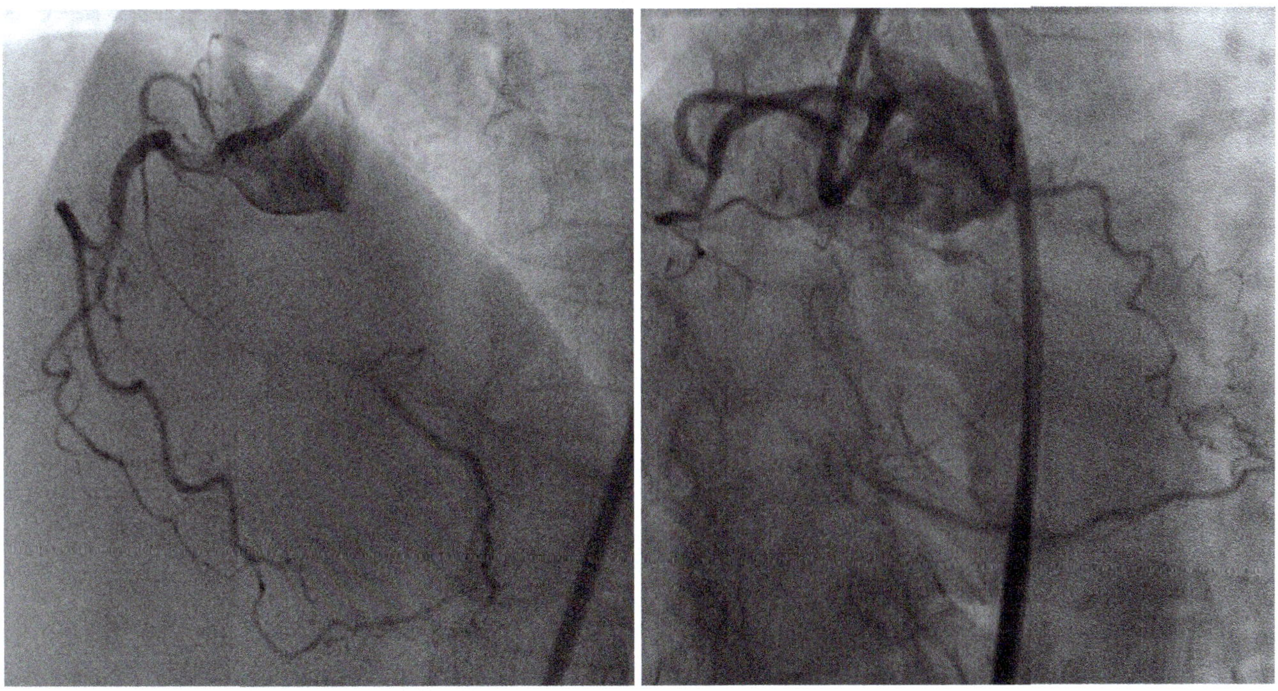

Fig. 1.39 Ipsilateral coronary collateral vessel. If there is a well-developed ipsilateral coronary collateral, contralateral imaging is not required because imaging of the target coronary artery provides sufficient information about the segment distal to the occlusion

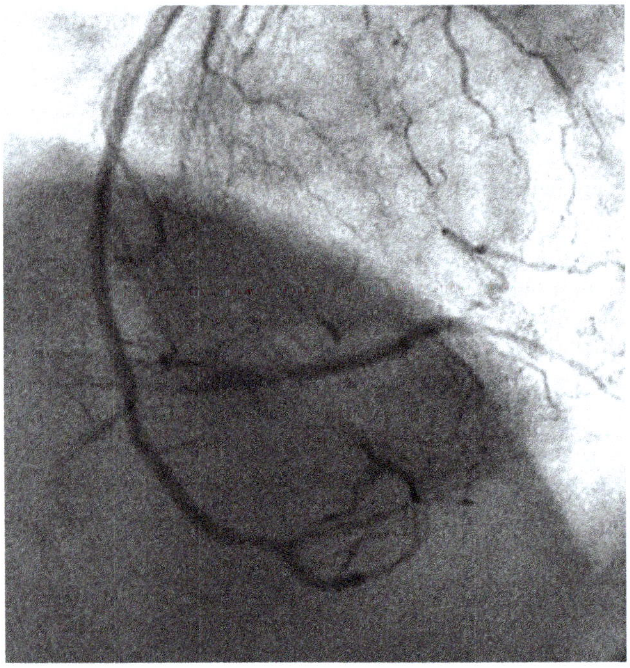

Fig. 1.40 In-stent occlusion in the distal RCA. Contralateral diagnostic imaging has delivered contrast medium to the target vessel distal to the stent. In this situation, you can smoothly advance a guidewire through the distal coronary artery segment from the end of the stent. You can also perform tip injection near the distal end of the stent to reconfirm the anatomy of the distal segment

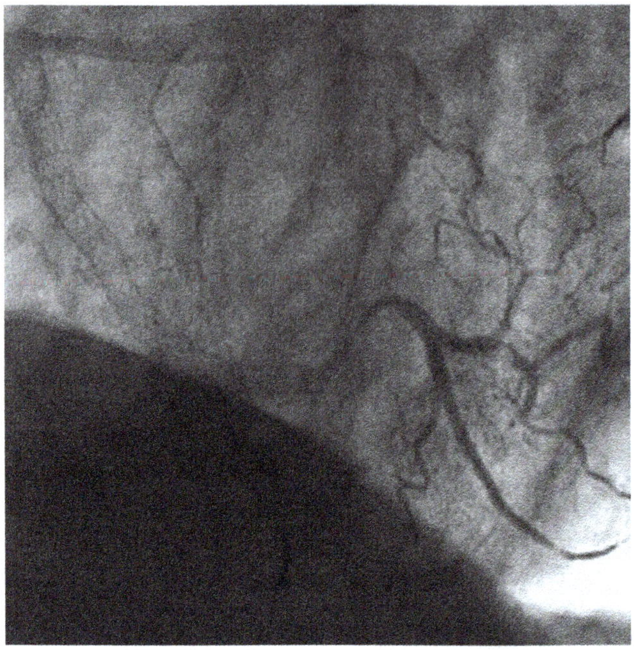

Fig. 1.41 In-stent occlusion in the RCA. Contralateral diagnostic imaging has not delivered contrast medium to the target vessel distal to the stent. After advancing a guidewire to the distal end of the stent, you need to find the distal cap of the lesion, and you will have to perform contralateral imaging to do so

Column 4 Rotational Angiography

Recent reports have demonstrated the benefit of rotational angiography for visualizing CTO lesions during PCI. Rotational angiography was originally used as a method for imaging examinations such as three-dimensional assessment of the cerebral vessels. This angiographic technique has subsequently attracted attention as a method for multidirectional observation of the coronary arteries during PCI for CTO where only monoplane imaging equipment is available. Although rotational angiography is useful in some respects, I do not employ it for the following reasons:

Rotational angiography is not compatible with biplane imagers. When performing PCI for CTO, I always use a biplane imager, and I do not think that rotational angiography is ever superior to simultaneous bidirectional (postero-anterior and lateral) imaging.

As mentioned in the text, to determine the optimal projections for checking whether the tip of a guidewire has entered the subintimal space or the true lumen (plaque), you only need to set one detector parallel with the longitudinal axis of the target vessel and then rotate the other detector at least 90 degrees around the vessel axis. Images obtained in these projections will clearly show whether the guidewire has deviated from the true lumen.

Nonetheless, imagers only permit rotation of the detectors around the body axis, rather than around the vessel axis. Many segments of the coronary arteries are parallel with the body axis in the vertical heart, but run at a wide angle or perpendicular to the body axis in the horizontal heart. Rotational angiography may be most useful when the target vessel axis is parallel with the body axis, but is virtually useless when the vessel axis is perpendicular to the body axis. At best, vascular movement with pulsation may provide some supporting information in the latter situation. Rotational angiography is of intermediate benefit in most other cases where the target vessel axis and body axis are at an oblique angle to each other.

Based on the above, rotational angiography is useful for confirming whether a guidewire is in the true lumen of a vessel that is parallel with the body axis. On the other hand, to correct the direction of a guidewire while using rotational angiography for guidance, it is necessary to check images obtained in the projection showing the greatest deviation and in a second projection perpendicular to the first, which means that you must search for the correct guidewire route in two nonsimultaneous projections that are not always parallel with the vessel axis. If you are not using rotational angiography, you can manipulate the guidewire while checking images obtained in two orthogonal projections that are parallel with the longitudinal axis of the target vessel, but it is impossible to manipulate a guidewire while obtaining images by rotational angiography. In contrast, biplane cineangiography provides simultaneous imaging of the target vessel in two orthogonal projections parallel with the longitudinal axis of the vessel, allowing the direction of the guidewire to be corrected in a real-time manner.

1.6 Antegrade Approach

I have always thought of antegrade PCI as the basic interventional method for CTO, even after introduction of the retrograde approach. Although retrograde PCI has undoubtedly led to new breakthroughs by allowing the recanalization of CTOs that are untreatable by antegrade PCI, there are still many CTOs that can be managed via the antegrade approach but not the retrograde approach. Therefore, interventionalists should first become familiar with antegrade PCI for CTO and should aim to develop sophisticated strategies and technical expertise in this setting.

1.6.1 Mechanism of CTO Formation and Changes After Occlusion

The mechanisms underlying coronary occlusion may be multifactorial, and occlusions that are caused by various mechanisms may evolve into CTOs over time. How successfully a particular guidewire can be used to cross a CTO will vary with the mechanism involved in formation of the occlusion. In addition to the underlying mechanism, the time since occurrence of occlusion and the properties of any preexisting plaque at the site of occlusion can influence success in crossing the CTO with a guidewire.

Here, I will discuss the possible mechanisms underlying the formation of coronary artery occlusion and the changes of the occlusion over time after it develops. I will also discuss changes of the surrounding plaque before occurrence of occlusion, in order to provide useful hints about how a guidewire can cross the CTO and how to select and manipulate the guidewire.

1.6.1.1 Occlusion Resulting from Tight Stenosis (Fig. 1.42)

In a patient without documented myocardial infarction, a CTO is most likely to result from gradually progression of tight stenosis (Fig. 1.42b). The final event that leads to complete occlusion may be thrombosis or plaque proliferation.

Functional CTO is characteristically accompanied by a relatively long tight stenosis that has progressed gradually. With progression of a long stenosis, the perfusion pressure in the stenosed segment may decrease until it is equal to that in collateral vessels, resulting in loss of both antegrade and retrograde perfusion at the site of a lesion that has not yet reached complete occlusion. In functional CTO, development of collaterals precedes the onset of occlusion, and the patient often remains unaware of the occurrence of occlusion since there are no or only mild symptoms. Therefore, it is often difficult to determine when occlusion actually occurred in patients with a CTO of this type. After occlusion, the occluded site and surrounding tissues undergo several changes over time, including (1) expansion of thrombus, (2) hardening of thrombus and plaque, (3) calcification of thrombus and plaque, (4) intra-thrombus/intra-plaque recanalization/angiogenesis, and (5) development of collateral circulation/arteriogenesis, and so on.

1. If there are no side branches near the site of occlusion, thrombus will extend to involve the nearest branch. If there is only a small amount of plaque at the nearest branch, the thrombus will become widespread and cause abrupt thrombotic occlusion (Figs 1.42c and 1.43). If a side branch (even a small one) is present near the proximal end of an occlusion resulting from tapered stenosis, a tapered type of occlusion will form (Fig. 1.44).
2. The thrombus occluding the vessel hardens over time, but remains softer than the surrounding plaque for a while. The difference in hardness between thrombus and plaque is particularly marked when the plaque is partially calcified. However, thrombus that extends to cover a nearly normal vessel wall may not necessarily be softer than the wall itself.
3. After more time has elapsed, the occluding thrombus may become fibrotic, organized, and sclerotic and can

undergo calcification. A calcified thrombus may be as hard as or even harder than the surrounding plaque. In particular, thrombus at the proximal end (entry) of an occlusion is likely to undergo fibrosis and sclerosis due to rheological stress.

4. The occluding thrombus may undergo local thrombolysis, leading to recanalization by a narrow channel through the thrombus or formation of a new capillary channel. If such recanalization or angiogenesis is visible on CAG and there is TIMI grade 1 flow, the lesion does not meet the definition of CTO. However, if competition with a gradually developing collateral results in loss of antegrade perfusion, such a new channel may be invisible on CAG, and TIMI grade 0 flow will be seen (functional CTO; Fig. 1.45). Functional CTO can also be due to a tight stenosis with no history of occlusion. Coronary artery occlusion that persists for at least 3 months basically meets the definition of CTO, but a small channel may still be visible on bilateral angiography. Without performing bilateral angiography, it is often difficult to determine whether there is a channel within a lesion. I routinely perform bilateral angiography if contralateral imaging shows any collateral, and I do not regard coronary occlusion accompanied by a visible channel as a CTO.

   However, a very small channel may not be detected, even if bilateral CAG is performed.

5. A CTO resulting from tight stenosis often has many collaterals and a clearly visible exit.

a
b
c

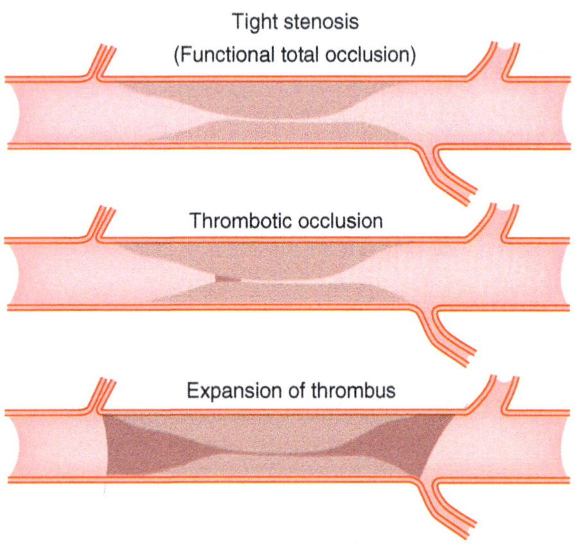

Fig. 1.42 Potential mechanisms of coronary artery occlusion (1). Thrombus formation in a functional CTO resulting from tight stenosis: In a vessel segment with a tight stenosis (**a**), thrombotic occlusion may occur (**b**). If the stenotic lesion is far from the nearest side branch, there will be no perfusion at the distal end of the occlusion, and the thrombus may extend as far as the first branch (**c**)

a
b
c

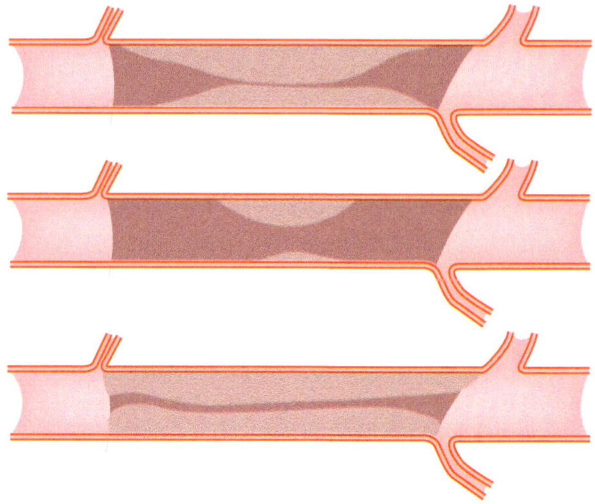

Fig. 1.43 Abrupt occlusion. Abrupt occlusion may occur if the occluding thrombus extends to the sites of branches (**a** or **b**) or if thrombus forms in an abruptly narrowed vessel (**c**)

a
b

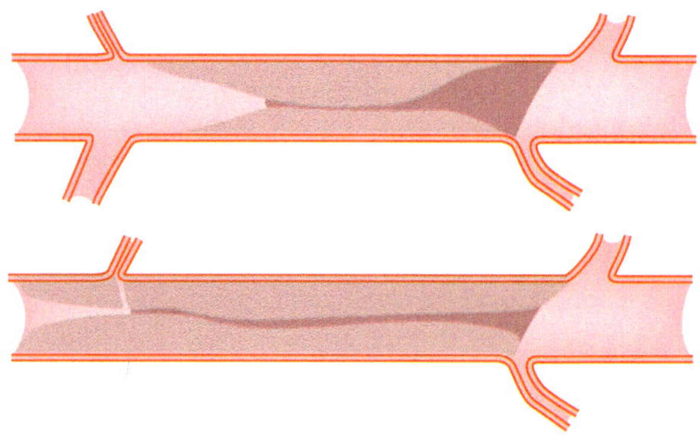

Fig. 1.44 Tapered occlusion. If a vessel is narrowed by tapered plaque and if there is blood flow (swirling) into the proximal blind end even after complete occlusion, thrombus will not form at the proximal end, and the occlusion will retain a tapered shape (**a**). If the plaque is originally tapered and the affected vessel becomes occluded just distal to a side branch, the occlusion will also be tapered (**b**)

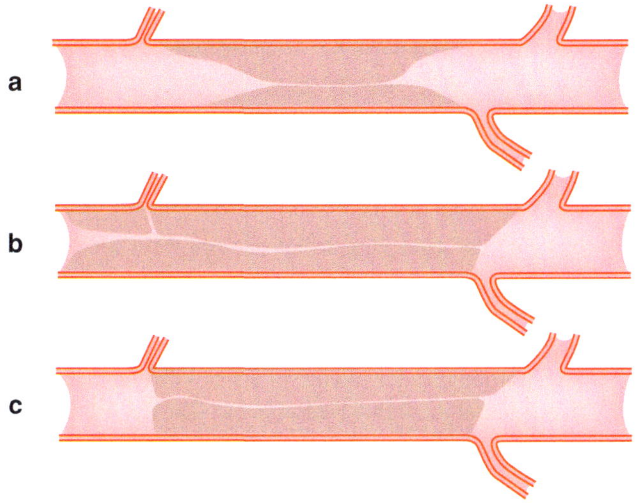

Fig. 1.45 Functional CTO (**a**, **b**, **c**). A vessel with a very tight stenosis (not complete occlusion) may appear to be occluded on diagnostic CAG. This occurs because development of collaterals reduces the pressure gradient across the stenotic region, leading to very poor blood flow between the proximal and distal ends of the tight stenosis. Functional CTO also includes occlusion with recanalization or with a microchannel that is not well developed enough to be detected by CAG. I consider that any occlusion with a channel recognizable on bilateral angiography should not be regarded as a CTO. Since many interventionalists do not perform bilateral angiography during PCI, the actual prevalence of functional CTO is unknown

1.6.1.2 Acute Thrombotic Occlusion (Fig. 1.46)

In patients with ST-elevation myocardial infarction, thrombotic occlusion occurs due to rupture of a plaque that has only caused mild stenosis (Fig. 1.46). In a patient with previous acute myocardial infarction or Q-wave infarction, a CTO is likely to have been caused by development of occlusion at such a site over time.

1. Like CTOs with other etiologies, the occluding thrombus expands until it reaches a branch vessel, i.e., the point where there is some blood flow (Fig. 1.46c), but thrombus is the predominant feature of the lesion, distinguishing this type of CTO from the others. For several months after the occurrence of occlusion, this type of CTO has a relatively soft central core for the full length of the lesion, and the wall of the occluded vessel is generally also soft.
2. The thrombus becomes more fibrotic and sclerotic over time, with the lesion largely being composed of relatively homogeneous tissue (Fig. 1.47). If the vessel wall also hardens, the thrombus in the lumen remains comparatively soft (refer to Column 5– Fig. 1.56. If the luminal thrombus hardens preferentially, it becomes harder than the vessel wall (refer to Column 5—Fig. 1.57.
3. Calcification of the thrombus/plaque may also occur, leading to a relatively homogenous lesion.
4. A recanalized channel due to thrombolysis is likely to appear early after thrombotic occlusion and is expected to have a relatively large diameter. In the later phase, angiogenesis may occur within the organized thrombus.
5. In many cases, collaterals are not fully developed immediately after acute thrombotic occlusion. While collaterals develop progressively over time, they are often not large enough to create a rim at the distal cap of the occlusion or to deliver blood to the distal lumen of the occluded vessel.

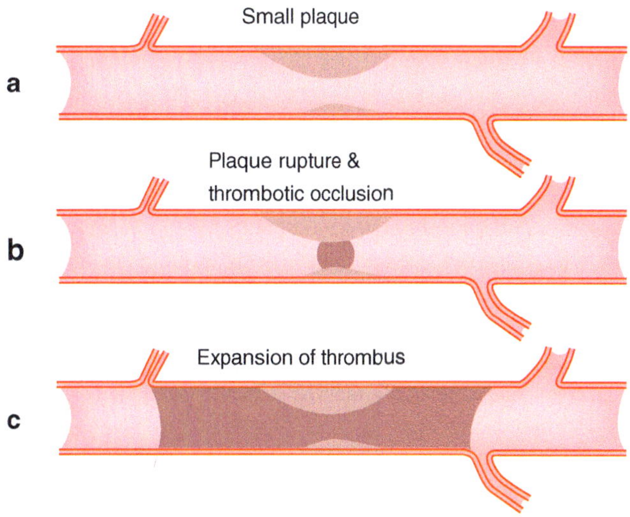

Fig. 1.46 Potential mechanisms of coronary artery occlusion (2). Another mechanism of coronary artery occlusion, which is associated with myocardial infarction, is rupture of a relatively small plaque (**a**) that results in thrombotic occlusion (**b**). When occlusion is due to this mechanism, the occluding thrombus often expands until it reaches the nearest side branch (**c**)

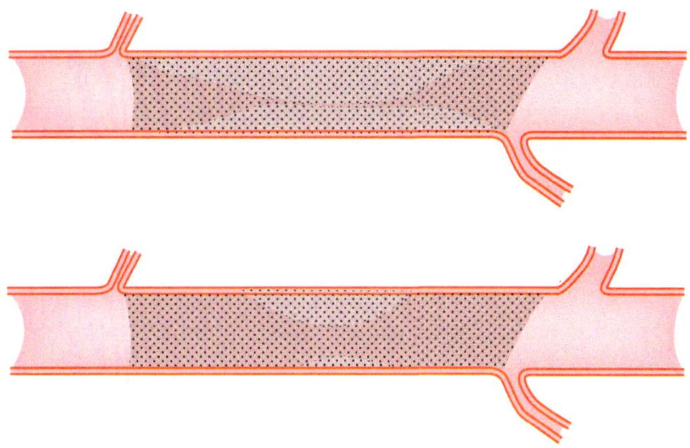

Fig. 1.47 Histological changes over time. Unlike an occlusion composed of heterogeneous tissue with a relatively small intraluminal channel (Fig. 1.42), a lesion created by acute thrombotic occlusion remains relatively homogeneous

1.6.1.3 Occlusions with Complex Etiologies

Theoretically, a tight stenosis and ruptured plaque can coexist in a vessel. Therefore, thrombotic occlusion due to ruptured plaque and occlusion of the stenotic lesion may occur either synchronously or metachronously.

1.6.2 Histological Features Before and After Occlusion

The condition of the coronary artery walls may differ before occlusion, and this can have various influences on guidewire crossing. Important factors that need to be considered include (1) the (extent of) tortuosity, the plaque burden, the hardness of the vessel wall and plaque, and the plaque characteristics (e.g., lipid content and severity of calcification) at the entry to the CTO and (2) the vessel tortuosity, plaque burden, plaque hardness, lipid core, and extent and distribution of calcification in the lesion itself.

The following changes may occur after occlusion: (1) thrombolytic or angiogenic recanalization; (2) fibrosis, sclerosis, and calcification at the entry of the occlusion; (3) fibrosis, sclerosis, and calcification of the lesion; and (4) fibrosis, sclerosis, and calcification at the exit of the occlusion.

Among these changes, calcification can have a major influence on the outcome of PCI, depending on its distribution. The extent of vascular calcification varies considerably among individuals and between anatomical regions, but it is well-known that dialysis patients often have very severe vascular calcification.

1.6.3 Guidewire Crossing Based on the Presumed Mechanism of CTO Formation and Changes After Occlusion

The outcome of PCI for CTO can be dramatically improved by prior knowledge of the properties of the culprit plaque, the mechanisms involved in CTO formation, and the post-occlusion changes of the lesion. However, we can only consider the possibilities before starting PCI and make the best conjecture from the final or interim outcome of the procedure. Information on how a guidewire was advanced through a vessel, whether there was an inflection point or whether it was blocked during intervention, is useful for estimating the route and the position of the tip within the occlusion. The interventionalist should modify his/her strategy while adjusting assumptions about the etiology based on these points.

My basic guidewire crossing strategies for use in antegrade PCI for various types of CTO are summarized below (the details are given later).

1. If there is a channel within the occlusion, you should slide a guidewire along the channel or advance a guidewire while exploring the channel (exploration strategy; Fig. 1.48).

   A channel may exist within an occlusion, even if it cannot be visualized by bilateral angiography or tip injection. Since standard coronary artery imaging has a resolution of 100 μm, a channel with a diameter less than 100 μm may not be visible on CAG.
2. If there is no channel within the occlusion, a guidewire must be used to penetrate it. In this case, you should advance the guidewire while exploring for a relatively soft point where the occlusion may be most recent (exploration with penetration strategy [Fig. 1.49]).
3. As in ST-elevation myocardial infarction, formation of a large thrombus after rupture of a small plaque may often be the initial event that leads to CTO. The thrombus often extends as far as the nearest relatively large side branch to form a large lesion that undergoes organization and fibrosis over time (Fig. 1.47). In this setting, the intrinsic hardness of the vessel wall as well as the extent of organization/fibrosis of the thrombus can determine the difficulty of crossing the CTO through the true lumen with a guidewire. For example, in a younger patient with old myocardial infarction, the vessel walls are relatively soft, but the occluding thrombus, if organized, will tend to block the guidewire inside the lesion and cause it to deviate into the subintimal space. In an older patient with arteriosclerosis and old myocardial infarction, the occluding thrombus, even if organized, may still be softer than the vessel wall (intimal sclerosis), potentially facilitating advancement of the guidewire through the true lumen.

   Thus, there may be no relatively soft region of a CTO created by acute thrombotic occlusion when the thrombus has undergone homogenous sclerosis. In such a situation, you will not find any softer region in the lesion compared with the surrounding vascular tissues. If the guidewire tip enters the lesion at the center of the lumen, it will advance through the true lumen, but it is sometimes difficult to make a clear distinction between the intraluminal and extraluminal tissues, and the absence of a dimple at the center of the lumen may make it difficult to find the true lumen. In a long CTO, initial success with directing the guidewire into the true lumen does not ensure that it will remain inside the lumen as it is advanced. To keep the wire in the true lumen, it must be advanced while exploring the route and checking the position of the tip with reference to various landmarks to verify that it has followed the presumed route of the lumen through the lesion. If this is not done, you cannot prevent deviation of the guidewire into the subintimal space. In this situation, extensive exploration may actually increase the risk of the guidewire deviating outside the true lumen. Since greater importance is placed upon penetration than exploration, this is termed the penetration with exploration strategy (Fig. 1.50).
4. If a guidewire has been blocked by hard tissue within the lumen and has slipped into the subintimal space, you should exchange it for another wire with a higher tip

load (to ensure greater crossability) and should find the point where the guidewire cannot easily be advanced further. Then you should explore the direction in which the guidewire can be advanced slowly without deviating into the subintimal space (penetration with exploration by the fixed point guidewire rotation strategy [Fig. 1.51]; see 1.4.6.3. "Fixed Point Guidewire Rotation").

5. In some cases, you cannot prevent the guidewire from slipping into the subintimal space. In this situation, you should pull the guidewire back to a point close to the entrance of the CTO and advance it in a different direction while attempting to follow the true lumen. If this also fails, you should orient the guidewire tip in the opposite direction to explore the site where it was blocked by hard tissue (Fig. 1.52). If no such site can be found, you should withdraw the guidewire to the entry and search for a dimple again. Alternatively, you can use the parallel wire technique. If the site of obstruction is found, you should keep the guidewire tip at that point and subtly direct it in the presumed direction of the true lumen. You should push the wire forward slightly while gently rotating it within ±90 degrees (see 1.6.4.3 "Fixed Point Guidewire Rotation"). If this maneuver leads to smooth advancement of the guidewire, there is a 90% probability that its tip is in the subintimal space. If the guidewire advances gradually without deviation, it is more likely to be in the true lumen.
6. If the guidewire is blocked by hard tissue inside the lesion despite these exploratory efforts, you should exchange it for another wire with a higher tip load (greater crossability) and explore the optimal direction for advancing the wire (exploration with penetration strategy).
7. You should set a landmark and then explore the optimal direction for advancing the guidewire with reference to the landmark (exploration with landmark strategy).

   I think that the basic guidewire crossing techniques can be summarized as (1) through (7) above, but it is also necessary to consider the variations described below.

8. A CTO can have the combined features of (2) and (3) if occlusion initially arises from a tight stenosis and thrombosis progresses to the nearest side branch at the proximal end of the occlusion (Fig. 1.46c). In such a CTO, a guidewire that is aligned with the center of the true lumen at the entrance to the lesion can be advanced smoothly through the true lumen.
9. There are many possible variations with regard to evolution of the lesion. If there is a fibrous cap at the proximal end of the occlusion, fibrosis and calcification will be more advanced at this site. Accordingly, a guidewire with a high tip load should be used to penetrate the proximal cap. After entering the true lumen, it may be reasonable to step down to a less stiff wire.
10. If a guidewire is blocked by a calcified region within the CTO, it may represent preexisting calcified plaque or may be calcification that occurred after occlusion (Fig. 1.53). In both cases, you should explore the optimal route by performing fixed point rotation of the guidewire in an exploratory manner (see 1.6.4.7 "Rotation").
11. Another tissue that can exist before occlusion is soft plaque, which is often associated with positive remodeling. When the guidewire is manipulated within soft plaque inside the lumen, the tip moves relatively freely, and you may feel as if the tip has gone outside the vessel wall (Fig. 1.54). Also, the distance between the guidewire tip and an available landmark in the lumen may be too long to allow estimation of the correct route for advancing the wire. In this situation, while the interventionalist expects the guidewire to pass through the subintimal space, post-crossing IVUS often demonstrates that the guidewire has actually crossed the lesion through the true lumen.
12. Sometimes, part of an occluded vessel may undergo extreme negative remodeling (Fig. 1.55), and the guidewire may enter the subintimal space at the end of such a region. You can only confirm this by post-crossing IVUS, so it is important to advance the guidewire according to the standard rules even at such sites.

    Some lesions show both positive and negative remodeling.

    When selecting the exploration strategy, you must keep the following in mind: "Always start guidewire manipulation with a feather touch and never push the guidewire so strongly as to deflect the tip" (see Chap. 5: "Mitsudo's Non-pushing PCI Technique"). Specifically, you should:

13. Always start exploration of the guidewire route with a feather touch.
14. Even when advancing a guidewire after the tip has entered a dimple, only the minimum force required to advance it should be employed.
15. Never push the guidewire forward strongly enough to deflect its tip.
16. If there is no route to advance the guidewire with a force that does not deflect its tip, exchange the wire for one with a higher tip load.
17. Start manipulation of the new guidewire with a feather touch, and explore the route that allows advancement with a force that does not lead to deflection of its tip.

It is uncommon to obtain information on the mechanisms involved in CTO formation and the histology of the lesion and surrounding tissues before starting PCI. However, you can make an estimate from the patient's medical history, age, and concomitant illnesses, as well as angiographic images of the lesion. After starting PCI, you may also obtain supporting information from the actual sensations as the guidewire is manipulated through the target vessel. For practical tips about fixed point guidewire rotation, please refer to 1.6.4.7 (page 58).

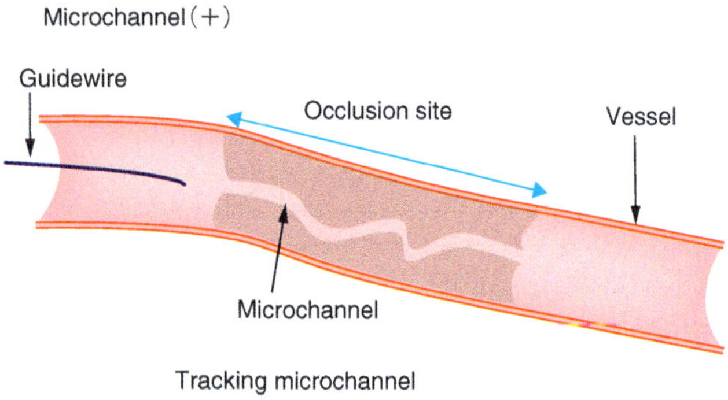

Fig. 1.48 Exploration strategy. If there is a microchannel within a relatively large occluded vessel, you should find its entrance and insert the guidewire. Once the entrance has been identified, the next step is to track the microchannel. You must not try to penetrate the CTO with a guidewire that was selected for tracking. When it is advanced forcibly in an attempt to cross the CTO, the guidewire often enters the subintimal space, even if it does not have a stiff tip

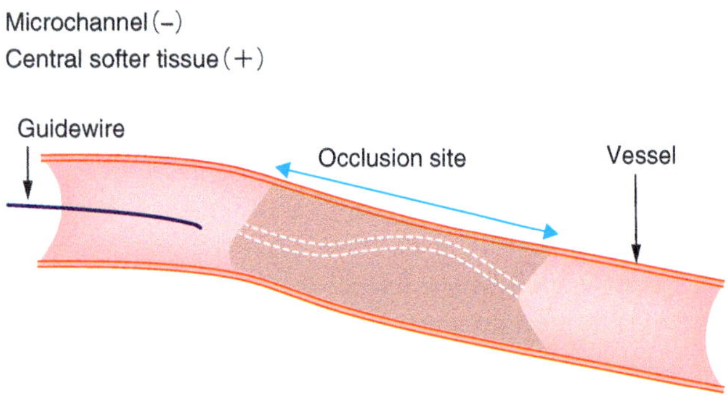

Fig. 1.49 Exploration with penetration strategy. The guidewire should be advanced while exploring to find a relatively soft site where occlusion would have occurred most recently. This strategy may be the same as "loose tissue tracking" (proposed by Sumitsuji). At the entry to the CTO, you should search for a point where the guidewire can penetrate the cap with as little pressure as possible. If exploration while pushing the guidewire strongly enough to slightly deflect its tip fails, you should exchange the guidewire for another wire with a higher tip load and repeat exploration. If the guidewire enters the lesion, you should then advance it with as little force as possible while exploring to find the correct direction

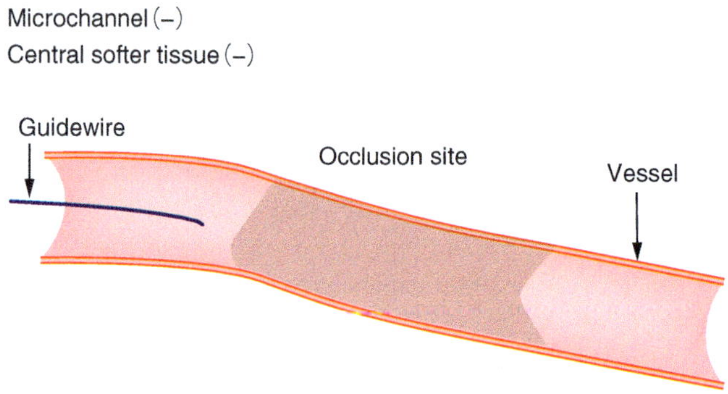

Fig. 1.50 Penetration with exploration strategy. The guidewire should be advanced through homogenous tissue within the CTO. The hardness of the plaque and the subintimal layer, as well as the distribution of plaque, may determine the correct direction for advancing the guidewire. If it is pushed forward forcibly, the guidewire will also deviate into the subintimal space in this setting, so you should advance the guidewire slowly with little force while exploring to find the correct direction

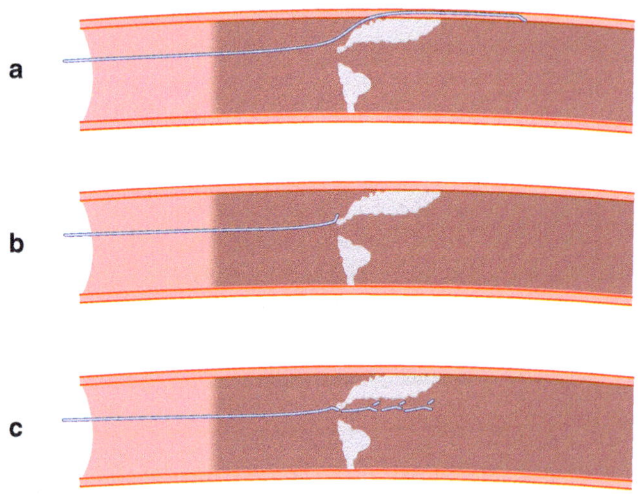

Fig. 1.51 Penetration with exploration by fixed point guidewire rotation. (**a**) If a guidewire becomes blocked by hard tissue within the lumen and then abruptly moves forward when pushed forcibly, its tip will usually have entered the subintimal space. (**b**) After slightly advancing the guidewire, either of the two projections will often show that it has been deflected. If so, you should pull the guidewire back nearly to the inflection point and search for the place where the wire was initially obstructed. (**c**) While keeping the guidewire tip at the blockage to prevent subintimal deviation, you should orient the tip in the opposite direction. Then you should explore to find the direction in which the guidewire can be advanced while rotating the tip within ±90 degrees

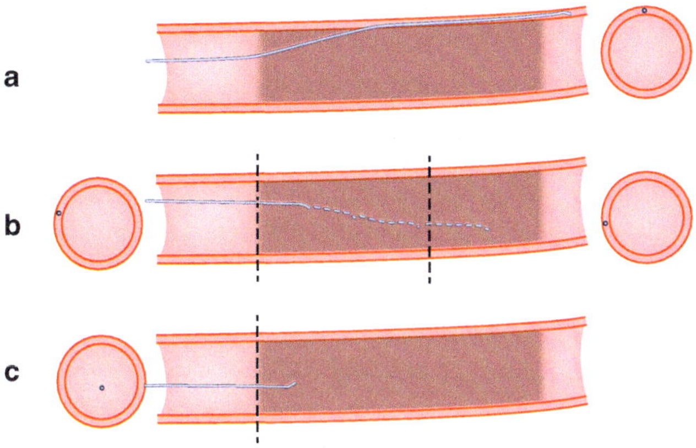

Fig. 1.52 If the guidewire enters the subintimal space relatively easily. (**a**) In this situation, the guidewire has been advanced into the subintimal space without any resistance, so the point at which the wire actually enters the subintimal space is difficult to determine. (**b**) If it is expected to be possible to track the true lumen from the entry of the CTO, you should pull the guidewire back to a most proximal point possible within the lesion and orient it in the opposite direction to explore for the correct route. (**c**) If this maneuver fails to advance the guidewire through the true lumen, you should completely withdraw the guidewire from the lesion and find a new entry point that is more likely to allow successful crossing of the CTO

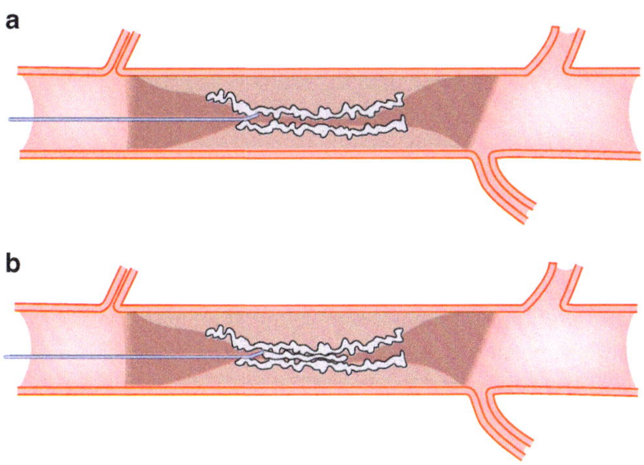

Fig. 1.53 Influence of calcified plaque at the occlusion. (**a**) The tip of the guidewire may enter preexisting plaque and become blocked by a calcified area of the plaque. (**b**) Alternatively, the tip of the guidewire may be obstructed by calcification at the core of the lumen where final occlusion occurred

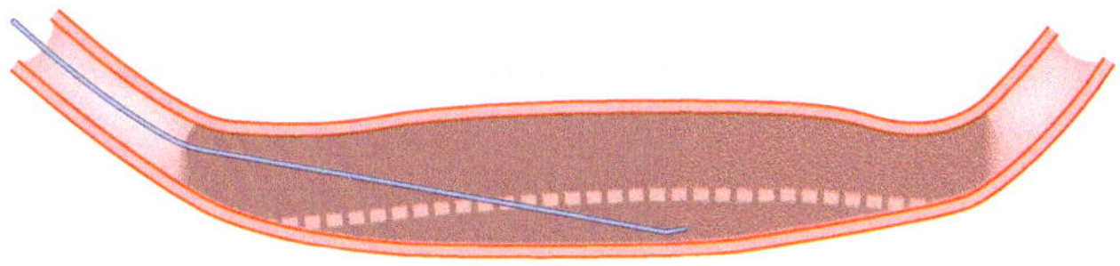

Fig. 1.54 Occlusion of a segment with positive remodeling. If there is marked positive remodeling, it may feel as if the guidewire is not crossing the lesion through the true lumen

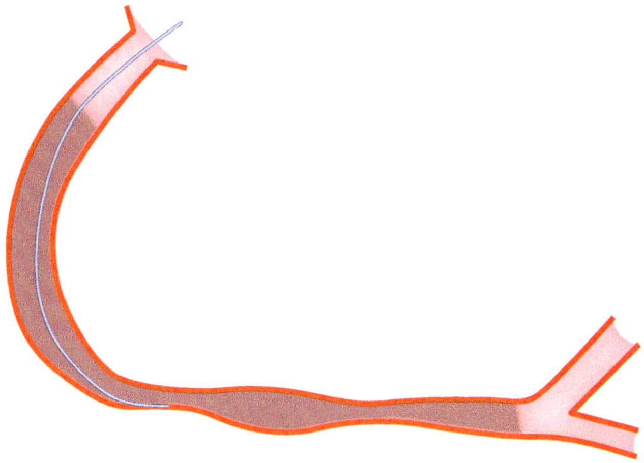

Fig. 1.55 Negative remodeling of the occlusion. This shows an occluded coronary artery with extreme negative remodeling, which means that a guidewire advanced through plaque readily deviates into the subintimal space

Column 5 Advancing the Guidewire and Influence of Tissue Hardness

Here, I will discuss how the hardness of tissue in the lesion influences advancement of the guidewire. This discussion is theoretical because we cannot accurately know the ultrastructure of each lesion. Nonetheless, we can often accomplish PCI successfully by devising strategies while simulating various scenarios during the procedure. Although the model used here has relatively soft tissue at the core, many of the lesions encountered in practice are homogeneous or heterogeneous with a mosaic structure. These latter two types may be modeled as homogeneous lesions and calcified lesions, respectively.

A guidewire with a tip that is stiff enough to penetrate the core tissue and not stiff enough to go through the surrounding plaque can readily follow the true lumen. A CTO with this histological architecture can be successfully crossed by drilling with a non-tapered guidewire of intermediate stiffness (Intermediate Miracle series; Fig. 1.56).

The hardness of the lesion will not necessarily be compatible with the stiffness of the guidewire selected. Of course, a guidewire that is less stiff than a CTO cannot cross it. Also, as the intima/media is unexpectedly soft, even a flexible guidewire is likely to enter the subintimal space. Since we usually do not know the exact hardness of the CTO, it is generally more economical to initially choose a moderately stiff guidewire, rather than stepping up from a more flexible wire. There are several tips for making the best use of stiff guidewires. If a stiff guidewire is advanced with a stronger force than is required for crossing the target plaque, it is likely to go through the plaque into the subintimal space (Fig. 1.57).

So, how should we manipulate the guidewire to avoid this outcome? The strategy to adopt is "exploration," and it is based on the following assumption. As seen in Fig. 1.57, the guidewire chosen is stiff enough to cross the occlusion and may be stiffer than required to penetrate the target plaque (which is considered to be hard). In order to advance such a stiff guidewire through relatively soft tissue rather than through hard plaque, you should start PCI by exploring to find the point where the guidewire can be advanced with as little force as possible. What is the optimal force for advancing the guidewire? I have measured the optimal force for advancing a Conquest Pro guidewire as "about 0.6 g" and "no more than 1.0 g" at maximum. When advanced using such force, the Conquest Pro guidewire often follows the soft core and does not penetrate hard plaque. If this exploration strategy using minimal force fails to advance the wire, it means that the core is not as soft as was expected. Then there is no choice other than to gradually increase the force applied to the wire until it enters the core, but it should never be pushed strongly enough to deflect the tip.

If even these efforts fail to identify the entry point or direction for crossing, you should exchange the guidewire for a stiffer one. Again start manipulation with minimal force, and gradually increase the force until crossing is successful. When a stiff guidewire is selected, you must not apply force strongly enough for its tip to be deflected.

This method of manipulation is applicable to all crossing guidewires, including those in the Conquest Pro and Gaia series (Fig. 1.58).

A lipid-rich plaque within the CTO may lead the guidewire into the subintimal space. If the guidewire enters the subintimal space, you should pull it back to the proximal part of the occlusion and try to advance it in the right direction again. However, subintimal guidewire deviation can only be verified by performing IVUS after recanalization. A lipid core in the plaque may be detected by CT, but is unlikely to provide an accurate landmark for deciding the optimal point to which the guidewire should be pulled back. You should retry crossing the CTO after pulling the guidewire back a long way if there is a possibility of success (Fig. 1.59).

A guidewire that is stiffer than the plaque at a CTO, but less stiff than a calcified or fibrosed region within the lesion, is likely to enter either the plaque or the subintimal space (Fig. 1.60).

Even if a guidewire is surrounded and blocked by hard tissue, you must not push it forward strongly enough to deflect it. If the presence of calcified plaque is suspected, you should explore to find a route that allows the guidewire to bypass the plaque, remembering that the gap between two calcified plaques will also be relatively hard. If a guidewire

is blocked by hard tissue, it is generally safer to exchange it for a stiffer wire. However, even a stiffer guidewire cannot penetrate the core of a calcified plaque, so it is necessary to try to advance the wire through the gap between two calcified plaques or near the rim of each plaque (Fig. 1.61).

Even while exploring with minimal force, you may accidentally advance a guidewire into the subintimal space and through the adventitia. If a guidewire advanced with minimal force has reached the artery distal to the occlusion but is in the adventitia, the wire must have entered the subintimal space at the entrance of the occlusion (Fig. 1.62). While leaving this guidewire in place, you should try to find another route through the CTO from the entrance with a second guidewire. If there is a side branch that can accommodate an IVUS catheter, you should perform IVUS to check that the second guidewire is located at the correct entry point before advancing it further (Fig. 1.63).

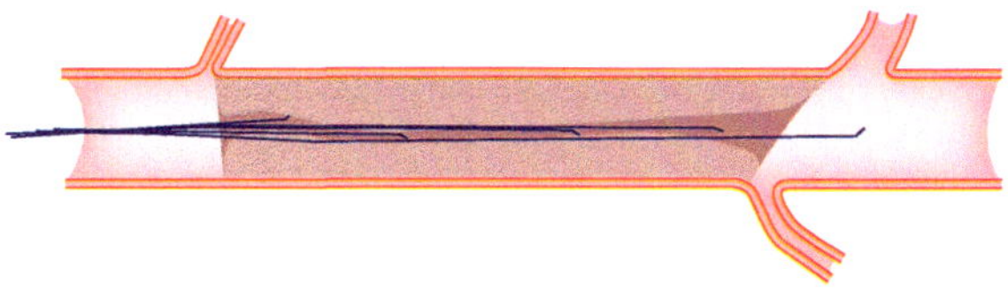

Fig. 1.56 Influence of tissue hardness on advancing the guidewire. $H_{CST} < S_{GW} < H_P$. H_{CST} hardness of the soft core, S_{GW} stiffness of the guidewire, H_P hardness of the surrounding plaque, H_{Ad} hardness of the adventitia, H_{Lip} hardness of the lipid core

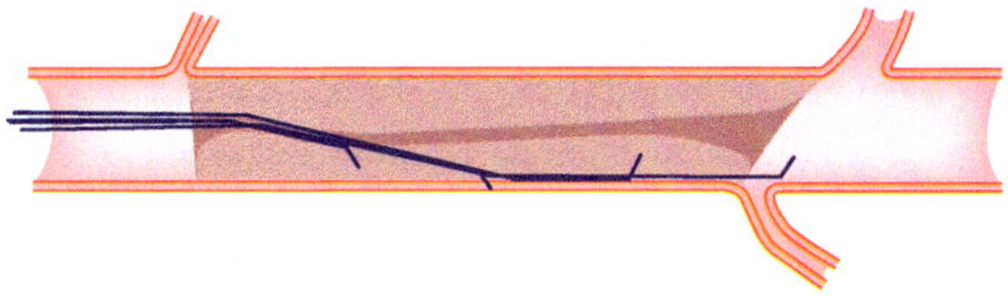

Fig. 1.57 If the guidewire is stiffer than the surrounding plaque. $H_{CST} < H_P < S_{GW}$

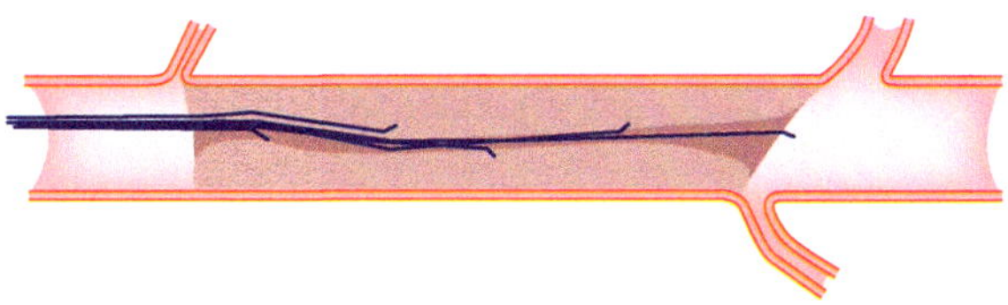

Fig. 1.58 If the guidewire is stiffer than the surrounding plaque. $H_{CST} < H_P < S_{GW}$

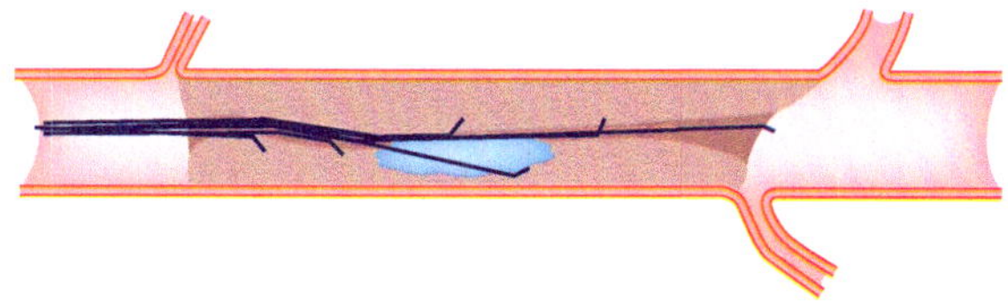

Fig. 1.59 If there is lipid-rich plaque within the occlusion. $H_{Lip} < H_{CST} < H_P < S_{GW}$. Lipid-rich plaque may lead the guidewire into the subintimal space

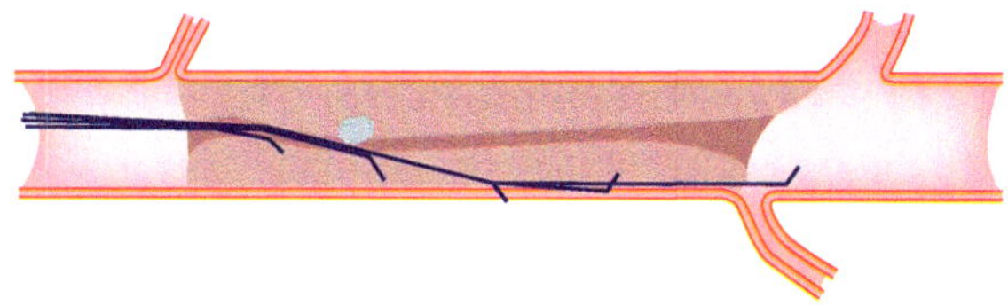

Fig. 1.60 If there is hard tissue within the occlusion. $H_P < H_{CST} < S_{GW}$. If there is calcified plaque, then $H_P < S_{GW} < H_{CST}$. The guidewire is blocked by the hard tissue and deviates into the subintimal space

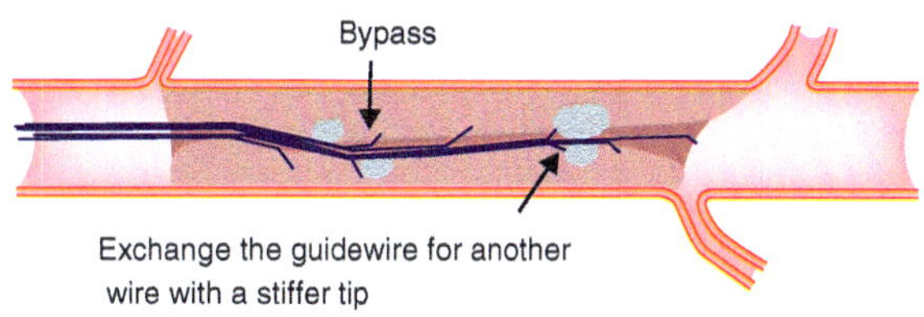

Fig. 1.61 If there is hard tissue within the occlusion. $H_P < H_{CST} < S_{GW}$. If there is calcified plaque, then $H_P < S_{GW} < H_{CST}$. Exploration should be performed to find another route that allows the guidewire to bypass the plaque

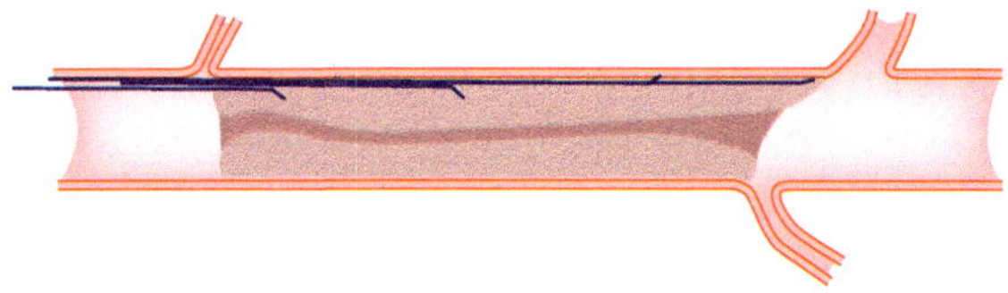

Fig. 1.62 If the guidewire has been advanced through the adventitia from the CTO entry point. $H_{Ad} < H_{CST} < S_{GW} < H_P$. If a guidewire advanced with minimal force has reached the vessel distal to the occlusion in the adventitia, the wire must have entered the subintimal space at the CTO entry

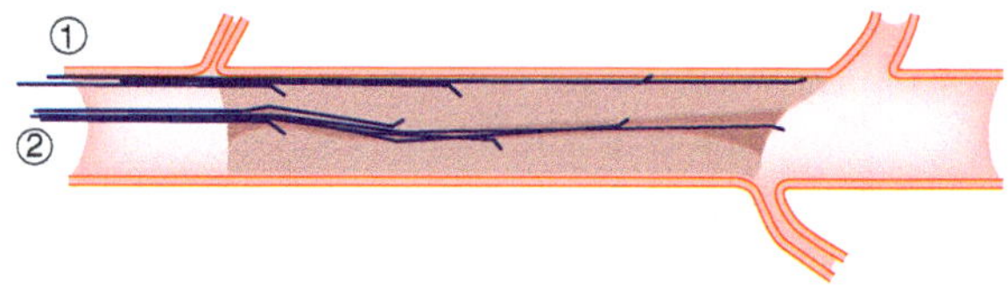

Fig. 1.63 If the guidewire has been advanced through the adventitia from the CTO entry. The guidewire may be inadvertently advanced through the subintimal space, even if it is pushed with minimal force throughout the procedure. Once the wire has entered the subintimal space, it is likely to advance while creating a dissection, even when very little force is applied. If the guidewire deviates from the true lumen into the subintimal space within the lesion, you will generally feel some obstruction during manipulation. It is reasonable to consider that the guidewire has entered the subintimal space at the CTO entry

1.6.4 Guidewire Strategies

1.6.4.1 Tip Load and Penetration Force: Why a Crossing Guidewire Is Needed to Perform Antegrade PCI for CTO

You may think that a non-tapered CTO guidewire with an intermediate tip load can more readily penetrate hard plaques and would be safer to use, i.e., less likely to deviate into the subintimal space or outside the vessel wall. It is true that a non-tapered guidewire can sometimes easily cross an occlusion even if it is not manipulated carefully.

However, a tapered guidewire has greater maximum penetration force per area unit compared to a non-tapered guidewire with an identical tip load, and thus less force needs to be applied for it to cross a lesion of a given hardness. The maximum penetration force is calculated as follows:

$$PF = G / TA$$

where PF is the penetration force, G is the tip load, and TA is the tip area. The ratio of the maximum penetration force of a crossing guidewire with a 0.009-inch tip relative to a guidewire with an identical tip load and a 0.014-inch tip is calculated as follows:

$$PF_{14} = G / \left(\pi 0.0014^2 / 4\right)$$

$$PF_9 = G / \left(\pi 0.0009^2 / 4\right)$$

$$\begin{aligned} PF_9 / PF_{14} &= G / \left(\pi 0.0009^2 / 4\right) / G / \left(\pi 0.0014^2 / 4\right) \\ &= 0.014^2 / 0.009^2 \\ &= 2.42 \end{aligned}$$

Thus, the penetration force of a guidewire with a 0.009-inch tip is about 2.5 times greater than that of a guidewire with a 0.014-inch tip. Conversely, to acquire equal penetration force, a 0.014-inch guidewire would need a tip load about 2.5 times higher than that of a 0.009-inch guidewire. Therefore, you do not need to push so hard on a tapered crossing guidewire to advance through a CTO. This is a great advantage of a tapered wire and is the chief reason why I use a tapered crossing guidewire when performing antegrade PCI for CTO.

However, please note that the penetration force of a guidewire during PCI also depends on the "pushing force" applied to it. For example, applying a force of "X g" (where $X < 9$ g) to the Conquest Pro 9-g and 12-g guidewires (both have a 0.009-inch tip) will result in exactly equal penetration force with both wires:

$$\begin{aligned} PF &= X / \left(\pi 0.009^2 / 4\right) \\ &= X / 0.00006362\, g / in^2 \end{aligned}$$

During PCI, the penetration force of a guidewire is a function of the pushing force and is independent of the intrinsic maximum penetration force, so it varies with the force applied to the wire. However, a guidewire with a tip load of 9 g must not be pushed with a force greater than 9 g (as explained later), while a guidewire with a tip load of 12 g can be pushed with a force of up to 12 g and therefore has a greater maximum penetration force.

A crossing guidewire usually has a hydrophilic coating, except at its tip. Friction between the shaft and the surrounding tissues increases the force needed to advance the guidewire through a lesion. To reduce friction and make "non-pushing PCI" practicable, a guidewire with a hydrophilic coating is required.

However, hydrophilic coating makes it more difficult to determine whether the guidewire has remained within the true lumen or is being advanced through the subintimal space. Certainly, the current CTO crossing wires do not produce sufficient friction to create a "rough" sensation. Of course, this "rough" sensation is subjective and cannot be quantified or

reported accurately. If possible, interventionalists should try to assess the outcome of PCI and transmit their own techniques to the next generation by using objective measures.

You do not need to use a guidewire with a hydrophilic coating on the tip when trying to catch a small dimple at the CTO entrance (Fig. 1.64) or when directing the tip of the wire in the desired direction within a lesion (Fig. 1.65). A coated tip may make the guidewire so slippery that it becomes hard to catch and penetrate a dimple or change direction inside the CTO. Therefore, the tip of the guidewire (at least the ball of the tip) should not have a hydrophilic coating.

If guidewires with different tip loads exhibited identical behavior, it would be possible to substitute a guidewire with a higher tip load for a wire with a lower tip load by using less force to advance the former wire. If so, gradually stepping up guidewires would be unnecessary, and a single guidewire would be enough to accomplish PCI, but this is not true in practice. In this subsection, I will discuss the structural and strategic factors affecting guidewire manipulation based on my empirical evidence and logical deduction.

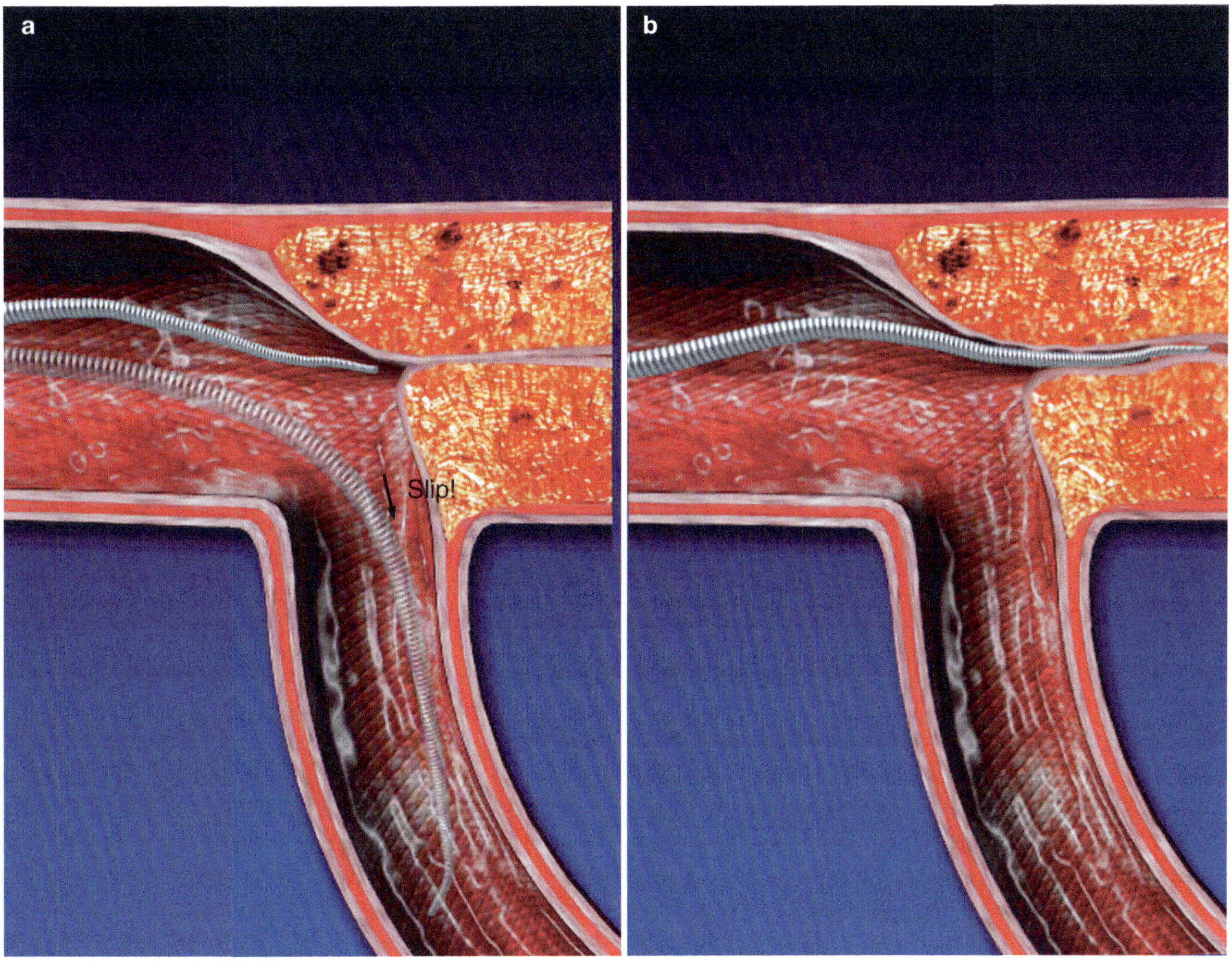

Fig. 1.64 Slipperiness of the guidewire. When manipulated to catch a small and shallow dimple, a guidewire with a smooth tip is likely to deviate into a side branch and fail to penetrate the dimple (**a**). On the other hand, a guidewire without a smooth tip is more likely to catch and penetrate the dimple (**b**)

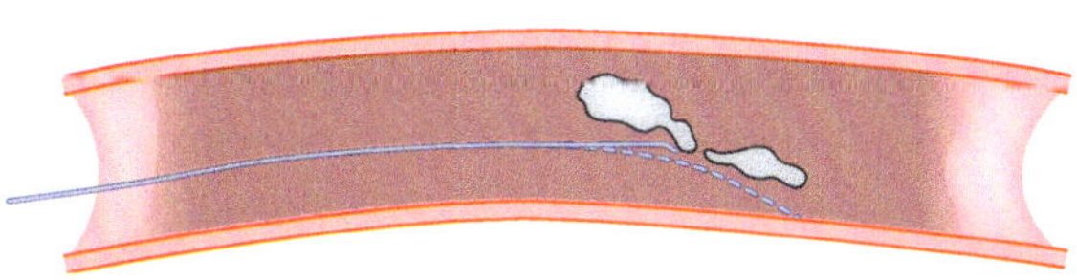

Fig. 1.65 Problem with hydrophilic coating. If a guidewire becomes blocked by calcified plaque, you may want to change direction. In this situation, a guidewire with hydrophilic coating on the tip may slide past the plaque and go in the wrong direction (dotted line)

1.6.4.2 Curve of the Guidewire Tip

A guidewire with a straighter tip has stronger penetration force. When a bench test is performed, the tip load of the guidewire is measured with its tip straight. However, you cannot control the direction of a guidewire with a straight tip when it is in a CTO (Fig. 1.66). What is the optimal size and angle for the curve of the guidewire tip? All patent (non-occluded) vessels have curves to a greater or lesser extent. For advancing a guidewire through a curved vessel, it is ideal if the distance between the tip and shaft of the wire is slightly greater than the inner diameter of the vessel (Fig. 1.67). It should optimally be 1 to 1.5 mm (30 to 40%) larger than the vessel diameter, although this depends somewhat on the curvature of the vessel. If the distance between tip and shaft is too short, the guidewire cannot be directed toward a side branch. If the distance is too long, it becomes difficult to control the wire at a sharp bifurcation.

A target vessel with a CTO corresponds to a vessel with an inner diameter of 0 mm. However, advancing a guidewire creates a new channel with an inner diameter of about 0.014 inches ($\approx$0.35 mm). When the abovementioned rule is applied, the optimal size of the curve at the guidewire tip is calculated to be about 0.5 mm and slightly larger than 0.35 mm. If the tip diameter is 0.009 inches (=0.225 mm), a guidewire with a curve slightly larger than 0.225 mm should be chosen.

While participating in the development of Conquest Pro guidewires around 1998 to 2000, I tried to minimize the curve of the tip. Using an inserter, I was able to shape a curve only 1 to 2 mm in size, as shown in Fig. 1.68, but I found that the curve was lost during intervention. I then tried to manually shape a curve at the tip of the wire with a 25-G needle or after extruding the tip from the top of the inserter, but failed to create a curve with a consistent shape and size. Since manual shaping also caused severe pain in my fingertips, I asked the manufacturer to make me a shaping device (Fig. 1.69).

I used this device to handcraft curves at the guidewire tip (Figs. 1.70 and 1.71). As can be seen in this photograph, these guidewires do not have a second curve, but I initially tried to cross CTOs with such guidewires. It could be suggested that a tapered guidewire with a high tip load might only go straight forward, but I thought that even such a wire could be deflected if advanced with minimal force after being blocked by a hard lesion (too hard to penetrate with a Conquest Pro). Because the tip load of a guidewire is measured with the tip straight, you may think that a guidewire with a tip load of 9 g cannot be deflected unless a force greater than 9 g is applied. However, a guidewire with a curved tip like that shown in Fig. 1.70 is deflected by even weaker forces. Dr. Osamu Kato referred to this as the "deflection" phenomenon and promoted this concept.

When manipulated within loose tissue, a guidewire with a high tip load and a small curve will go straight toward the lateral wall of the vessel at a bend. However, if such a guidewire becomes blocked by tissue that is too hard to penetrate, the curve of the tip will be increased whenever the wire is pushed, and its tip will be oriented medially in the desired direction (Fig. 1.72). The guidewire can be advanced through a CTO in the desired direction if its tip, even if deflected, can find the optimal route. Thus, I found it possible to control the direction of the tip of a guidewire when the tip load and curve had been optimized with reference to the hardness of the target lesion, even if the tip was stiff and tapered as with the Conquest Pro series.

Subsequently, I only used guidewires from the Conquest Pro series with a small tip curve for a while, and these guidewires were deflected from hard tissues inside many CTOs. However, I found that I could not direct a guidewire without a second curve toward the CTO entry in some tortuous vessels.

Therefore, I handcrafted a guidewire with a gentle second curve (Fig. 1.73). I found that this modification sometimes led to successful crossing of the CTO, but the second curve was easily lost during prolonged manipulation, making the tip straighter and leaving only the first curve. To prevent this, the second curve must be created by bending the guidewire. I initially thought that bending the guidewire at 5–8 mm from the first curve (Fig. 1.74a) would create a gentle second curve, but I found that a guidewire curved in this way produced severe whipping artifacts and was difficult to control. By reducing the distance between the first and second curves, I gradually overcame problems with whipping. Finally, I found that the optimal distance between the two curves was about 2 mm (Fig. 1.75b) to minimize the frequency of whipping while preserving a functional second curve.

At present, I set an almost constant distance between the two curves at the tip of a tapered CTO crossing guidewire, but I slightly modify the angles of the curves according to the diameter of the target vessel just proximal to the occlusion, the type of stump (abrupt or tapered), the tortuosity of the vessel, and the hardness of the occlusion (Fig. 1.75).

As mentioned later, the guidewire needs a sufficiently large curve at its tip to orient it toward the entry of a bifurcation occlusion or an occlusion in a large tortuous vessel. In such circumstances, a gentle curve at the tip of a guidewire with a low tip load (e.g., an XT-R or XT-A) can prevent it from becoming straight during manipulation, whereas a guidewire from the Gaia series or any other series with a higher tip load should desirably have multiple staggered curves (Fig. 1.76b) rather than a single gentle curve (Fig. 1.76a).

The optimal size and acuteness of the curve at the tip will depend on the features of the lesion, which are often demonstrated during IVUS-guided PCI. If a guidewire with the tip shape shown in Fig. 1.77a cannot remain inside the true lumen at a point distal to the CTO entry, penetration should be reattempted after the curve of the tip has been made slightly smaller and slightly more acute (Fig. 1.77b). This second attempt is often successful.

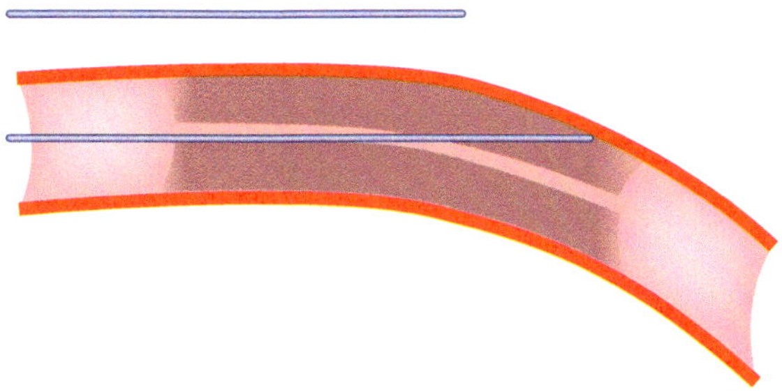

Fig. 1.66 Guidewire with a straight tip. A guidewire with a straight tip has the greatest penetration force, but its direction is difficult to control

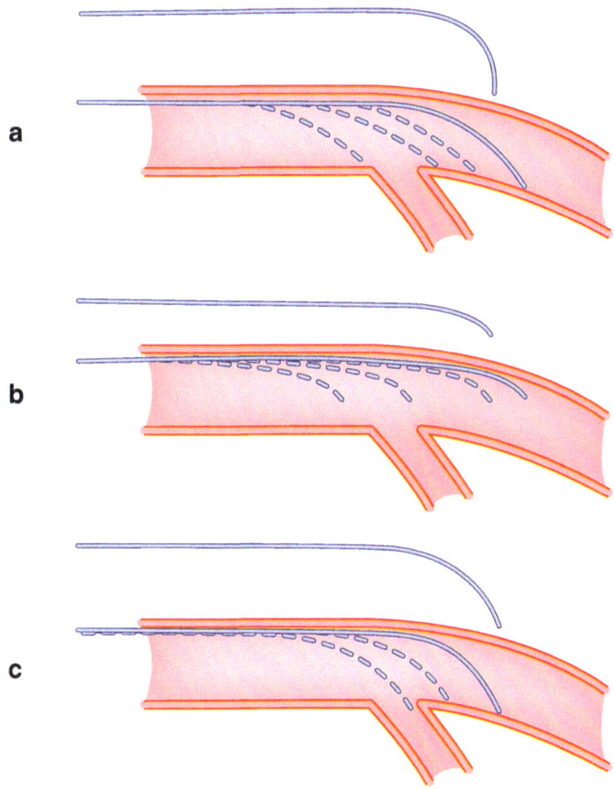

Fig. 1.67 Guidewires with tip curves of various sizes in non-occluded coronary arteries. While the vessel diameter changes continually, the relationship between diameter and the size of the guidewire tip curve at critical points is considered here. (**a**) If the curve of the guidewire tip is too large for the vessel diameter, it is difficult for the guidewire to enter a small side branch arising at an acute angle (particularly if a larger curvature is required to enter the branch). (**b**) On the other hand, if the curve of the guidewire tip is too small for the vessel diameter, the guidewire cannot reach the ostium of a side branch arising at an acute angle for which a smaller curve is needed or is likely to enter another side branch that requires a larger curve. (**c**) It is optimal for the curve of the guidewire tip to be slightly larger than the vessel diameter

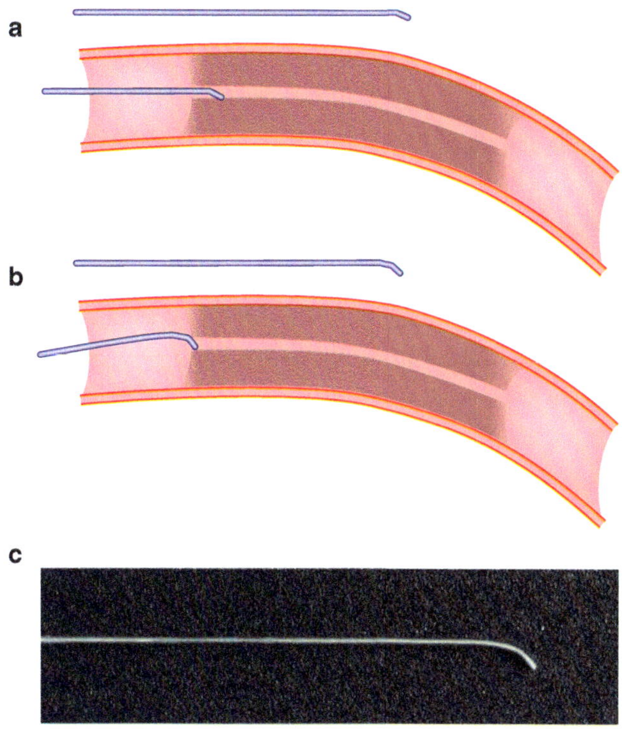

Fig. 1.68 Optimal guidewire tip curve for crossing a CTO. (**a**) If the plaque is hard, a guidewire with a tip curve slightly larger than the diameter of the new channel created by advancing the guidewire (0.009 to 0.014 inches = 0.22 to 0.35 mm) should be used. (**b**) A guidewire with too large a tip curve is difficult to control. (**c**) Conquest Pro guidewire with a tip curve shaped by using an inserter

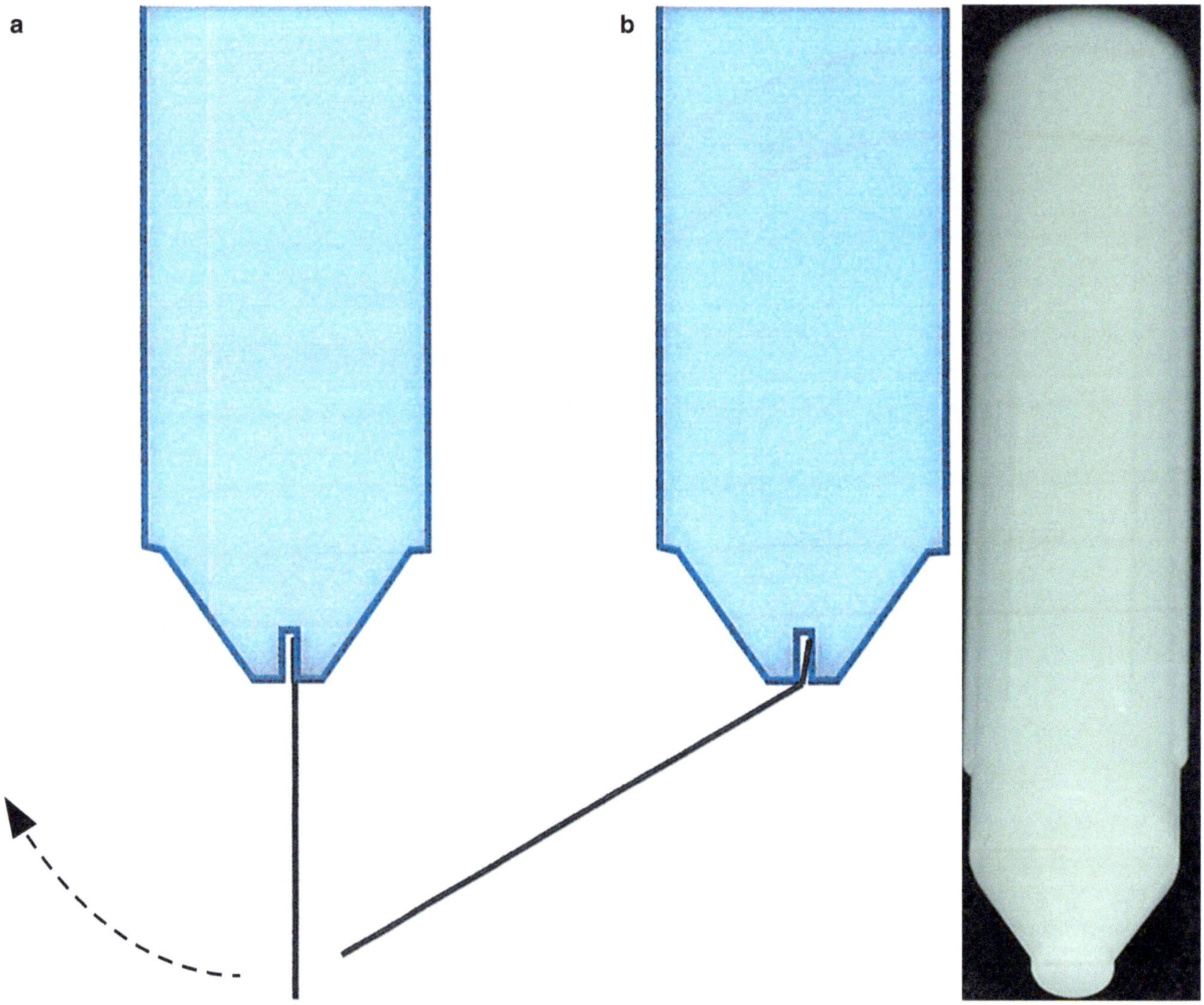

Fig. 1.69 Shaping device. To shape a curve at the tip of a guidewire, insert the tip into the hole at the top of the device (**a**), and bend the tip (**b**). This simple device is useful for creating small curves at the tips of guidewires, including wires in the Conquest Pro and Gaia series. The smallest curve that can be created with this device is around 0.5 to 0.6 mm. While there is no device or method available to shape even smaller curves at the guidewire tip, curves of this size are sufficient for manipulation

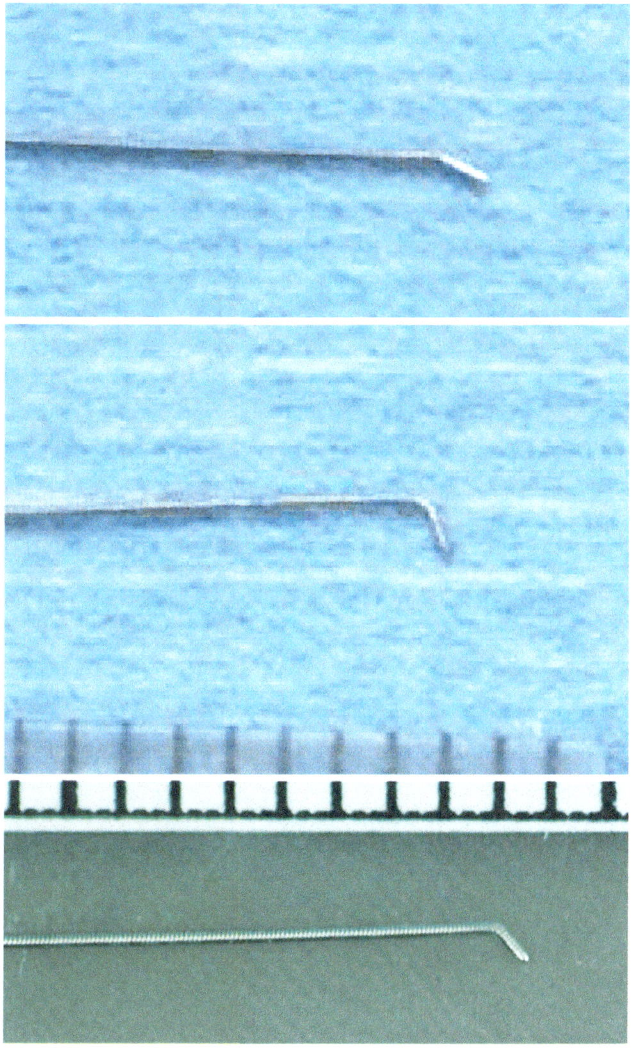

Fig. 1.70 Tip curves for crossing guidewires. For some time, the tip curves shown in this figure were recommended for the prototype Conquest Pro guidewires. Many interventionalists complained that these guidewires could go only straight forward, but I and others knew that even these guidewires could be deflected in an occlusion once the tip was blocked and bent by a hard lesion. In fact, we knew that a guidewire of intermediate stiffness (the first choice at the time) would be trapped ("deflected" according to current concepts) without going straight forward if it was unable to cross the CTO. Absence of hydrophilic coating at 1 mm from the tip made it easier for the guidewire to catch a dimple at the CTO entrance and to be deflected when penetrating a tortuous lesion. To obtain optimal deflection and advance the guidewire in the desired direction, I think that it is important to rotate the guidewire tip clockwise and counterclockwise within the range of 90 degrees. This point was also taken into account when recommending the shapes and angles of the tip curve. Nonetheless, guidewires with these tip curves sometimes fail to reach the entry of a curved lesion in a relatively large vessel

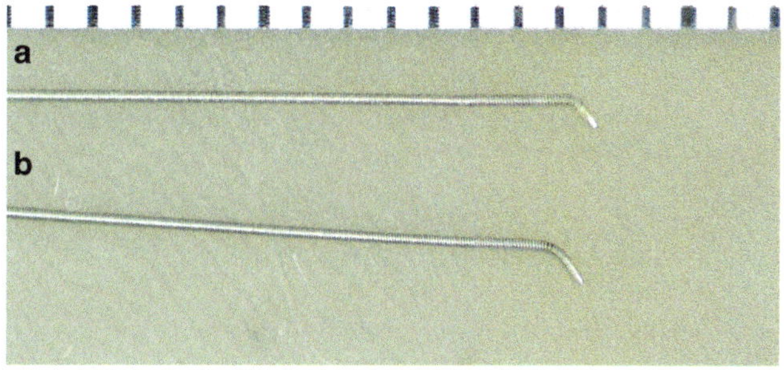

Fig. 1.71 Tip curves for Gaia guidewires. (**a**) A custom-made curve created with the shaping device. This curve is about 0.6 to 0.7 mm. (**b**) A pre-shaped curve slightly larger than 1 mm

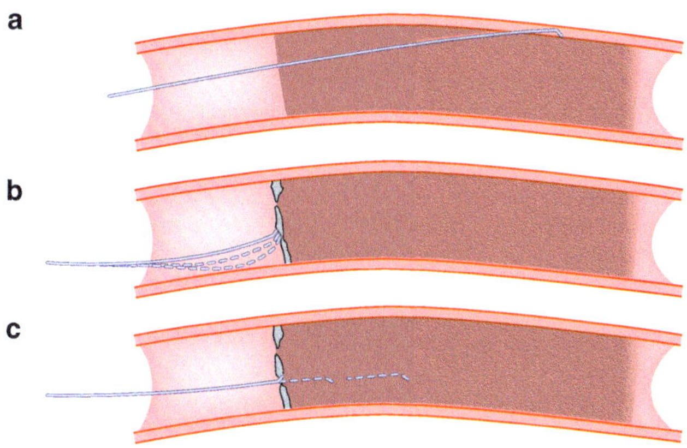

Fig. 1.72 Advancing a guidewire with a high tip load and a small curve at the tip. (**a**) A guidewire with a high tip load and a small curve at the tip will go straight through a soft lesion. (**b**) If it is blocked by hard tissue in the lesion, even a guidewire with a small tip curve will deviate medially when it is pushed forward. (**c**) If it is rotated at the point where it was blocked by hard tissue in the occlusion, the guidewire will go forward and force its way into the lesion

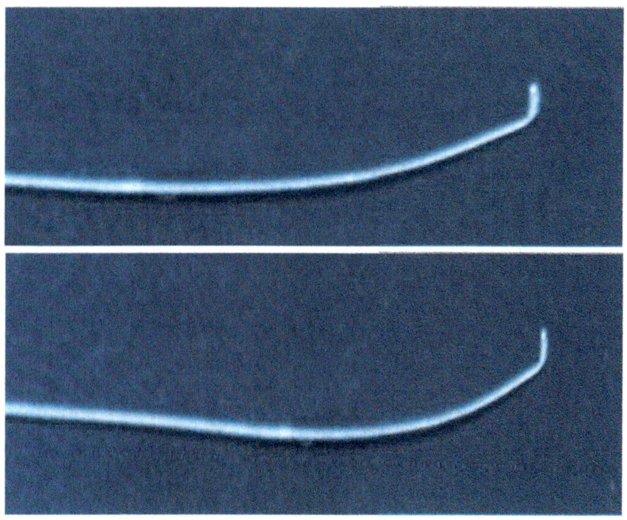

Fig. 1.73 Guidewires with a second curve. If the entry point to a CTO is located at a bend of the target vessel, a guidewire without a second curve will sometimes fail to reach the dimple. I used guidewires with a gentle second curve for some time, but I found that a gentle second curve at the tip of a Conquest Pro guidewire was straightened again soon after starting intravascular manipulation

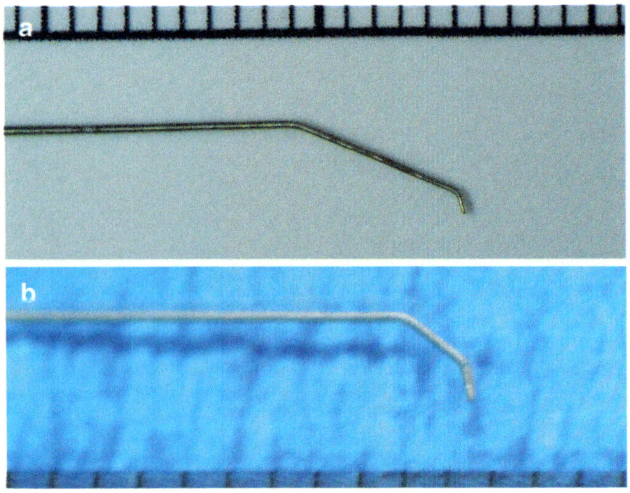

Fig. 1.74 Shaping the second curve of a Conquest Pro guidewire. Although I knew that whipping was more frequent when the guidewire was shaped with a more acute curve than the gentle curve shown in the previous figure, creating an acute second curve was necessary to maintain its shape. Whipping is more likely to occur as the second curve becomes longer (**a**). Therefore, the length of the second curve was restricted to about 2.5 mm at maximum (**b**), leading to the currently recommended shape for the second curve. Some interventionalists may suspect that a guidewire with such a second curve will be difficult to control or not have sufficient pushability. However, a guidewire with a second curve of this size is easier to control during advancement in a slightly tortuous lesion. In practice, I often use a guidewire with a more acute second curve than that shown in this figure, and the curve may be modified according to the tortuosity of the lesion

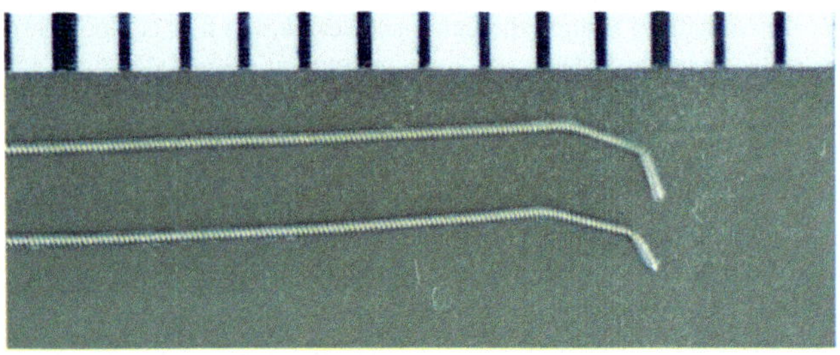

Fig. 1.75 Tip curves for Gaia guidewires. Gaia guidewires exhibit virtually the same behavior as Conquest Pro guidewires, and therefore the second curve is shaped according to the characteristics of the lesion. I sometimes use a Gaia guidewire with a third (or even fourth) curve

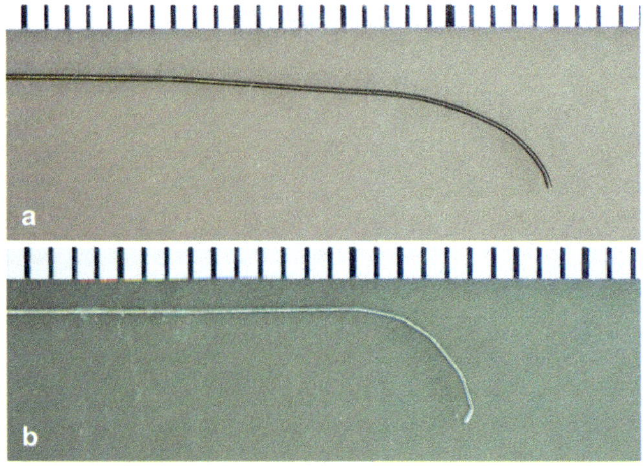

Fig. 1.76 Guidewires with a large curve at the tip. (**a**) Curve at the guidewire tip handcrafted with a 25-G needle. A CTO crossing guidewire with a tapered tip and a higher tip load than a Gaia wire is likely to show straightening of the tip during manipulation in a hard vessel lumen, resulting in failure to reach the entrance of the lesion. (**b**) A guidewire with multiple staggered curves (each 1 to 2 mm long) at the tip is more likely to maintain its curvature

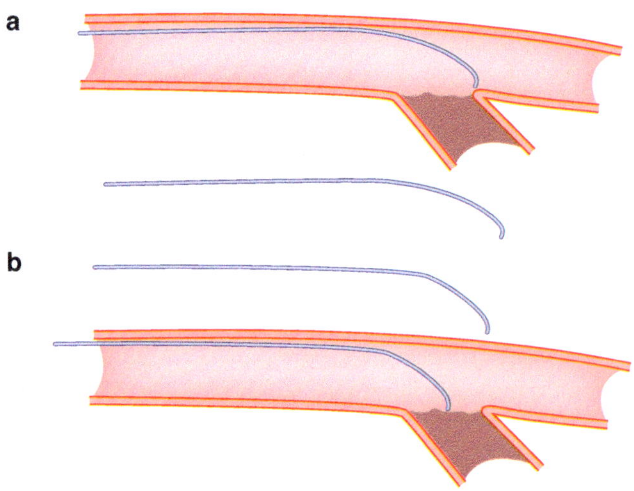

Fig. 1.77 Optimal tip curve of a guidewire for bifurcation CTO. While exploring the entry point of the occlusion under IVUS guidance, you may find that the guidewire can only be advanced into the subintimal space or the boundary between the true lumen and subintimal space (**a**). If you reshape the curve at the tip so that it is slightly smaller and slightly more acute, it will be easier for the guidewire to catch a proximal dimple (**b**)

1.6.4.3 Fixed Point Guidewire Rotation

A guidewire that has entered the true lumen at the entry of a CTO and then has been advanced through the subintimal space on the way to the exit often shows an inflection point (refer to 4. "Guidewire Trapping and Inflection" [page 52]). If the guidewire is suspected to have entered the subintimal space, you should pull it back to a site just proximal to the inflection point and explore to find the direction in which the guidewire can go straight forward without deviation. If the guidewire advances in the same direction again, you should manipulate a second guidewire with a tip load one level higher while using the first wire as a landmark (parallel wire or seesaw wiring technique) and attempt to find the direction in which it can advance without deviation. In most cases, the first guidewire has been blocked by hard plaque and has deviated toward the adventitia through softer tissue. The best solution is to advance the second stiffer guidewire to the site where the first wire was blocked, direct its tip in the opposite direction to the deviation of the first wire, and rotate the second guidewire around a fixed point. Rotation should be performed very slowly and through a limited arc, or the second guidewire will probably deviate into the same subintimal space. A guidewire with a smaller curve at the tip can be rotated more stably around a fixed point, while a guidewire with a large curve may be unsuitable for fixed point rotation (Fig. 1.78).

If the occluded coronary artery is tortuous and stiff at a bend, a guidewire with a small curve at the tip sometimes cannot be advanced in the desired direction, even if "deflection" of the tip is utilized (Fig. 1.79a). If this happens, do not make the first curve larger because this will severely reduce manipulability of the guidewire. If the second curve is made larger instead, it often becomes possible to direct the guidewire toward a hard dimple (Fig. 1.79b). Once a dimple has been caught at the CTO entrance, rotate the guidewire around a fixed point to penetrate the lesion.

If the tip of the guidewire that has caught a dimple slips out of the dimple when fixed point rotation is initiated, you should exchange the guidewire for another wire with a stiffer tip. Then the new guidewire can be rotated at the fixed point without slipping out of the dimple.

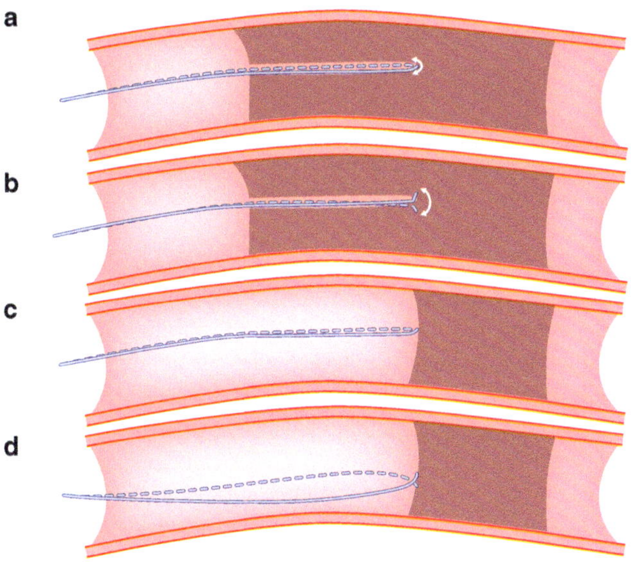

Fig. 1.78 Fixed point rotation of a guidewire. (**a**) Rotating a guidewire with a small curve at its tip. (**b**) A guidewire with a large curve at its tip requires greater torque for rotation. When rotated, the tip of such a guidewire will move through a curve with a large radius. If the wire enters the subintimal space, it will create a large dissection. (**c**) When rotating a blocked guidewire with a small tip curve at the point of obstruction in order to alter its direction and help the wire to penetrate the lesion, it is relatively easy to shift the wire from one direction (solid line) to another direction (dotted line). (**d**) It is sometimes difficult to redirect a guidewire with a large tip curve, even by utilizing deflection, because the wire is unable to effectively catch a dimple of a hard lesion

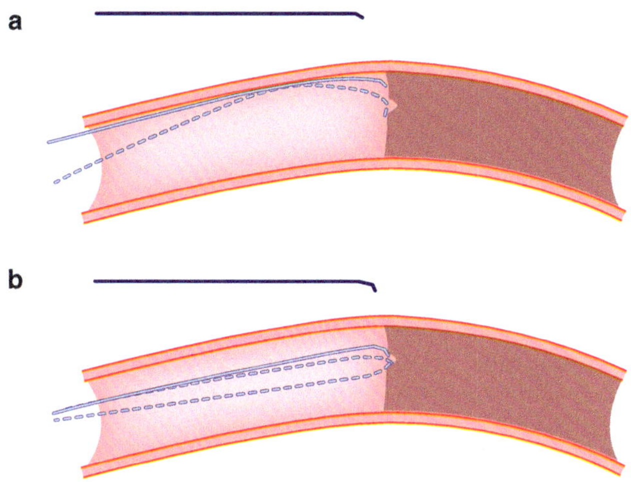

Fig. 1.79 Guidewire with a tip curve that is too small. (**a**) A guidewire with a curve at its tip that is too small may be difficult to navigate to a dimple at the CTO entrance, even by utilizing deflection. (**b**) If the guidewire is reshaped with a small second curve, it can readily catch a dimple. Once the guidewire has caught a dimple, the wire should be advanced while rotating it around a fixed point and keeping the tip in the desired direction

Column 6 Mechanisms of Guidewire Penetration

In an attempt to elucidate the mechanisms involved in guidewire penetration, I will discuss the behavior of guidewires in various types of coronary artery occlusion.

To pass through an almost normal coronary artery, it is desirable for the guidewire to have a tip curve slightly larger than the vessel diameter. A guidewire with too small a tip curve cannot isolate a side branch for which a smaller curvature is needed, while a guidewire with too large a tip curve cannot enter a side branch arising at an acute angle. To pass through a coronary artery that has been narrowed by plaque, the guidewire should also have a tip curve slightly greater than the inner diameter of the vessel (see Fig. 1.67).

To pass a guidewire through the main vascular trunk, it should be advanced with to-and-fro rotation, so that it will advance without being deflected against the vessel wall. This is natural in a patent blood vessel, since a moving guidewire with a soft tip can clearly distinguish between the completely open lumen and the vessel wall. What about in a CTO?

The situation will vary according to the mechanism underlying formation of the occlusion. Let us assume that the CTO was formed by occlusion of a central channel in a gradually progressive stenosis (see Fig. 1.44). There will be a clear difference in hardness between the central tissue of the lesion that actually caused occlusion and the surrounding plaque responsible for the preceding chronic stenosis. A CTO that develops in this way has a softer central region. You will be able to penetrate such an occlusion by repeated rotation of a guidewire with a tip that is stiff enough to allow free rotation in the soft central core without penetrating the surrounding hard plaque and with a tip curve smaller than the diameter of the soft core. While the soft central core of the occlusion is expected to have a small diameter, the actual diameter cannot be estimated. To allow the tip of the guidewire to move relatively freely within the central core, its tip curve should optimally be slightly smaller than the diameter of the core. For this reason, a guidewire with a small tip curve should be employed.

Next, consider a guidewire penetrating a homogenous CTO (see Fig. 1.47). If occlusion has persisted for more than 1 year, the thrombus will be organized and will never be softer than the vessel wall; it is likely to be as hard as or harder than the wall. To cross such a lesion, you must use a guidewire stiff enough to penetrate the organized thrombus. This type of occlusion is unlikely to have tapered ends, so the guidewire should be focused on the center of the lumen revealed by CAG. It is often relatively easy for the guidewire to cross this type of CTO unless it is long or the coronary artery lumen distal to the occlusion has a small diameter. However, you can easily imagine that tracking the center of the organized thrombus becomes more difficult if the occlusion is very long and/or the arterial lumen distal to the occlusion is too narrow. In this case, you cannot visually confirm whether the tip of the guidewire is within the true lumen or in the subintimal space. In practice, you advance the guidewire in the direction in which it goes forward with minimal force while rotating it, moving through the predicted central part of the lumen of the occluded vessel whenever possible. Despite performing plane rotation of the guidewire, it may deviate into the subintimal space because the subintimal tissue is softer than the organized thrombus. In this case, a guidewire with a small curve at its tip will create a smaller dissection when rotated and cause less subintimal injury. On the other hand, a guidewire with a small tip curve is difficult to redirect after it enters a soft occluding plaque. A Gaia guidewire has a relatively large tip curve of about 1.20 mm because this was found to be optimal for redirection within the E-TOS model simulating a relatively soft CTO. To penetrate harder plaque, you should use a guidewire with a smaller curve at the tip. Using the shaping device, I create a customized curve of about 0.6 mm at the tip of the guidewire by bending the point (see Figs. 1.69 and 1.70). A guidewire with a small tip curve is likely to advance straight through a relatively soft lesion. If such a guidewire is given a small second curve (see Fig. 1.76b), it becomes easier to reorient it in the desired direction, even inside a soft lesion. This is another reason why I create a second curve at the tip of the guidewire. Under some circumstances, a single relatively large curve (0.7 mm) at the guidewire tip seems to exert an equal effect to that of a very small first curve plus a small second curve.

1.6.4.4 Guidewire Trapping and Inflection

While attempting to cross a relatively long CTO, you often find that the guidewire becomes trapped within the lesion. The guidewire may be trapped by severe calcification or deformation (kinking), but trapping is unrelated to the extent of calcification in most cases. Although the mechanisms involved in guidewire trapping remain to be elucidated, I suggest that the following factors may be involved based on insights from IVUS findings.

To enter the subintimal space, a guidewire that was in the true lumen at the CTO entry must cross the tunica media. I think that the tip of the guidewire will not be trapped in the

media if it enters this layer at a large angle (Fig. 1.80a), but the tip can be trapped if it enters this layer at a small angle and then is advanced for some distance parallel to the vessel wall (Fig. 1.80b).

If you find that a guidewire can no longer be advanced into a CTO, its tip may be trapped. If further advancement is impossible, you should withdraw the guidewire a little to determine whether the tip is trapped. If the tip has been trapped for a long time, the wire is difficult to withdraw and must not be pulled back directly or forcibly. If a trapped guidewire is pulled back forcibly, its shaft core may be ruptured, and the coil spring may be stretched. Therefore, before attempting to withdraw a trapped guidewire, you must first rotate it clockwise and counterclockwise several times with minimal force. Upon withdrawal of the guidewire, the microcatheter holding the wire may advance to the point of trapping. This is often unavoidable and can be rather convenient in most cases.

If the tip of the guidewire has been trapped within the tunica media, it is likely to return to the true lumen at a site 1 to 2 mm proximal to the point of trapping. Therefore, you should pull the guidewire back slightly and advance it in a new direction (Fig. 1.81). If the guidewire was in the true lumen at the entry of the CTO and it reaches the lumen distal to the occlusion without being trapped again, it will probably have crossed the occlusion through the true lumen.

However, a trapped guidewire does not always return to the true lumen at a point just proximal to the site of trapping. For example, the tip of a guidewire that has been advanced outside the media may be directed medially and then become trapped in the media (Fig. 1.82), but the interventionalist cannot distinguish this scenario from the one mentioned above. In the latter case, if the guidewire is pulled back from the point of trapping and advanced in a new direction, it will eventually return to the subintimal space and advance outside the media. This emphasizes the importance of targeting the true lumen at the entry of a CTO.

Guidewire trapping is almost the only information other than fluoroscopic images that suggests deviation from the true lumen into the media and provides the interventionalist with a chance to redirect the wire into the true lumen under fluoroscopic guidance. Tight trapping of a guidewire may result in fracture of the wire and/or intracoronary retention. If you feel even a little difficulty in advancing the guidewire when crossing a CTO, you should pull the wire back to check if it has become trapped. If it is not pulled back carefully, a guidewire that is trapped will be freed abruptly and will jump out. If there is even slight resistance when withdrawing a guidewire that may have become trapped in a lesion, you should advance a microcatheter over the wire toward the entry of the occlusion and then slowly pull the wire back while rotating it. If you try to pull back a tightly trapped guidewire while advancing a microcatheter, the catheter will often enter the lesion as far as the point where the wire is trapped and then also become trapped itself (Fig. 1.81a). In this situation, forcible withdrawal of the guidewire will lead to dissection of its tip. Instead, you should slowly pull the guidewire back while rotating it, but note that excessive rotation in one direction will lead to fragmentation of the guidewire core. Therefore, it is important to free the tip of the guidewire by performing several alternating clockwise and counterclockwise rotations (to-and-fro rotation) until unforced withdrawal becomes possible.

A guidewire that has gone outside the media without being trapped often moves smoothly. If the guidewire penetrates the media at a large angle and abruptly enters soft subintimal tissue, it tends to advance through the adventitia toward the larger curvature of a curved vessel. A guidewire taking such a course will often show an inflection point at the curve, if viewed in a lateral image. If you try to correct the direction of a guidewire that has advanced through the adventitia based on imaging in a single projection, the guidewire will remain in the adventitia and take a spiral course along the vessel wall. On CAG, the inflection point is where the guidewire begins this spiral course. If an inflection point cannot be recognized in one projection, it is often seen in another projection that is orthogonal to the first one.

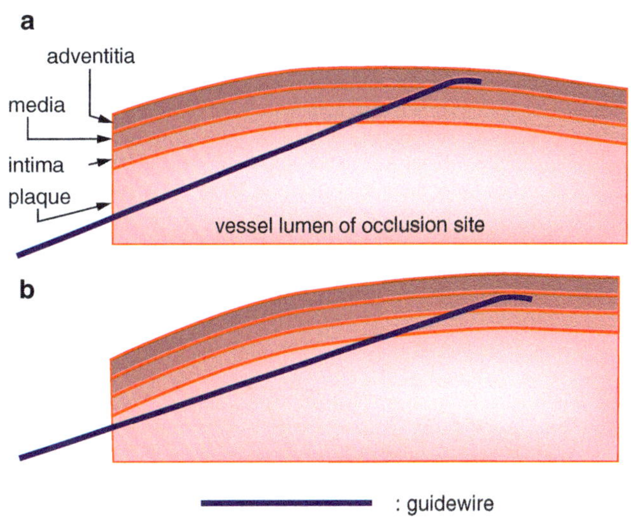

Fig. 1.80 Trapping of the guidewire tip. (**a**) A guidewire does not encounter much resistance when it crosses the media at a large angle. Once it enters the subintimal space, the guidewire can be advanced with minimal force, easily creating a dissection. (**b**) If a guidewire enters the tunica media at a small angle, it will remain within the media and will become trapped after it has been advanced for a certain (long) distance

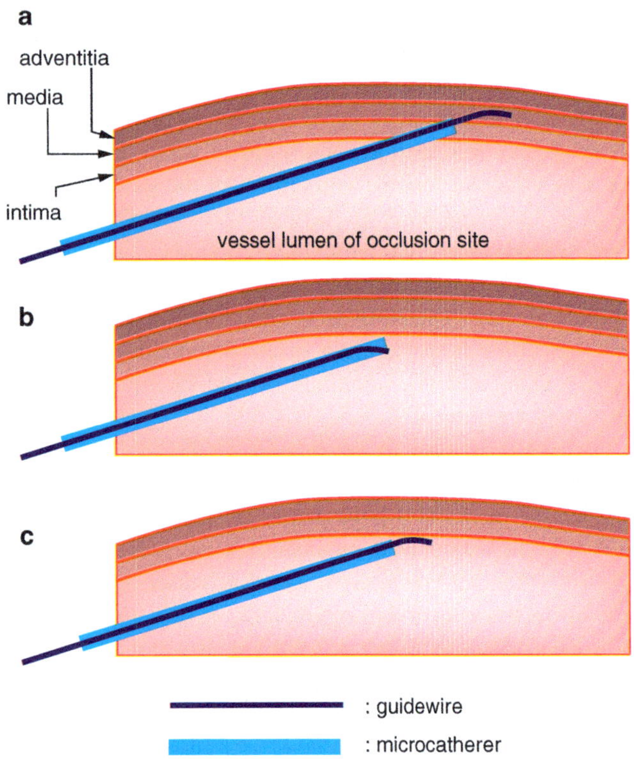

Fig. 1.81 Countermeasures for guidewire trapping. Slightly withdraw the trapped guidewire, and advance it in a new direction where trapping does not occur. (**a**) If the tip has been trapped, a guidewire is often difficult to withdraw. Efforts to withdraw the trapped guidewire will cause the microcatheter holding the wire to advance to a point at least 2 to 3 mm proximal to the guidewire tip. While keeping the microcatheter at this point, perform to-and-fro rotation of the guidewire, and attempt to pull it back slowly. It may take several minutes to withdraw a guidewire that has become tightly trapped. Never pull the trapped guidewire forcibly or rotate it excessively in one direction because this will lead to fragmentation of the shaft core and stretching of the coil spring. (**b**) After retracting the guidewire into the microcatheter, pull the wire back together with the catheter for a distance of 2 to 3 mm. The tip of the microcatheter is likely to remain in the true lumen. (**c**) While keeping the microcatheter at this point, slowly advance the tip of the guidewire, and find the direction in which the wire can cross the CTO through the true lumen without being trapped again

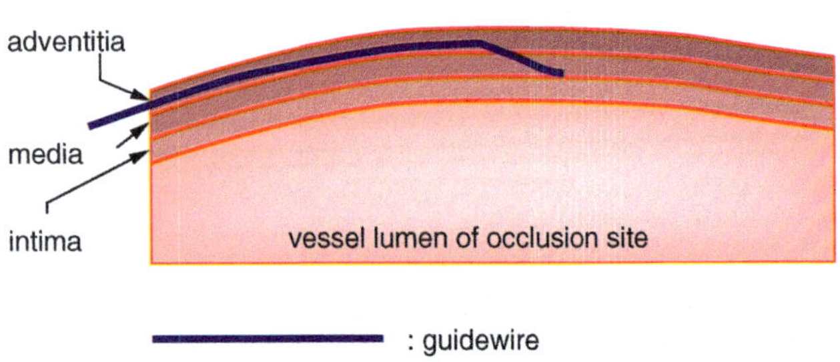

Fig. 1.82 Guidewire advanced outside the media while crossing a CTO. The guidewire can be advanced easily while creating a dissection. If the guidewire is redirected medially and enters the tunica media, its tip can become trapped

1.6.4.5 Does a Stiff Guidewire Only Advance Toward the Larger Curvature in a Curved Vessel?

Interventionalists often complain that a stiff guidewire is not very useful because it can only advance toward the larger curvature at a bend in a curved vessel. If the interventionalist is well-known, this comment is accepted as the truth and becomes a widespread belief, but it is a "myth."

In fact, a guidewire with a high tip load relative to the hardness of the occlusion and the wall of the target vessel (i.e., a guidewire with a small curve at its tip that can be advanced within the lumen or soft tissue with little force while maintaining the shape of the curve [Fig. 1.83a]) will go straight forward and then will follow the larger curvature at a bend of the vessel after being blocked by the harder adventitia. However, if the guidewire is only slightly stiffer relative to the tissue of the lesion so that its tip is deflected when blocked, the wire can take a course medial to the larger curvature at the bend of the vessel (Fig. 1.84). Of course, the guidewire has to be stiff enough to penetrate the lesion. If the guidewire does not have sufficient stiffness, its tip will deviate into the soft subintimal tissue and go toward the adventitia despite being advanced carefully. Thus, the stiffness (tip load) of a CTO crossing guidewire should be adequate to cope with the hardness of the lesion, but it should not be stiff enough to maintain the shape of its tip curve during advancement. In other words, the guidewire should have a tip load that is well balanced between penetrability and deflection. This balance largely depends on the hardness of the target occlusion. Penetration of softer tissue is more sensitive to changes in the tip load of the guidewire, while altering the tip load will have little influence if the hardness of the target lesion is above a certain threshold. In that situation, you will need to carefully manipulate the guidewire while making the best use of deflection and fixed point rotation.

Anyway, please bear in mind that the tendency of a guidewire to go straight forward does not only depend on its tip load. For this reason, if you expect the hardness of the tissue in a CTO to show significant heterogeneity, you should consider exchanging the guidewire as required to maintain the optimal tip load for each part of the occlusion. For example, if a guidewire with a relatively high tip load (e.g., a Conquest Pro 12) is needed to penetrate the very hard entry point of a CTO, but the distal segment of the occlusion is not so hard, it is safer and reasonable to exchange the guidewire for another with a lower tip load after entering the lesion. If the exit of the occlusion is hard, you may want to exchange the guidewire again for another with a higher tip load.

This is the basic concept of selecting a guidewire based on its tip load relative to the hardness of the target lesion. Now let us consider a tortuous occlusion near the origin of the RCA, in which the guidewire is likely to enter the adven-

titia at the larger curvature of the bend in the vessel. In this case, the balance between the tip load of the guidewire and the hardness of the target lesion will not solely determine the likelihood of guidewire deviation toward the larger curvature and the risk of vascular dissection. When performing PCI for a hard tortuous occlusion, as shown in Fig. 1.84, a CTO crossing guidewire with a small curve at its tip will enter the subintimal space despite every effort to achieve deflection. Once it enters the subintimal space, a guidewire with a higher tip load will create a larger subintimal dissection (Fig. 1.85), based on the assumption that a wire with a higher tip load will have a stiffer shaft. Naturally, a guidewire with a stiffer shaft will advance more laterally toward the adventitia. To penetrate the entry point of such a CTO, you should use a guidewire with a larger curve at its tip and find the optimal entry point. Optimizing the size and shape of the guidewire curve provides the key to successfully entering such a lesion. The tip of the guidewire should have a very small first curve with a small angle, and the second curve should be located about 2 mm from the first curve (see Fig. 1.75), so that the shaft is pressed against the larger curvature of the vessel wall when the tip catches a dimple at the CTO entrance (Fig. 1.84b & c). The optimum angle of the guidewire tip relative to the surface of the occlusion is slightly less than 90 degrees. As mentioned above, you should ensure the correct direction of the guidewire tip by performing biplane cineangiography and then apply fixed point rotation for successful entry into the CTO.

Employing these techniques and optimizing the curve of a stiff CTO crossing guidewire can allow it to be navigated in the appropriate direction along the curve of the target vessel.

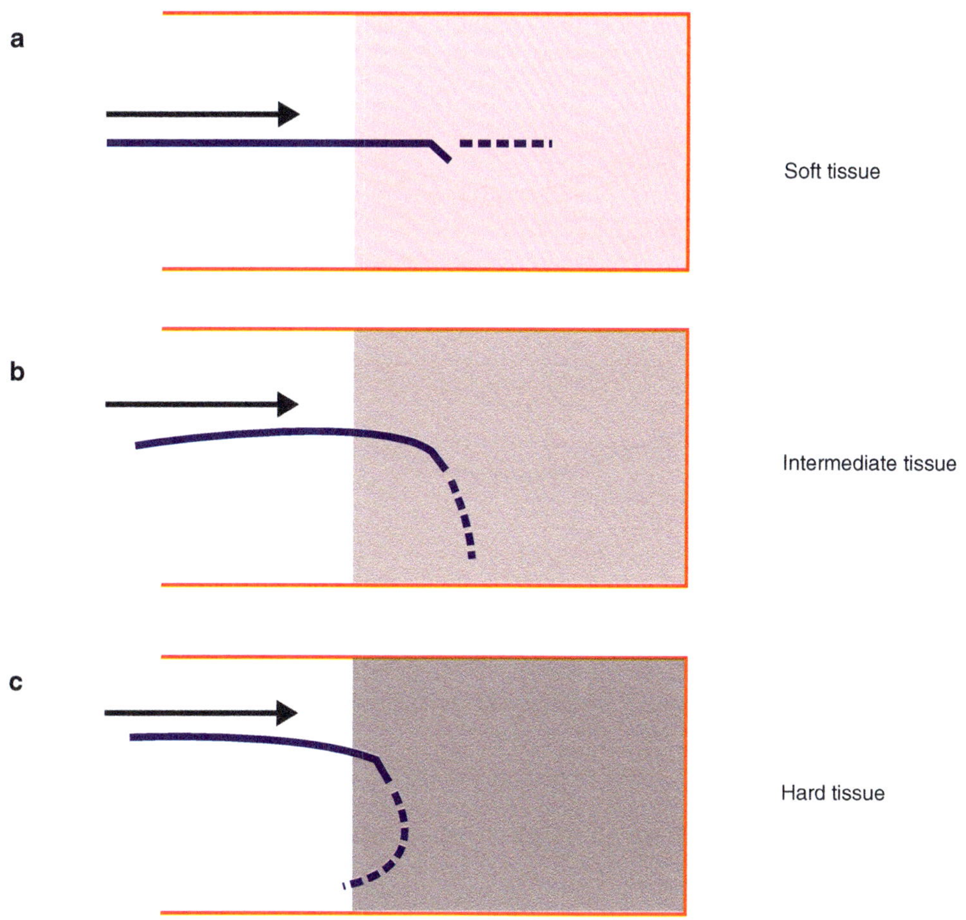

Fig. 1.83 Effect of tissue hardness on the course of the guidewire. When pushed forward without rotation into a heterogeneous occlusion, a guidewire with a small shallow curve at its tip will advance in a straight line if the tissue composing the lesion is soft (**a**). If the tissue is so hard that it prevents advancement of the guidewire after entry is achieved, the wire will curve back in the wrong direction (**c**). If the tissue is of intermediate hardness, the guidewire will show behavior between these two extremes (**b**)

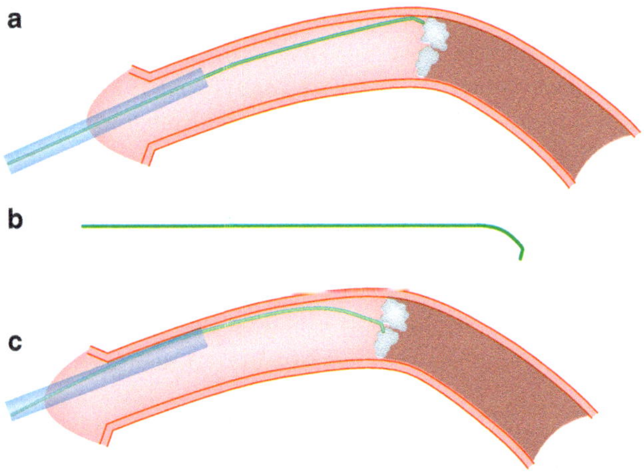

Fig. 1.84 Effect of the tip curve on the course of the guidewire. If the entry of a CTO is located at a bend in the target vessel, a guidewire with a single curve at the tip cannot reach the dimple at the entrance (**a**). If forcible penetration of the occlusion is attempted, the guidewire will inevitably be deflected outside the media. To catch the dimple at the entrance, a guidewire should be designed with second and third curves at the tip (**b**), so that the tip can reach the dimple when the shaft of the wire is running along the larger curvature of the vessel (**c**)

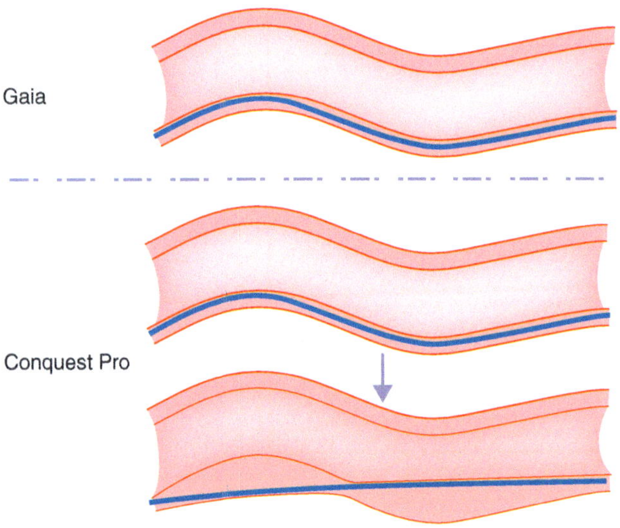

Fig. 1.85 Risk of dissection after a guidewire enters relatively soft subintimal tissue. A Gaia guidewire is less likely to cause dissection because the shaft is flexible near the tip, allowing it to follow a tortuous vessel. In contrast, the shaft of a Conquest Pro guidewire is stiff even near the tip, and this wire straightens as it is advanced, creating a large dissection. Therefore, once a Conquest Pro guidewire has entered the subintimal space of a relatively soft vessel, you would usually hesitate to retry wiring with the same guidewire because it would be expected to enlarge the dissection. If a second wire is manipulated parallel to the first wire, it is also likely to enter the subintimal space and cause narrowing of the vessel lumen distal to the occlusion, which can prevent imaging. On the other hand, a Gaia guidewire does not create a large dissection, so repeated attempts with the same wire are feasible

1.6.4.6 Straightening of the Guidewire Tip

A guidewire may gradually become uncontrollable as it is advanced through a relatively long and hard CTO. The usual reason is that the curve at the tip of the guidewire (Fig. 1.86a) has been lost because the tip has been stretched and straightened (Fig. 1.86b). It is natural for a guidewire to become difficult to control once the tip is straightened. If this problem is suspected, you should advance a microcatheter over the guidewire to an appropriate point and then withdraw the wire to check the tip. If the tip has lost its curve, you can reshape the curve or replace the guidewire with a new one. Fluoroscopy can also help to determine whether the tip of a guidewire has lost its curve. If neither biplane angiography nor multidirectional imaging can confirm a curve at the guidewire tip, or if monoplane angiography does not show rotation of the tip during rotation of the wire, it should be concluded that the curve has been lost.

As mentioned above, I used to bend the tip of a Conquest Pro guidewire with an original shaping device because it was difficult to manually produce a small curve at the tip and because a curve created manually was easily lost. However, even a curve shaped using the device can be straightened. As it is advanced and withdrawn through a very small channel that only just permits the passage of the guidewire through a hard occlusion, the curve at the tip of the wire will gradually become shallower, and the wire will eventually be straightened.

If the occlusion is relatively soft, the guidewire will retain the curve at its tip. If the tissue of the occlusion is hard enough to straighten the guidewire tip as it crosses the CTO, it is unavoidable for the curve to be straightened to some extent. Increasing the frequency of forward and backward movements of the guidewire and performing more to-and-fro rotations will increase the risk of straightening the tip.

While manipulating a guidewire, you should always be thinking about whether the tip has retained its curve or not. The following events or findings during guidewire manipulation suggest straightening of the tip: (1) loss of contact with a hard object that was previously caught by the guidewire tip, (2) loss of control of the guidewire tip and a tendency for it to go straight forward, (3) no detectable curve at the tip with imaging in two orthogonal views, and (4) failure to rotate the guidewire tip or change its direction even when rotating the torquer. If any of these events occurs, you should advance a microcatheter over the wire to an appropriate point and then withdraw the guidewire to check the shape of its tip. Fluoroscopy does not always confirm straighten-

ing of the guidewire tip. Passing the guidewire through a relatively small and hard occlusion may cause straightening of the tip, but the curve can reform if the tip has only been stretched within the limit of its deformability. Even if fluoroscopy shows that the tip of the guidewire appears to have been straightened, you may continue PCI with the same wire if you can optimize its direction through blocking by hard tissue.

If there are many risk factors for guidewire tip straightening and if the wire is trapped, there may be no good solution other than replacing it. When pushed forcibly, a guidewire with a straightened tip becomes hard to control and eventually enters the subintimal space. Under the same circumstances, a guidewire with a higher tip load is less likely to undergo straightening than a wire with a low tip load. Prompt crossing of a hard lesion without repetitive forward and backward movement of the guidewire prevents straightening of the tip. For these reasons, it is useful to replace the guidewire with a new one having a tip load one level higher.

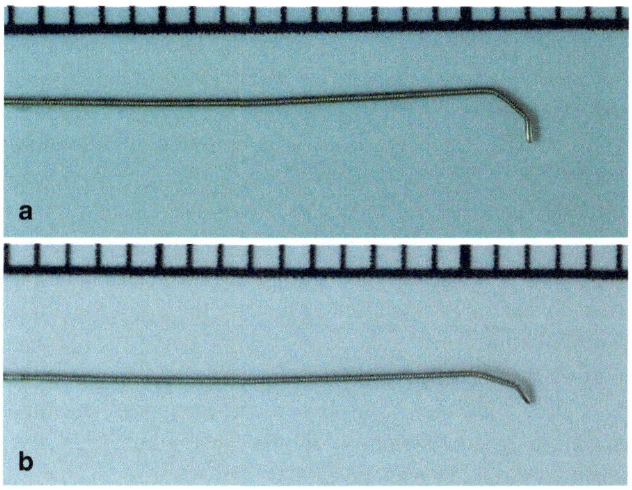

Fig. 1.86 Loss of the curve at the guidewire tip. After the tip of a guidewire has been shaped into a curve (**a**), the tip may become straightened again as it is advanced through a relatively hard lesion (**b**). If the guidewire becomes difficult to control, it should be withdrawn to check the curve at its tip

1.6.4.7 Basic Techniques for Manipulating a CTO Guidewire

A CTO guidewire can only be manipulated actively in three ways, i.e., it can be "pushed," "pulled," or "rotated." There is also one important guidewire manipulation that does not involve active movement, which is fixing the tip.

Pushing (Advancing) the Wire

The purposes of pushing a guidewire forward include (1) advancing the guidewire tip toward a distal segment of the vessel, (2) penetrating the entry point of an occlusion or penetrating hard plaque/thrombus, (3) deflecting the guidewire tip, and (4) advancing the guidewire tip to find a route that can bypass hard plaque/thrombus.

You should only advance a guidewire without rotation before it has reached the entrance of the CTO or after it has entered the vessel lumen distal to the occlusion, or with the intention of just advancing it slightly while orienting the tip medially to a bend in the target vessel (Fig. 1.87).

A guidewire can easily be advanced through the softer core of a relatively hard occlusion if you apply minimal force while performing to-and-fro rotation of the tip. This mimics the situation where a guidewire with a soft tip can easily pass through a non-occluded vessel while avoiding plaques on the walls if it is advanced with to-and-fro rotation. If the guidewire is blocked by hard plaque on the vessel wall, continuous rotation of the tip helps to return the wire to the lumen (soft core) and allows it to be advanced with little force.

Of course, many CTOs do not have a soft core due to the mechanism underlying formation of the occlusion. A guidewire may be able to cross a short CTO that lacks a soft core if it is advanced in the right direction. However, many CTOs are long, and their precise anatomy cannot be determined. To cross such occlusions, the guidewire should be advanced with minimal force when its tip is oriented in the desired direction while continuously performing to-and-fro rotation of the tip ("plane rotation"; see "Rotation" in this subsection).

Pulling the Wire

The guidewire is pulled back in preparation for the next manipulation (i.e., pushing), and this may be done for two purposes. One is to withdraw the guidewire and change the position of its tip (Fig. 1.88a), while the other is to reduce stress on the tip without moving it in order to eliminate or attenuate deflection (Fig. 1.88b).

A guidewire is withdrawn if its tip has entered the subintimal space. In this situation, the guidewire should be withdrawn to the point just before it entered the subintimal space, and exploration should be performed to find a new direction for the wire. When the tip of the guidewire is blocked by hard tissue in the occlusion, you should push the tip forward slightly to check whether it can be advanced. The tip of the guidewire will be deflected by hard tissue and will be deflected further when the wire is pushed forward. If the guidewire will not advance any further, you should just pull back on it slightly while keeping the tip at the same position to lessen its deflection. Then you should redirect the guidewire with minimal force at an angle within 90 degrees of the desired direction while performing slow to-and-fro rotation to find a route that can bypass the hard tissue in the occlusion.

Fixing the Tip

If the guidewire is blocked by hard tissue in the lesion and it enters a side branch or the subintimal space when advanced, you should fix the tip at the point where it was blocked and push the wire forward slightly with the tip oriented in the desired direction. The guidewire should be rotated within ±90 degrees of the right direction. It is important to keep the tip at the point of obstruction while pushing and rotating the wire (fixed point rotation; see "Rotation"). In both of the situations illustrated in Fig. 1.89, the guidewire is blocked by hard tissue in the lesion and deviates rightward into the subintimal space or a side branch. If you feel the guidewire tip change direction after being blocked by hard tissue in the occlusion, you should rotate the wire within ±90 degrees in the opposite direction with the tip fixed at the point of obstruction (see "Rotation"). This manipulation is aimed at increasing the penetration force of the guidewire (so as to cross the lesion without pushing the wire) and finding the direction in which the wire can easily be advanced. If the guidewire slips to the right and its tip cannot be oriented to the left, you may increase the angles of the first and second curves at the tip to enhance its ability to remain at the point, but it is better to exchange the wire for another with a higher tip load. A guidewire with a higher tip load can be expected to cross the hard part of the occlusion when advanced with a force that is not strong enough to deflect its tip.

Rotation

The tip of the guidewire can be rotated by rotating the attached torque device. It should be noted that rotation of the guidewire tip includes fixed point rotation (rotation of the extreme tip; Figure 1.90a) or plane rotation (rotation of the entire first or second curve at the tip; Figure 1.90b). For example, fixed point rotation is performed when attempting to catch a dimple and penetrate the CTO entry point, while rotating a guidewire within a soft lesion is plane rotation. In practice, the interventionalist can advance a guidewire by making optimum use of these maneuvers as appropriate. If the target CTO is a soft occlusion surrounded by hard fibrosed/calcified tissue, you should intentionally employ plane rotation of the guidewire to ensure safe crossing of the lesion with minimal force. If the CTO is a soft occlusion surrounded by soft tissue, a guidewire that is not advanced in the correct direction is likely to enter the subintimal space, so you should rotate the guidewire within ±90 degrees to obtain the effect of fixed point rotation.

Rotating a guidewire in a lesion composed of somewhat harder tissue than its tip will generate stronger fixed point rotation. This can be understood from the fact that even a guidewire with a high tip load (stiff tip), such as a Conquest Pro, can lose its tip curve while being advanced through a long hard occlusion. As mentioned above, if the tip of the guidewire is straightened (especially the first curve), it becomes impossible to change direction within the occlusion, and the wire should therefore be reshaped with an appropriate curve at the tip. If straightening of the reshaped guidewire occurs easily, it should be exchanged for a new wire.

I would like to re-emphasize here that a CTO crossing guidewire must not only be rotated in a single direction. As mentioned above, to-and-fro rotation is important, so if five clockwise rotations have been performed, the guidewire must then be given five counterclockwise rotations. If a guidewire is rotated too much in a single direction, it will easily be damaged when its tip becomes trapped. With regard to withdrawing a guidewire after its tip has been trapped, please refer to 1.9: "Troubleshooting."

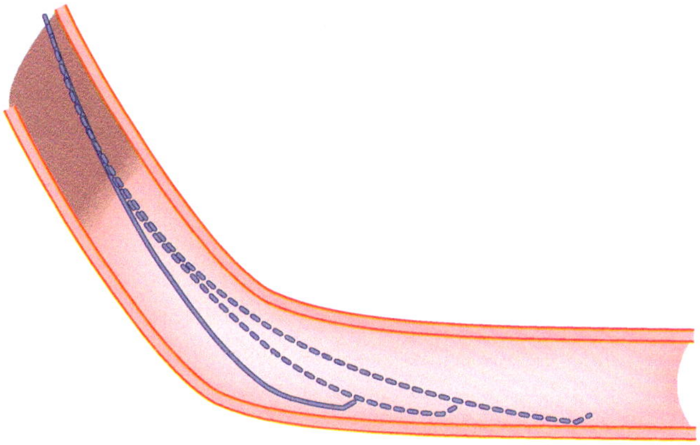

Fig. 1.87 When the guidewire reaches the vessel lumen distal to the occlusion. You should advance the guidewire into the distal lumen with very little force (feather touch) and without rotating it while orienting the tip toward the smaller curvature of the vessel. If the guidewire is within the true lumen and there is no distal stenosis, it will go forward without deflection of the tip. However, the tip will be deflected if the guidewire enters the subintimal space or is blocked by something hard

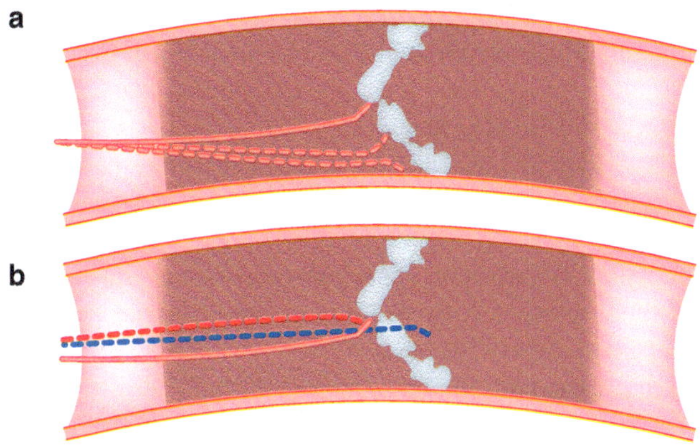

Fig. 1.89 Deviation of a blocked guidewire into the subintimal space. (**a**) When pushed forward at the point of blockage by hard tissue in the lesion (solid line), the guidewire deviates downward (dotted line) and eventually enters the subintimal space. (**b**) The direction of the guidewire tip should be changed (but not its position) and the wire should be rotated within ±90 degrees (fixed point rotation; red dotted line) to find a route that can bypass the hard tissue in the occlusion, until the guidewire can be advanced further (blue dotted line)

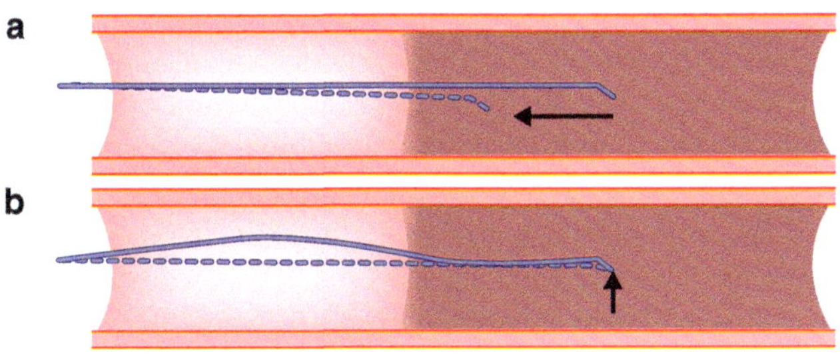

Fig. 1.88 Pulling the guidewire back. (**a**) Withdrawing a guidewire that has entered an occlusion (arrow) to change the position of its tip. (**b**) Pulling back a guidewire that has entered an occlusion without changing the position of its tip to reduce or eliminate deflection

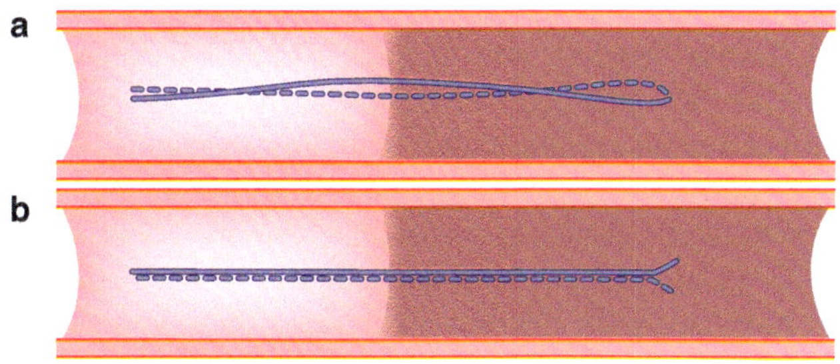

Fig. 1.90 Fixed point rotation versus plane rotation. (**a**) Fixed point rotation means rotation of the guidewire while its tip is fixed at a certain point. Because of fixing the tip, the shaft is deflected during rotation (dashed line). However, the tip will not remain fixed at a single point if rotation of the guidewire is too vigorous and the arc is too large. (**b**) Plane rotation means rotation of the guidewire tip while the shaft is not deflected along its axis. Such rotation may be relatively vigorous, consisting of several alternating clockwise and counterclockwise rotations

1.6.4.8 Selection and Manipulation of Guidewires in Various Situations

Role of the First Guidewire

In antegrade PCI for CTO, the first guidewire has the following two roles:

To Allow Advancement of a Microcatheter to the Entry of the Occlusion Without Injuring the Proximal Coronary Artery Segment

If there is a long distance from the ostium of a coronary artery to the entry of the CTO, a tapered guidewire with a tip load equal to or greater than that of a Gaia First wire may inadvertently penetrate the intima and enter the subintimal space.

At the ostium of the RCA, it may not be possible for the guiding catheter to be engaged coaxially with the artery. If a guidewire with a stiff tip is advanced carelessly into the RCA through the guiding catheter in this situation, there is a high risk of causing dissection. When advancing a guidewire into the RCA ostium from a guiding catheter, you should very slowly move the tip of the guidewire forward with minimal force while checking the position and shape of the guidewire tip in the LAO projection or any other view that allows visualization of the ostium along its longitudinal axis. If the guidewire enters the RCA without resistance, you may then follow the standard procedure for manipulation. If the guidewire is blocked by the vessel wall at the ostium, you should never try to advance it forcibly, but instead undertake the following procedures: (1) withdraw the guidewire and try to advance it into the RCA from the guiding catheter via another route, or (2) change the orientation of the tip of the guiding catheter by to-and-fro rotation and other movements, and then try to advance the guidewire through the catheter again.

For the latter maneuver, it is better to use a guidewire with a soft tip to ensure safe advancement to the entrance of the occlusion, while a tapered CTO crossing guidewire with a high tip load is absolutely unsuitable. Accordingly, I use a 0.014-inch soft-tipped guidewire.

Exploration for Microchannels That May Exist in an Occlusion

Even if bilateral angiography fails to visualize microchannels in a CTO, the possibility of the existence of such channels cannot be completely ruled out. A tapered guidewire is suitable when exploring for microchannels. The guidewire does not need a stiff tip to track a microchannel. However, it requires a tip with good shape memory because it often has to pass through tortuous channels and be steered exquisitely in the right direction.

To perform these functions, a guidewire needs to meet the following criteria: (1) a tapered tip, (2) a low tip load, (3) a tip with good shape memory, and (4) good slipperiness. I usually choose an XT-R guidewire for this purpose, while other similar guidewires include the XT-A and Wizard 78. You might think that a guidewire with a stiffer tip is more effective for tracking a tortuous channel. However, after failing to isolate the microchannel with an XT-R guidewire, I always replace it with a Gaia or another crossing guidewire because I think a crossing guidewire is needed to track a channel that cannot be followed by the XT-R.

Even if it is invisible, a microchannel should connect with the distal true lumen to perfuse the peripheral myocardium. If advancement of an XT-R guidewire through a microchannel is blocked, this suggests that the channel may be very tortuous, that it may branch into even smaller channels, or that it may not be a true microchannel. In all of these circumstances, a crossing guidewire will be needed to track the microchannel.

I also think that attempting to pass a Gaia First guidewire through a microchannel in a CTO is not associated with a significant risk of subintimal tracking.

Non-tapered Guidewire with a Soft Tip

To navigate a microcatheter up to an occlusion with no detectable microchannels, you should use a non-tapered guidewire with a soft tip. This guidewire should only be used to bring the microcatheter as far as the entry of the occlusion and not to cross it. A non-tapered guidewire with a soft tip should also be used if dissection might be caused by advancing a tapered guidewire into the coronary artery (e.g., RCA) through a guiding catheter that is not coaxial with the ostium.

Column 7 Author's Selection and Rationale: Part 1

[Non-tapered guidewire with a soft tip]

If I need a non-tapered guidewire with a soft tip, I choose one with a tip load of no more than 1.0 g and without a hydrophilic polymer jacket. This is because such a guidewire can be retained in the lumen after it crosses the lesion with little risk of causing coronary perforation. To minimize the risk of perforation, a guidewire with as low a tip load as possible is preferred at the cost of slightly less slipperiness.

To facilitate delivery of devices after crossing the CTO, a guidewire with a shaft that provides relatively strong support is preferable. If delivery of multiple devices will be required (e.g., stenting with the kissing balloon technique or culotte stenting for multiple bifurcation lesions), a guidewire with a tip that has good shape memory and easily regains its curve(s) is preferred.

[First guidewire in antegrade PCI for CTO]

To perform antegrade PCI for CTO, I currently choose the XT-R first and not the XT-A. This is because the XT-R meets the abovementioned requirements and is suitable for both exploration and for tracking a microchannel. It would also be reasonable to choose the XT-A as the first guidewire because it can be used to expand and track a small microchannel that cannot be crossed by the XT-R.

As I always try to perform "non-pushing PCI" to prevent subintimal wire entry or tracking, I prefer to minimize the force exerted on the guidewire when crossing an occlusion. For this reason, I choose the XT-R initially and then the Gaia First.

Manipulation at the CTO Entry

Selection and manipulation of a guidewire for penetrating the entry point of a CTO will depend on the pattern of occlusion, the expected hardness of the lesion, and the expected ease of catching a dimple. For example, if you expect a soft tapered-type occlusion, there is no need to seek for a dimple. You should advance a tapered guidewire with a soft tip (e.g., an XT-R or Wizard 78) while performing to-and-fro rotation. Push the guidewire into the occlusion slightly when its tip is oriented in the direction of the expected course of the vessel. If resistance to the guidewire increases (and there is fluoroscopic evidence of blocking of the guidewire tip), you should withdraw the wire for a distance of several millimeters or just pull it back and change the direction of the tip. Then you should move the guidewire forward again while exploring for a route along which it can be advanced with minimal force.

If the CTO entry is located at the ostium of a main branch (or a side branch), the diameter of the proximal segment of the main branch (main trunk), the branching angle, and the hardness of the entry point will all influence the optimal shape of the guidewire tip and the method of manipulating the wire.

However, the general principle is to create a curve at the guidewire tip that keeps the tip coaxial with the ostium of the occluded vessel and rotate the wire within ±90 degrees while the tip is fixed at a dimple (fixed point rotation) until it starts to advance (Fig. 1.91). If the tip of the guidewire deviates into a side branch without prolapsing, a more acute tip curve is required. If the tip of the guidewire prolapses, the curve should be made less acute (Fig. 1.92). If the guidewire tip is still unable to catch the dimple after the curve has been modified in this way, you should exchange the guidewire for one with a higher tip load. Then the new guidewire is manipulated in the same manner.

For example, when performing PCI for an LAD ostial occlusion, the optimum guiding catheter is a short-tipped Judkins catheter (see 1.3. "Guiding Catheter"). You should previously introduce a floppy guidewire into the LCX to ensure prompt countermeasures against insufficient LCX perfusion resulting from unexpected injury of the LMT or LCX ostium by the guidewire, to facilitate IVUS-guided PCI, and to permit use of the Crusade microcatheter. You should then seek for a dimple at the entrance by using a guidewire with a staggered curve at the tip (see Fig. 1.75). The curve should be designed so that the tip becomes coaxial with the longitudinal axis of the LAD ostium when it catches a dimple (Fig. 1.93). After the tip of the guidewire has caught the dimple, you should rotate the wire within ±90 degrees while its tip is fixed at the dimple (fixed point rotation) to penetrate the entrance of the CTO. After successful penetration, you should advance the guidewire for a short distance in the direction of the longitudinal axis of the LAD while maintaining the large curve at its tip. This will require a little patience. To ensure that the guidewire is advanced in the same direction as the longitudinal axis of the LAD, you should keep the tip almost coaxial with the LAD by fixed point rotation and alternately advance and withdraw the wire to control deflection. Since the guidewire tip is likely to become straightened while crossing the CTO, you should advance the guidewire slowly so that its markedly curved tip stretches out gradually (Fig. 1.94). After confirming by IVUS that the guidewire has been advanced within the true lumen and that a microcatheter advanced over the guidewire will reliably penetrate the

CTO entry point, it is reasonable to exchange the wire for one with a lower tip load and a regular tip curve (Fig. 1.95).

When performing PCI for an LCX ostial occlusion, the optimum guiding catheter is the EBU (Voda) or a similar catheter (see 1.3. "Guiding Catheter"). Basically, you should try to penetrate the CTO entry point by the same procedure as that employed for an LAD ostial occlusion. If the LCX branches at an acute angle, the guidewire can easily prolapse into the LAD (Fig. 1.96a). You should make efforts to prevent guidewire prolapse, such as pulling up the guiding catheter so that it is easier to keep the guidewire coaxial with the LCX and advancing a microcatheter over the guidewire to the LCX ostium (Fig. 1.96b & c). Using a Crusade microcatheter may also be helpful for preventing guidewire prolapse (Fig. 1.96d).

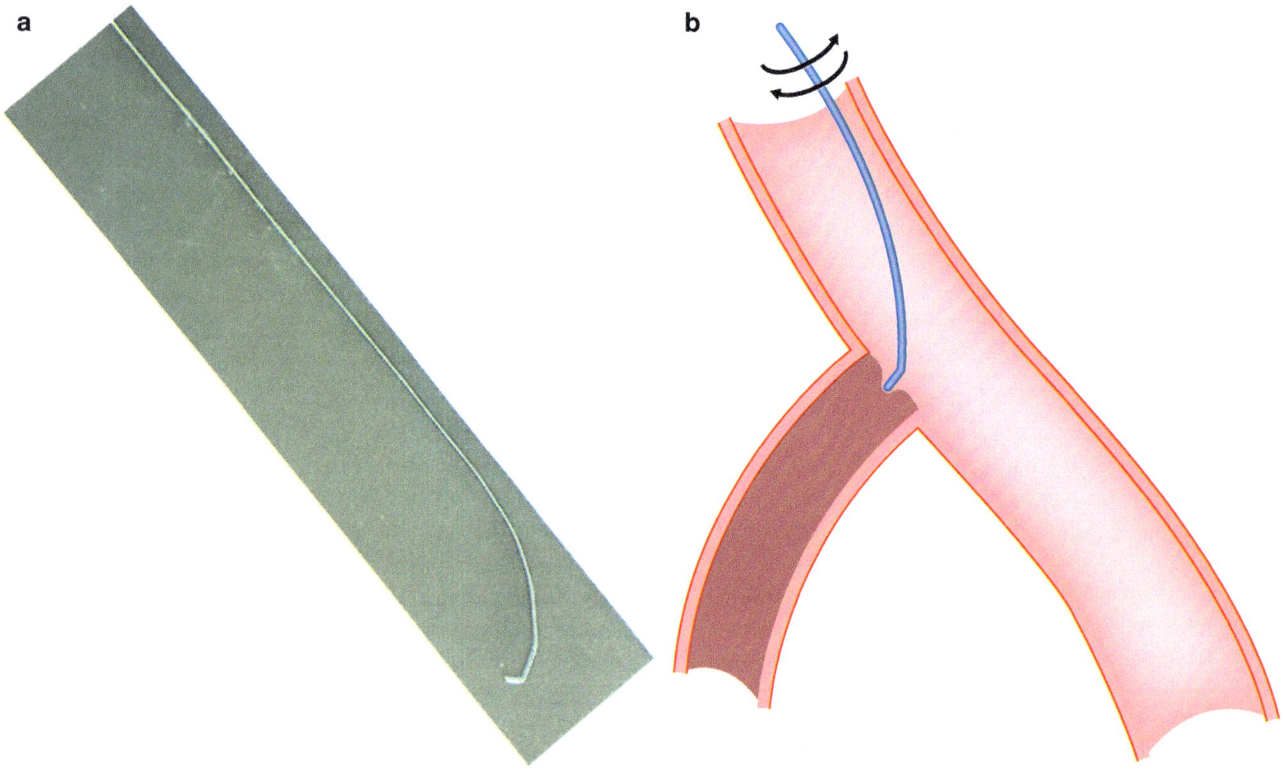

Fig. 1.91 CTO entry at the ostium of a branch. The curve at the guidewire tip should be shaped so that the tip is oriented in the direction of the occluded branch (**a**). Then the guidewire should be used to catch a dimple and should be rotated while keeping the tip concentric with the occlusion (fixed point rotation) until penetration of the CTO entry is achieved (**b**)

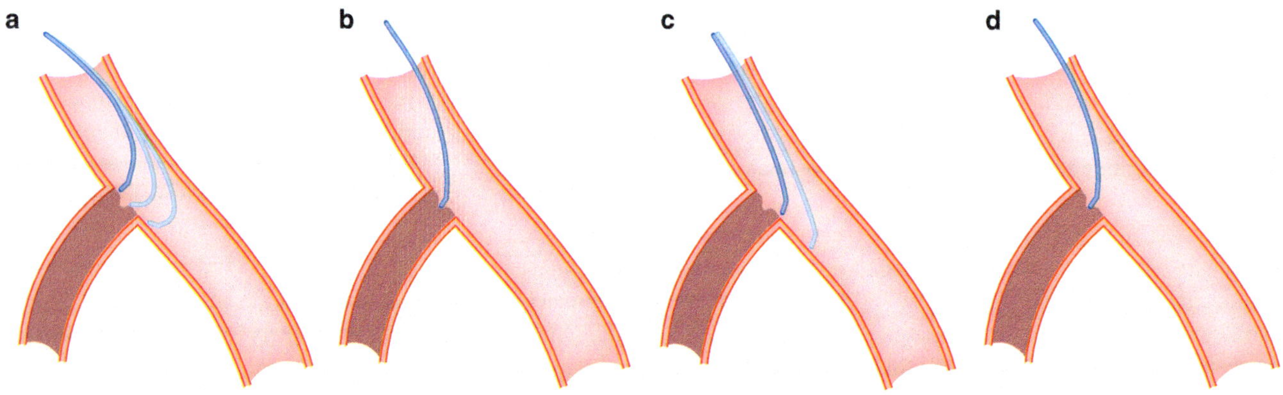

Fig. 1.92 Optimum guidewire tip shape for a bifurcation occlusion. (**a**) If the guidewire catches a dimple but then prolapses into the non-occluded branch when pushed with minimal force, the tip curve is too large and its angle is too acute. (**b**) The tip curve should be reshaped to a less acute angle so that the guidewire shaft is supported by the vessel wall contralateral to the bifurcation when the tip catches a dimple and so that the tip is perpendicular to the non-occluded branch (concentric with the occluded branch) when pushed in slightly. (**c**) If the guidewire fails to reach a dimple or slips into the non-occluded branch after catching a dimple, the tip curve is too small. (**d**) The tip curve of the guidewire should be enlarged so that the shaft and tip take the positions described in b

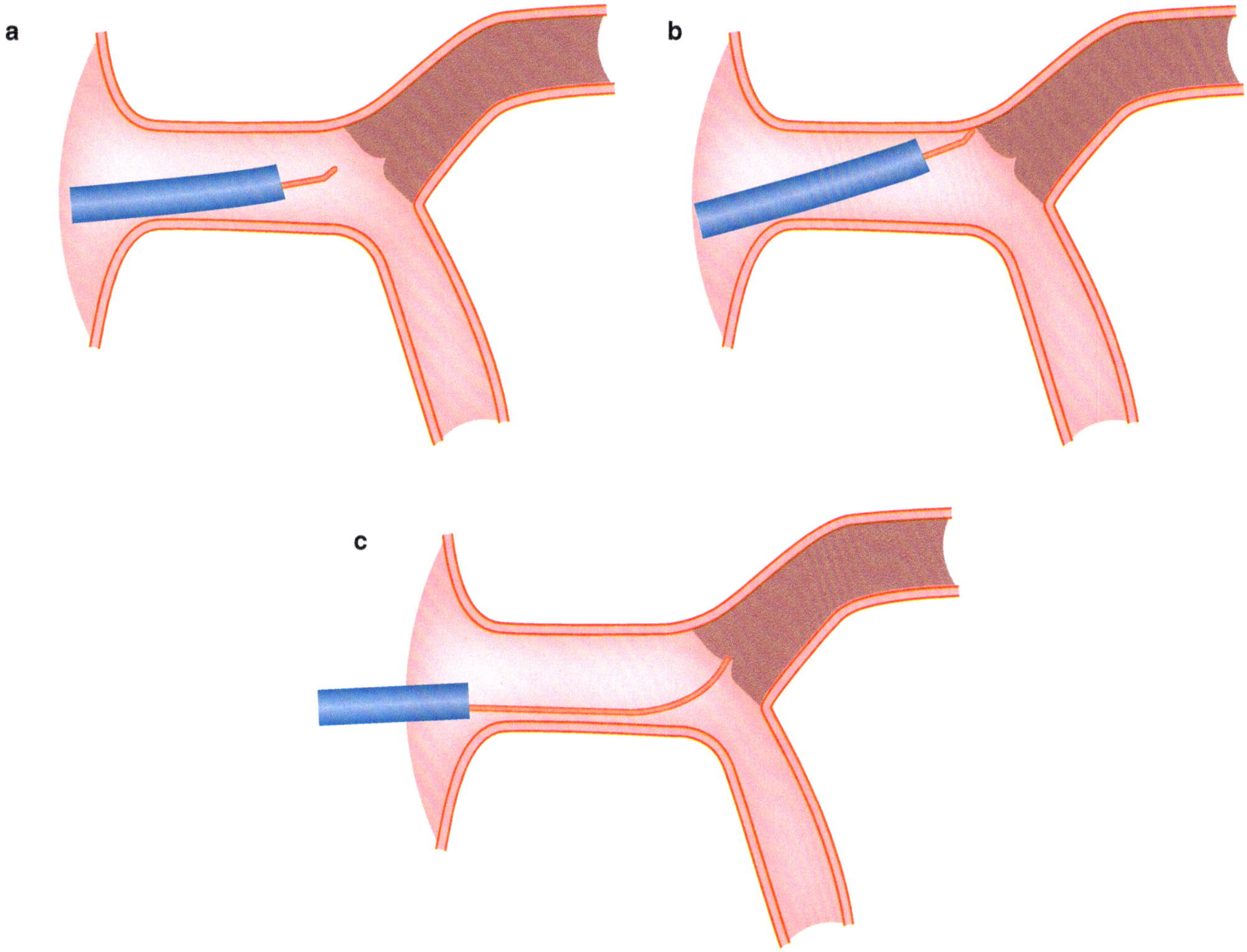

Fig. 1.93 Approach to an LAD ostial occlusion. (**a**) When performing PCI for an LAD ostial occlusion, the tip curve of the guidewire should be shaped so that the shaft is supported by the contralateral LMT wall and the tip is coaxial with the occluded branch (LAD). This may be difficult if the LMT is too short. (**b**) It is better not to bring the tip of the guiding catheter too close to the occlusion because the catheter is not always coaxial with the LAD ostium. (**c**) If the LMT is too short to maintain some distance between the guiding catheter and the LAD ostium, but has a sufficiently large diameter, the tip curve of the guidewire needs to be large with an acute angle. That is, the guidewire tip has to be curved more acutely than the angle of the LAD ostial axis

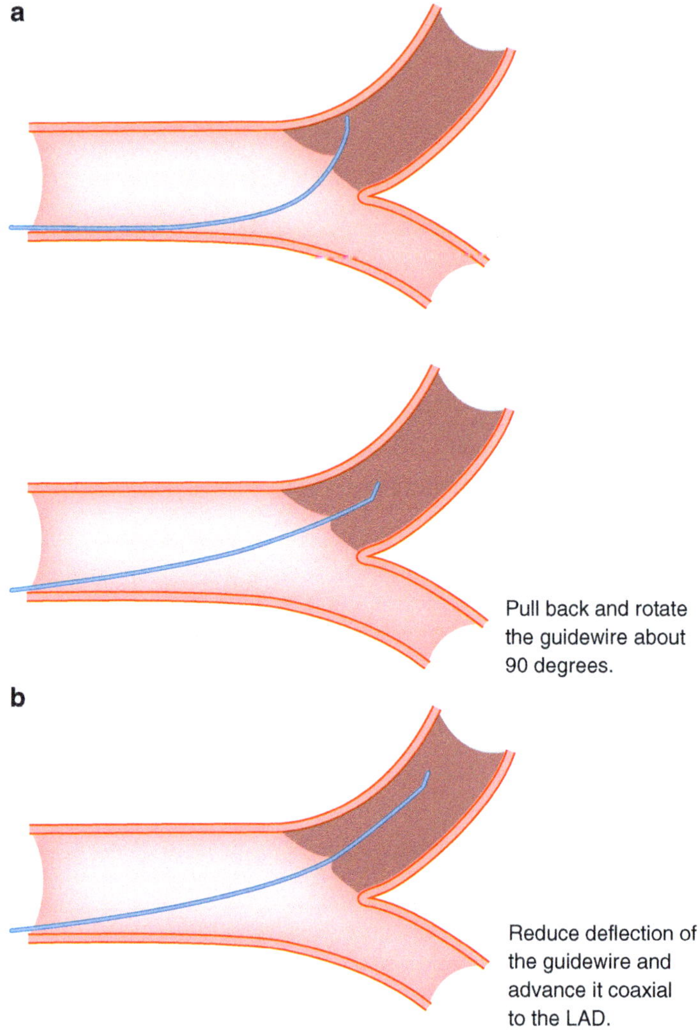

Fig. 1.94 Achieving guidewire coaxiality. (**a**) After penetrating the entry point to the CTO, a guidewire that is not coaxial with the LAD ostium may go upward at the first large bend. If this happens, you can try to correct the guidewire direction by fixed point rotation, but such attempts are not always successful. (**b**) Since the guidewire tip will gradually straighten over time, you should withdraw the wire to a point just distal to the CTO entry and redirect it. The guidewire is then more likely to advance into the LAD while remaining coaxial with the vessel

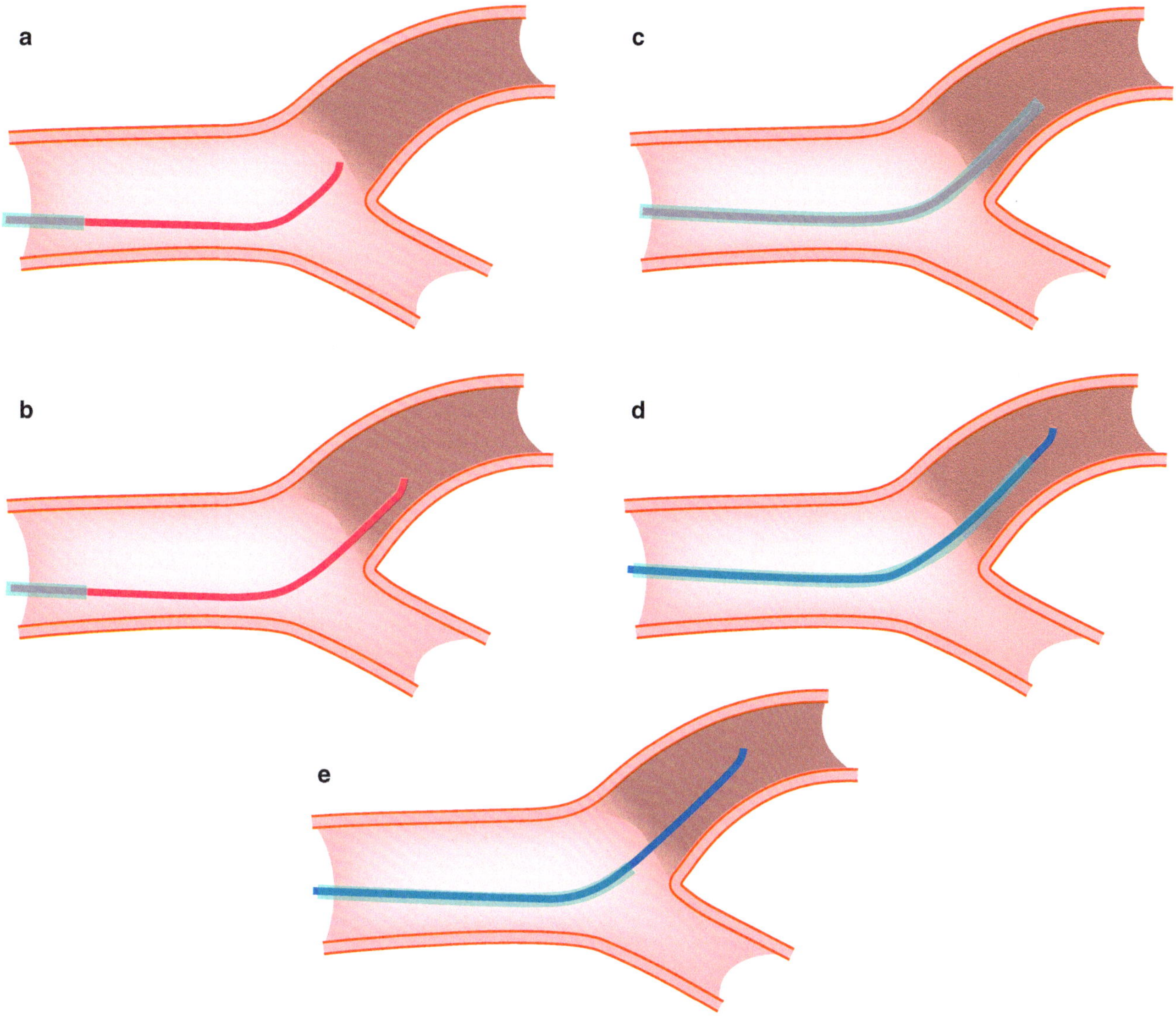

Fig. 1.95 Advancing a guidewire into a bifurcation occlusion. If the proximal cap is hard and the CTO entry point is located at an acute bend, a guidewire with a high tip load will often be needed to penetrate the cap (**a**). After the guidewire has entered the CTO (**b**), a microcatheter is advanced over the guidewire (**c**), and then the guidewire is exchanged for one with a lower tip load and a smaller curve at the tip (**d** & **e**)

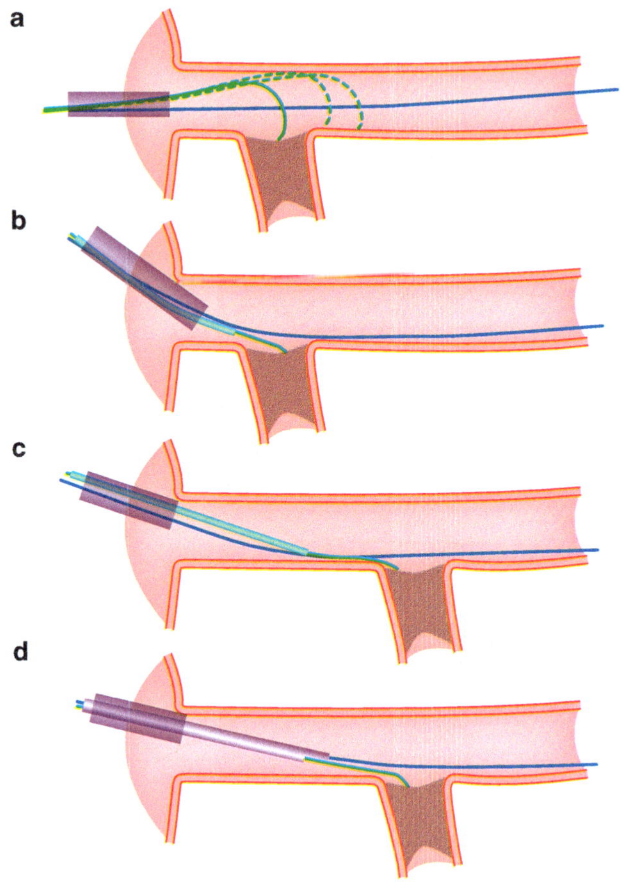

Fig. 1.96 Approach to an LCX ostial occlusion. (**a**) A suitable guidewire for an LCX ostial occlusion must have a large acute curve at its tip because the LCX branches at an acute angle. It is easy for the guidewire to prolapse into the LAD, which has a larger diameter than the LCX. (**b**, **c**) The guiding catheter should be pulled back and its tip oriented downward so that even a guidewire with a small tip curve can catch a dimple and be pushed in with minimal force. A microcatheter may also be advanced over the guidewire to the CTO entry (c). (**d**) A Crusade microcatheter may facilitate advancement of the guidewire into an LCX ostial occlusion

Manipulation Within the Occlusion

When manipulating a guidewire within an occlusion, you should appropriately utilize one or more of the four basic manipulation techniques described in the previous subsection (page 57) according to the status of the lesion. If the CTO is short (10 mm or less), you can easily estimate the correct direction for the guidewire. Therefore, the main method of manipulation is rotating the guidewire within ±90 degrees while advancing it in the desired direction.

This discussion will be focused on manipulating a guidewire in longer occlusions ranging from ≥20 mm to >10 cm. First, consider a CTO such as that shown in Fig. 1.97. A relatively radiolucent lesion is sandwiched by two clusters of calcification along the coronary artery wall. This suggests that the target vessel may have almost circumferential calcified plaque and that complete occlusion was caused by thrombosis of the central lumen (Fig. 1.98). In such an occlusion, a guidewire can track the true lumen if it is advanced with to-and-fro rotation (plane rotation) after entering the soft central tissue of the lesion. However, the guidewire may deviate toward a side branch or toward the adventitia if it comes into contact with calcified plaque or may deviate after it enters preexisting soft plaque (Fig. 1.99a). If this occurs, you should pull the guidewire back and correct the direction of the tip while rotating it within ±90 degrees, after which you can advance the guidewire in the desired direction (Fig. 1.99b & c).

The guidewire should also be manipulated in this way if the CTO is composed of hard plaque with a soft central core, even if there is no obvious calcification. How can you determine whether the target occlusion has a central core that is softer than the plaque on the vessel wall? This type of occlusion is predicted by detection of heterogeneous calcification on CAG and by the presumed CTO being associated with tapering of the coronary artery to some extent (see Fig. 1.44).

If the CTO does not have these features, it is difficult to determine from CAG findings whether it has a relatively soft central core or whether the entire vessel lumen is filled with homogenous tissue (see Fig. 1.43). If the homogeneous tissue forming the occlusion is softer than the vessel wall, you may be able to achieve intraluminal tracking with a guidewire by rotating the tip to-and-fro (plane rotation). However, if the homogeneous intraluminal tissue is harder than the vessel wall, it may often be impossible to prevent guidewire deviation into the subintimal space. Subintimal tracking is often unavoidable when PCI is performed for a long occlusion without any landmarks. If the guidewire has deviated into the subintimal space, you should use the parallel wire technique or seesaw technique to search for a different route so that the first guidewire or another wire can enter the true lumen and follow it. In this situation, you should rotate the guidewire within ±90 degrees (exploratory fixed point rotation) to determine whether it can be advanced along the predicted path of the lumen. If the guidewire begins to advance in this direction, you should perform to-and-fro rotation (plane rotation) to identify a route by which it can continue to cross the occlusion.

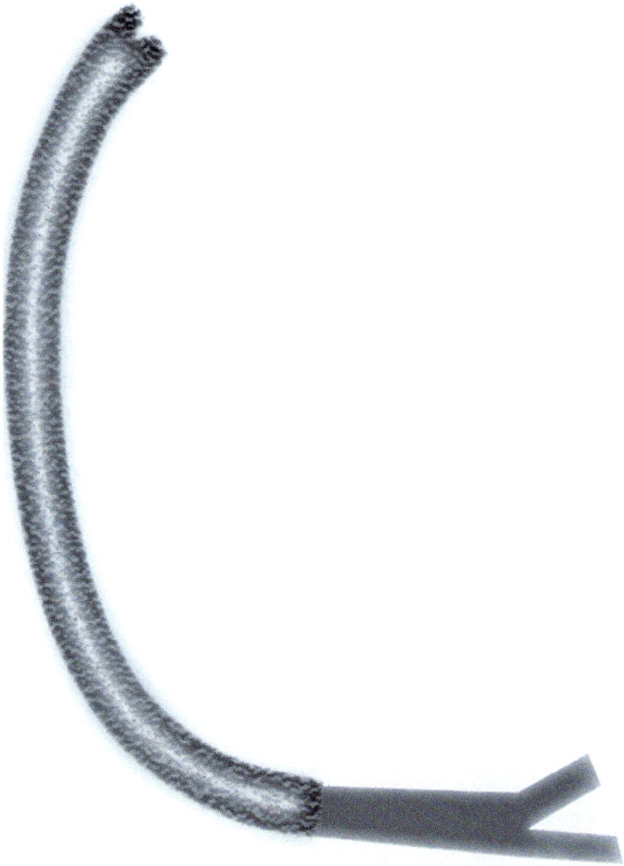

Fig. 1.97 Handling a long occlusion. Illustration of a long, partially calcified occlusion from a stationary cineangiographic image. A long occlusion may have a relatively radiolucent central core sandwiched between calcification along the vessel walls. The distal segment is filled here to show how it appears on an angiogram

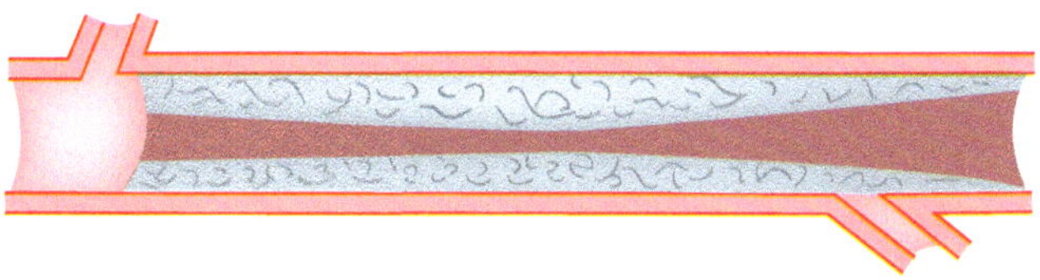

Fig. 1.98 CTO resulting from luminal occlusion at a site of chronic stenosis due to calcified plaque. At a site of chronic stenosis, the residual central lumen may become occluded, and old plaques may develop calcification

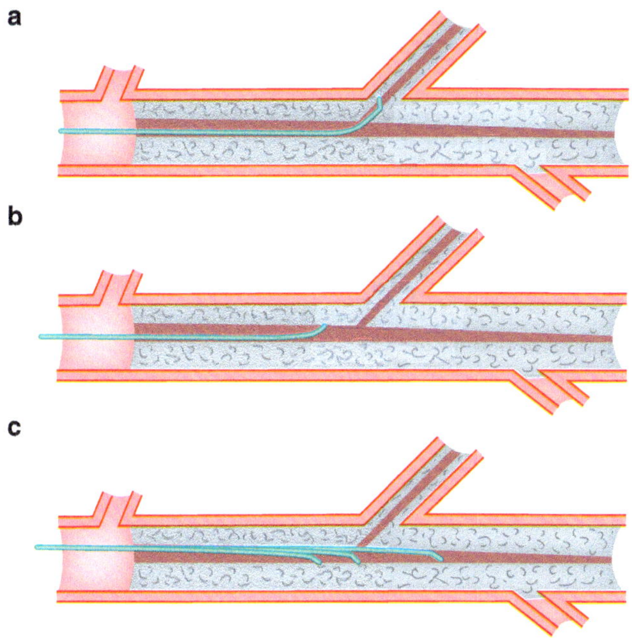

Fig. 1.99 Deviation of the guidewire from the central core of a calcified lesion toward the vessel wall (adventitia). The guidewire may deviate toward a side branch (**a**) or toward the adventitia when an occlusion is formed from a mosaic of calcified plaque, fibrous plaque, and soft plaque. If deviation of the guidewire is suspected, the wire should be withdrawn to a point just proximal to the site of branching (**b**), and its tip should be oriented in the opposite direction to that of the branch vessel. Then fixed point rotation of the guidewire should be performed until it passes the branching point, after which the wire is subsequently advanced with plane rotation (**c**)

Desired Direction of the Guidewire

A tapered guidewire will usually advance straight across a CTO, although it will sometimes bend, probably following the course of the target vessel. How the distal part of the guidewire (including the tip) bends will depend on the stiffness of the shaft at the tip, the tortuosity of the target vessel, the extent of curvature of the microchannel, soft central core, and the hardness of plaque within the occlusion.

As a representative guidewire with a soft and tapered tip, the XT-R may strictly follow a tortuous channel (Fig. 1.100a) because of its flexible tip. When advanced through thrombus that has not yet organized completely, the XT-R may thread its way among relatively hard sections of the thrombus and the vessel wall. Advancing the guidewire through soft thrombus is very similar to subintimal tracking. The tip of the guidewire will be bent at many points as it passes through the occlusion, whereas the curve will be stretched out (flattened) after the stiff shaft of the wire enters the lesion.

A guidewire with a higher tip load and a stiffer shaft is less likely to undergo bending at many points during passage through the common types of occlusions, so multiple bends are unlikely to develop with the Gaia Second wire, Gaia Third wire, and Conquest Pro series.

Even if multiple bends do not occur, the guidewire may still develop an abrupt bend or change direction. I call the point where the radius of curvature of the guidewire changes abruptly the "inflection point." Please note that use of the term "inflection point" here is different from that in mathematics. Why can an inflection point develop even if the guidewire has a stiff shaft that can flatten its curved tip? This may be explained as follows: (1) the route through the occlusion may be hard and tortuous enough to overcome the tendency of the guidewire to straighten its curved tip (Fig. 1.101a); (2) the guidewire may have deviated from the true lumen into the subintimal space (Fig. 1.101b); or (3) the guidewire may be constrained as it advances through the subintimal space since the subintimal route follows the vessel wall (Fig. 1.101c).

Thus, the formation of an inflection point is a multifactorial process and does not always suggest that the guidewire has entered the subintimal space. Conversely, a guidewire that deviates into the subintimal space does not always display an inflection point. However, if the tip of the guidewire is in the subintimal space near the exit of an occlusion and if cineangiography performed in multiple projections (usually two orthogonal projections) detects an inflection point in one projection, it is reasonable to think that the guidewire has entered the subintimal space at that point (Fig. 1.102a). If the guidewire is withdrawn to that point (Fig. 1.102b) and then slowly advanced in the opposite direction to the inflection (Fig. 1.102c), after which it becomes blocked and cannot go forward, it is reasonable to conjecture that hard tissue at this location has caused the wire to deviate into the subintimal space from the true lumen. Accordingly, the guidewire tip should be navigated in an appropriate direction while performing exploratory fixed point rotation so that it either penetrates or bypasses the hard region of the occlusion (Fig. 1.102d). If the guidewire is still blocked by hard tissue and deviates toward the subintimal space despite exploratory fixed point rotation (Fig. 1.103a), effective measures can include reshaping the tip of the wire to create a more acute curve (for a CTO located at a large bend) and exchanging the guidewire for one with a higher tip load (Fig. 1.103b).

Guidewire "blocking," as referred to here (Fig. 1.104a), should be distinguished from trapping of the guidewire. A guidewire that has been trapped will not advance in the direction of the inflection point (Fig. 1.104c), even if the tip is oriented in this direction (Fig. 1.104b). In this situation, you should withdraw the wire until it is 1 to 2 mm proximal to the site of obstruction and reorient it in the desired direction while performing fixed point rotation of the tip.

You may be able to correct the direction of a guidewire that has not actually been blocked and bypass the blockage if the hard region of the occlusion is limited in size. However, you may not be able to correct the direction of a guidewire with no inflection point or obstruction. In this case, the guidewire must have entered the subintimal space at a more proximal site, most likely at the entry of the CTO.

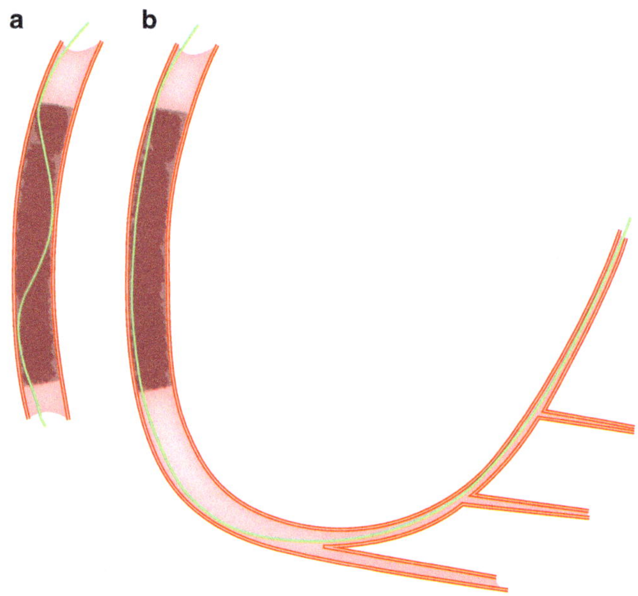

Fig. 1.100 A guidewire with a flexible tip showing multiple bends. In a patient with acute myocardial infarction and thrombotic occlusion at a site of mild stenosis, the guidewire may pass between the thrombus and the intima. The guidewire may also wind its way around the thrombus like passing through the subadventitia (**a**). On fluoroscopic images, a guidewire taking such a course is seen to have multiple bends. After the stiffer shaft of the guidewire enters the occlusion, the wire spontaneously straightens or becomes less bent either within or outside this pseudo-dissection (**b**)

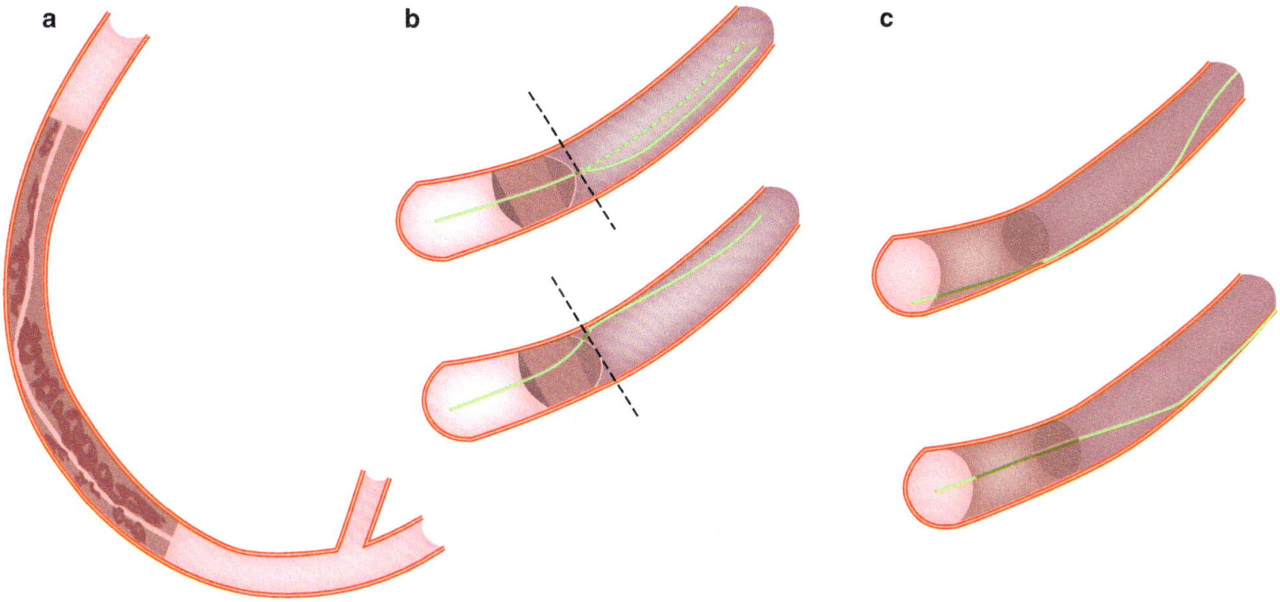

Fig. 1.101 Reasons for formation of an inflection point. (**a**) An inflection point forms in a guidewire when it passes through a winding microchannel in a CTO, especially if the channel is lined with calcified tissue. (**b**) In an orthogonal projection, a guidewire that leaves the true lumen inside a CTO and enters the subintimal space will be viewed as deviating from the predicted course of the target vessel. Once it has entered the subintimal space, the tip of the guidewire will only advance tangentially to its initial direction. If you attempt to return such a guidewire to the predicted course of the target vessel, it changes direction to the right or left when viewed in an orthogonal projection. This is why an inflection point is formed near the site where the guidewire enters the subintimal space. (**c**) If a guidewire enters the subintimal space at the entry of an occlusion, an inflection point will also be formed if an attempt is made to return it to the true lumen. Imaging in two projections is useful (essential) for detecting the inflection point

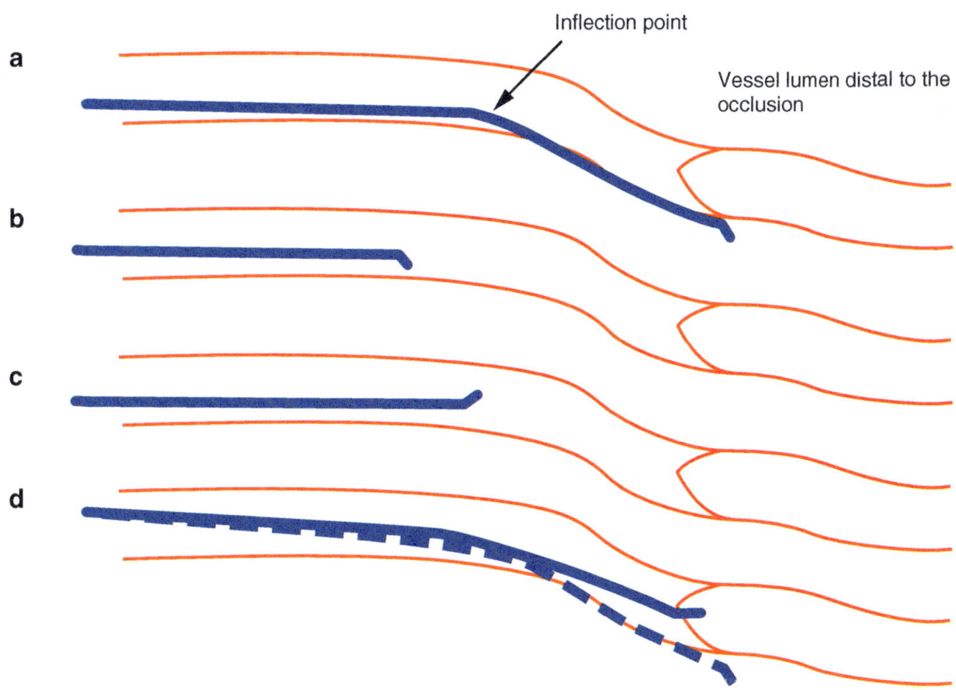

Fig. 1.102 If the guidewire enters the subintimal space. (**a**) A guidewire that is outside the true lumen at the exit of a CTO is found to have abruptly changed direction (inflection point) within the occlusion. (**b**) You should withdraw the guidewire to the inflection point and explore to find a new direction in which the guidewire can be advanced without inflection. (**c**) If the guidewire is blocked by hard tissue when its tip is oriented in the direction opposite to that of inflection, you should fix the tip at that point and perform small fixed point rotations until the wire advances. (**d**) If the wire advances without deviation or inflection, it is likely to remain in the true lumen. If the guidewire cannot be advanced, you should replace it with another one that has a higher tip load and manipulate the new guidewire in the same way

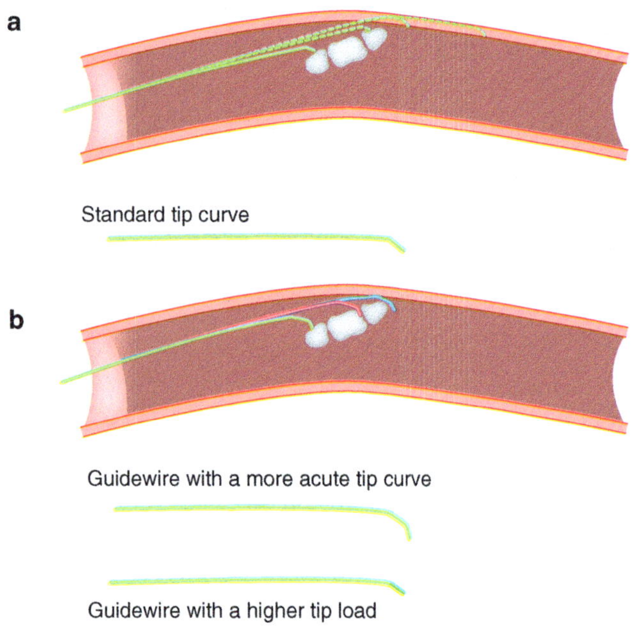

Fig. 1.103 If the guidewire enters the subintimal space despite fixed point rotation (**a**). (**b**) Penetration should be reattempted after the guidewire tip is reshaped with a more acute second curve of the same size. If this retry also fails, exchange the guidewire for one with a higher tip load

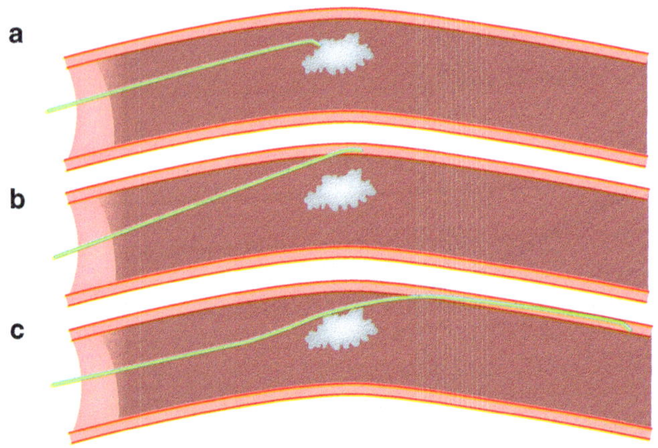

Fig. 1.104 Blocking (**a**) versus trapping (**b**) of a guidewire tip. A guidewire that is trapped can no longer be advanced, but will not enter the subintimal space as shown in (**c**). After prolonged manipulation, a trapped guidewire becomes difficult to withdraw, and forcible attempts to withdraw it may cause disruption and retention of the coil within the occlusion. Therefore, never persist with manipulation of a trapped guidewire

Selection of the Parallel Wire Technique or Retrograde Approach and Timing for Switching to These Strategies

If the first guidewire has reached the vessel distal to the CTO (but is outside the true lumen) or if the first guidewire cannot be advanced further within a long occlusion, you should then use the parallel wire technique or switch strategies to the retrograde approach. Which strategy should be chosen and when antegrade PCI should be switched to either of these strategies largely depends on the interventionalist's expertise and on the angiography equipment that is available (monoplane or biplane). My opinions on these issues are summarized below.

1. If you are using monoplane angiography equipment, you should switch from the antegrade approach to the retrograde approach earlier. With monoplane imaging equipment, it is necessary to rotate the detector through 90 degrees repeatedly to assist fine guidewire manipulation. Even if a retrograde channel appears to be a little difficult to track, you should try collateral channel tracking and attempt to cross the CTO by the retrograde approach, with the expectation that the guidewire can be advanced through the true lumen even when manipulated with guidance by monoplane angiography. It is safer to try to accomplish PCI by the kissing wire technique or the reverse CART technique using a continuous landmark.
2. If a calcified region can be used as a landmark, you can continue trying to cross the occlusion with a single wire for a longer time. If obvious calcification is found during PCI, you should be more likely to switch to the retrograde approach. If the calcification is obscured during prolonged PCI, you should try to use a second guidewire as a new landmark.
3. If there is no calcification to use as a landmark, you should try to correct the guidewire route several times. If these attempts fail, you should then use the parallel wire technique. Since a guidewire with a stiff shaft, such as the Conquest Pro, is likely to create a large dissection in a relatively soft vessel wall, you should switch to the retrograde approach earlier whenever possible (after a favorable collateral channel is found).
4. When it becomes difficult to obtain good images of the vessel lumen distal to the occlusion on fluoroscopy, you should start retrograde PCI.
5. If a guidewire being manipulated in an old RCA ostial occlusion enters a small side branch and goes outside the vessel wall just distal to the entry point, you should directly switch to retrograde PCI without considering the parallel wire technique.
6. If a guidewire being manipulated in a long occlusion of the RCA enters a small side branch and then goes outside the vessel wall around Segment #3, where the anatomy of the target vessel is absolutely unknown, it is better to choose the retrograde approach.
7. If there is no accessible collateral channel whatsoever, you will have no choice but to use the parallel wire technique via the antegrade approach. If there is only a very difficult collateral channel, you should generally try for longer to succeed with antegrade PCI. If collateral channel tracking fails, there is no choice but to resume antegrade PCI.

8. If both the retrograde approach and parallel wiring are unsuccessful, you should attempt IVUS-guided crossing of the CTO.

Manipulation in the Vessel Lumen Distal to the Occlusion

When a tapered CTO guidewire reaches the vessel lumen distal to the occlusion, you will usually feel a sudden decrease of resistance. A guidewire that has entered the distal true lumen will advance without deflection of the tip when pushed forward slightly with its tip oriented medially relative to the curvature of the vessel. If the tip is deflected when the guidewire is advanced slightly, the tip must have deviated into the subintimal space or been blocked by protruding plaque, since the tip will never be deflected if it remains within the true lumen. Because of the shape of its tip, a tapered CTO guidewire creates resistance when passing through a hard occlusion, and this may make it difficult to determine whether the guidewire is in the true lumen or has gone outside it. If you become unsure of this, you should push the guidewire forward slightly while rotating it within ±90 degrees with its tip oriented medially against the curvature of the vessel. If the guidewire can be advanced without deflection of the tip, it must be within the true lumen. If the tip is deflected, it must be in the subintimal space or blocked by hard plaque, and you should reattempt intimal tracking.

If the guidewire has successfully crossed a CTO through the true lumen, but is likely to damage a tightly stenosed segment distal to the occlusion (Fig. 1.105a), you can perform tip injection and guidewire exchange without damaging the distal segment if a microcatheter can be advanced to the distal lumen before the guidewire tip reaches the stenosis (Fig. 1.105b). If the microcatheter is vigorously pushed forward or pulled back over the guidewire, the tip of the guidewire will also move forward and backward, potentially causing damage to the stenosed distal segment. Therefore, you should advance the microcatheter with a steady force while rotating it to-and-fro until it crosses the lesion. To facilitate penetration by the microcatheter, you may use a very small balloon, but you should minimize its vibration to suppress forward and backward movement of the guidewire tip. If a Tornus microcatheter has crossed the occlusion, guidewire exchange can be performed, but not tip injection.

You should use the anchoring technique to stabilize the guiding catheter and consolidate backup.

Using a child catheter (e.g., a GuideLiner) or deep engagement of a guiding catheter as small as 5 Fr may help to improve pushability.

The situation is the same if there is a subtle island of contrast medium within an occlusion. If the guidewire has definitely reached the island, you should advance a microcatheter over the guidewire to the island and then perform tip injection and guidewire exchange through the microcatheter.

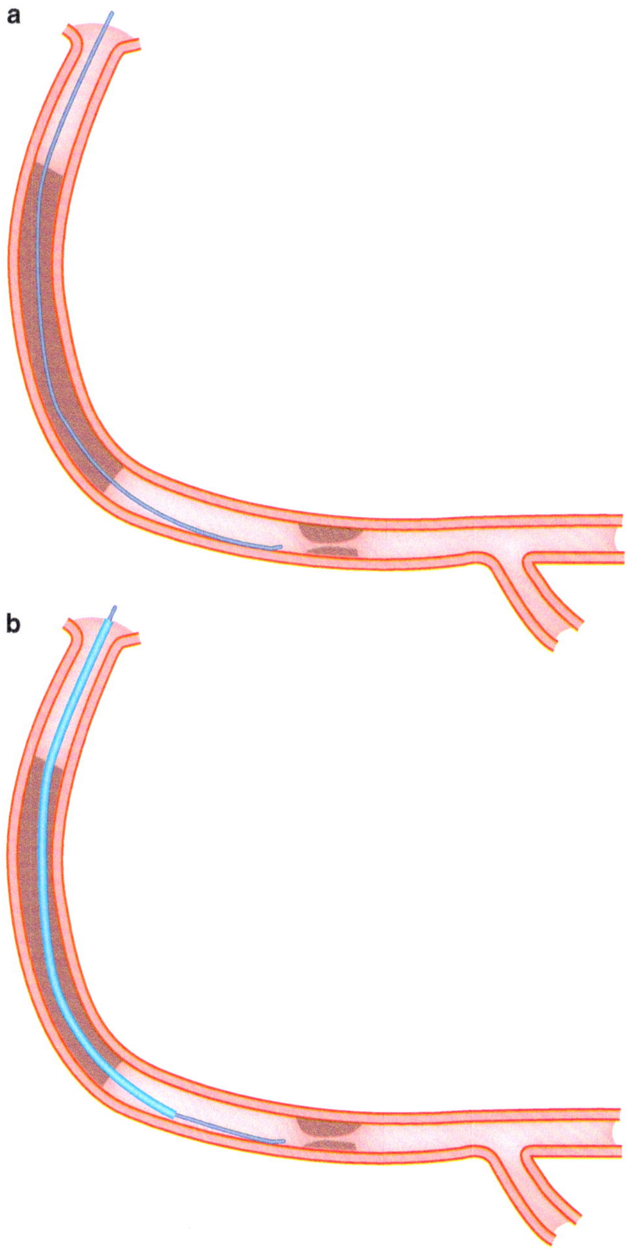

Fig. 1.105 If a guidewire that has crossed a CTO through the true lumen might injure a distal stenosed segment (**a**). A microcatheter should be advanced over the guidewire to the coronary artery lumen distal to the occlusion (**b**), and the guidewire should be exchanged for one with a lower tip load and an appropriate tip curve

1.6.4.9 Setting a Landmark

Whether you are performing antegrade or retrograde PCI, the presence of a landmark can provide assistance for assessing the anatomy of the target vessel and makes guidewire manipulation much easier. Therefore, setting a landmark is an important key to the success of antegrade PCI.

Calcification and subtle islands of contrast medium are some of the landmarks that are often available within or around coronary arteries (Table 1.6). Other potential landmarks that become visible with injection of contrast medium are collateral channels connected to the vessel distal to the occlusion and side branches arising from the occluded segment. Devices that are advanced toward the occlusion and can be used as landmarks include a parallel wire and the tip of a retrograde guidewire. Among these possibilities, calcification, a parallel wire, and the tip of a retrograde guidewire are permanent landmarks that will always remain visible and help to determine the distance from the guidewire being manipulated. I frequently employ such permanent landmarks because of their great usefulness.

The principle methods of manipulating a guidewire are to orient its tip in the direction of the route through the occluded target vessel determined from a landmark, rotate it within ±90 degrees (fixed point rotation), and push it forward with minimal force while seeking the direction in which it can be advanced. If there is a soft central core inside a relatively hard vessel or plaque, you should perform to-and-fro rotation (plane rotation) of the guidewire.

Table 1.6 Possible landmarks

Landmarks	Natural	Continuous
Calcification	○	○
Collateral angiography	○	×
Subtle islands of contrast	○	×
Side branch from the occlusion site (collateral flow)	○	×
Parallel wire (seesaw wiring)	×	○
Retrograde wire	×	○

Landmarks, Imaging Equipment, and Fluoroscopy Angle

To maximize the detection of calcification, a high-resolution cineangiography apparatus must be available and must be calibrated appropriately. I think that biplane cineangiography is essential, and viewing in at least two orthogonal projections is necessary for this purpose. Some sites of calcification can be clearly viewed in one projection, but are hardly visible in another projection that is orthogonal to the first one. If the main vessel and its side branch can be clearly distinguished in one projection, the two vessels will overlap each other in another projection that is orthogonal to the first one.

Let us consider this point using the LAD as an example.

When the midportion of the LAD is viewed in two orthogonal projections, the AP + CR and LL + CR projections (see Figs. 1.32 and 1.33), calcification is clearly visualized in the AP + CR projection and easily distinguished from the Dg and SB. Therefore, calcification can be readily used as a landmark in this projection. In the LL + CR projection, the LAD and the Dg overlap, as does calcification in these arteries. The difficult fluoroscopic conditions of this projection also make it hard to demonstrate calcification, but a calcified area may still be used as a landmark, if recognizable. If there is no recognizable calcified landmark, you can only check whether the guidewire has deviated from the vessel lumen distal to the occlusion based on the estimated route of the true lumen. It is easier to navigate the tip of the guidewire toward the coronary artery lumen distal to the occlusion in the AP + CR projection. However, if the guidewire cannot reach the true distal lumen, deviation from the true lumen can often only be recognized in the LL + CR projection (Fig. 1.106). When using the parallel wire technique, you should attempt to advance the second guidewire parallel to the route of the first guidewire in the AP + CR projection and should use the LL + CR projection to explore whether the second guidewire can be advanced through the true lumen from the proximal segment of the occluded vessel (Fig. 1.106).

Conversely, if the first guidewire appears to be outside the true lumen in both projections (Fig. 1.107), you should change the projections so that the guidewire is viewed as being inside the true lumen in one projection, while it will deviate more markedly from the true lumen in the other new projection (Fig. 1.108). If the direction of the guidewire is corrected while using the latter projection, successful crossing of the lesion through the true lumen is more likely to be achieved.

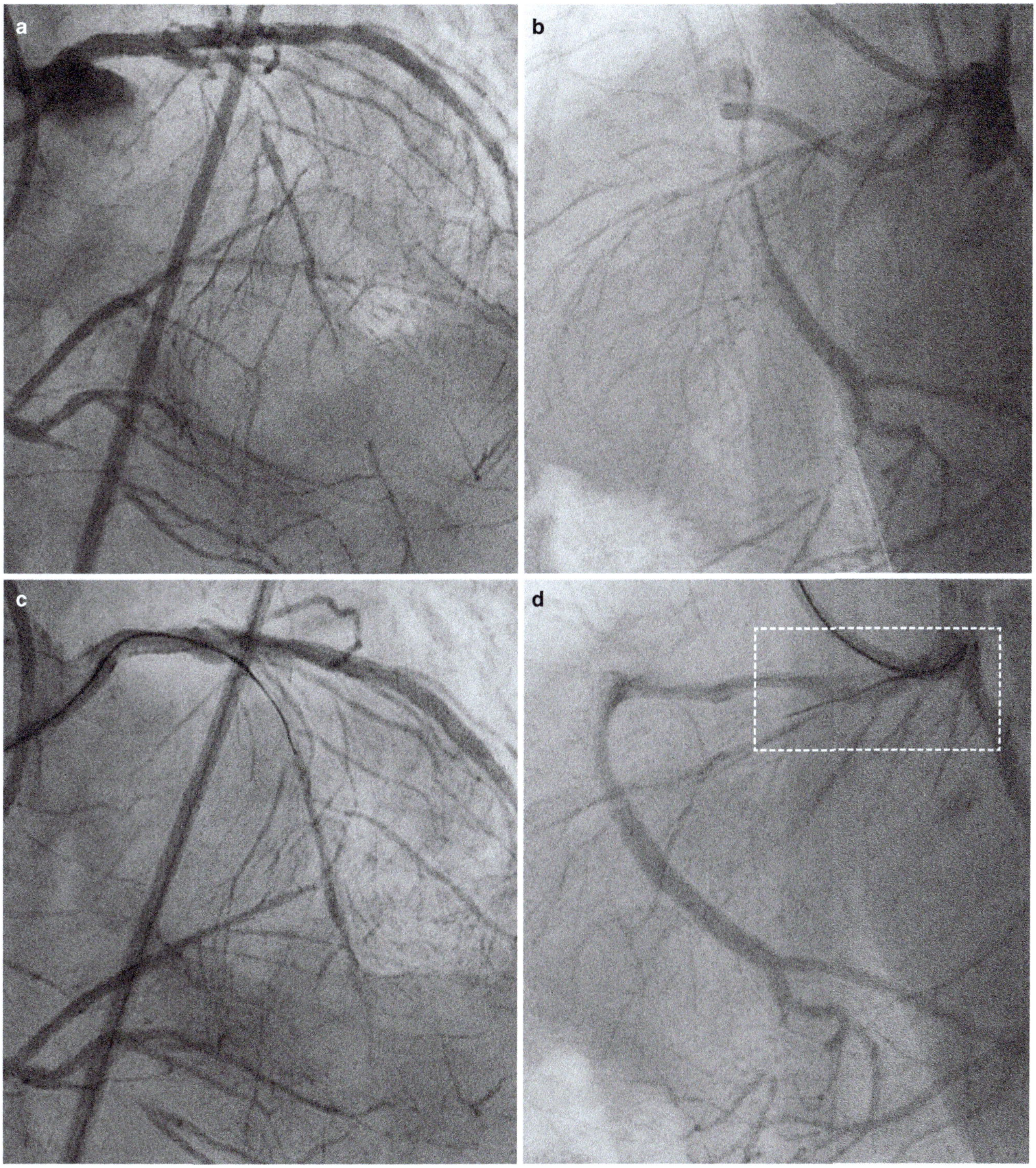

Fig. 1.106 Occlusion of the proximal LAD. (**a**) AP + CR image. (**b**) LL + CR image. The first guidewire was manipulated under fluoroscopic guidance in the AP + CR view. The guidewire seemed to have reached the LAD lumen distal to the occlusion in the AP + CR view (**c**), but it was seen to have deviated upward considerably in the LL + CR view (**d**). In this view, an inflection point (arrow) can clearly be recognized (**e**). Using the seesaw wiring technique, a second guidewire was advanced along the first guidewire to a site just proximal to the inflection point. In the AP + CR view, the second guidewire that was advanced in parallel with the first guidewire was seen to be crossing the occlusion through the true lumen (**f**). In the LL + CR view, the second guidewire was advanced around the inflection point with the tip oriented downward while performing fixed point rotation to explore for a blockage. After this manipulation, the guidewire was also seen to cross the occlusion through the true lumen in the latter projection (**g**). An enlarged view (**h**) clearly shows that the second guidewire has been advanced without creating non-inflection point, like that in the first guidewire

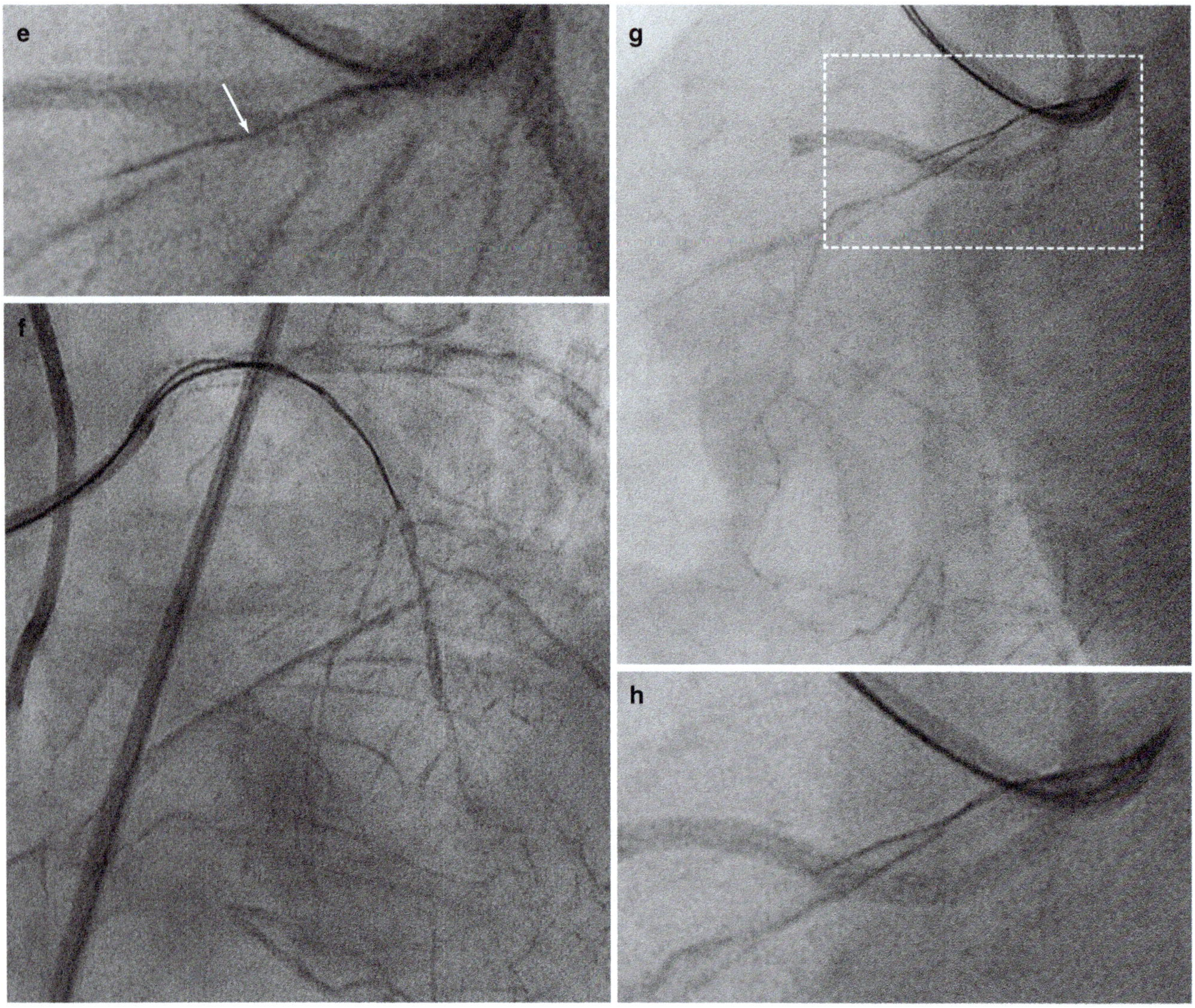

Fig. 1.106 (continued)

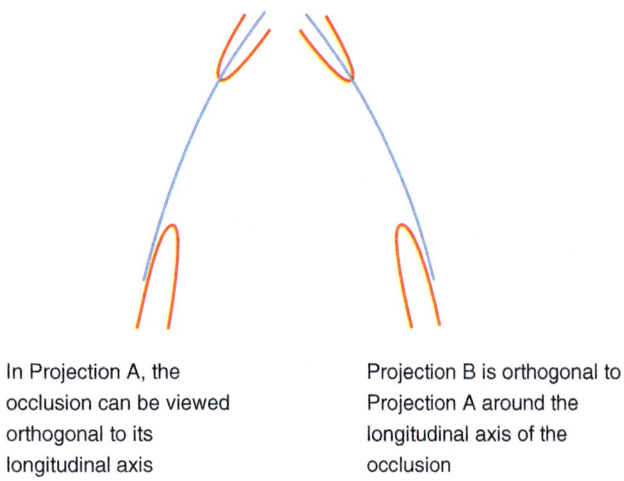

Fig. 1.107 Guidewire direction relative to the distal true lumen. Projections A and B are orthogonal to each other around the longitudinal axis of the occluded target vessel. In both projections, the guidewire deviates from the true lumen. These two projections cannot show the maximum deviation of the guidewire or the accurate location of the inflection point and therefore will not be useful for correcting the direction of the wire

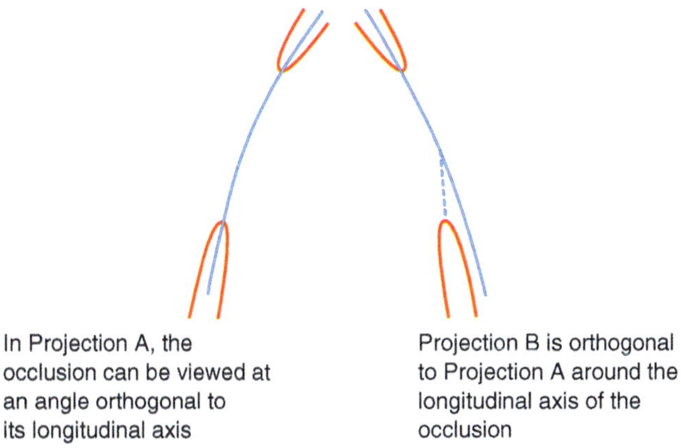

Fig. 1.108 Guidewire direction relative to the distal true lumen. Projections A and B are orthogonal to each other. These two projections may be obtained by modifying the projections shown in Fig. 1.107. Unlike the previous figure, the guidewire appears to be inside the true lumen in Projection A, but is outside the true lumen in Projection B. The maximum deviation of the guidewire from the true lumen can be viewed in Projection B, and the inflection point is more clearly recognizable. Using two such projections makes it easier to correct the direction of the guidewire, irrespective of whether you are employing a single guidewire or the parallel wire technique. While keeping the first guidewire in Projection A or advancing the second guidewire along the first one in this projection, you should explore for a new route that runs to the left from near the inflection point in Projection B

1.6.4.10 Parallel Wire Technique

Choice of the Second Guidewire **(Figs. 1.109, 1.110, 1.111, 1.112, 1.113, and 1.114)**

If the first guidewire runs through the subintimal space and fails to reach the distal true lumen, you should use it as a landmark and try to cross the occlusion with another guidewire. As the second guidewire, I always choose one with a higher tip load than that of the first wire. This is because it is generally accepted that obstruction by hard tissue (calcified or fibrous plaque) in the true lumen often causes a guidewire to deviate into the relatively soft subintimal tissue. While this concept is not supported by scientific evidence, it has the following empirical background.

After being blocked by hard tissue, a guidewire may slip and then go forward when pushed. This can suggest to the interventionalist that it has penetrated a hard cap and advanced into the distal true lumen. Although a guidewire exhibiting such behavior occasionally does enter the distal true lumen as expected, angiography almost always shows deviation of the wire into the subintimal space. If the tip of a stiffer guidewire is pressed up against the obstruction and fixed point rotation within ±90 degrees is performed, the wire can often follow an intraluminal route through the occlusion and eventually reach the distal true lumen.

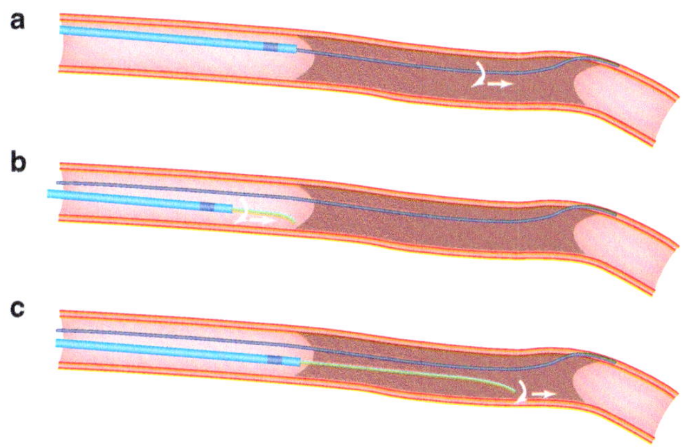

Fig. 1.109 Parallel wire technique. (**a**) The first guidewire has deviated into the subintimal space. You should only withdraw the microcatheter by using Nanto's technique or a Kusabi catheter. (**b**, **c**) You should insert another guidewire into the microcatheter and attempt to find the true lumen with the second wire while using the first guidewire as a landmark

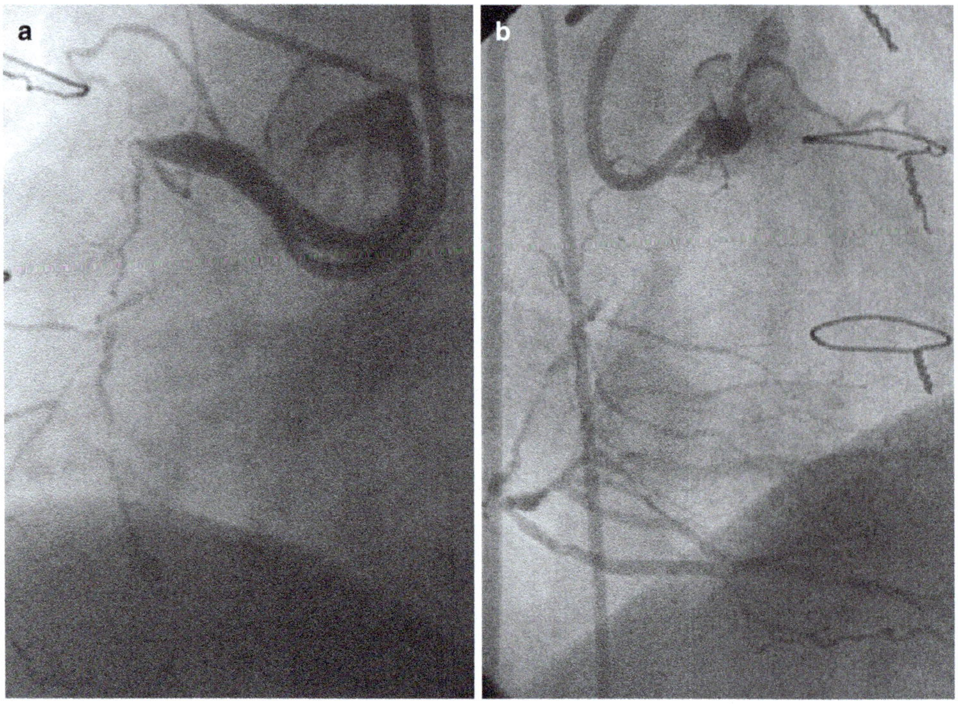

Fig. 1.110 CTO of the RCA (Segment #1). Imaging of the RCA segment distal to the occlusion via a bridging collateral. (**a**) LAO view. (**b**) RAO view

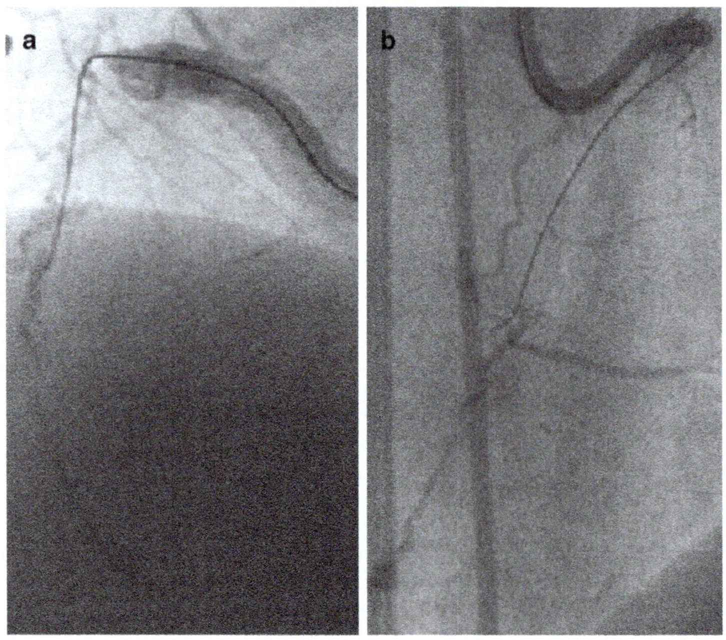

Fig. 1.111 The first guidewire. At the exit point, the first guidewire deviates slightly rightward in the LAO view (**a**), while it deviates leftward in the RAO view (**b**)

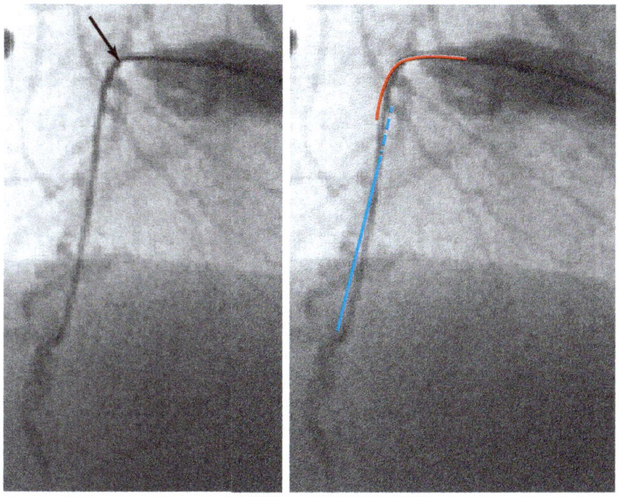

Fig. 1.112 Enlargement of the LAO image shown in Fig. 1.111. The guidewire is suspected to have undergone inflection near the point indicated by an arrow. The optimal guidewire route from the distal side of the occlusion (solid blue line) probably starts from the distal true lumen parallel with the first guidewire and runs toward the proximal part of the occlusion. It will cross the first guidewire at some point and then will approximate and reach the first wire in the proximal true lumen. The optimal guidewire route from the proximal side of the occlusion (solid red line) is most likely to run downward just proximal to the inflection point, after which it will form an arch, cross the first guidewire, and then run slightly leftward

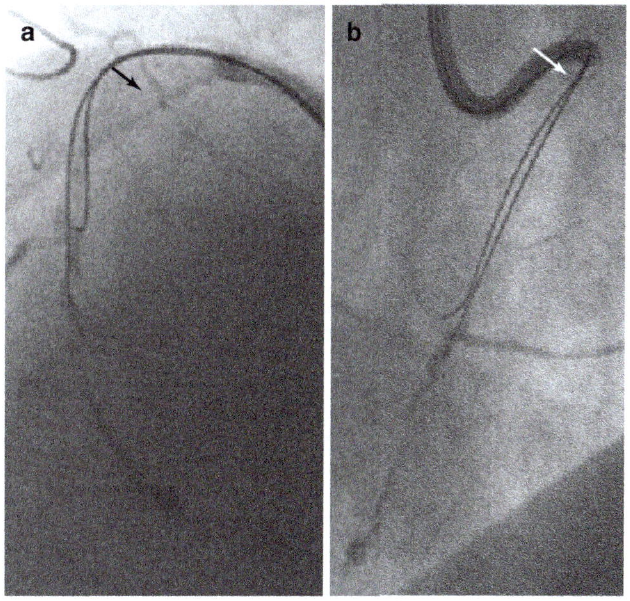

Fig. 1.114 The same PCI procedure shown in Fig. 1.111. From Point 1 in the RAO (**b**), the second guidewire could be advanced within the true lumen. It crossed the first guidewire around the inflection point in the LAO (**a**), as expected. Thus, a guidewire that deviates into the subintimal space often enters it at the most proximal inflection point

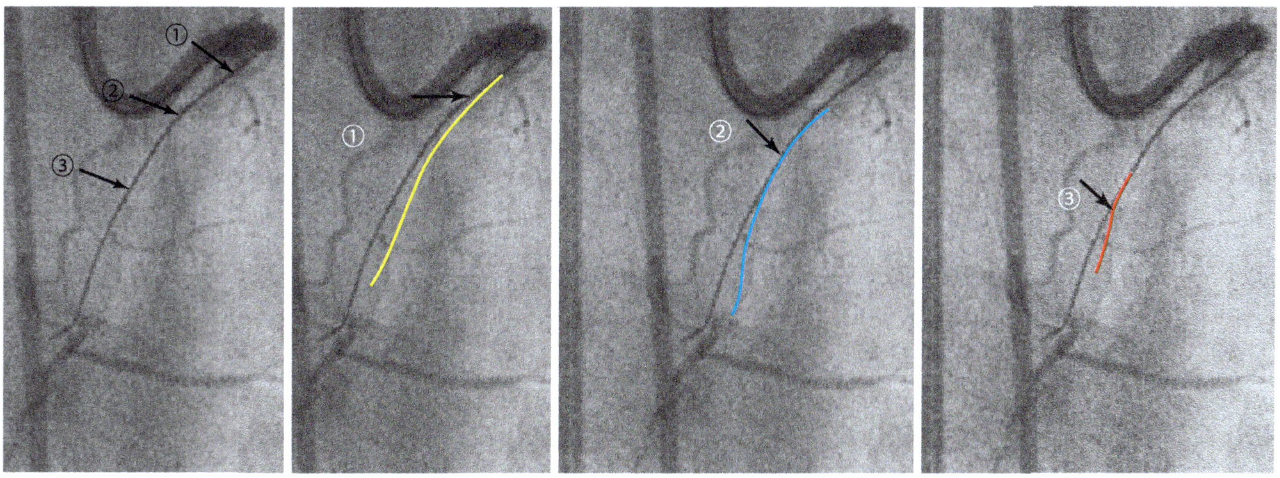

Fig. 1.113 Enlargement of the RAO image shown in Fig. 1.111. The first guidewire may have undergone inflection at any of three points (arrows). The optimal guidewire route will follow the yellow line if the first guidewire underwent inflection at Point 1, while the blue line indicates the optimal route for inflection at Point 2, and the red line indicates the optimal route for inflection at Point 3

Seesaw Wiring (Fig. 1.115)

If the first guidewire eventually fails to penetrate a hard obstruction in an occlusion, you should use it as a landmark and attempt to penetrate the obstruction with a slightly stiffer guidewire. Instead of the parallel wire technique, which involves withdrawing the microcatheter over the first guidewire and using it to advance the second guidewire, you may advance the second guidewire through a second microcatheter while leaving the microcatheter of the first guidewire in place (seesaw wiring). If the second guidewire is also blocked by the obstruction, you should exchange the first guidewire for an even stiffer wire and then advance it through the first microcatheter to cross the CTO by using the second guidewire as a landmark.

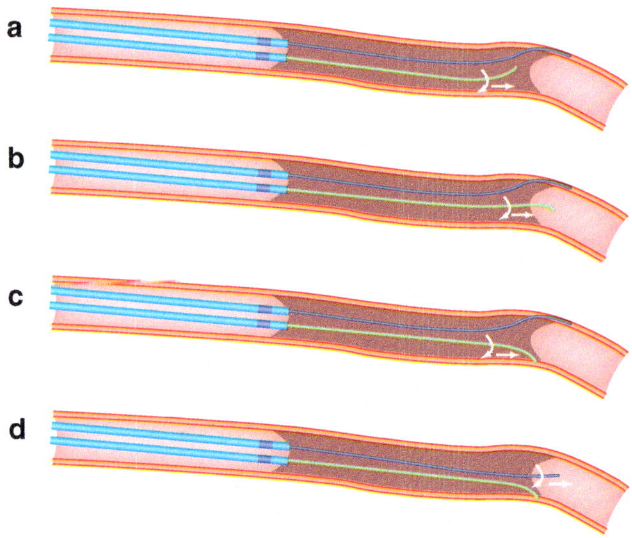

Fig. 1.115 Seesaw wiring, a parallel wire method using a second microcatheter. The first guidewire has deviated into the subintimal space. You advance a second guidewire through a second microcatheter (**a**). Seesaw wiring is successful if the second guidewire enters the distal true lumen (**b**). If the second guidewire also deviates into the subintimal space (**c**), you can easily try to advance the first guidewire through the true lumen (**d**). Before attempting this, you may want to exchange the first guidewire for one with a higher tip load if the first wire is thought to have an insufficient tip load

Parallel Wiring Through a Crusade Microcatheter

Here I will discuss the circumstances and reasons why a Crusade microcatheter is useful for parallel wiring or for penetrating the entrance of a CTO located in a side branch. First, a Crusade microcatheter helps a second guidewire to easily track a tortuous vessel. Second, the stiffness of a Crusade microcatheter which has accommodated the first guidewire provides stronger backup for a second guidewire (Fig. 1.116a). Third, if the side hole of the catheter happens to be oriented toward the side branch, the catheter can help to control the direction of the second guidewire and provide stronger backup to facilitate successful entry into the occlusion in the branch vessel (Fig. 1.116b).

However, the short tip and great stiffness of the Crusade tend to bias this microcatheter and make it rather difficult to control (Fig. 1.116c–f). Accordingly, you may have to carefully adjust the curve at the guidewire tip when using a Crusade microcatheter. You may sometimes have to adjust the curves at the tip of both the Crusade microcatheter and the guidewire.

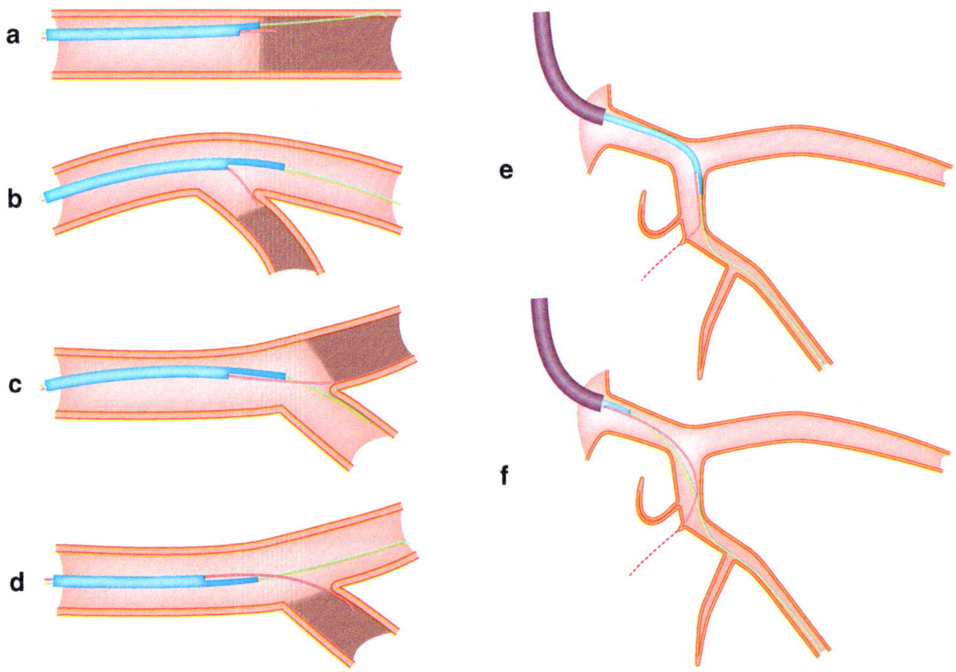

Fig. 1.116 Guidewire manipulation through a Crusade microcatheter. (**a**) A Crusade microcatheter provides good backup in a relatively straight occlusion. (**b**) The side hole of a Crusade microcatheter is often medial to the first guidewire that has entered a curved main branch. If the side hole faces the ostium of the branch, it will provide considerable assistance for a second guidewire to penetrate an occlusion in the branch. However, if the side branch originates from the larger curvature of a bend in the main vessel, the side hole of the Crusade microcatheter will not always face the ostium of the branch (**c** & **d**). If the side hole is oriented toward the occlusion, a second guidewire can be easily controlled through a Crusade microcatheter (**e**). If this is not the case, the second guidewire becomes difficult to control as it needs to be manipulated from a more proximal point (**f**)

1.6.4.11 Correcting the Guidewire Route by Using a Landmark

If there is strong evidence that subintimal deviation of the guidewire has occurred, the next step is usually to reorient the wire toward the true lumen by using a landmark.

In the days when I used a 0.014-inch less slippery non-tapered guidewire, I could feel the resistance to its tip and use the magnitude of resistance to decide whether the wire was in the true lumen or had deviated into the subintimal space. Since the recent CTO crossing guidewires create less resistance, the interventionalist cannot rely on subjective judgment of resistance alone to make a reliable assessment. Currently, visual evidence is absolutely required to determine whether a guidewire is in the true or false lumen.

However, when imaging shows the interventionalist that the tip of a guidewire is unable to advance further in a vessel, the tip may actually have been trapped within the occlusion. Trapping, which makes the guidewire difficult to withdraw, seems to occur when the tip of the wire has been advanced through the media parallel with the vessel wall for a certain distance (see 1.6.4.4 "Guidewire Trapping and Inflection" [page 52]). If a guidewire has become trapped, you still have a good chance to correct the route of the wire and to ensure that it follows the true lumen. However, if the guidewire remains trapped for too long, it will become extremely difficult to withdraw. Therefore, you should suspect guidewire trapping and attempt to correct it at an early stage. You should promptly pull the guidewire back slightly if it becomes impossible to advance further and check that the tip can be pulled free and moved before attempting to correct the route of the wire by using a landmark.

Since confirmation of guidewire trapping is a basic procedure, I will discuss here how to use a landmark to correct the guidewire route after trapping has been confirmed. I would like to emphasize that the methods for correction described under [1] and [4] in "Parallel Wire Technique" (page 75) are also applicable to retrograde PCI.

First, I would like to review the basics of correcting the guidewire route. Under what circumstances and when should you correct the route of a guidewire that has deviated into the subintimal space? In general, if the tip of the guidewire is near the distal true lumen, but collateral imaging indicates that it will not enter the distal lumen, the wire is a candidate for correction unless you can verify that it is coaxial with the target vessel and directed toward the distal lumen. If the guidewire has been advanced as far as the distal true lumen, but its tip is actually outside the lumen, it is also a candidate for correction. The tip of the guidewire may deviate from the true lumen in various ways. For example, it may deviate toward the larger curvature (Fig. 1.117a) or toward the smaller curvature (Fig. 1.117b) of the bend in a vessel in only one projection (Fig. 1.118a) or in both of two projections (Fig. 1.118b), or it may deviate in a non-coaxial manner (Fig. 1.119). The mode of guidewire deviation from the true lumen influences the method of correcting it.

To correct a deviating guidewire, it is recommended to search for an inflection point in the wire as the site from which to start correction and/or use two orthogonal projections, one of which shows the guidewire outside the true lumen (Figs. 1.108, 1.118a, and 1.120). In a long CTO with no natural internal landmarks, if the tip of the guidewire is outside the true lumen distal to the occlusion, the wire will not always have a definite inflection point within the occlusion (Fig. 1.121). You should suspect that the guidewire is winding through the subintimal space. If the guidewire is found to show slight deviation in a certain direction in both projections, it is worth pursuing that direction (Fig. 1.121). This is especially true if there is an obstruction in that direction.

Using monoplane angiography, most guidewires that have deviated from the true lumen are visualized as remaining within the lumen in one projection and exhibit maximum deviation from the lumen in another projection that is orthogonal to the first.

Figure 1.122 shows a typical occlusion of the proximal LAD. When performing PCI for CTO of the proximal LAD, the interventionalist usually advances a guidewire under fluoroscopic guidance, primarily employing the AP + CR view. In this case, the guidewire is seen to follow the LAD in the AP + CR view, but deviates from the course of the target artery in the LL + CR view. If the guidewire enters the distal true lumen in one, but not in the other, of two orthogonal projections obtained with the detector surfaces parallel to the longitudinal axis of the occluded vessel, the latter projection is very useful for correcting the position of the guidewire. When performing the parallel wire technique, you should advance another guidewire along the first guidewire using the projection in which the first wire seems to remain in the true lumen and should attempt to find the right direction to avoid deviation of the second guidewire in the other projection (Figs. 1.123 & 1.124).

If the occlusion is not so long, the inflection point of the first guidewire can often be identified easily in the projection which displays maximum deviation of the wire from the distal true lumen.

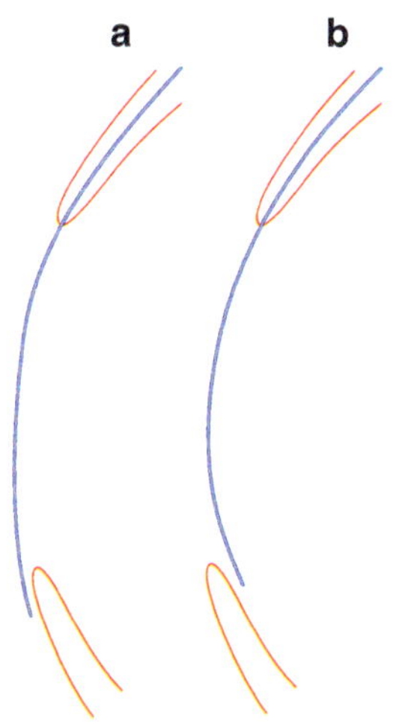

Fig. 1.117 Guidewire direction relative to the distal true lumen. (**a**) Guidewire deviating from the distal true lumen toward the larger curvature of the vessel. (**b**) Guidewire deviating from the distal true lumen toward the smaller curvature of the vessel

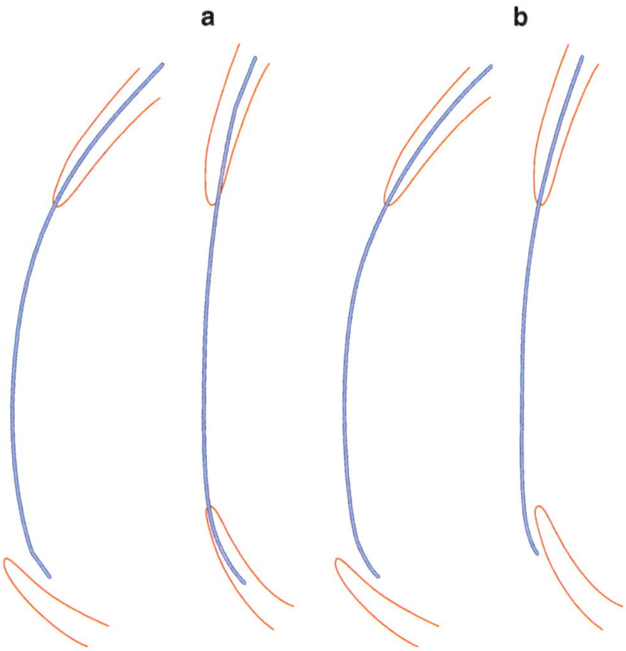

Fig. 1.118 Guidewire direction relative to the distal true lumen. (a) Guidewire deviating from the distal true lumen in only one of two orthogonal projections. (b) Guidewire deviating from the distal true lumen in both of two orthogonal projections

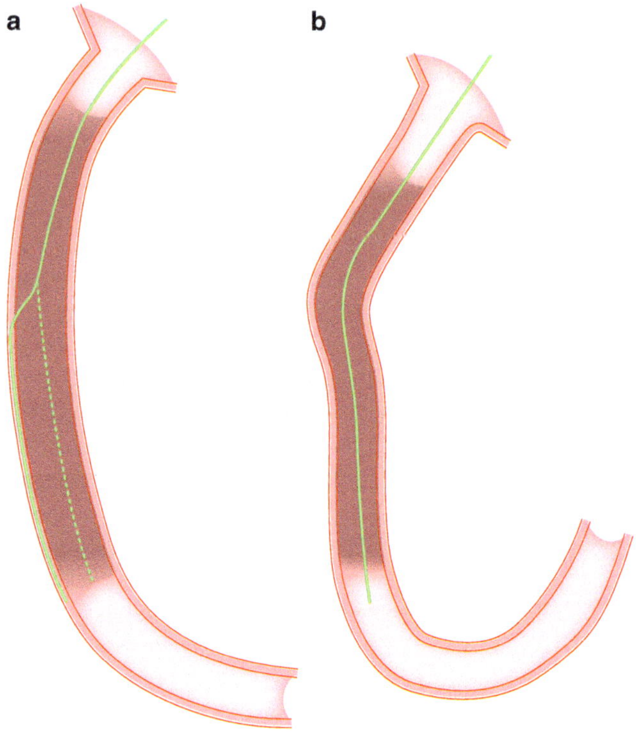

Fig. 1.120 Two orthogonal projections. Deviation of a guidewire advancing along the vessel wall is difficult to identify. However, a guidewire that is viewed as following the center of the distal true lumen in one projection (b) is viewed as deviating from the true lumen in another projection orthogonal to the first (a)

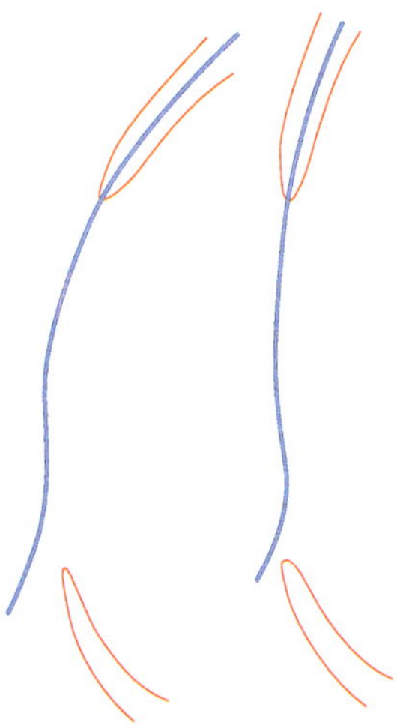

Fig. 1.119 Guidewire direction relative to the distal true lumen. The guidewire is not directed toward the distal true lumen due to loss of coaxiality and deviates from the lumen in both of two orthogonal projections

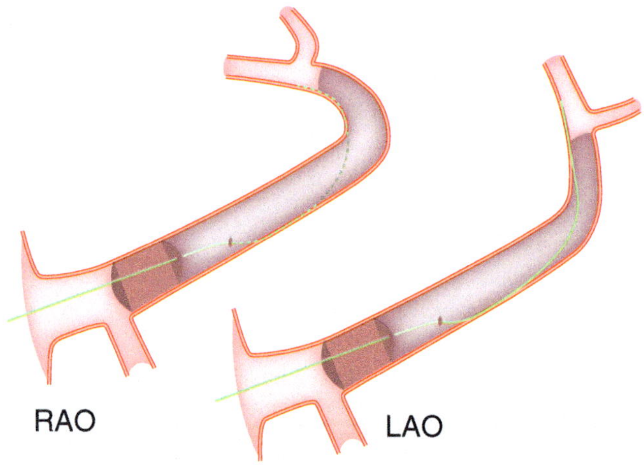

Fig. 1.121 Guidewire deviating into the subintimal space in a long occlusion. If the guidewire deviates into the subintimal space and follows a winding course within a long occlusion, the inflection point of the guidewire is difficult to identify, even using two orthogonal projections

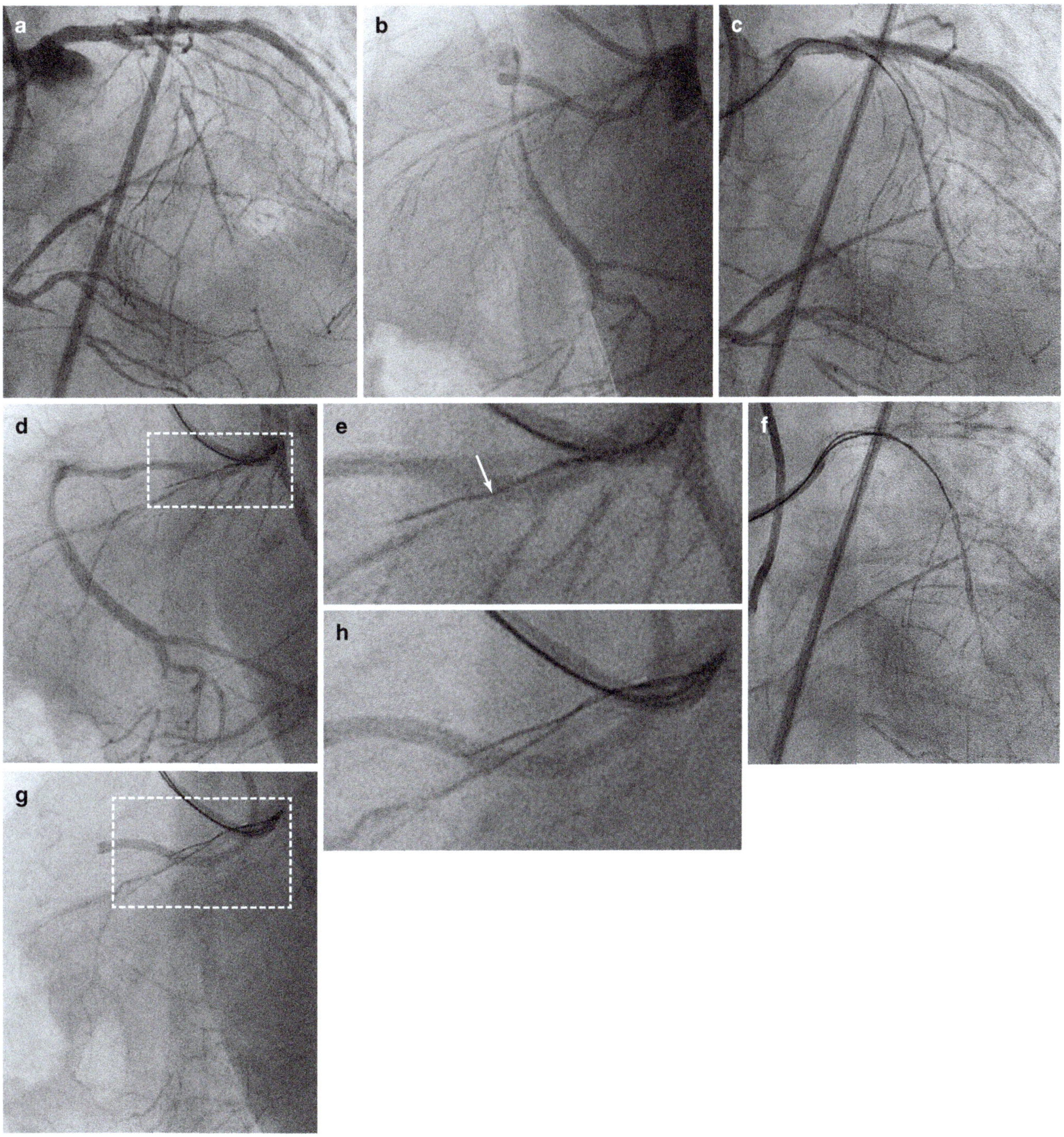

Fig. 1.122 Occlusion of the proximal LAD: the same procedure as shown in Fig. 1.106. (**a**) AP + CR view. (**b**) LL + CR view. The first guidewire was manipulated under fluoroscopic guidance in the AP + CR view. In the LL + CR view, which is almost orthogonal to the AP + CR view, the coronary artery branches overlap considerably, and precise guidewire manipulation is impossible. Biplane angiography shows that the guidewire reaches the distal true lumen in the AP + CR view (**c**), but deviates considerably upward from the true lumen in the LL + CR view (**d**). In this view, an inflection point (arrow) can be clearly recognized (**e**). Using the seesaw wiring technique, the second guidewire was advanced along the first guidewire to a site just proximal to the inflection point. In the AP + CR view, the second guidewire advanced in parallel with the first guidewire was seen to be crossing the occlusion through the true lumen (**f**). The second guidewire was advanced in the LL + CR view with its tip oriented downward around the inflection point while applying fixed point rotation to explore the site of obstruction. After this manipulation, the guidewire was also seen to be crossing the occlusion through the true lumen in the latter projection (**g**). An enlarged image (**h**) clearly shows that the second guidewire has been advanced without undergoing inflection like that observed in the first guidewire

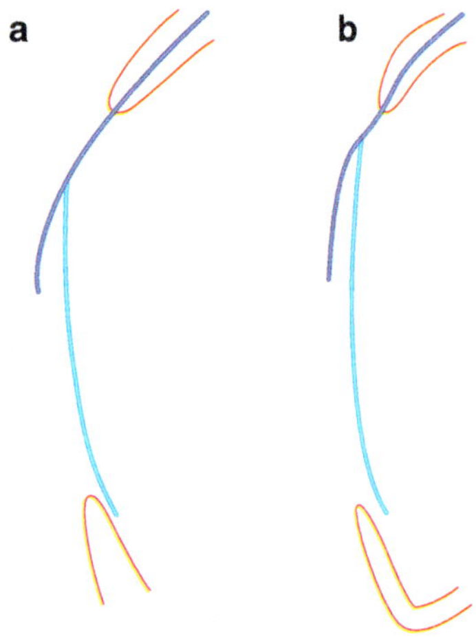

Fig. 1.123 Finding the route for the second guidewire with the parallel wire technique. (**a** & **b**) Two orthogonal views. If the anatomy of the occluded vessel is unclear, the second guidewire should be advanced along a route that initially diverges from the first guidewire, but then goes parallel to it without increasing divergence between the two wires

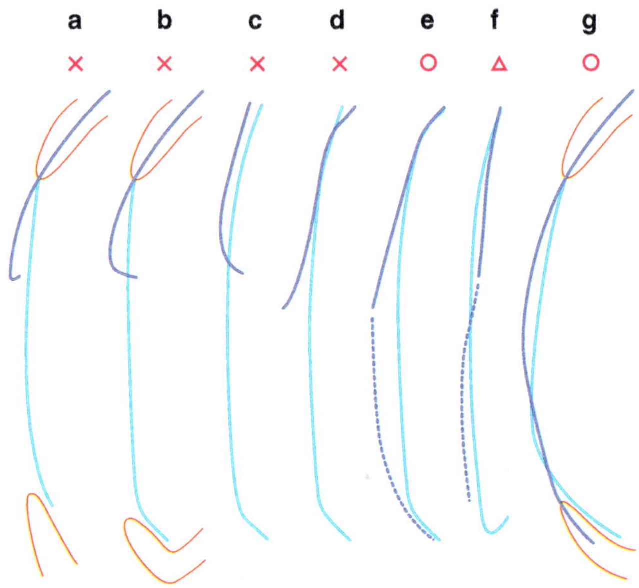

Fig. 1.124 Correcting the direction of the second guidewire relative to the landmark guidewire. The second guidewire is considered to have been successfully corrected if it eventually becomes parallel with the first guidewire, even if it initially deviates considerably from the other wire (**e**). If the second guidewire is not parallel with the first guidewire and is advanced in the wrong direction (**a**, **b**, **c** & **d**), it will not reach the true lumen distal to the occlusion. If the second guidewire initially deviates from the first guidewire, but then takes a parallel course, it is worth advancing the second wire further in that direction of (**e**). If the two guidewires are parallel but very close to each other in both orthogonal projections, it may be doubtful that the second wire is in the true lumen (**f**). It is often seen that the second guidewire crosses the first wire one or more times and then eventually goes toward the distal true lumen (**g**). This is probably the result of the first guidewire winding through the subintimal space

Using Calcified Plaque as a Landmark

When advancing a guidewire toward the distal true lumen by using calcified plaque as a landmark, you may obtain a fluoroscopic view of the calcified plaque like that shown in Fig. 1.125a. When performing PCI under fluoroscopic guidance, the guidewire is manipulated toward the distal true lumen that has been visualized by collateral imaging, and it eventually appears to have reached the lumen in this view. However, using calcified plaque as a landmark does not allow us to determine the accurate anatomy of the occluded vessel, which may be like that shown in Fig. 1.125b or c. In Fig. 1.125c, the guidewire appropriately follows the curve of the vessel and appears to remain within the true lumen. However, Fig. 1.125d displays a guidewire following the course shown in Fig. 1.125b within an occluded vessel having the same curvature as in Fig. 1.125c. In this view, the guidewire appears to deviate into the subintimal space, at least at the midportion of the occlusion. Thus, a guidewire that apparently follows the course shown in Fig. 1.125b, c, or d in one projection may have an unexpectedly different course in another projection orthogonal to the first projection.

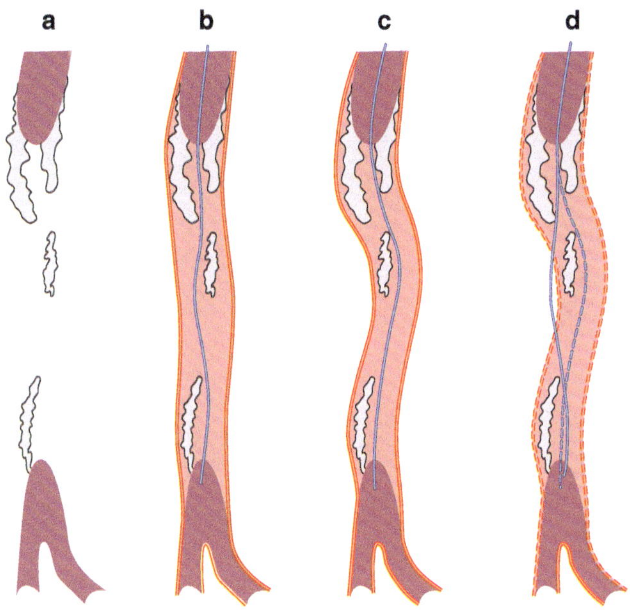

Fig. 1.125 Using calcified plaque as a landmark. In (**a**) CTO with areas of calcification as shown in a, the anatomy of the occluded vessel may be as shown in (**b**) or (**c**). It can often be predictable from the movement of the vessel, but not until the start of guidewire manipulation. If (**b**) and (**c**) represent the predicted and actual anatomy of the vessel, respectively, a guidewire advanced through the CTO will inevitably deviate into the subintimal space (**d**)

Using the Distal True Lumen Visualized by Contralateral Imaging as a Landmark

If the distal true lumen visualized by contralateral (collateral) imaging is the only landmark available, it can only be seen temporarily during imaging and is not a sufficient guide for accurate correction of the guidewire route with the single-wire technique. However, if the inflection point of the guidewire can be clearly identified, you can withdraw the guidewire to a site just proximal to that point and then slowly advance it in the opposite direction to the direction of inflection. If the guidewire advances along the predicted route of the true lumen, you may continue in that direction and advance it further while performing fixed point rotation. If favorable guidewire advancement continues, you may switch from fixed point rotation to plane rotation.

You can try to correct the guidewire route several times using a single crossing guidewire, but if these attempts fail, it is better to switch your strategy to parallel wiring or retrograde PCI. If attempts at correction are repeated too often, the guidewire may deviate into the same subintimal space repeatedly and create a large dissection. A Conquest Pro guidewire has a stiffer tip than a Gaia guidewire and readily causes dissection if it deviates into the subintimal space and is advanced through that space (see Fig. 1.85). To prevent creation of a large dissection, you should proceed to the next step at an early stage.

Parallel Wire Technique

As mentioned above, the parallel wire technique involves using one guidewire as a landmark to advance another guidewire. You should bear in mind that the first guidewire is a secondary landmark compared to the distal true lumen visualized by collateral imaging, since the exact point where the first guidewire deviates into the subintimal space is unknown. However, the following five signs may indicate the point of guidewire deviation:

1. Inflection point: If there is an inflection point, investigate whether inflection of the second guidewire can be avoided and the wire can be advanced in an appropriate direction from that point (Fig. 1.102).
2. "Blocking" point: If there is a point where "blockage" occurs, press the tip of the second guidewire against the obstruction, and apply fixed point rotation to identify the direction in which the guidewire can be advanced (see Fig. 1.89).
3. Divergence point: If the tip of the guidewire is outside the true lumen, explore a new direction by the second guidewire from any point of slight divergence of the two wires, even if they are parallel with each other (Fig. 1.123). There are several patterns of divergence (Fig. 1.124). If advancement of the guidewire is blocked, also perform fixed point rotation at that point and attempt to find the direction in which it can go forward.

4. Trapping point: The guidewire is usually trapped at the boundary between the true lumen (inside plaque) and the subintimal tissue, i.e., in a layer very close to the true lumen (see 1.9.1 "Guidewire Entrapment"). You should pull a trapped guidewire back by a distance of 1 to 2 mm and then advance it again while exploring to find a direction in which it does not get trapped again.
5. Entry point: A guidewire may deviate into the subintimal space or go outside the vessel wall via a small side branch at the CTO entry. In this situation, try to penetrate the entry at a different point or explore a different route for advancement of the wire from the entrance (Fig. 1.126). If the guidewire seems to have penetrated a hard proximal cap and then passed through the occlusion smoothly without obstruction to reach the exit, but fails to enter the distal true lumen, it may have deviated into the subintimal space just near the entry. Subintimal deviation at the CTO entry should also be suspected if the guidewire returns to the distal subintimal space without being blocked while crossing the occlusion after it has been withdrawn from this space and advanced again in an attempt to find the correct route.

Deviation of the guidewire outside the vessel wall just at the CTO entry can easily be detected by a sudden marked reduction of resistance and unrestricted movement of the wire after it has passed through a hard obstruction.

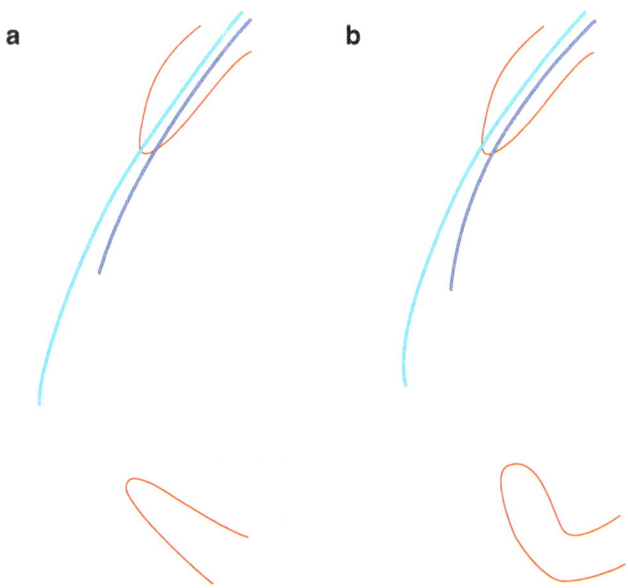

Fig. 1.126 Correcting the guidewire direction from the CTO entry. Two orthogonal projections (**a** & **b**). If the first guidewire is suspected to have deviated into the subintimal space or outside the vessel wall, you should explore another route from the CTO entrance (another point of penetration) with the second guidewire

Contralateral Guidewire Technique (See 1.7.13 "Kissing Wire Technique")

If a guidewire has been advanced retrogradely into an occlusion, the guidewire will be in the true lumen at least at the exit of the CTO. Therefore, you should advance an antegrade guidewire toward the retrograde guidewire at the exit point, but it is unclear how far the retrograde wire remains in the true lumen. The antegrade guidewire should be advanced according to the abovementioned rules [1] through [5]. If it comes into contact with the retrograde guidewire (Fig. 1.127), it can then reach the distal true lumen by being advanced to the exit point alongside the retrograde wire. It does not matter where the two guidewires come into contact with each other, whether in the subintimal space or inside a plaque. In both cases, the second (antegrade) guidewire should be able to follow the track created by the first (retrograde) guidewire. To ensure this, you should use a Gaia Second or stiffer CTO guidewire.

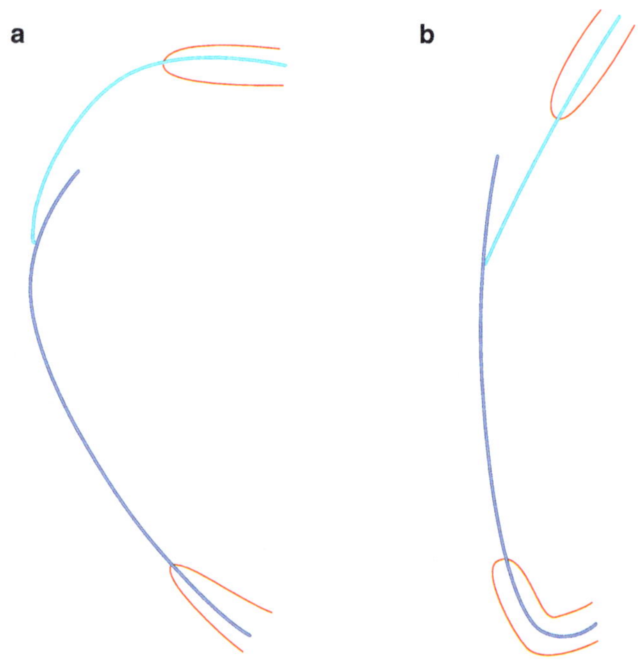

Fig. 1.127 Correcting the direction of an antegrade guidewire with a retrograde guidewire as the landmark. Two orthogonal projections (**a** & **b**). Using a retrograde guidewire (whether in the true lumen or subintimal space) that cannot be advanced further as a landmark (kissing wire technique), you should exchange the antegrade guidewire for another wire with a higher tip load and attempt further advancement through the occlusion to the distal true lumen. If the antegrade guidewire comes into contact with the retrograde guidewire at any point on its way to the exit, you should attempt the reverse CART technique

1.6.4.12 IVUS-Guided Wiring: Side Branch Technique

A guidewire that is confirmed to be in the subintimal space at the exit of a CTO has often gone into the subintimal space at the entry of the occlusion. Many guidewires fail to track the true lumen at the CTO entry and are located in the subintimal space at the exit. If you are manipulating a stiff CTO guidewire toward the entry of an occlusion and there is a side branch that can accommodate an IVUS catheter near the entry, you should introduce an IVUS catheter into the side branch to check if the guidewire tracks the true lumen at the CTO entry.

When penetrating the proximal cap with the guidewire, you should focus attention on the fluoroscopic image rather than the IVUS image. The fluoroscopy angle should be set so that the guidewire can be viewed en face on the plane that includes the axis of the side branch and the putative line at the entry of the occlusion. You should advance the guidewire toward the entry with its tip oriented in the opposite direction to the side branch and manipulate the wire to catch a dimple at the entry by slightly altering the direction of the tip (Fig. 1.128). During manipulation, you should check the IVUS screen to determine whether the tip of the guidewire is oriented in the correct direction at the bifurcation and is located at an appropriate entry point and to make fine adjustments to these parameters. If an assistant can relay the IVUS findings, the interventionalist can continuously focus on the fluoroscopic image without the need to alternately check the IVUS screen.

If the tip of the guidewire cannot catch a dimple at the CTO entry, you should create a more acute curve at the tip. If the guidewire still fails to catch a dimple after being reshaped in this way, you should exchange it for another guidewire with a higher tip load.

If the tip of the guidewire goes into the subintimal space from the main vessel distal to the entry of the occlusion, you should make the tip curve more acute (Fig. 1.128b). In contrast, if the tip of the guidewire enters the subintimal space from the main vessel proximal to the CTO entry, you should make the curve at the tip larger and less acute (Fig. 1.128c). While keeping the IVUS probe at the CTO entry, you should advance the tip of the guidewire into the side branch and then pull the wire back with its tip oriented in the opposite direction. Then you should perform fine adjustment to direct the guidewire tip toward the true lumen at the entry of the occlusion using the IVUS image. With the tip oriented toward the true lumen, you should push it forward slightly to find a dimple. If the tip catches a dimple, you should check the IVUS image to determine whether the tip is still oriented toward the true lumen.

It is almost impossible to penetrate calcified plaque capping the entry of an occlusion (in a main branch). In this case, you will need to find a non-calcified part of proximal cap that can be penetrated, but entry at such a site often leads to subintimal tracking. If you fail to achieve reentry of the guidewire into the true lumen, it becomes necessary to attempt the reverse CART technique (described later).

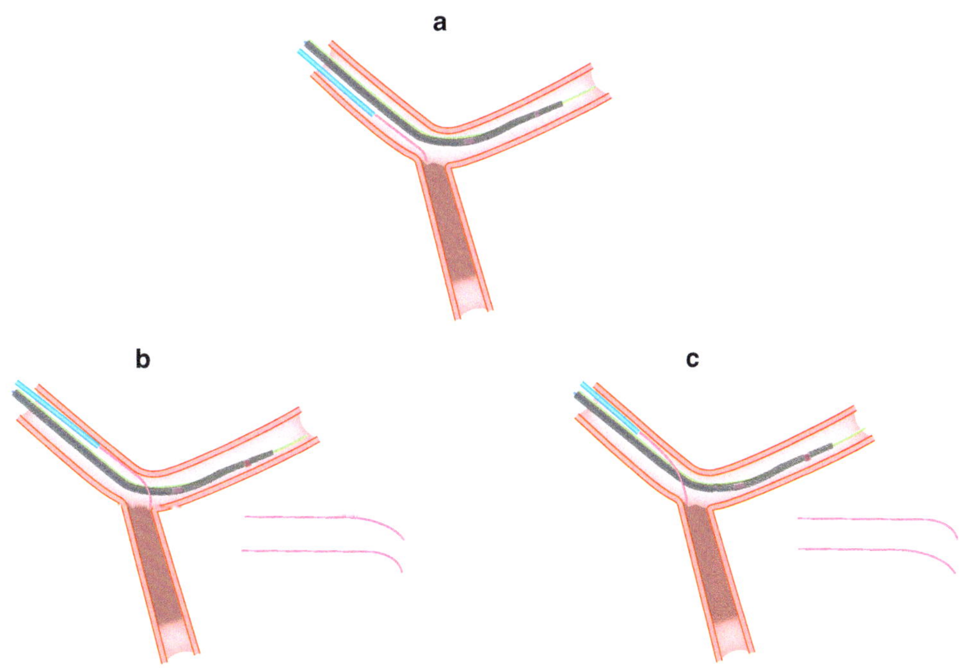

Fig. 1.128 IVUS-guided penetration of the entry to a CTO at the ostium of a side branch. This is a typical example of a target vessel with a CTO branching from the larger curvature of the patent main vessel. A guidewire can be advanced smoothly to the entry of the occlusion (**a**). Then the guidewire tip may be advanced to a point distal to the dimple, so that it enters the subintimal space on the distal side of the occlusion (**b**). If the guidewire tip is curved as shown in the upper figure, it should be reshaped with a slightly smaller and more acute curve, as shown in (**c**), to catch the dimple

1.6.4.13 IVUS-Guided Wiring: False Lumen Technique

When the guidewire is found to be in the subintimal space at the exit of an occlusion, there may be no side branch available, and parallel wiring may fail. It may also be impossible to attempt retrograde PCI because of the lack of a trackable collateral channel. In this situation, you should attempt IVUS-guided tracking of the true lumen by introducing an IVUS catheter into the existing subintimal space from the entry of the occlusion (Fig. 1.129). You should explore the site of obstruction at the CTO entry with the tip of a guidewire oriented toward the true lumen and parallel with the IVUS catheter/guidewire. In this situation, it is best to manipulate the guidewire toward the predicted true lumen based on fluoroscopic images and to confirm the direction of the lumen by IVUS. On fluoroscopic images, the true lumen is usually present on the smaller curvature of the occluded vessel. In general, a guidewire deviates from the hard true lumen into a false lumen in the direction of the larger curvature of the occluded vessel, as indicated by the finding that an IVUS catheter or other device tends to easily run along the larger curvature of a curved occlusion.

If there is a blocking point (obstruction), you should patiently rotate the guidewire within ±90 degrees at that location (fixed point rotation) until it enters the occlusion. This is to ensure penetration of the guidewire into the true lumen because previous guidewires presumably deviated into the subintimal space at this point. After penetration into the lesion, you should advance the guidewire within the true lumen if there is no intimal calcification and if the lumen is clearly visible on IVUS. If there is intimal calcification, you cannot use IVUS to confirm that the advancing guidewire remains within the true lumen. In the first window without calcified plaque that is found as the IVUS catheter is advanced, you should confirm the position of the true lumen and estimate the course for the guidewire to follow. Then you should advance the guidewire toward the predicted point parallel with the IVUS catheter/guidewire to find a direction in which it can easily go forward. When the guidewire is about to reach the plaque window, you should check if it is still in the true lumen. If it is, you should further advance the IVUS catheter/guidewire and repeat your IVUS check until the guidewire is advanced into the true lumen at the exit.

If the guidewire is found to be outside the true lumen at the window, you should pull it back to the previous window where it was confirmed to be in the true lumen and then try to advance it through the true lumen up to the next window.

For IVUS-guided wiring by the false lumen technique, it is better to use an IVUS catheter with a short nose. The Eagle Eye (Volcano) was commonly used at one time, and the double R type NaviFocus WR (Terumo) has also become popular in recent years (Fig. 1.130). Currently, I also use the latter catheter.

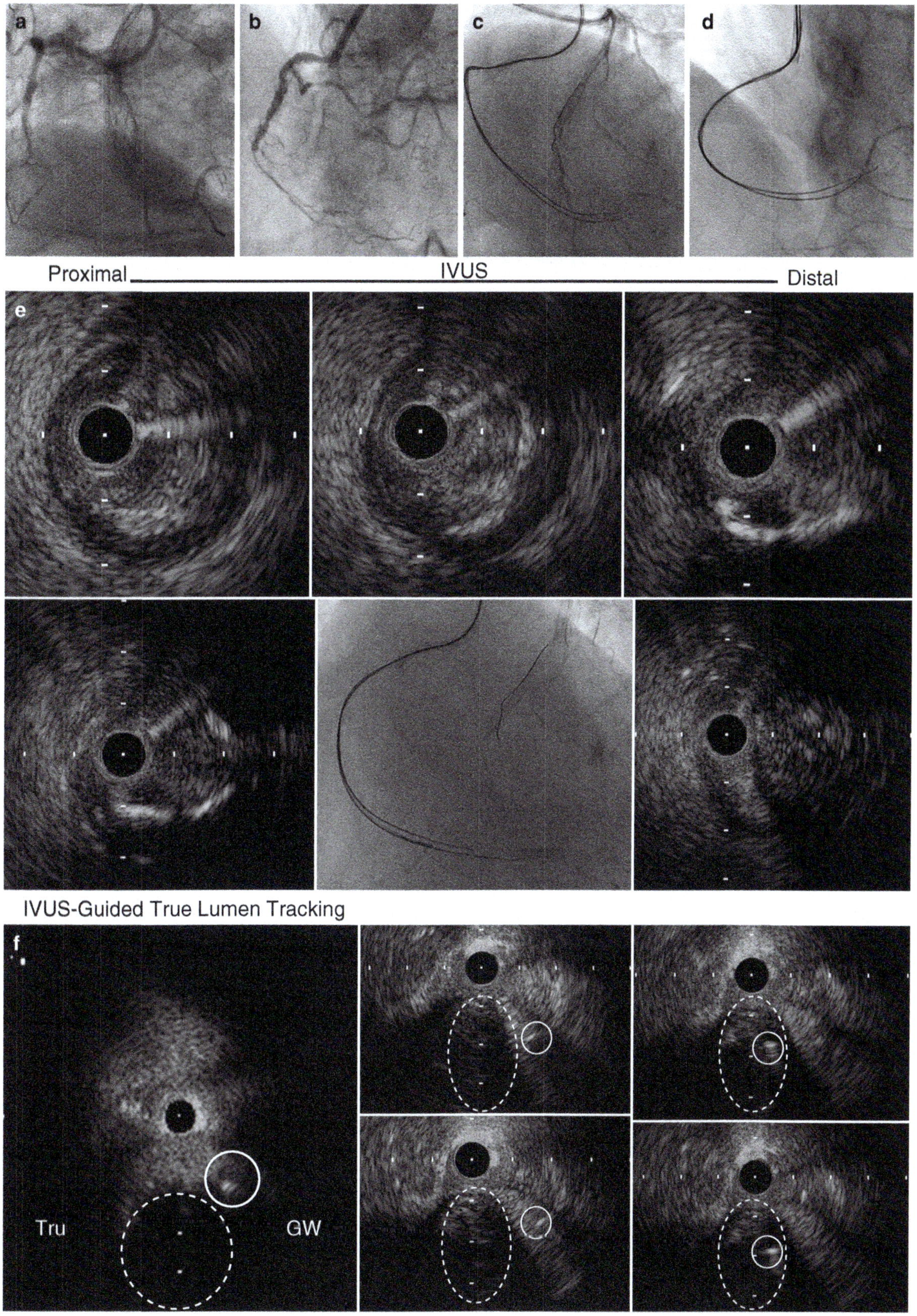

Fig. 1.129 IVUS-guided wiring: False lumen technique. (**a** & **b**) CTO of the RCA (Segment #3), with reattempted IVUS-guided wiring by the false lumen technique. (**c** & **d**) Antegrade PCI resulted in deviation of the guidewire into the subintimal space, so the strategy was switched to retrograde PCI, but attempts at collateral channel tracking failed. A second antegrade guidewire manipulated by the parallel wire technique also failed to reach the true lumen. (**e**) IVUS showed that the guidewire was in the subintimal space. (**f**) While the position of the true lumen was checked by IVUS, a guidewire was advanced along the predicted correct route. (**g**) After the guidewire reached the exit, it was confirmed to be in the true lumen, and PCI was completed by stent implantation

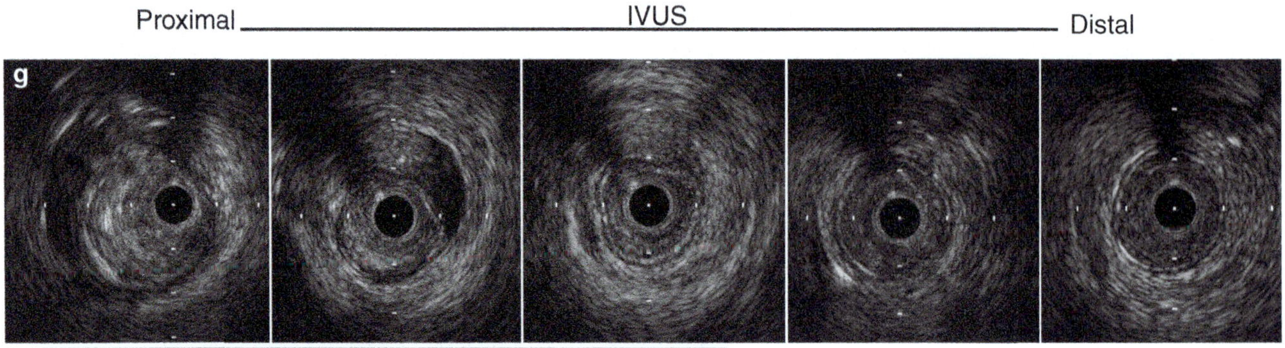

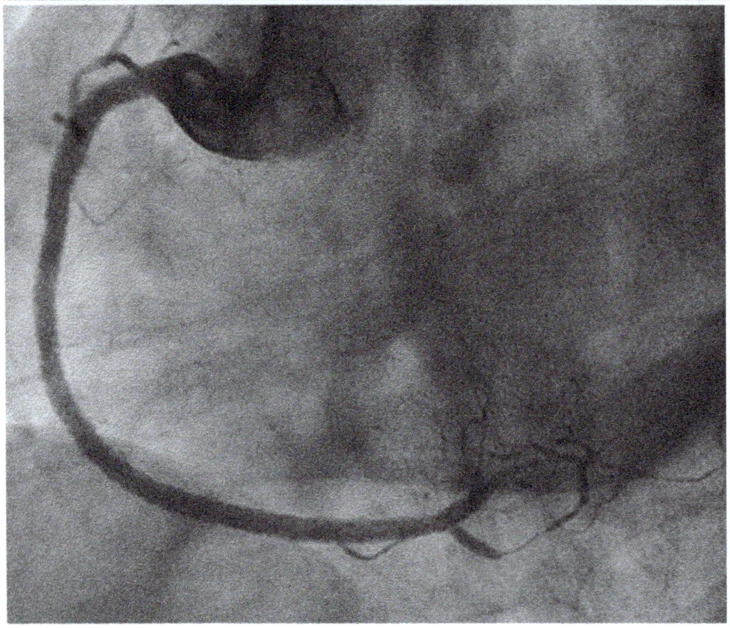

Fig. 1.129 (continued)

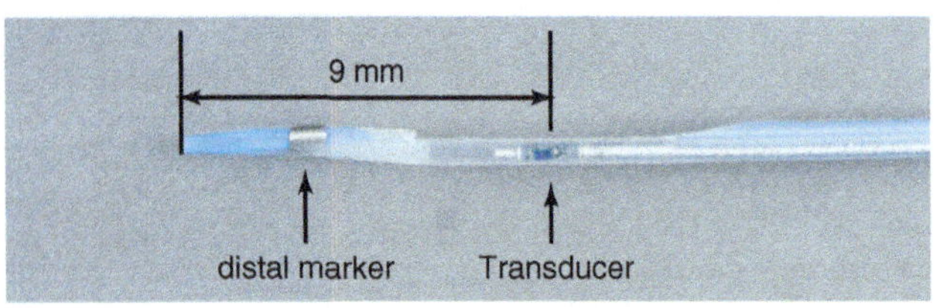

Fig. 1.130 Photograph of the NaviFocus WR. The NaviFocus WR has a short nose, with a distance of only 9 mm between the tip and the transducer

1.6.4.14 Confirmation of Crossing the True Lumen and Points to Be Considered After Crossing

As mentioned above, crossing the true lumen with a guidewire is first recognized by a sudden reduction of resistance and almost spontaneous advancement of the wire. However, this also occurs when the guidewire has gone outside the vessel wall. These two different situations can usually be distinguished easily on the basis of the movement and route of the guidewire, but sometimes may be confused. Crossing through the true lumen has to be confirmed by collateral (usually contralateral) imaging.

After a stiff tapered CTO guidewire enters a relatively soft false lumen, resistance to advancing the wire is reduced considerably, which may lead to the misunderstanding that the guidewire has entered the true lumen. The guidewire is tracking the true lumen if it does not show deflection when advanced slowly without rotation and with the tip oriented medially to the curve of the occluded vessel. However, subintimal tracking must be suspected if there is even slight deflection of the tip when the guidewire is advanced a little. To check whether the guidewire is in the true or false lumen, it must be advanced without rotation, since a guidewire that is advanced with tip rotation may move forward in a false lumen without showing deflection in response to even light pressure.

After the guidewire has reached the exit of the occlusion, you should perform collateral imaging to determine whether it is inside or outside the true lumen. If the guidewire has crossed the CTO in a false lumen, you should choose from the following strategies: (1) attempt to cross the occlusion through the true lumen with the same guidewire, (2) attempt to cross through the true lumen with a second guidewire (parallel wiring or seesaw wiring), or (3) switch the strategy to the retrograde approach.

If you can confirm that the guidewire has crossed the occlusion through the true lumen, you should advance a microcatheter over the guidewire, exchange the guidewire for another with a less stiff tip, and deliver the appropriate devices to dilate the lumen. If collateral imaging fails to provide clear confirmation that the guidewire has crossed the occlusion through the true lumen, you should check for free backflow of blood from the microcatheter after withdrawing the guidewire and then perform tip injection. After confirming that the guidewire crossed the CTO through the true lumen, you should record the confirmation.

1.6.5 Microcatheter

You must always use a microcatheter to assist the guidewire in crossing a CTO. Using a microcatheter allows you to exchange guidewires and to finely adjust the orientation, movement, and backup of the guidewire.

1.6.5.1 Selection of the Microcatheter

Which microcatheter should be chosen for antegrade PCI? The minimum requirement to be met may be the ability to improve the manipulability of the guidewire more. In particular, friction between the microcatheter and guidewire needs to remain relatively constant, even after passing through a very tortuous vessel (Fig. 1.131).

In addition, the microcatheter needs to have a tip that can easily enter an occlusion when advanced over a guidewire. To meet this requirement, the microcatheter should have a tip that is as small as possible and a shaft that is as slim as possible. A microcatheter with superior crossability even with rotation is better. A desirable microcatheter can be used to advance a Conquest Pro 12 or another guidewire that has a high tip load without perforation of the microcatheter by the guidewire tip, even when the tip is located at a curve of the target vessel. There is no ideal microcatheter among the many currently available, so the optimal microcatheter should be selected depending on the morphology and hardness of the target lesion.

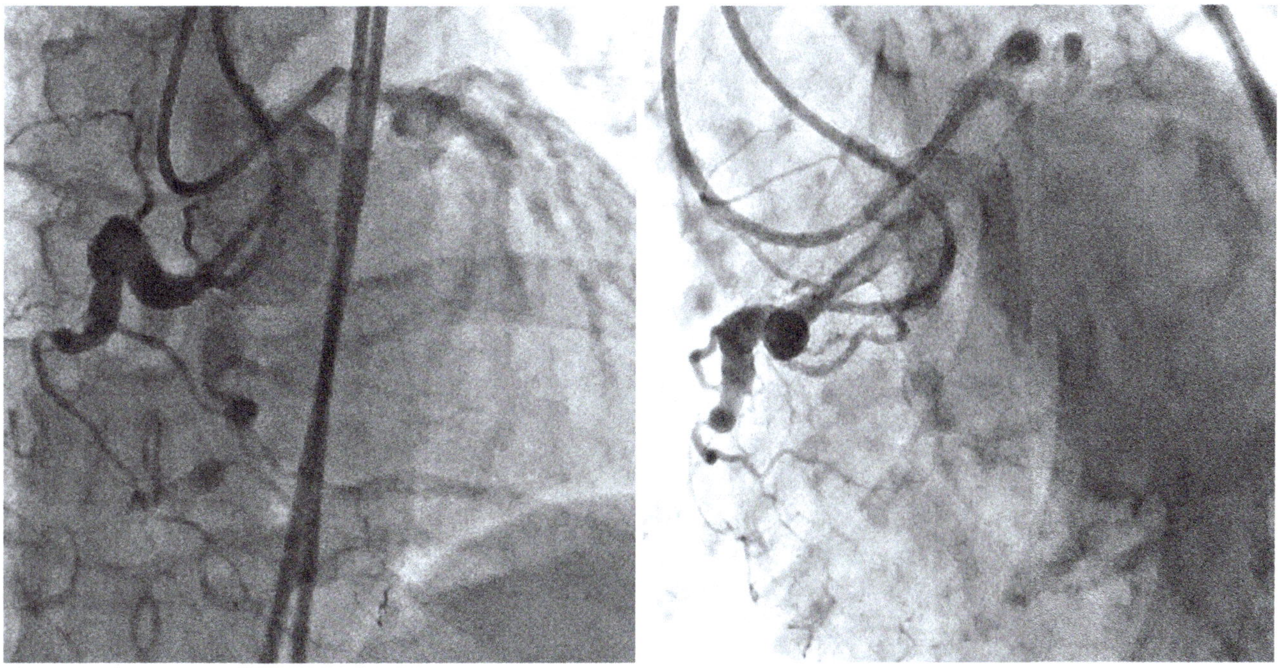

Fig. 1.131 CTO of an RCA with a very tortuous proximal segment. In this situation, using a soft microcatheter will cause greater friction with the guidewire and reduce its manipulability

1.6.5.2 Position of the Microcatheter Tip

When manipulating a guidewire toward a CTO through a microcatheter, you should place the tip of the microcatheter near the entrance of the occlusion. Positioning the tip of the microcatheter about 5 mm from the entry will improve backup for the guidewire. However, if the distance is too short, the microcatheter will bias the guidewire toward the larger curvature of a curved vessel and increase the risk of guidewire whipping. You may approximate the microcatheter tip to the CTO entry if stronger backup is absolutely necessary, but you should usually position the catheter tip at 1 to 1.5 cm from the entry to ensure good manipulability of the guidewire.

1.6.6 Device Delivery Strategy

After a guidewire has crossed a CTO through the true lumen, you can deliver devices along the guidewire. To reduce the risk of injury or perforation of the coronary artery segment distal to the occlusion during device delivery, you should exchange the CTO crossing guidewire for another guidewire. Before performing guidewire exchange, you should first advance a microcatheter along the guidewire.

Advancing this device is the only procedure during PCI for which an interventionalist may use a strong pushing force.

1.6.6.1 Microcatheter

For the reasons mentioned above, a microcatheter with good crossability should be selected. The crossability of a microcatheter is a function of the characteristics of the lesion and the properties of the microcatheter tip. Here, I will discuss a phenomenon that is particularly notable with balloon catheters, but is also applicable to microcatheters. In brief, it is difficult to cross a hard (e.g., calcified) occlusion using a microcatheter with a soft tip. This is because the tip of a microcatheter tends to flare out when blocked by a hard obstruction (Fig. 1.132a) and it will be deformed if pushed forcibly (Fig. 1.132b). These changes substantially increase the profile of the tip and make it more difficult for the microcatheter to cross the occlusion. In contrast, if the microcatheter has a stiff tip that is not easily deformed, it can be advanced while deforming the lesion instead.

Because of good trackability, a microcatheter with a soft tip may be able to cross a tortuous lesion that is relatively hard, while a microcatheter with a stiff tip often fails to do so, since the latter type of catheter can be advanced into a hard CTO but cannot track a tortuous vessel.

The crossability of a microcatheter also depends on the diameter of its shaft. A microcatheter with a slimmer shaft can cross an occlusion more easily. One may think that a microcatheter with a stiffer shaft provides stronger backup. Considering the importance of reducing friction by rotating the microcatheter to facilitate its advancement, a stiffer shaft is better as it provides superior torque and greater resistance to twisting deformation. Nonetheless, a microcatheter may only be rotated to-and-fro several times.

Once a microcatheter has become wedged in an occlusion or tight stenosis and cannot be rotated further, continued attempts to rotate it in the same direction will cause deformation of the shaft. It is very difficult to slide the guidewire through such a deformed microcatheter. To withdraw the microcatheter, it is also necessary to withdraw the guidewire that has successfully crossed the lesion.

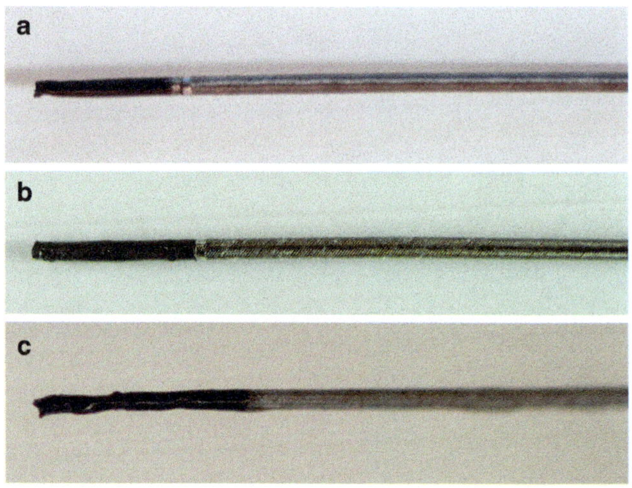

Fig. 1.132 Microcatheter with a small soft tip. When a microcatheter with a small soft tip is pushed forward into a severely calcified hard occlusion, the tip may flare out (**a**) or be deformed (**b**). If the microcatheter crosses such a hard occlusion, its tip may be stretched when the catheter is withdrawn from the lesion (**c**). The appropriate microcatheter for a severely calcified hard lesion should have a small stiff tip

1.6.6.2 Balloon Catheter

If a microcatheter fails to cross the occlusion, you should try to deliver a semi-compliant balloon catheter with the smallest diameter feasible. As is the case for microcatheters, a balloon catheter with a stiff tip is more suitable for crossing a hard straight occlusion, while a balloon catheter with a soft tip is desirable for a tortuous lesion.

If a balloon catheter that has been advanced with sufficient backup fails to cross the occlusion, you should consider the next strategy. Before proceeding to the next step, you should withdraw the balloon catheter and inspect its tip. If the tip is even slightly flared, cut off about 0.3 mm using sharp scissors (Fig. 1.133), since the balloon catheter may cross the occlusion without its flared tip. Instead of using a new balloon catheter, I modify the first catheter in this way to save limited medical resources (see Chap. 2.3.4 "Delivery of a Balloon Catheter for the Kissing Balloon Technique" [page 186]).

1.6.6.3 Anchoring

As mentioned in Sect. 1.3 ("Guiding Catheter"), anchoring is very effective for stabilizing a guiding catheter, which can easily become disengaged when a balloon catheter is pushed in through it. I use an Amplatz left-type guiding catheter (e.g., AL 1 ST) when performing PCI for CTO of the RCA, and anchoring is sometimes necessary to stabilize this catheter because its curve does not always fit the size of the sinus of Valsalva. In this setting, the side branch used for anchoring may be the conus branch, sinoatrial node branch, right ventricular branch, or atrial branch. The anchoring balloon should be slightly oversized and should be inflated at a low pressure of about 4 to 6 atm.

1.6.6.4 Tornus Crossing Catheter

If the occlusion is too hard to cross with a balloon catheter, you can often use a Tornus crossing catheter instead. If the guiding catheter is unstable even when using a Tornus cath-

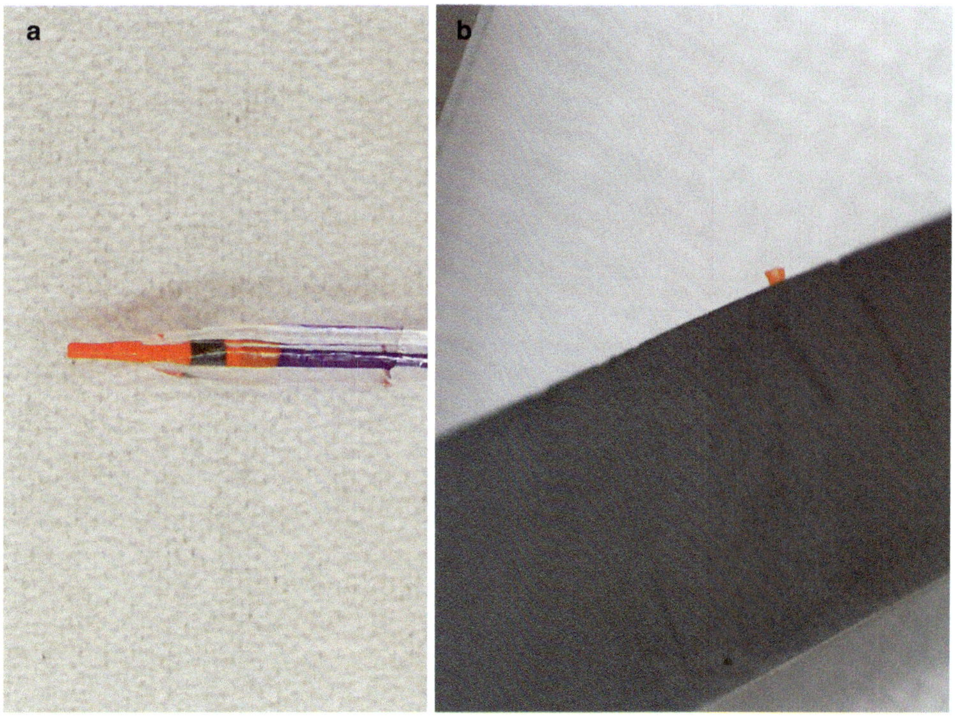

Fig. 1.133 Modifying a balloon catheter with a flared tip. During attempts to penetrate a severely calcified hard occlusion with a balloon catheter or to enter a side branch through a stent strut, the tip of the catheter may become flared (**a**), and even slight flaring can interfere with delivery. After the flared tip is cut off with scissors (**b**), the balloon catheter may become able to cross the lesion or pass the stent strut

eter, you should maintain the anchoring balloon at its previous position to stabilize the guiding catheter. An anchoring balloon with a diameter of 2 mm or more can be used as a trapping balloon during delivery and removal of the Tornus catheter.

After delivering the Tornus catheter, you should exchange the guidewire for a 0.014-inch extra support-type guidewire and try to advance a balloon catheter over the wire. (Alternatively, you can exchange the guidewire for a floppy RotaWire in order to perform rotablation.) If the balloon catheter fails to cross the lesion, you should exchange it for a Tornus catheter again and exchange the 0.014-inch guidewire for a floppy RotaWire to start rotablation (see Chap. 5.1.3 "Tornus Catheter" [page 245]).

1.6.6.5 Excimer Laser Coronary Angioplasty (ELCA)

If a retrograde guidewire has crossed the occlusion, a loop can be formed between the antegrade and retrograde guiding catheters, which will almost definitely ensure successful delivery of the devices. If an antegrade guidewire has crossed the occlusion, a loop cannot be formed until guidewire exchange, so a balloon catheter or Tornus catheter may be unable to cross the lesion. In such cases, a laser catheter with a diameter of 0.9 mm can be used to perform angioplasty (excimer laser coronary angioplasty: ELCA). However, ELCA is not effective for recanalizing a severely calcified lesion, and there is often no choice other than to perform rotablation for this purpose.

1.6.6.6 Rotablator

To perform rotablation before device delivery, you have to exchange the guidewire for a RotaWire through a microcatheter with its tip fixed at the CTO entry point. If the microcatheter is advanced too far, its tip will become bent upon withdrawal of the guidewire from the catheter (Fig. 1.134), and it will be impossible to orient the tip toward the entry point. Therefore, when exchanging guidewires before rotablation, it is important to only press the tip of the microcatheter lightly against the CTO entry point.

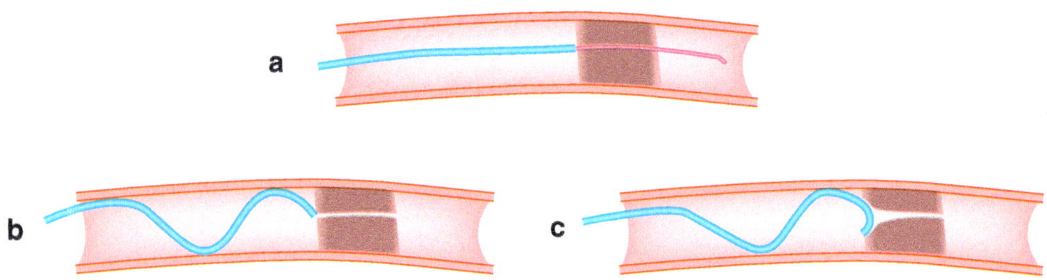

Fig. 1.134 If a microcatheter is advanced into an occlusion, its tip becomes bent on withdrawal of the guidewire. A microcatheter with a guidewire inside it is relatively straight (**a**). Upon withdrawal of the guidewire, the microcatheter (and its tip) becomes curved due to the release of accumulated force (**b**). When advanced through a microcatheter with a slightly bent tip that has lost coaxiality with the occlusion, it will be difficult for a RotaWire to follow the correct route. A microcatheter with a slightly bent tip can be reused after withdrawing it and straightening the tip. However, a microcatheter with a severely deformed and folded tip (**c**) can hardly be returned to its original shape. Therefore, after its tip has been pushed into the occlusion, you should pull a microcatheter back slightly to release the accumulated force before withdrawing the guidewire from the catheter

1.6.6.7 Double or Triple Wires

In the past, I would deliver a device to the occlusion through a lumen that was enlarged by using two or even three CTO crossing wires. However, I have not employed this strategy recently because the CTOs that I encounter have not required or permitted it.

1.6.7 From Balloon Inflation to Stent Placement

After device delivery has been achieved, balloon inflation may be performed. In general, you should dilate an occlusion by inflating a small balloon (1.0 to 1.5 mm in diameter) and then perform observation by IVUS. The ballooning and stenting procedures employed for CTOs are largely the same as those for non-occlusive lesions, except that special care is needed in case of crossing a false lumen and for preserving a small side branch when treating double CTOs of the main trunk and a larger branch. Please refer to IVUS-guided wiring in Sect. 1.7 "Retrograde Approach."

1.7 Retrograde Approach

The "retrograde approach" is a term that has become widely used since 2005, when Dr. Osamu Kato proposed a breakthrough strategy that he referred to as "controlled antegrade and retrograde subintimal tracking (CART)." However, Dr. Kato and colleagues actually started to employ retrograde guidewires around 2000 to track a collateral channel and reach the vessel distal to a CTO for use as a landmark when navigating an antegrade guidewire through the occlusion.

Here I summarize the strategies that I include in the category of retrograde PCI for CTO.

1. Direct retrograde crossing: This involves retrogradely advancing a guidewire through a collateral channel to reach the lumen of the target coronary artery distal to a CTO and directly crossing the occlusion by using a retrograde CTO guidewire with the support of a microcatheter for the proximal true lumen (Fig. 1.135a).
2. Reverse CART technique: This involves navigation of a retrograde guidewire to a space within a CTO that was previously reached by an antegrade guidewire and enlarged by a balloon and using the retrograde wire to cross the occlusion (Fig. 1.135b).
3. CART technique: This involves navigation of an antegrade guidewire to a space in the distal part of an occlusion that was previously reached by a retrograde guidewire and enlarged by a balloon and using the antegrade wire to cross the occlusion (Fig. 1.135c).
4. Antegrade CTO crossing: This involves placing the tip of a retrograde guidewire in the distal part of a CTO and using it as a landmark while crossing the CTO antegradely (Fig. 1.135d).
5. Kissing wire technique: This involves advancing an antegrade or retrograde guidewire into a CTO and using it as a landmark to navigate another guidewire across the occlusion from the opposite direction (Fig. 1.135e).

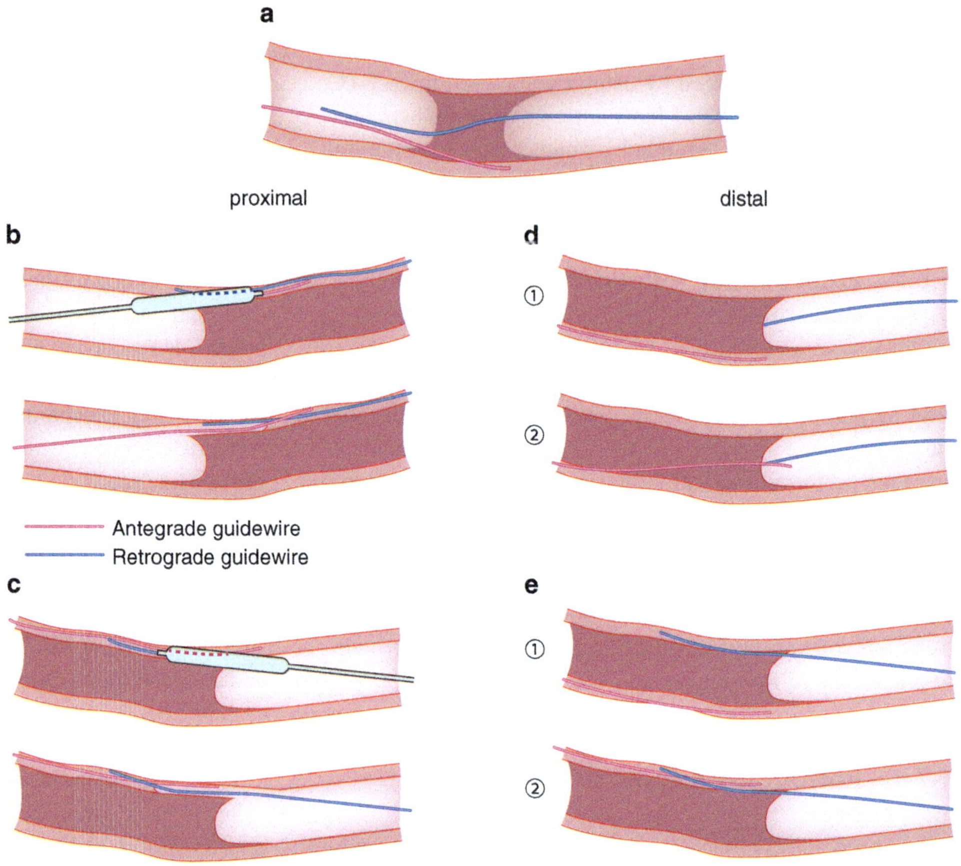

Fig. 1.135 Techniques for the retrograde approach. (**a**) An antegrade guidewire (landmark) is not always required to perform direct retrograde crossing. As I attempt antegrade PCI for CTO before switching to the retrograde approach whenever possible, I always leave the antegrade guidewire in position as a landmark for direct retrograde crossing. (**b**) Reverse CART technique. (**c**) CART technique. (**d**) Antegrade CTO crossing: A retrograde guidewire is used as a landmark for the distal true lumen. The tip of the retrograde guidewire is positioned just beyond the distal end of the occlusion, (1) and an antegrade guidewire is advanced toward it (2). (**e**) Kissing wire technique using a retrograde guidewire as a landmark for the distal true lumen. A retrograde guidewire is advanced into the occlusion (1), and then an antegrade guidewire is navigated toward the retrograde wire (2)

1.7.1 Indications for the Retrograde Approach

As mentioned above, I consider antegrade PCI to be the "primary intervention for CTO." However, I think that retrograde PCI can be indicated if there is a collateral channel that can be tracked and if any of the following requirements are met:

1. If a large dissection (false lumen) has been created in a CTO after failure of antegrade PCI (Fig. 1.136): You may be lucky enough to find a route that leads to the true lumen at the end of the occlusion, but an antegrade CTO crossing guidewire will readily enter the large false lumen in most cases. Therefore, you should consider early switching to retrograde PCI.

   Before switching to retrograde PCI, you should advance a relatively soft antegrade CTO guidewire. This wire may possibly be able to cross the occlusion through the true lumen, and it can serve as a landmark to facilitate retrograde wiring if crossing fails.
2. If the proximal cap of a CTO is located at a large coronary ostium and is inaccessible from the ostium (Fig. 1.137): Such a CTO cannot be recanalized by antegrade PCI. If possible, an antegrade guiding catheter should be positioned at the proximal end of the lesion to serve as a landmark. PCI is contraindicated for occlusions resulting from coronary ostial atresia. To rule out this possibility, you must perform CT angiography if there is no dimple at the proximal end of an ostial occlusion, since a diagnosis of ostial atresia can only be established by CT angiography (Fig. 1.138).
3. If the distal end of an occlusion is at a branching point and both branches require recanalization despite having small luminal diameters (Fig. 1.139): Even if an antegrade guidewire crosses such an occlusion through the true lumen, it often penetrates plaque at the branching point and enters the true lumen distal to the carina. In this situation, the side branch may not be isolated even after dilation by a small balloon. In contrast, a guidewire advanced retrogradely to the branching point always enters plaque proximal to the carina, so the side branch will not be occluded by inflating a balloon in the occlusion.
4. If an antegrade guidewire fails to enter the distal true lumen (Fig. 1.140).
5. If an antegrade guidewire undergoes deviation into the subintimal space after being blocked by a hard obstruction (Fig. 1.141): When an antegrade guidewire with a very high tip load (e.g., a Conquest Pro 12) is blocked by a hard obstruction within a CTO and cannot be advanced

further through the true lumen, you should advance another guidewire retrogradely. If the retrograde guidewire can reach the site of the obstruction, you may then bypass the obstacle relatively easily with the antegrade guidewire. Eventually, this may lead to successful crossing of the CTO by the reverse CART technique (reverse CART) with a short false lumen passage.

6. If an antegrade guidewire undergoes extravascular deviation while being advanced through a long occlusion with anatomy unclear: In this situation, you should promptly switch to retrograde PCI. If a retrograde guidewire fails to enter the true lumen, you may try to advance an antegrade guidewire again using the retrograde guidewire as a landmark (kissing wire technique). This often leads to successful intimal/subintimal tracking and allows reverse CART.

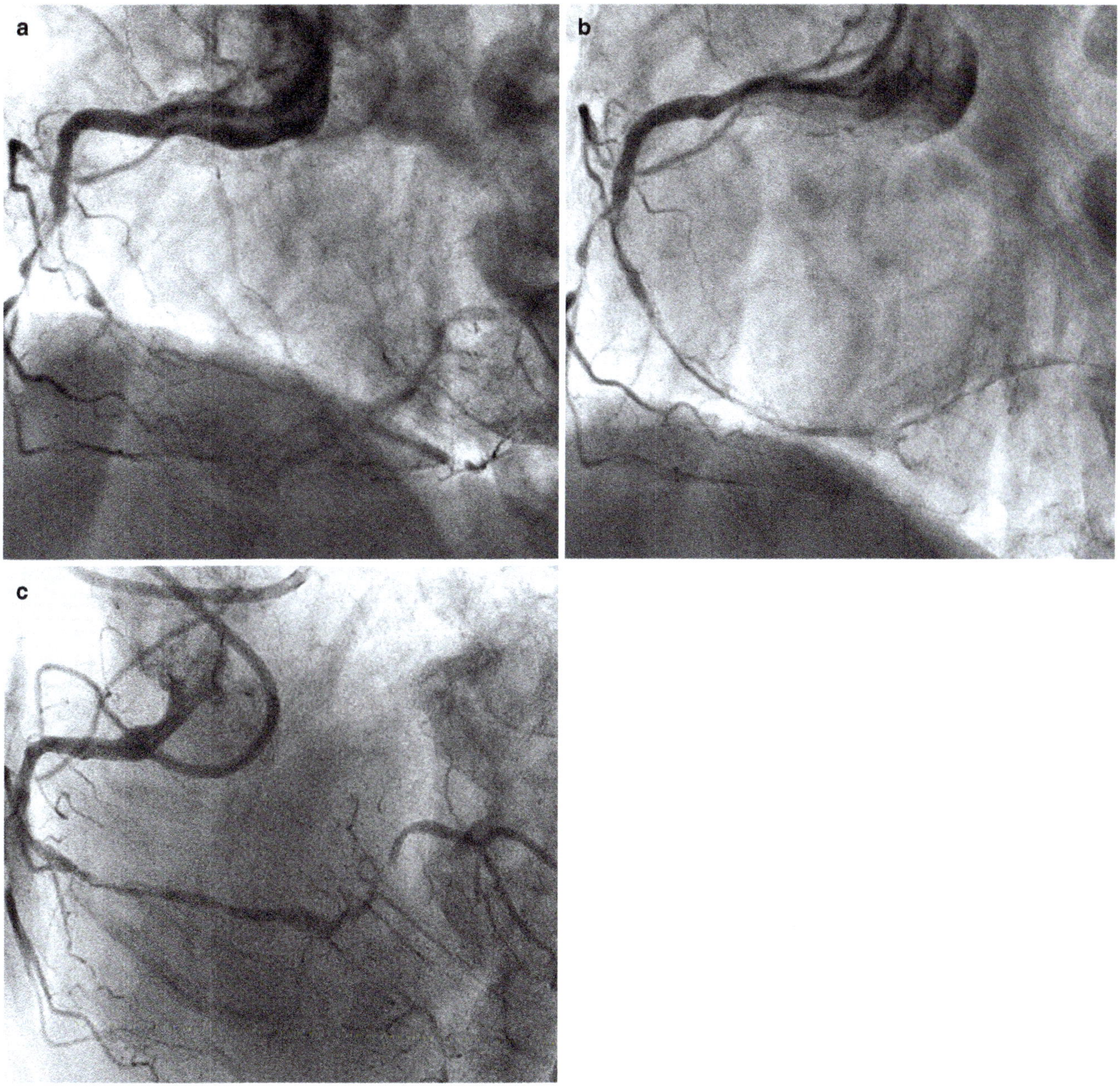

Fig. 1.136 CTO of the distal RCA (Segment #3) (**a**). (**b**) An antegrade guidewire has reached the distal true lumen, but has tracked through a false lumen on its way to the exit. After completion of PCI, the posterior descending branch was still occluded. (**c**) Imaging immediately before reattempting PCI showed a large false lumen in Segment #3. A guidewire could easily track the posterolateral branch, so the posterior descending branch was approached retrogradely, and the CTO was successfully recanalized without side branch occlusion

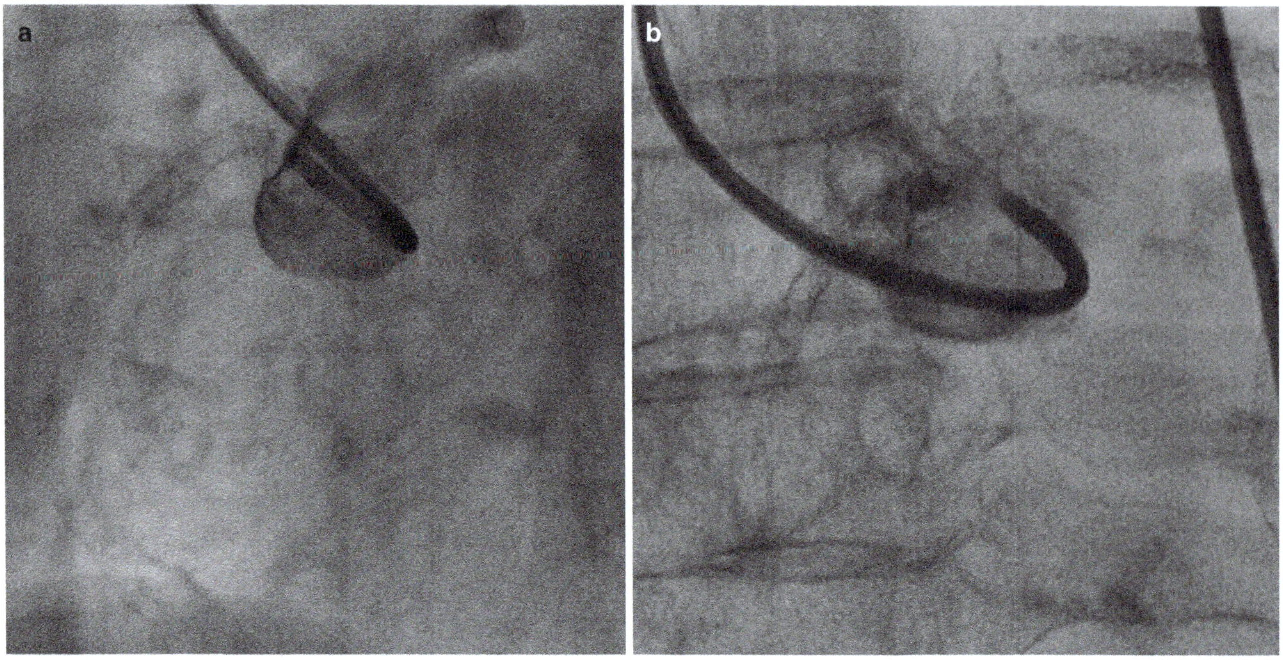

Fig. 1.137 In-stent occlusion in the proximal RCA. A stent previously implanted from the ostium of the RCA precluded sufficient backup by the guiding catheter and diagnostic contrast imaging

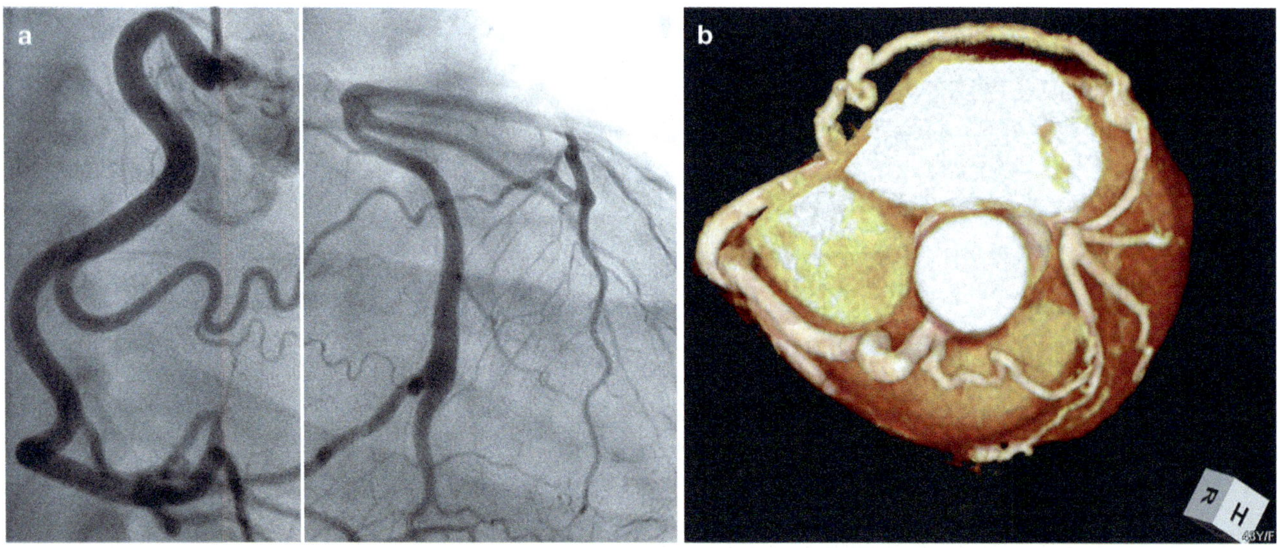

Fig. 1.138 Coronary ostial atresia. (**a**) CAG. (**b**) CT angiogram. RCA angiography provides good visualization of the LCA. CT angiography shows no findings suggestive of LCA ostial atresia

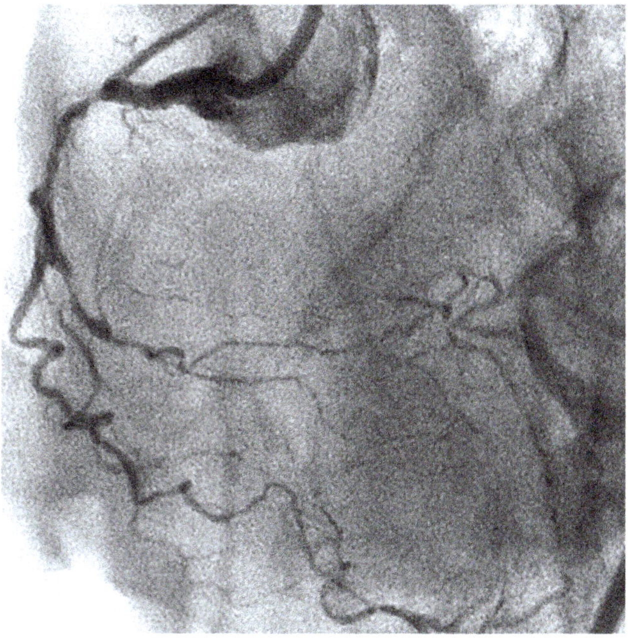

Fig. 1.139 CTO of the distal RCA (Segment #3). Antegrade PCI was attempted, but the CTO could not be crossed. Subsequently, retrograde PCI via the LCX was successful

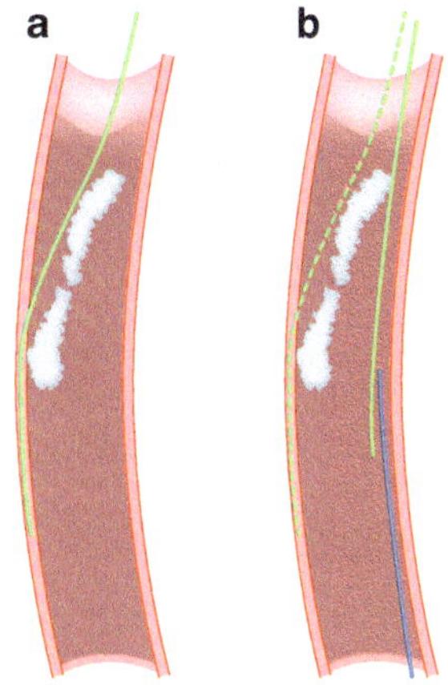

Fig. 1.141 Antegrade guidewire blocked by a hard obstruction (**a**). (**b**) After a retrograde guidewire has entered the occlusion in the true lumen, it may become easier to direct the antegrade guidewire toward the true lumen

Fig. 1.140 CTO of the LAD (**a**) (Segment #7). After failure to cross the CTO antegradely (**b**), the retrograde approach via the RCA was successful (**c**)

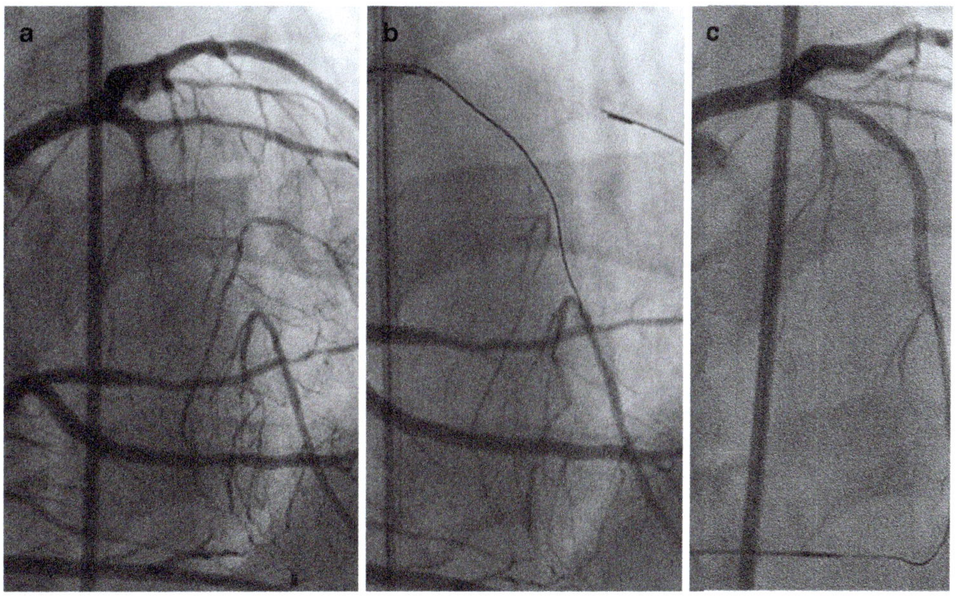

1.7.2 Collateral Channels

Whether the retrograde approach can be performed is dependent on the availability of accessible collateral channels. General knowledge of the collateral channels that usually exist may help you to discover obscure channels on CAG. In addition, understanding the anatomy of these channels facilitates selection of the optimal fluoroscopy angles for viewing the longitudinal axis of each channel, as well as assisting with assessment of the accessibility of each channel and devising the optimal tracking strategy.

Here, I present the collateral channels that I have successfully tracked when performing retrograde PCI, although this list may not include all types of channels that could potentially exist.

Collateral channels that can be used for the retrograde approach to CTOs of the RCA, LAD, and LCX are presented in Figs. 1.142, 1.143, and 1.144, respectively.

Diagnostic CAG images and control CAG images obtained immediately before switching to retrograde PCI should be reviewed to identify every possible collateral channel and determine their accessibility.

Continuity of a channel may be obvious in a certain view, but not in another view. Performing tip injection of contrast medium with a microcatheter will eventually lead to a conclusion regarding channel continuity. However, the anatomy of collateral channels generally follows certain rules. An epicardial channel does not cross another channel without communication, i.e., it does not jump over a nearby vessel to join another more distant vessel. As a result, collateral channels that connect the anterior and posterior sides of the heart run on the surface of the atria or through the atrial septum, or through the ventricular septum, or on the surface of the apex. Even if two channels running through the ventricular septum appear to cross each other, they will actually run on the left and right ventricular sides of the septum and not in the same plane (i.e., overhead crossing). You must not miss such channels that appear to cross each other on CAG. A guidewire may be able to track a channel that is invisible on CAG and reach the lumen of the target vessel distal to the occlusion. This is particularly true for septal channels, and it should be remembered that a guidewire may be advanced beyond the visible end of a channel (Fig. 1.145).

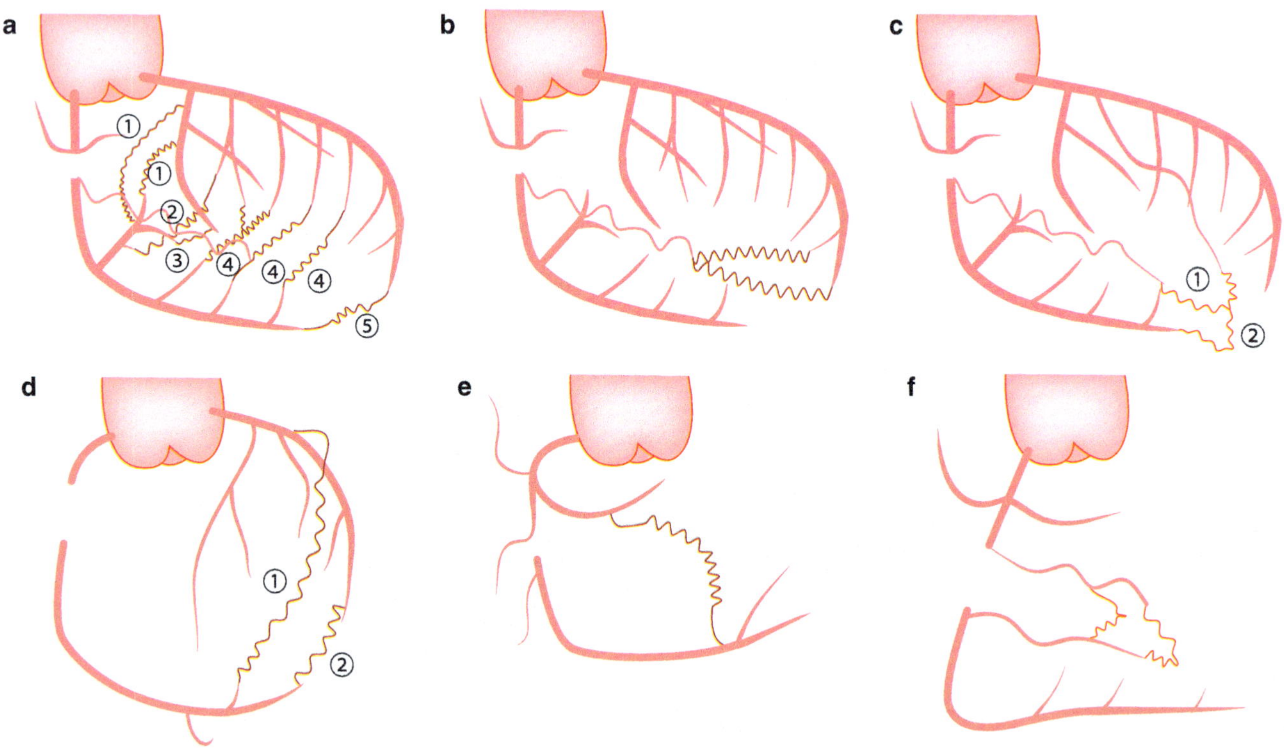

Fig. 1.142 Collateral channels available for the retrograde approach to CTO of the RCA. (**a**) RAO. (1) LCX → ACC → AVB. (2) SB → AVB. (3) PL → FWEp→RCAPL. (4) SB → 4PD. (5) LAD apex→4PD. (**b**) RAO. RVB → SB and RVB → LAD. (**c**) RAO. (1) Dg → Apex→RVB. (2) Dg → Apex→4PD. (**d**) LAO. (1) LCX → ACC → AVB. (2) LCX → FWEp→AVB. *ACC* atrial circumflex channel, *AVB* atrioventricular branch, *FWEp* free wall epicardial channel. (**e**) LAO. Intracoronary collateral; Right atrial branch (SNA) → Kugel anastomosis→AVB (AVNA). *SNA* sinoatrial node artery, *AVB* atrioventricular branch, *AVNA* atrioventricular node artery. (**f**) RAO. Intracoronary collateral; RVB → RVB. RVB: right ventricular branch

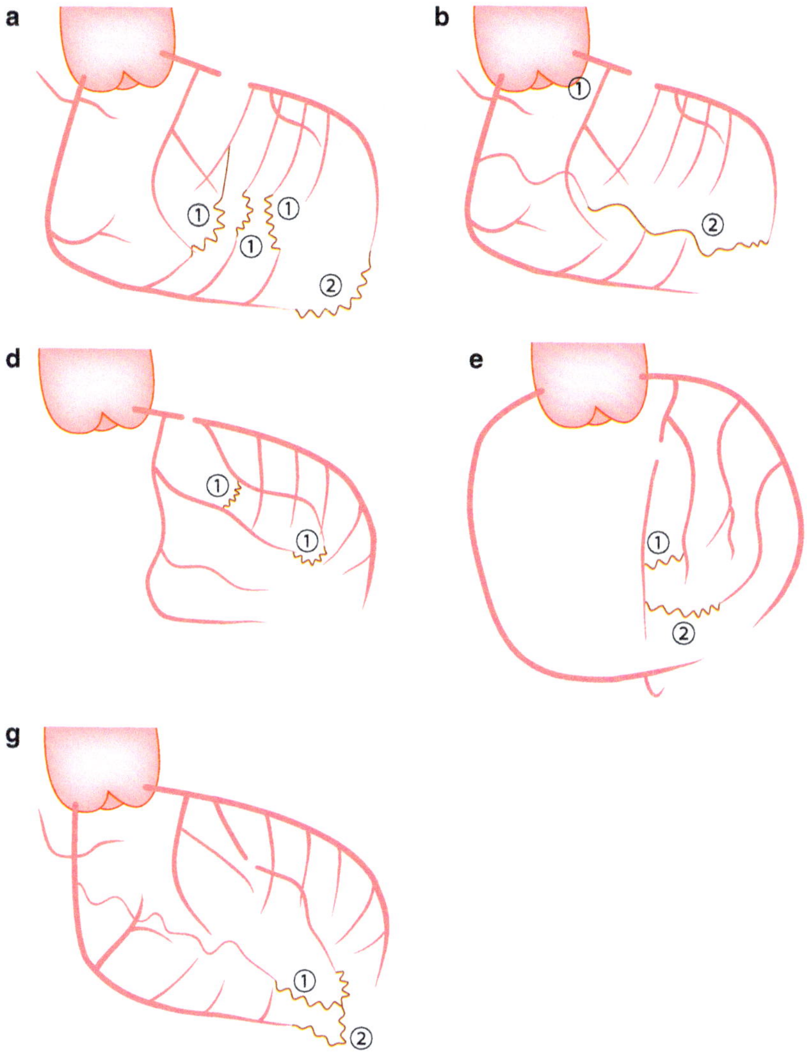

Fig. 1.143 Collateral channels available for the retrograde approach to CTO of the LAD. (**a**) RAO. (1) PDA → SB → LAD. (2) PDA → Apex→LAD. (**b**) RAO. (1) Conus branch→Vieussens anastomosis→LAD prox. (2) RVB → LAD distal or apex. (**c**) RAO. Intracoronary collateral; LAD→SB → SB → LAD. (**d**) RAO. Intracoronary collateral; (1) OM → FWEpi→first Dg → LAD. If the LAD is occluded between the first and second diagonal branches, another channel (first Dg → FWEpi→second Dg → LAD) may be used. (**e**) LAO. (1) Dg → FWEpi→LAD. (2) PL (OM) → FWEpi→LAD. (**f**) If the Dg is occluded; (1) OM → FWEpi→Dg. (2) LAD→FWEpi→Dg. (3) LAD→Apex (FWEpi) → Dg. (**g**) RAO. (1) RVB → Apex→Dg. (2) PDA → Apex→Dg

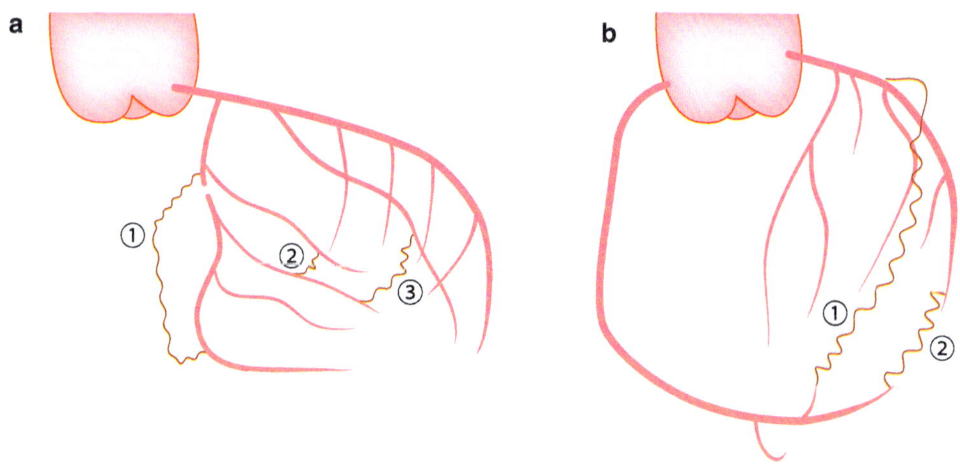

Fig. 1.144 Collateral channels available for the retrograde approach to CTO of the LCX. (**a**) RAO. (1) LCX prox→ACC → LCX distal. (2) OM → FWEpi→PL. (3) Dg → EWEpi→PL. (**b**) LAO. (1) AVB → ACC → LCX main trunk. (2) AVB → FWEpi→LCX

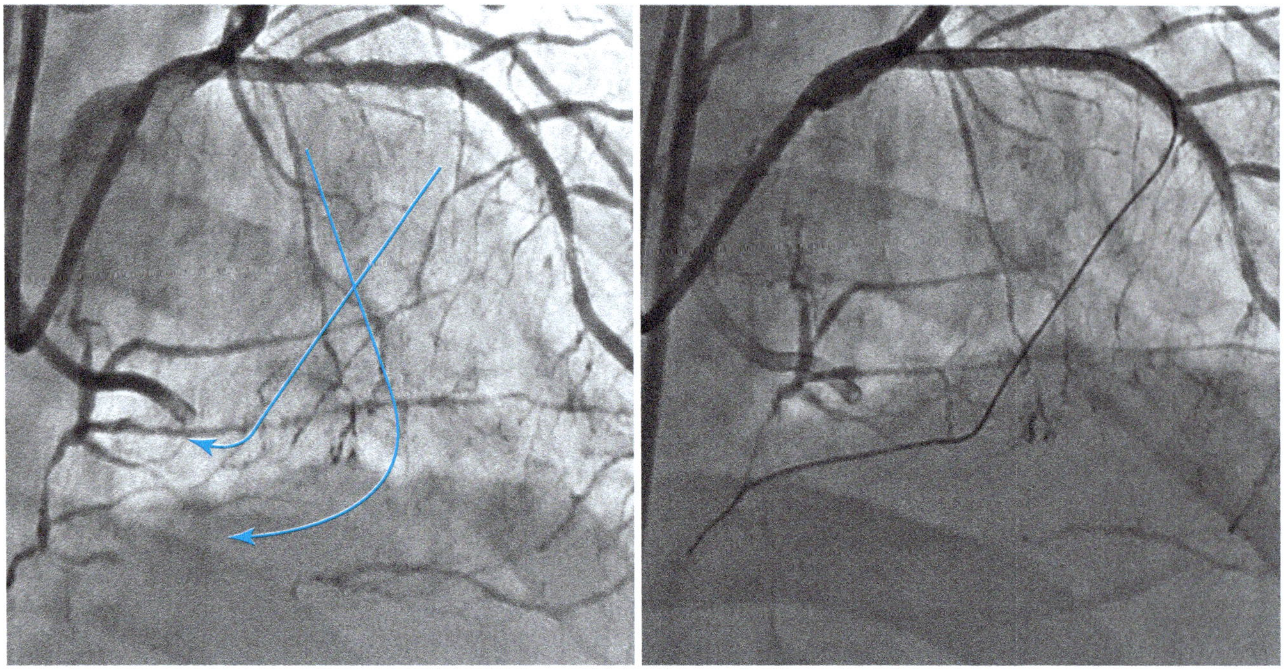

Fig. 1.145 Two crossing septal branches. On CAG, two septal branches appeared to cross each other and to give rise to channels leading to the posterolateral branch of the RCA. The channel originating from the first septal branch is very tortuous, whereas that from the second septal branch is relatively straight. The latter channel was selected for wiring and was tracked successfully

1.7.3 Selection of a Collateral Channel

Before selecting a channel, you should assess the anatomy of all available channels. To do this, you should carefully review the diagnostic CAG images. Using the list of channels presented in the previous subsection for reference, be careful not to miss any of the channels that may be present. Note that diagnostic CAG images may not be obtained at angles that are suitable for following all possible channels or may visualize two small vessels crossing at two levels as if they formed one continuous channel. Therefore, immediately before starting retrograde PCI, you should obtain a contrast image at the angle which provides the best view of the route of the channel selected.

Then, I select the collateral channel for retrograde PCI according to the following rules:

1. Select a septal channel before an epicardial channel: A septal channel should be chosen first, even if its diameter is rather small. There is a low risk of cardiac tamponade after perforation of a septal channel, which is the most important reason for preferring this type of channel. Other reasons for preferentially selecting a septal channel include less tortuosity and easier tracking.

   If the distal end of the occlusion is at a bifurcation of the RCA, you may consider using an epicardial channel that leads to the atrioventricular branch, if there is no other accessible retrograde route to the distal RCA (Segment #3) and if the posterior descending branch comes off the distal RCA at a large angle (Fig. 1.146).

   A collateral channel running toward the RCA from the first septal branch often joins the atrioventricular branch (Fig. 1.147). If such a channel is found, you can safely advance a guidewire from a septal branch directly toward the distal RCA through the channel and penetrate the distal cap of the occlusion.

   Even if there is no visible collateral channel from a septal branch and another channel is prominent, you may still be able to achieve successful tracking by advancing a guidewire into a septal branch (Fig. 1.148). In such cases, the other prominent channel presumably reduced the pressure gradient between the donor artery of a relatively small septal channel and the distal true lumen, thus preventing visualization of the channel. Since you cannot distinguish such invisible channels from the actual absence of channels by performing CAG, you cannot verify the absence of septal channels without first exploring the septal branches. This may be a good reason for performing septal surfing.

   Sometimes, no collateral channels are visible even when there is delayed visualization of the distal true lumen, presumably via several collateral channels with a large pressure gradient between the donor artery of the collaterals and the distal true lumen. If this happens, it is reasonable to consider that the collateral channel is too small for tracking by a guidewire to reach the distal true lumen and it is no use performing septal surfing blindly.
2. Select a channel with fewer severe bends: Contrast imaging in two projections is useful for determining if a channel has any severe bends. It is best to view the channel in two orthogonal projections that are perpendicular to its longitu-

dinal axis. If two orthogonal projections that are not completely perpendicular to the longitudinal axis of the channel show severe tortuosity at the same point (Fig. 1.149), it will be very difficult to track the channel with a guidewire and/or microcatheter (Fig. 1.150). A corkscrewing channel can easily be tracked if the diameter of the spiral is small (Fig. 1.150b), but not if it is large (Fig. 1.151a & b).

3. Select a larger channel: A non-tortuous septal channel visualized by CAG can often be tracked successfully, even if very small. On the other hand, a tortuous epicardial channel is easier to track when it has a diameter of about 1 mm than when it is a fine thread, but may conversely be rather difficult to track when the diameter is too large. Even a large epicardial channel can be tracked if its proximal part is straightened by advancing a guidewire or microcatheter (Fig. 1.152), but will be difficult to track if the proximal part is not straightened (Fig. 1.151c).
4. Avoid a channel that joins the target vessel just distal to the occlusion (Fig. 1.153a & b): After tracking such a channel, a retrograde CTO guidewire is likely to create a dissection from the distal end of the occlusion. When performing retrograde PCI, a small balloon is used to dilate the lesion. If the diameter of the balloon is larger than that of the channel tracked, inflation of the balloon can lead to dissection of a channel that is too close to the occlusion. If dissection occurs in the proximal segment or in a side branch, it may be impossible to advance a guidewire to the distal true lumen even through a Crusade® microcatheter.

Therefore, it is preferable for there to be a certain distance between the point where the channel joins the target vessel and the distal end of the occlusion.

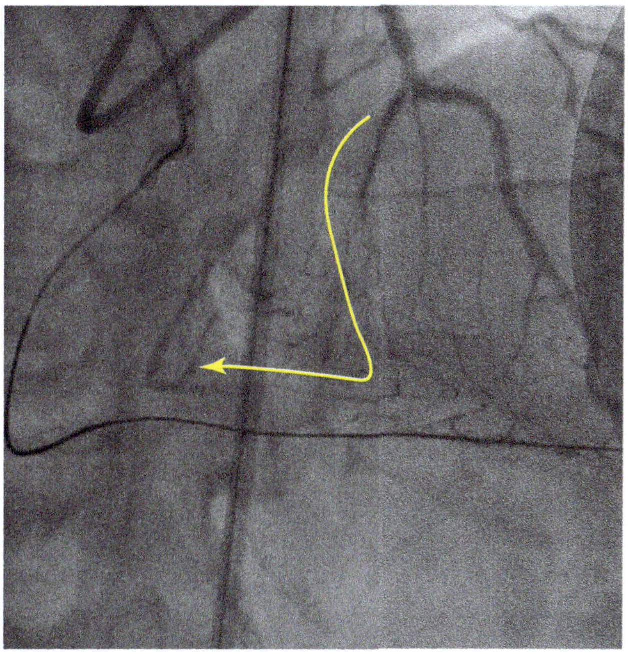

Fig. 1.147 Channel arising from the first septal branch. A collateral channel from the first septal branch runs into the posterolateral branch and not into the posterior descending branch

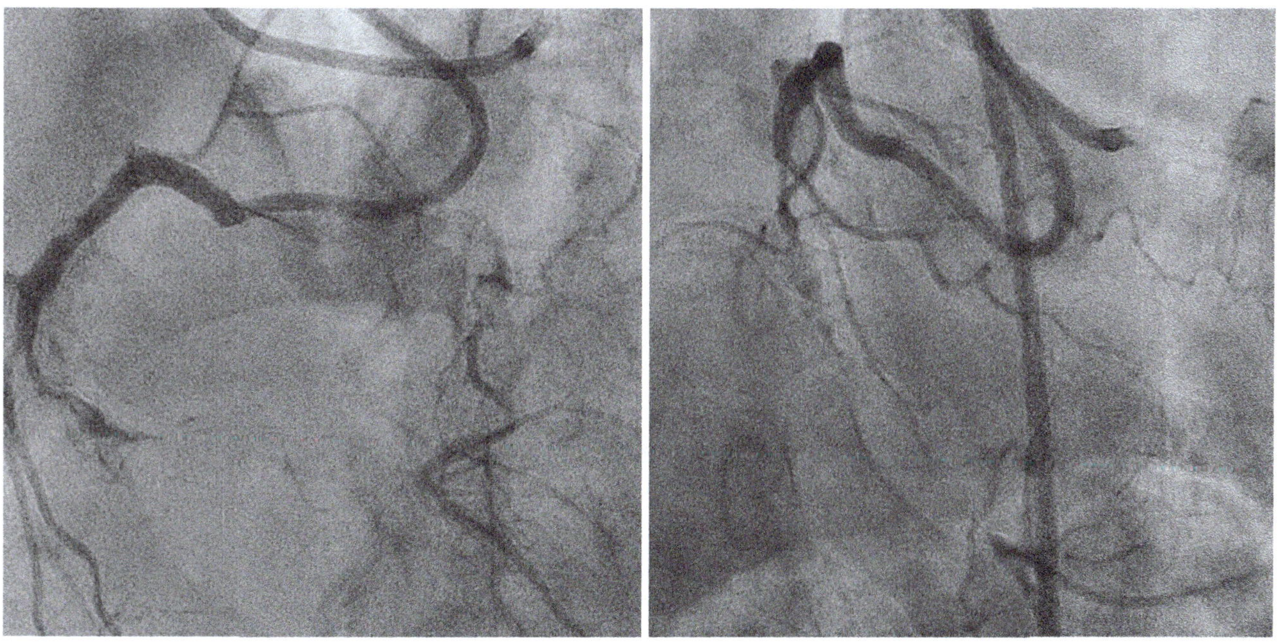

Fig. 1.146 CTO with its distal end at the bifurcation of the distal RCA (Segment #3). The posterior descending branch arises at too large an angle to be tracked retrogradely, whereas the posterolateral branch is parallel and straight. An AC collateral channel arising from the LCX is visible

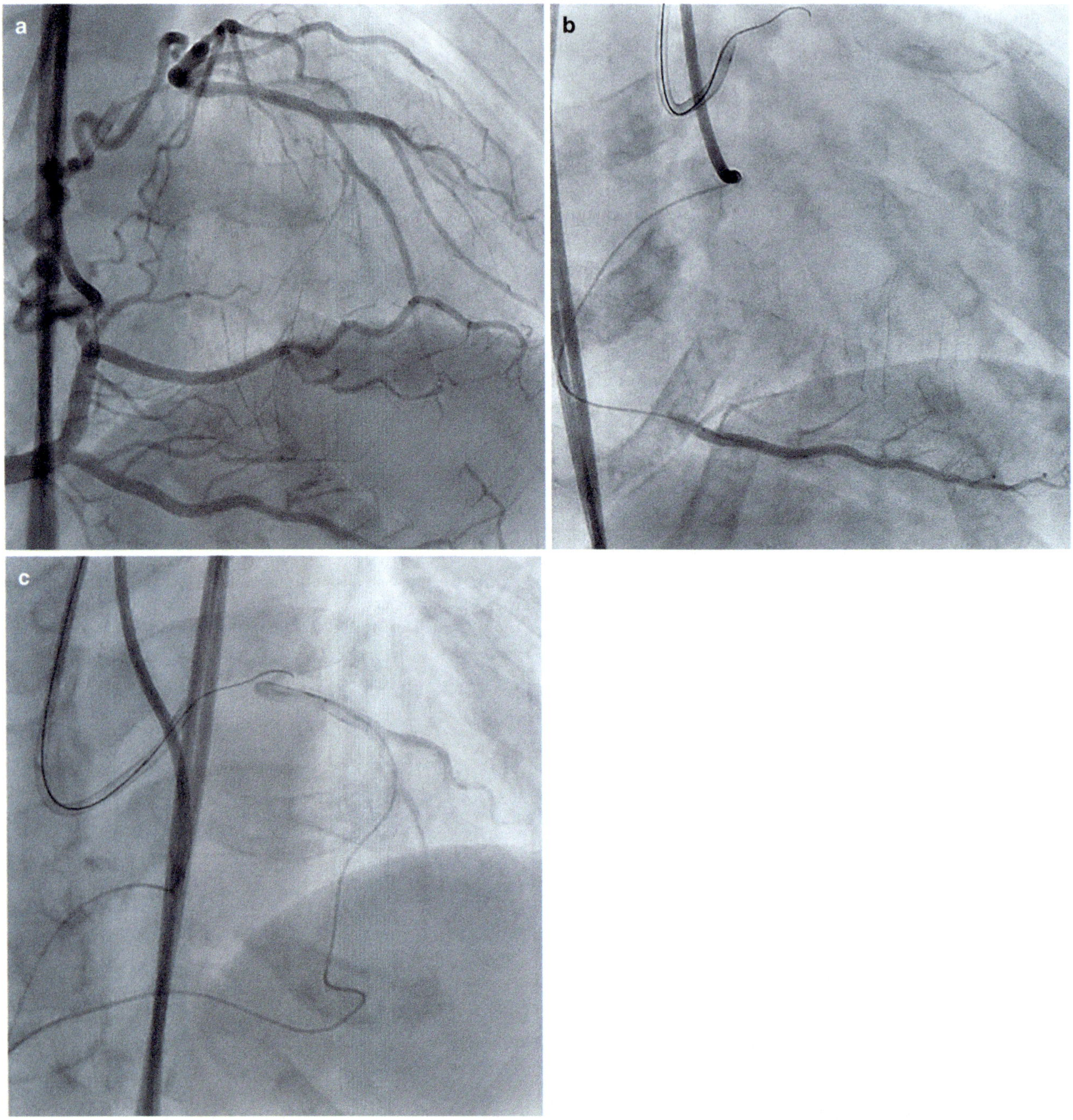

Fig. 1.148 CTO of the LAD. There is a good collateral channel running from the atrioventricular branch (**a**). Tip injection in the posterior descending branch also shows a collateral channel from a septal branch (**b**). Retrograde PCI was performed via this septal branch (**c**)

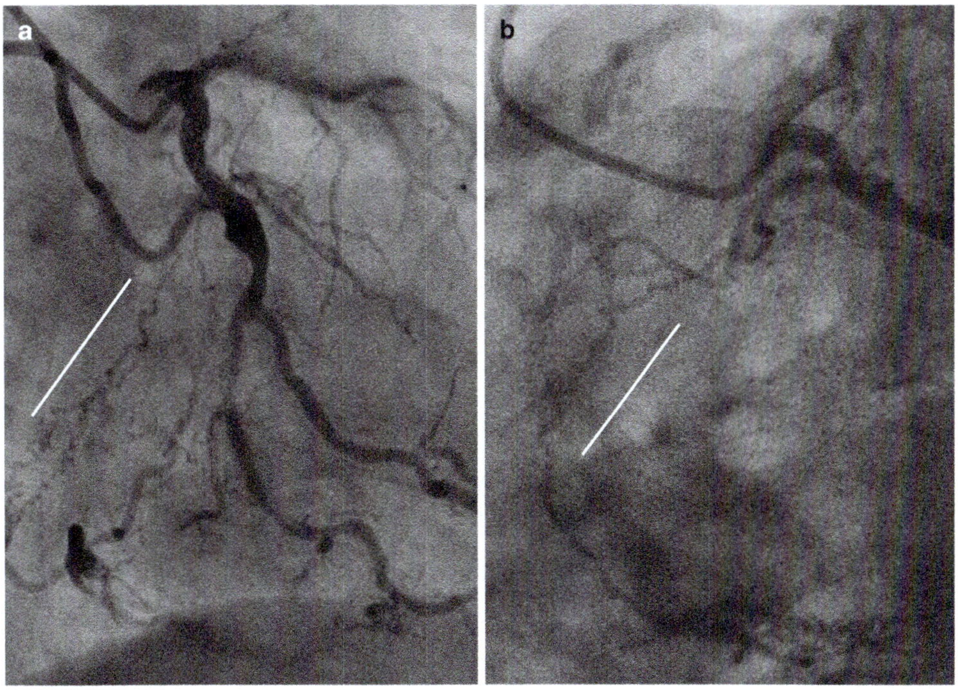

Fig. 1.149 Tracking a very tortuous channel. (**a**) RAO + CA. (**b**). LAO + CA. The part of the channel indicated by a white line appears very tortuous in both of two orthogonal projections

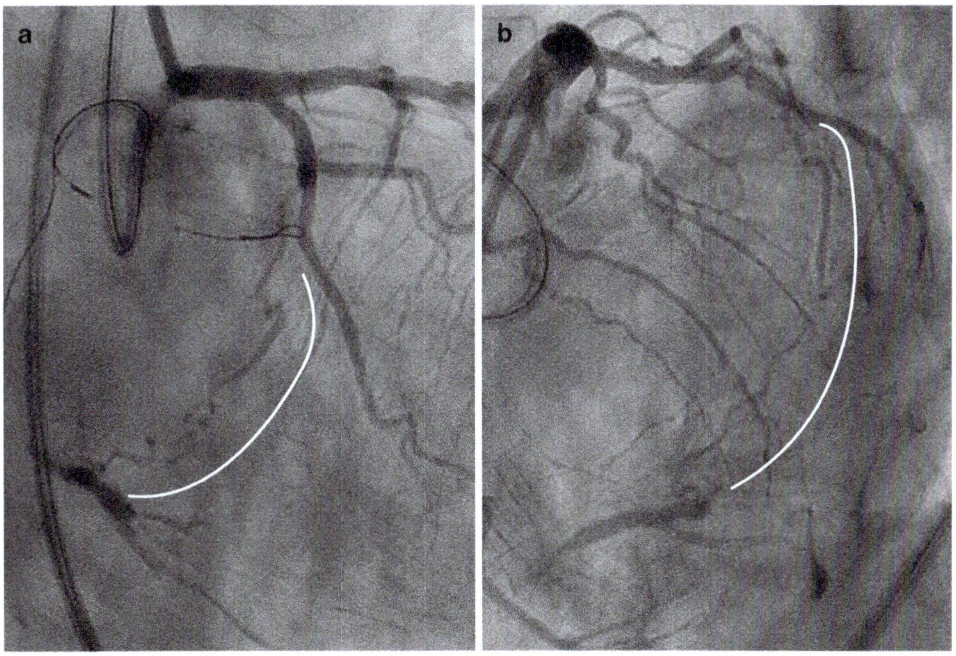

Fig. 1.150 Tracking a corkscrewing channel. This channel appears very tortuous in the RAO + CA view (**a**), but is less tortuous and partially straight in the LAO + CA view (**b**). The corkscrew spiral of this channel has a small diameter

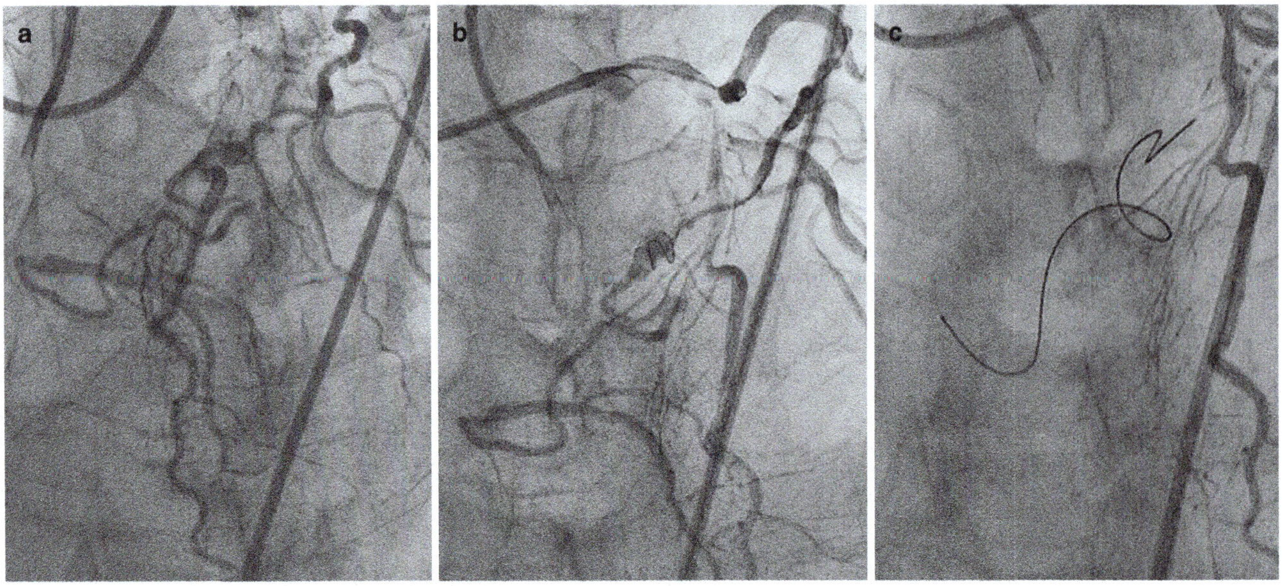

Fig. 1.151 Tracking a corkscrewing channel with a large spiral diameter. The corkscrew spiral of this channel has a large diameter (**a**), and it was difficult to track with a guidewire (**b**). Even after passage of a microcatheter/guidewire, the channel was not straightened (**c**). A guidewire is much less manipulable in such a channel, but attempts to forcibly straighten the channel may injure its walls

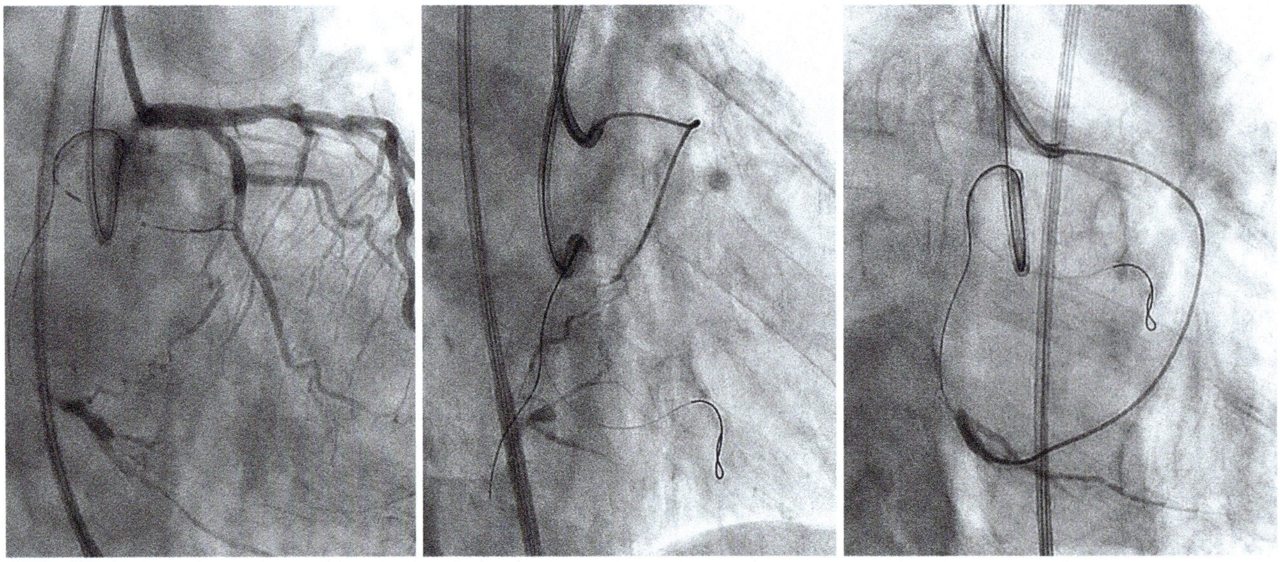

Fig. 1.152 Tracking a bending channel. This bending channel was straightened by advancing a microcatheter

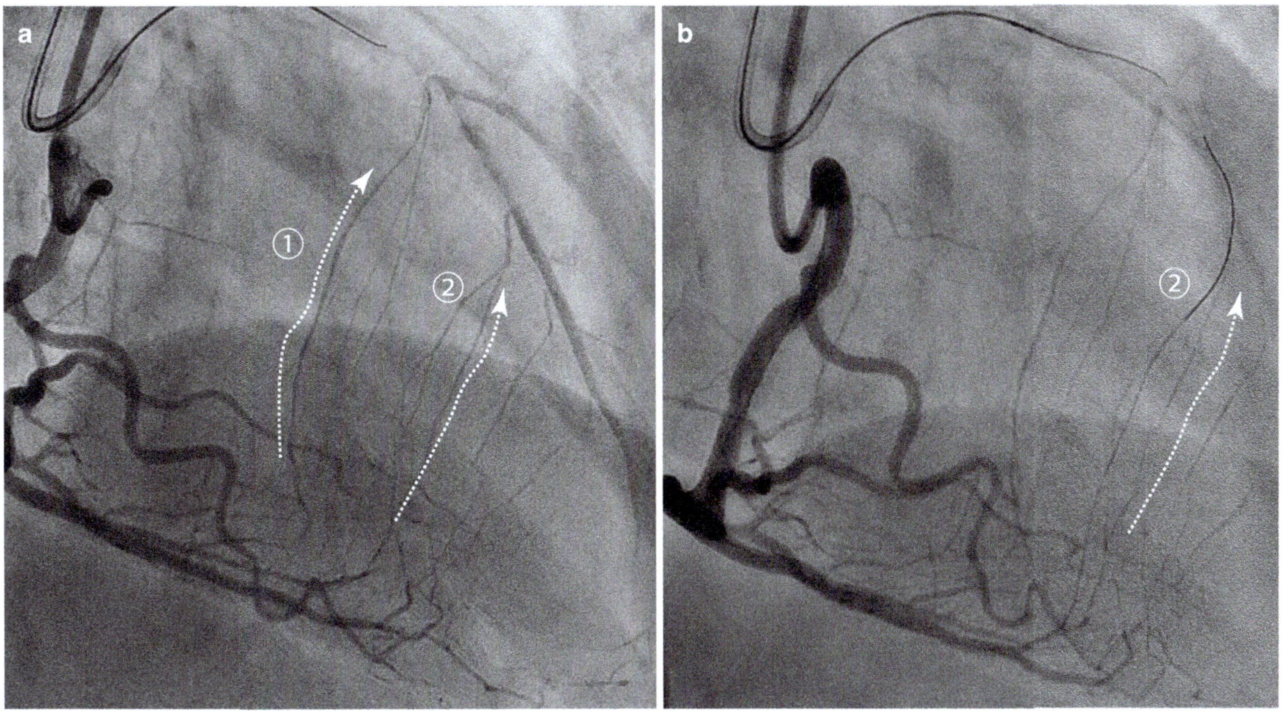

Fig. 1.153 Optimal distance between the channel and the distal end of the occlusion. (**a**) Several possible septal channels arise from a posterior descending branch. Among them, channel (1) joins the target vessel too close to the distal end of the occlusion, so channel (2) or another channel should be tried first. (**b**) Channel (2) was chosen because it joined the target vessel at an appropriate distance from the distal end of the occlusion

1.7.4 Guiding Catheter

A guiding catheter for the retrograde approach does not require particularly strong backup. Like the antegrade approach, you should only use a guiding catheter with a shape that ensures stable coaxial engagement. To accommodate the possible need for anchoring, the guiding catheter should be 6 Fr or larger in size. For the retrograde approach, I usually employ a 7-Fr guiding catheter, but I use a 6-Fr catheter for introduction into the internal thoracic artery (ITA).

After tracking a long collateral channel (e.g., a channel running beyond the apex or starting from the ITA), the tip of a 150-cm-long microcatheter may not be able to reach the antegrade guiding catheter.

To solve this problem, I recommend using a short (85- to 90-cm-long) retrograde guiding catheter. Alternatively, you can shorten a 100-cm-long regular guiding catheter by cutting off the proximal part and connecting the cut ends with a sheath (Fig. 1.154). While doing this, you should keep the guiding catheter engaged in the coronary artery to prevent excessive shortening of the catheter that may preclude its engagement.

If a retrograde microcatheter advanced through a 100-cm-long regular guiding catheter fails to reach the antegrade guiding catheter after successful introduction of a retrograde guidewire into the antegrade catheter, you should trap the guidewire before withdrawing the retrograde microcatheter and then withdrawing the retrograde guiding catheter. You should shorten the guiding catheter, as mentioned above, and reintroduce the shorter catheter. Before withdrawing the guiding catheter, you should estimate the amount of shortening that is required from its engagement in the coronary artery.

After the tip of the retrograde microcatheter reaches the antegrade guiding catheter, you should use a 300-cm-long guidewire (e.g., an RG-3) to introduce the microcatheter into the antegrade guiding catheter and to push it through for externalization.

If the tip of the retrograde microcatheter cannot reach the antegrade guiding catheter despite your efforts, you may also introduce an RG-3 guidewire into the antegrade guiding catheter for direct externalization.

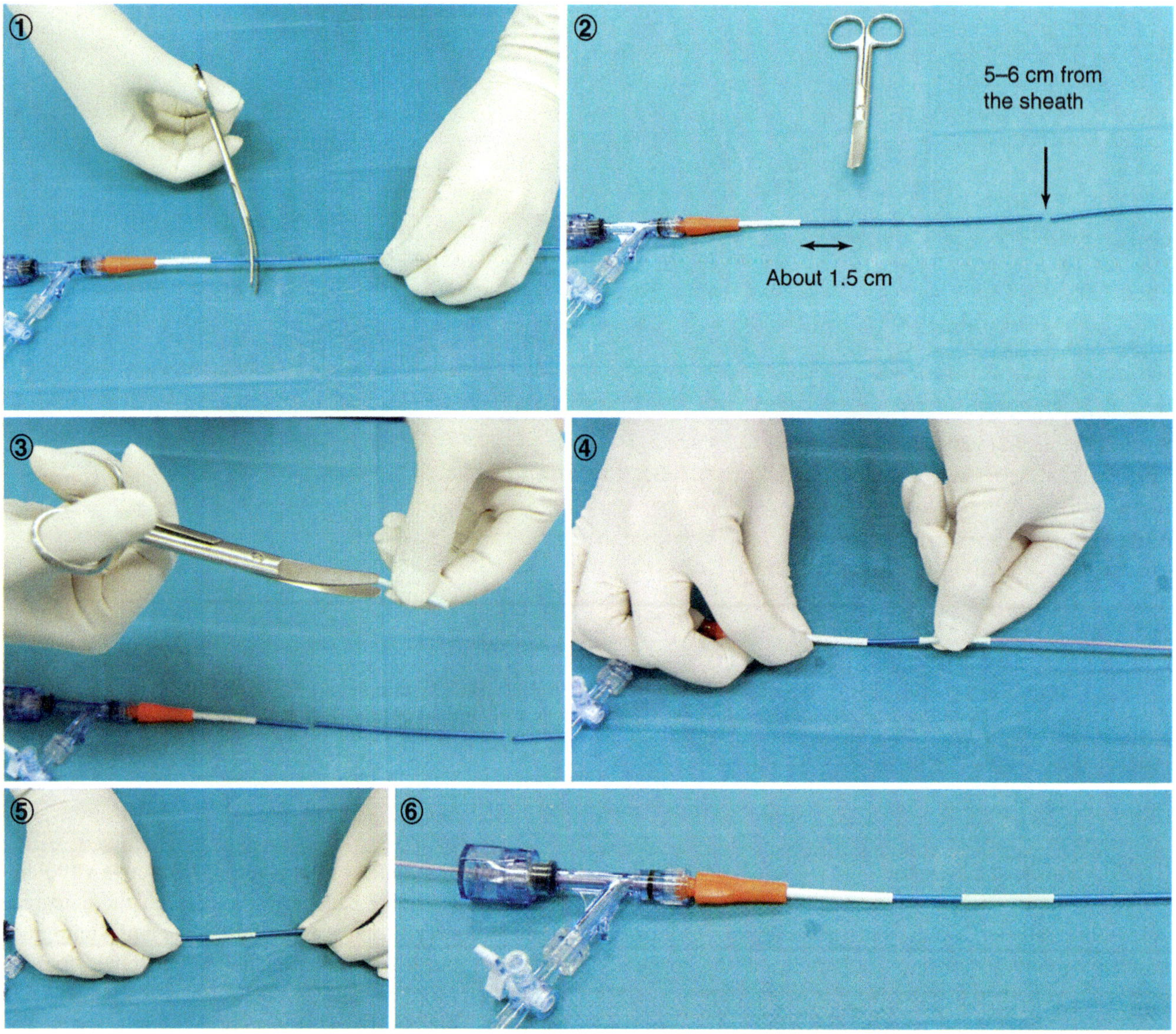

Fig. 1.154 Shortening a retrograde guiding catheter. The retrograde guiding catheter should be cut short while keeping it engaged in the coronary artery so as to determine the exact distance from the sheath. You should withdraw the retrograde guiding catheter before cutting it, if this is being done to pass a retrograde microcatheter through the lesion after a crossing it with a retrograde guidewire (1 & 2). I use a 6-Fr outer sheath to connect the cut ends of a 7-Fr guiding catheter. Using scissors, you should make two cuts about 1.5 mm in length at 180 degrees apart on the rim of each end and spread the ends out (3). Then you should tightly connect the two ends with a 0.035-inch wire and a 5-Fr inner sheath (4, 5, 6)

1.7.5 Microcatheter

A retrograde microcatheter should have a length of 150 cm. To ensure safe tip injection in a small tortuous collateral channel, the retrograde microcatheter should have a tip that is as small and soft as possible. Currently, a Caravel microcatheter is always my first choice for retrograde PCI.

For advancing into a septal branch just distal to a stent in the LAD, a tapered microcatheter with a soft tip (such as a Corsair or Caravel) is useful.

1.7.6 Fluoroscopy and Contrast Imaging Angles

You should obtain contrast images at the optimal angles for visualizing the branching and tortuosity of the collateral channel you intend to track, as well as to clearly distinguish between branches and the main vessel (Tables 1.7 and 1.8).

In general, a septal channel originating from the LAD is best separated from the LAD in the AP or RAO + CR views, while a channel near the ostium of the PDA is often seen best in the RAO or RAO + CA views.

To separate the atrial circumflex branch from the LCX, the AP + CA or RAO + CA view (together with the LAO + CA view for double projection) is optimal. The midportion of a channel running from the atrial circumflex branch to the RCA is often seen best in the LAO (RAO) view, and while the LAO + CR (RAO + CR) view is often optimal for the part of the channel near the atrioventricular branch of the RCA. These projections may be used in a reverse order to view channels running from the RCA to the atrial circumflex branch of the LCX.

To find the best view of a septal channel originating from the posterior descending branch of the RCA, you will often have to search among the RAO, RAO + CR, and RAO + CA projections for the optimum separation of the channel from the branch.

Table 1.7 Optimum projections for en face viewing of collateral channels

Donor	Recipient	Angle
Conus branch	LAD	AP + CR
RV branch	LAD RCA distal	RAO— AP + CR
RSA	4-AV	LAO
4-PD (Sept)	LAD	RAO
4-AV (AC)	LCX prox LCX distal	LAO (+CR) LAO + CR

Table 1.8 Optimum projections for en face viewing of collateral channels (continued)

		Angle	
Donor	Recipient	Entry	Channel
Septal branch	4-PD LAD distal	AP—RAO + CR	RAO
RV branch	RCA distal LAD distal	AP—RAO + CR	RAO—AP + CR
Diagonal	LAD distal LCX PL	AP—RAO + CR	LAO (+CR)
LAD apex	4-PD	LAO + CA	RAO (+CR)
LCX prox AC	RCA 4-AV	AP + CA	LAO (+CR)
LCX distal AC	RCA 4-AV	RAO (+CA—CR)	LAO + CR
LCX PL	RCA PL LCX PL	RAO (+CR)	RAO (+CR)

1.7.7 Tip Injection

For successful tracking of a collateral channel, you should introduce a guidewire into the channel from the donor vessel and advance it with minimal force to see whether it passes into the channel. If the guidewire enters the channel but cannot pass through it smoothly to reach the lumen of the artery distal to the occlusion, you should advance a microcatheter into the channel and perform tip injection to confirm that the channel reaches the distal true lumen and whether it is tortuous or branched. You should use a syringe with a Luer lock connector for tip injection and should always confirm backflow of blood into the syringe under negative pressure before injecting contrast medium. Note that if there are multiple collateral channels and if the tip of the microcatheter is kept coaxial with the channel to be tracked, backflow of blood will be noted even if the catheter has wedged the target channel and blocked antegrade blood flow.

The backflow volume indicates the size of the lumen distal to the microcatheter that can accommodate contrast medium. This means that, when the backflow volume is small, vigorously injecting contrast medium will increase the peripheral intraluminal pressure and cause leakage of contrast into the surrounding tissue or create vascular dissection and/or perforation. Conversely, if the backflow is very large, it is necessary to inject contrast medium more rapidly to obtain good images of the channel.

As with radiographic assessment of the occlusion, the fluoroscopy angles should be selected to provide the longest possible view of the channel to be tracked, especially its most tortuous part, or to allow the tortuous part to be viewed en face so that the bends of the channel are opened up most widely. When viewed in a projection orthogonal to the first, the tortuous part of the channel will appear to be either straight (Fig. 1.155a) or corkscrew-like (Fig. 1.155b). You should manipulate the guidewire while looking at images obtained in the projection which opens up the bends most widely. If a side branch originates from the most tortuous part of the main vessel and/or if such a side branch is subsequently tracked, it may be difficult to separate the branch from the main vessel, and you may be unable to track the channel with a guidewire until separation becomes possible. After failing to isolate the channel at a branching point, you should search for a projection perpendicular to the course of the main vessel that provides the best separation of the side branch (Fig. 1.156).

It is sometimes difficult to isolate a channel from the main vessel, e.g., to isolate a septal branch from the posterior descending artery. This may occur under the following circumstances:

1. The channel originates from a branch of the main vessel, and the channel and the branch overlap on CAG images (Fig. 1.157).
2. Despite actually communicating with the proximal part of the channel, it appears that two independent branches arise from the main vessel due to overlapping (Fig. 1.158).
3. The channel branches in a direction that is not always the same as the course of its distal segment (Fig. 1.159).
4. A branch from the main vessel does not actually connect to another vessel, but appears to do so because of overlapping another channel (Fig. 1.160).
5. The main vessel is very tortuous, and the channel branches in the direction where the tortuosity is most severe, precluding isolation of the channel.

If you fail to enter a visible channel, you should perform tip injection in the main vessel with imaging at an appropriate angle to obtain more insight into the anatomy of the channel.

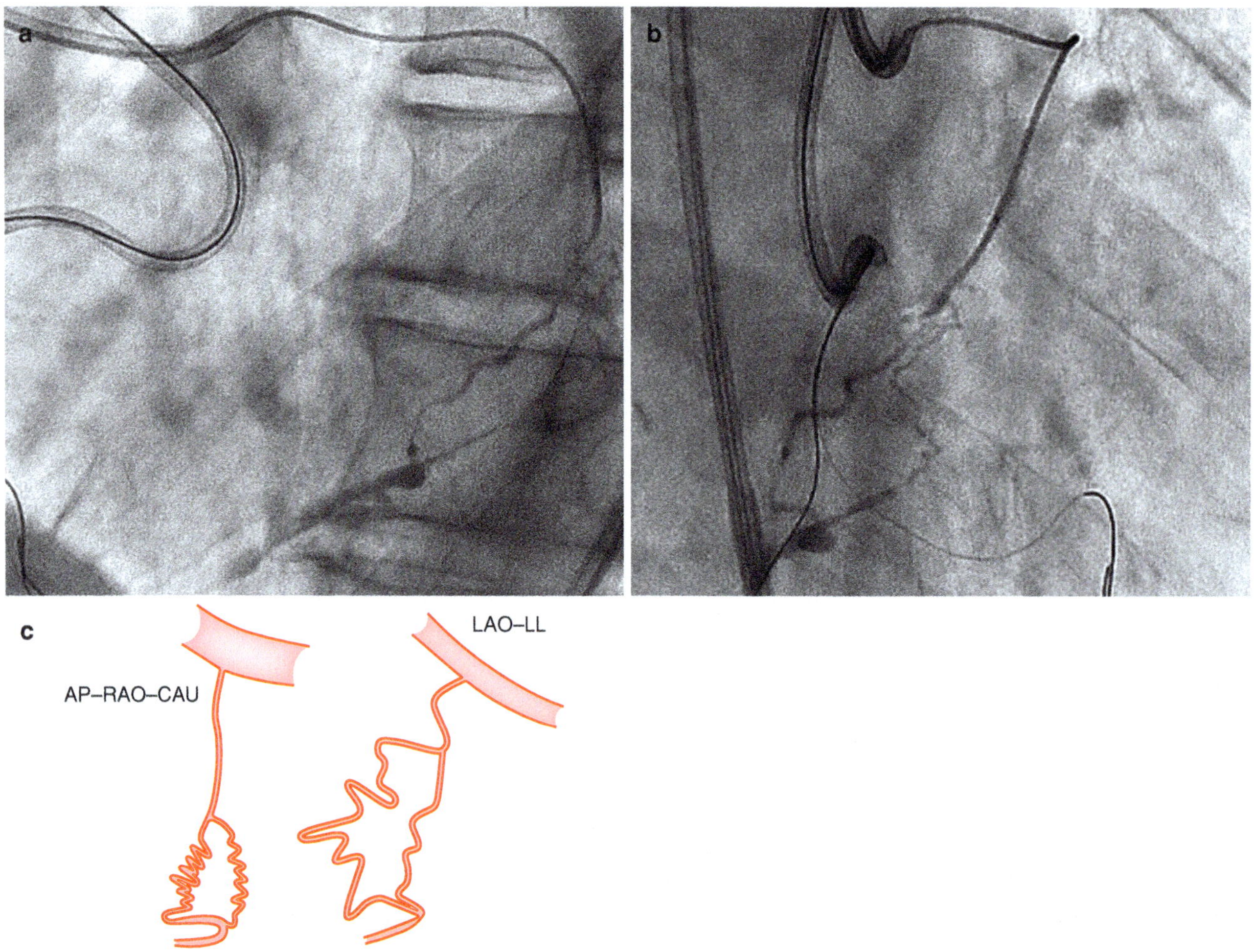

Fig. 1.155 Contrast imaging of an epicardial channel from the LCX to the RCA. (**a**) RAO. b. LAO. (**b**) The LAO projection provides the longest view of the target channel. (**c**) Views of a tortuous channel in two projections

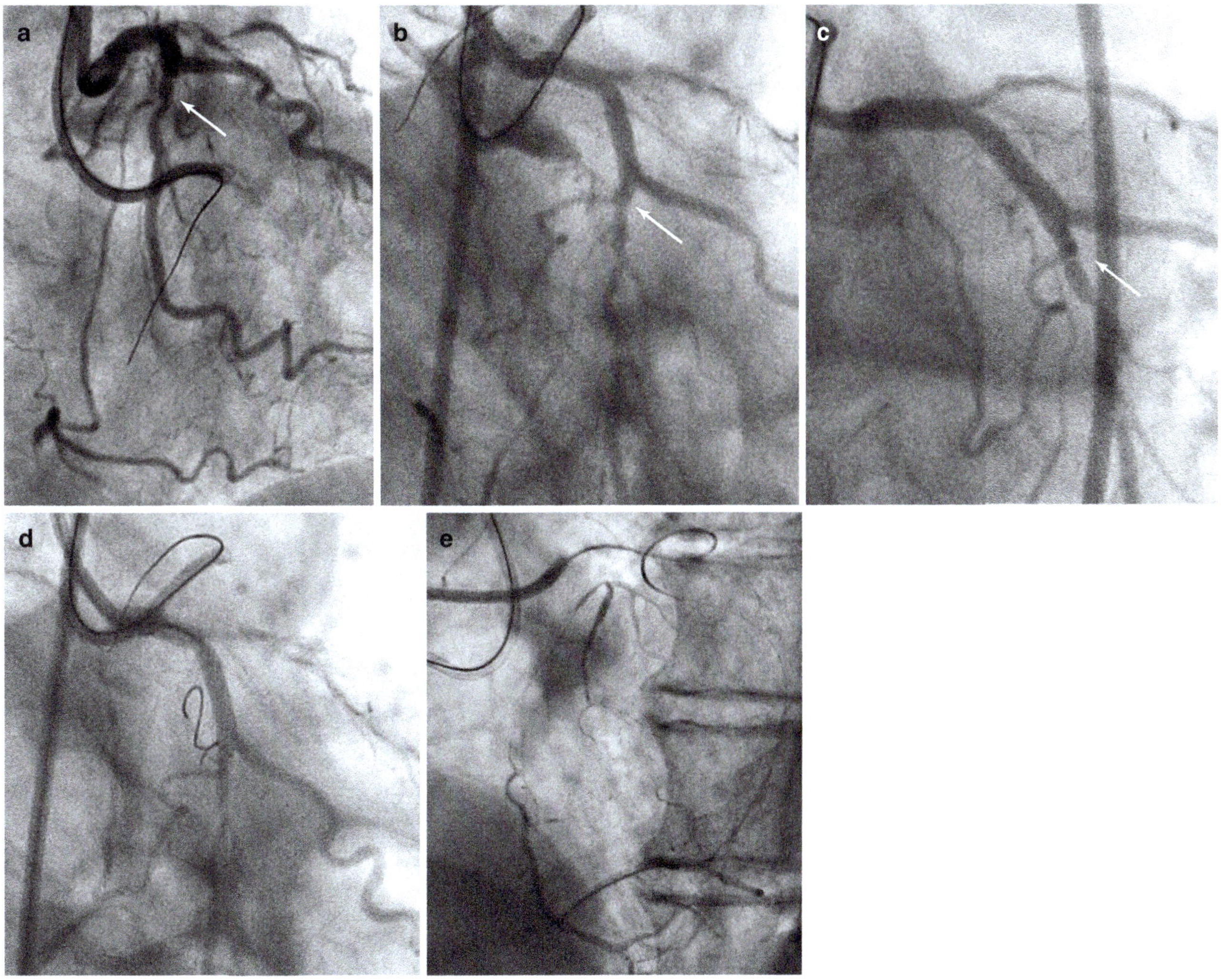

Fig. 1.156 CTO of the RCA. An epicardial channel runs from the atrial circumflex branch of the LCX to the RCA. At a bifurcation, overlapping branches are difficult to separate in the RAO (**a**) and AP + CA (**b**) projections. In the RAO + CA projection (**c**), good separation was obtained, and a guidewire could be advanced into the channel. The guidewire (**d**) and a microcatheter (**e**) successfully tracked the channel

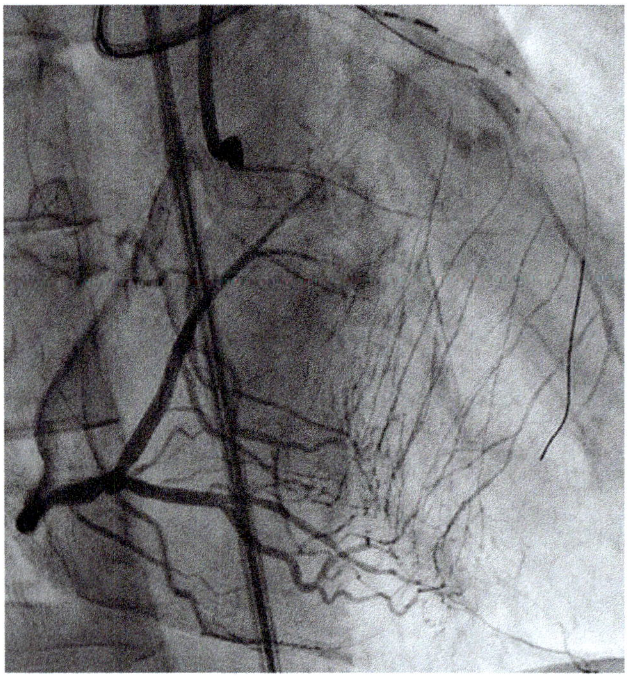

Fig. 1.157 Multiple septal channels to the LAD. It was difficult to identify or isolate the best channel because multiple channels crossed and overlapped each other

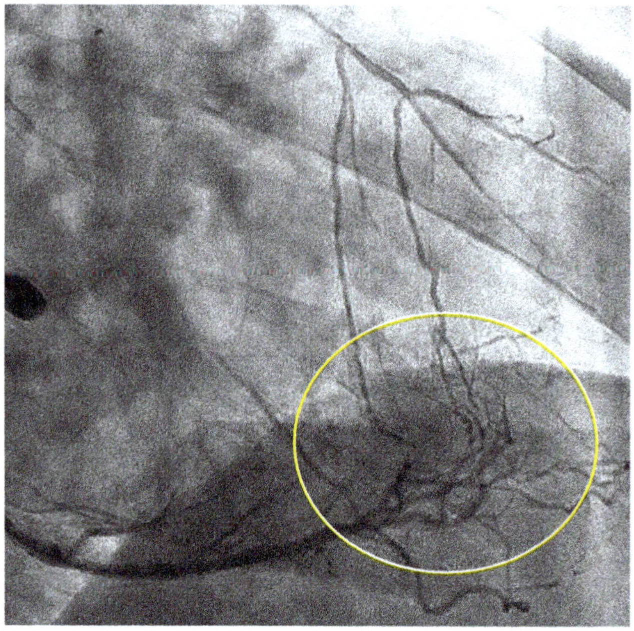

Fig. 1.159 A tortuous channel between septal branches arising in different directions, one from the posterior descending branch of the RCA and the other from the LAD

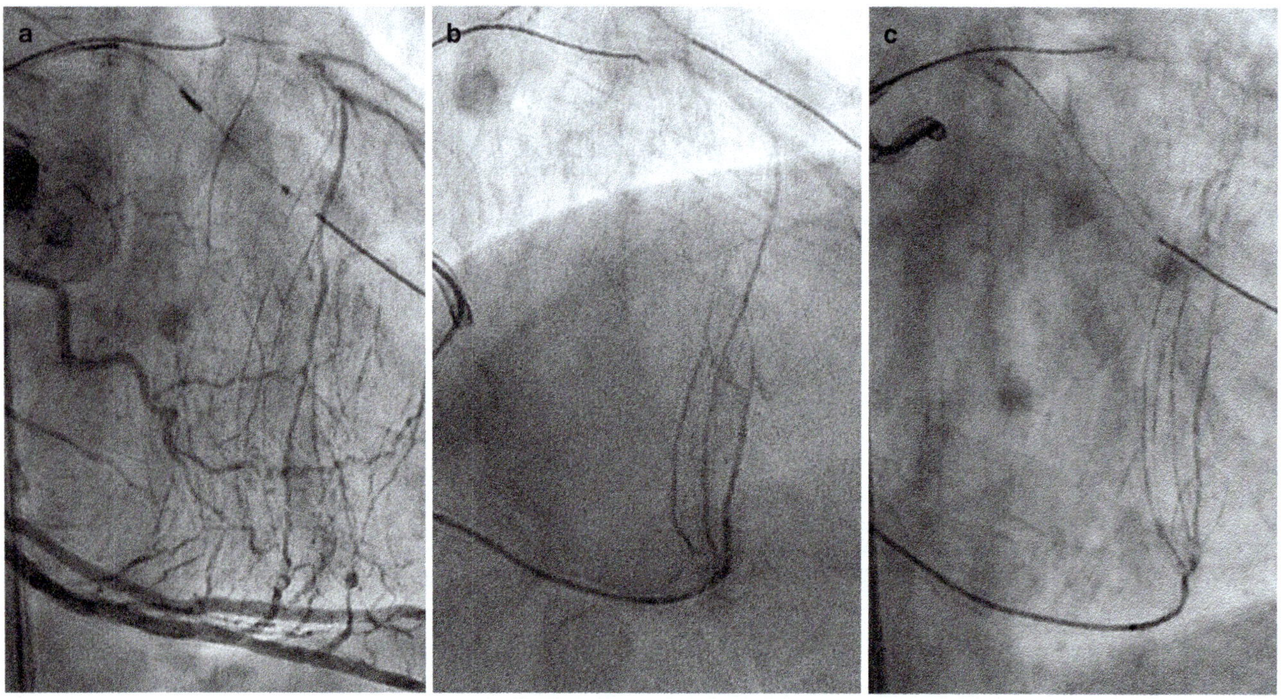

Fig. 1.158 Two apparently independent branches. (a & c) RAO. b. AP + CR. Multiple channels are seen, but all of them overlap the main vessel for most of the route (**a**). You should isolate a channel in a different projection that permits better separation from the main vessel (**b**) and then return to the original projection that gives the longest view of the channel (**c**)

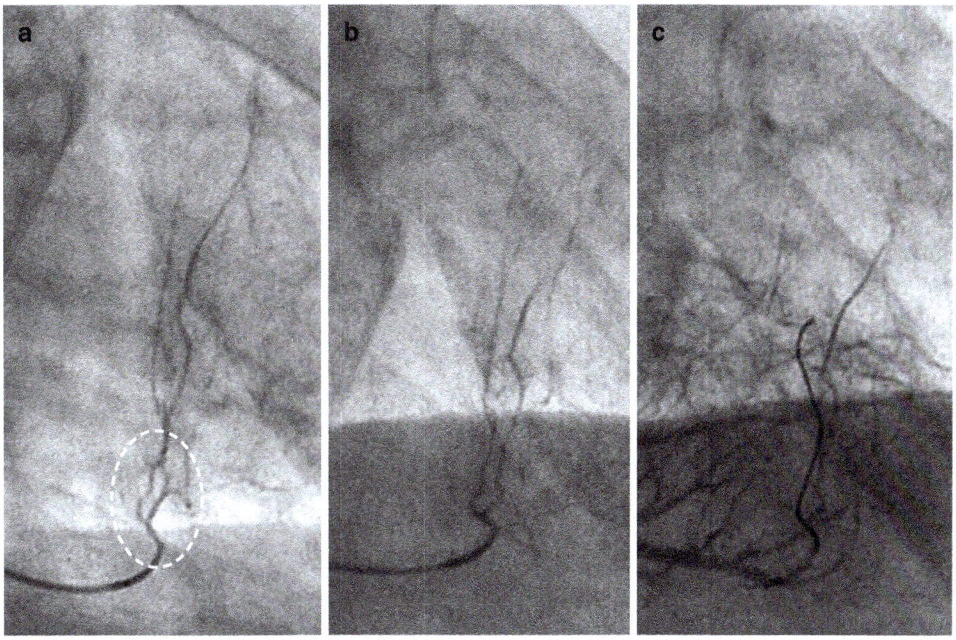

Fig. 1.160 A vessel that is seen to not be a channel in a different projection. In the RAO + CA projection, the two vessels encircled by a dotted line appear to form channels between common donor and recipient vessels (**a**). In different projections, one of these vessels loses continuity (i.e., it is not a channel) (**b** & **c**)

1.7.8 Guidewire Selection and Handling for Each Channel Type

For tracking a collateral channel, it is better for a guidewire to have a very low tip load, as soft a shaft as possible, and good slipperiness. Currently, a Sion guidewire is my first choice.

Until the entrance of the channel is reached, a retrograde guidewire needs a tip curve of a sufficient size for introducing it into the channel (Fig. 1.161). Once the retrograde guidewire has reached the entrance of the channel, you advance it further with minimal force and attempt to track the channel to reach the artery distal to the occlusion. However, the guidewire will often fail to track a small tortuous channel and reach the distal true lumen because the tip curve is too large or the wrong shape. Therefore, it is often necessary to advance a microcatheter into the channel for an appropriate distance and exchange the guidewire for another wire with a different tip curve.

It is very useful to perform tip injection through the microcatheter after withdrawal of the first guidewire because it can confirm tortuosity of the channel and continuity with the distal true lumen without interference by overlapping vessels (Fig. 1.162).

For retrograde tracking of a collateral channel, the tip of the guidewire should ideally be curved according to the tortuosity and branching of the channel (Fig. 1.163), but a guidewire with a small tip curve is generally satisfactory (Fig. 1.161c).

To prevent entry into a side branch at the vertex of a small acute curve when tracking a collateral channel, the guidewire may need to have a tip curve that is smaller and more acute than the curve in the channel. A very small and tortuous channel may be difficult to track with a guidewire that has a 0.014-inch tip. Such a channel can often be tracked by a tapered polymer-jacketed guidewire (e.g., an XT-R) if the tip is shaped into a very acute curve. However, a tapered guidewire has the potential to cause intimal injury, particularly during the phase of the cardiac cycle when the tip of the guidewire whips to and fro extensively. Accordingly, you should take great care when manipulating a tapered guidewire to track a collateral channel.

To track a channel with multiple small corkscrew-type bends (Fig. 1.164), it is recommended to make the tip flexible by forming a small curve using a guidewire inserter (Fig. 1.165a & b) and to reshape the wire by using a 25-G shaping mandrel to obtain the optimal curve at the tip (Fig. 1.165a→c).

When tracking a collateral channel, I generally keep the following points in mind:

1. Use minimal force when advancing the guidewire into the channel, and never push it hard.
2. Primarily view the channel in a projection perpendicular to its longitudinal axis.
3. Always keep the tip of the guidewire parallel to the channel while advancing it, especially as it passes through an acute bend.
4. Advance the guidewire with as little force as possible and only when it is oriented in the correct direction.
5. Exchange the guidewire for another with more slipperiness if the resistance is too great to advance it without employing strong force.

Of these points, (3) and (4) should especially be followed if it becomes difficult to advance the tip of the guidewire

in the correct direction. Obtaining images from different fluoroscopy angles often provides new information. Part of the collateral channel that appears straight in one projection may be seen to be tortuous in another projection orthogonal to the first (Fig. 1.166), or it may be found that the guidewire has entered a small side branch. Moreover, the actual branching point and direction of a collateral channel may be different from those expected initially (Fig. 1.167). Under fluoroscopic guidance in the optimal views for assessing channel tortuosity and branching, you should optimize the tip curve of the guidewire by viewing the reference image and advance the wire in the desired direction with minimal force while performing rotation to help it pass through the channel.

In order to advance the guidewire when it has become difficult to move forward through the channel, you will need to determine the correct course for the wire by viewing images in other projections and intentionally orient its tip in that direction. You should always remember never to forcibly push a guidewire that has become difficult to advance.

Fig. 1.161 Optimal guidewire tip curves for channel selection. (**a** & **b**) To advance a guidewire from the main vessel into a collateral channel, the wire should initially have a tip curve that is of an appropriate size for the diameter of the main vessel. (**c**) After reaching the entrance of the collateral channel, the guidewire should be reshaped to create a smaller tip curve in order to track the channel with a smaller diameter

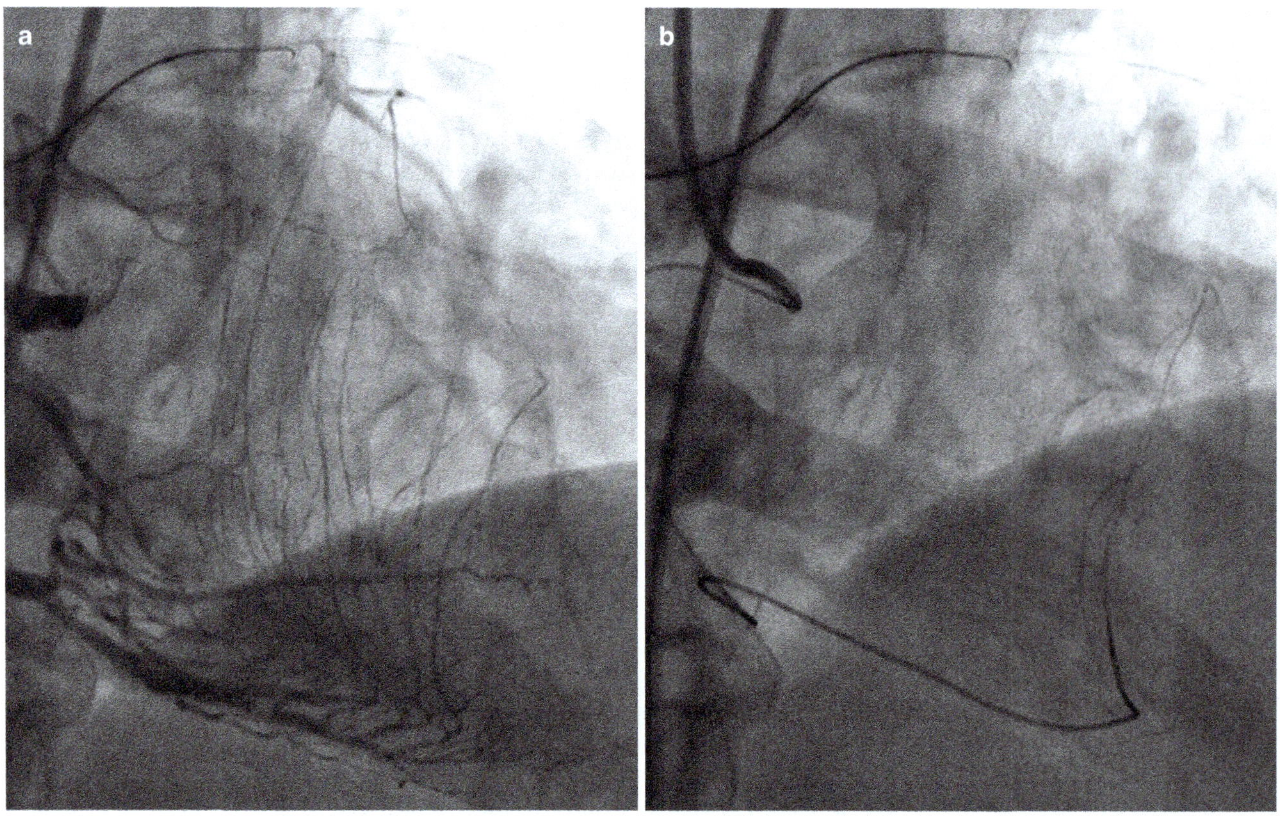

Fig. 1.162 Tip injection. Injecting contrast medium from the guiding catheter provides little information on the anatomy of the target channel because many other overlapping vessels are also visualized (**a**). However, tip injection from a microcatheter clearly visualizes the target channel (**b**)

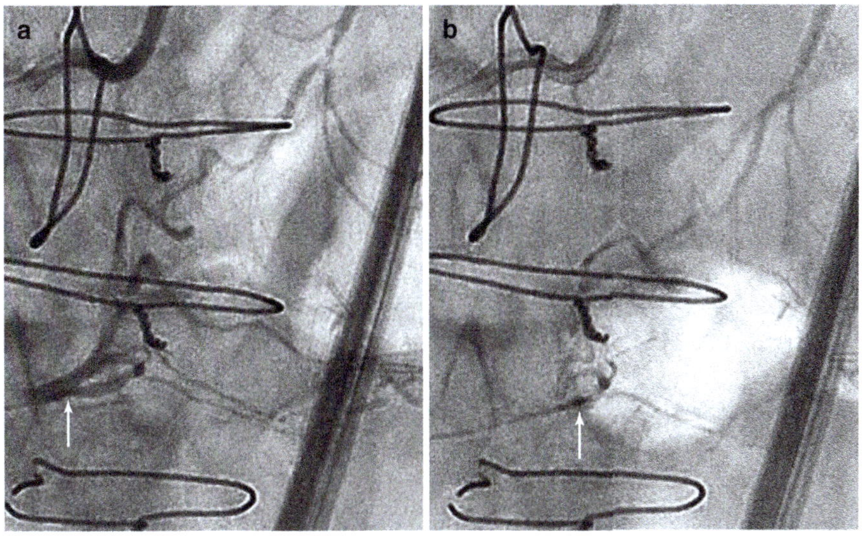

Fig. 1.163 Epicardial channel from the posterolateral branch of the RCA. The tip of a microcatheter is indicated by the arrow. The guidewire needs to be reshaped to have appropriate tip curves for the diameter and tortuosity of the branch/channel to be tracked. Initially, the guidewire needs a relatively large curve at the tip to select the right branch (**a**). When advanced further, the guidewire needs a small tip acute curve (**b**). Imaging by tip injection provides clear information about these requirements

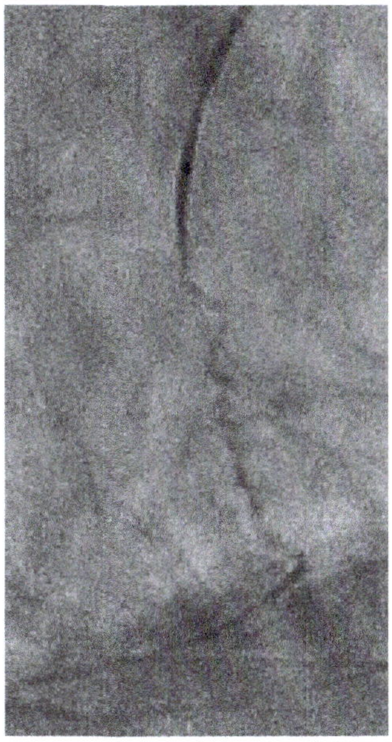

Fig. 1.164 Corkscrew-type collateral channel. This channel could not be tracked by a regular guidewire, but was tracked by a broken-tipped guidewire (shown in the next figure)

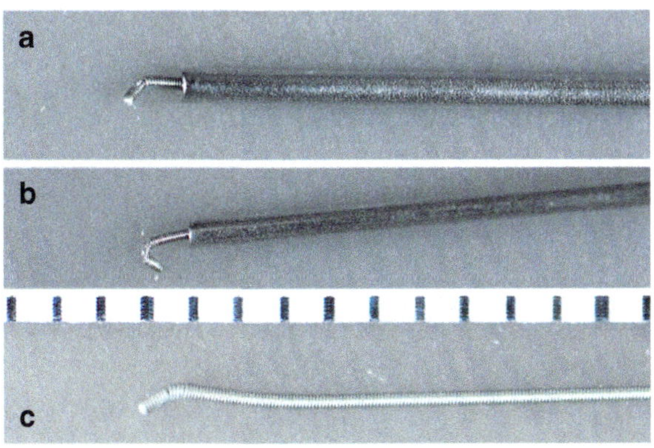

Fig. 1.165 Making a broken-tipped Sion guidewire. (**a**) A regular curve is formed using the tip of a guidewire introducer. (**b**) The curve is altered to a J-shape. (**c**) The curve is made less acute again by using a 25-G shaping mandrel

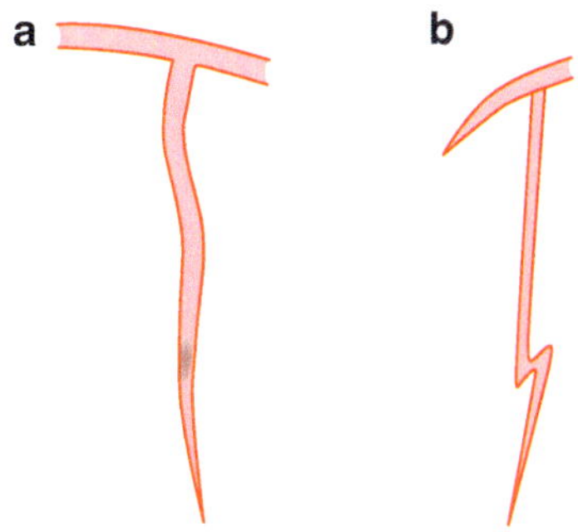

Fig. 1.166 Variation of channel appearance in different fluoroscopy projections. A channel that appears linear in one projection (**a**) may be tortuous in another projection (**b**)

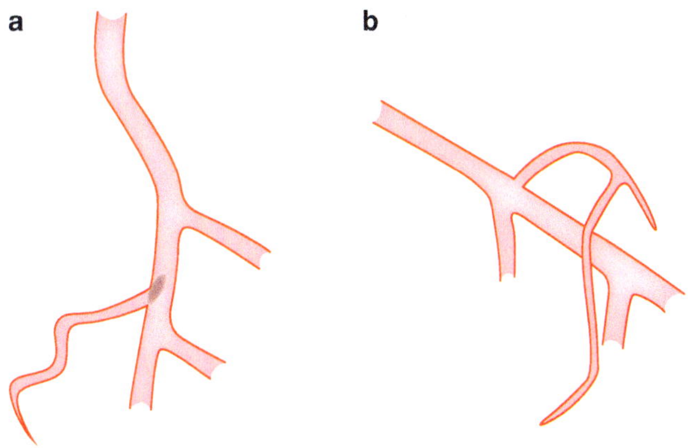

Fig. 1.167 Variation of channel appearance in different fluoroscopy projections. A channel that appears to have no branches in one projection (**a**) may show a branch in another projection (**b**)

Column 8 Sion Guidewire

As of March 2015, the Sion is the best guidewire for the abovementioned collateral channel tracking technique. A Sion guidewire can successfully track a tortuous collateral channel as the shaft of its several centimeters long tip has optimal flexibility and slipperiness. To track a tortuous channel with tight bends, the guidewire needs to be flexible up to the tip if possible. Unfortunately, the actual tip of every guidewire is not flexible as it has a brazed part about 1-mm-long. If the tip of a guidewire is broken by bending it excessively (see Fig. 1.165b), only 0.6–0.7 mm of the tip remains inflexible, so the guidewire becomes able to track even a corkscrew-type channel with tight bends. Simply bending the tip of the guidewire into a J shape would rather increase the risk of causing vascular injury. Therefore, the bent tip is straightened again, and the angles are smoothed to form a natural curve at the tip (see Fig. 1.165c), creating a safe and effective guidewire for collateral channel tracking. Figure 1.168 shows an example of successfully tracking a tortuous channel with a broken-tipped Sion guidewire.

A new guidewire with a completely flexible tip has been proposed. This wire would have no core at its tip, and consequently the spring coil would be much more flexible, so it would have an overwhelming advantage over existing guidewires for tracking a non-branching tortuous channel. However, if the channel has a side branch at the vertex of one of its curves, would it be possible to control the guidewire and prevent entry into the side branch? In such circumstances, a guidewire with a core at its tip usually seems to have better performance. As is known by every interventionalist and is expected from the reason a vessel becomes tortuous, a tortuous vessel (especially an epicardial artery) often has a side branch at the vertex of one of its curves. Recognizing such a side branch and navigating the guidewire through the channel across the branching point are the keys to successful collateral channel tracking.

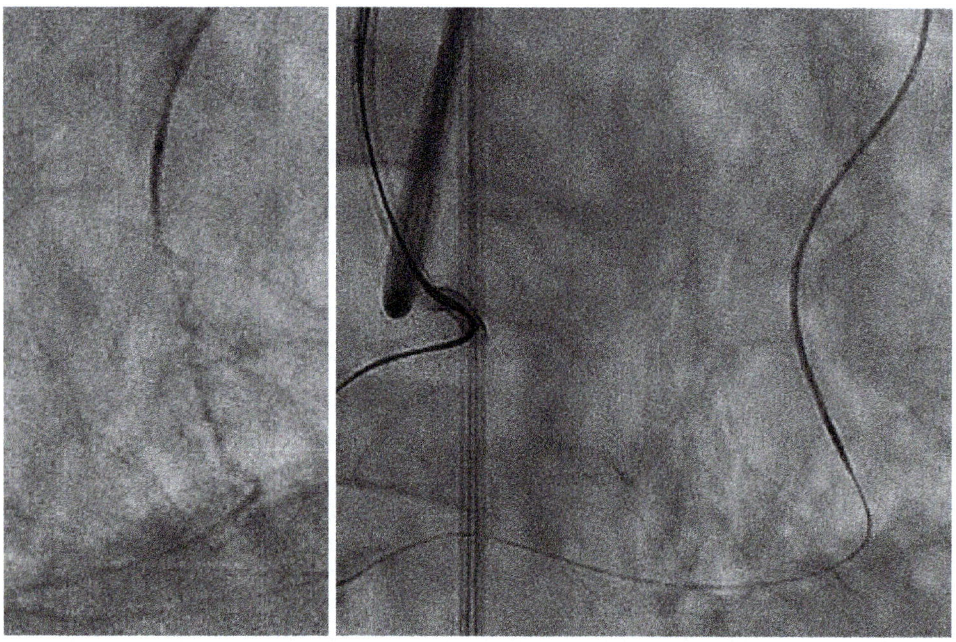

Fig. 1.168 Successful tracking of a tortuous channel by a broken-tipped Sion guidewire

1.7.9 Confirmation of Channel Penetration

When you think that the retrograde guidewire has reached the lumen of the target coronary artery distal to the CTO, you should perform retrograde imaging via other collateral channels to confirm that the tip of the wire is in the distal true lumen. A retrograde guidewire quite often enters a vein or a cardiac ventricle (Fig. 1.169a & b), probably via a pre-existing fistula. In particular, you may think a guidewire has entered the artery lumen distal to the CTO although it has actually entered a vein if the vein and the target coronary artery have similar anatomy. In this case, advancing a microcatheter along the guidewire without confirming that the wire has reached the distal true lumen will cause arteriovenous disruption at the fistula, resulting in pericardial hemorrhage.

A guidewire that has tracked a collateral channel may reach the lumen of a small vessel with very similar anatomical features to the distal true lumen. Although you may be almost certain that a retrograde guidewire has reached the distal true lumen without performing angiography, you should never fail to perform contralateral imaging to confirm this before advancing a microcatheter along the guidewire.

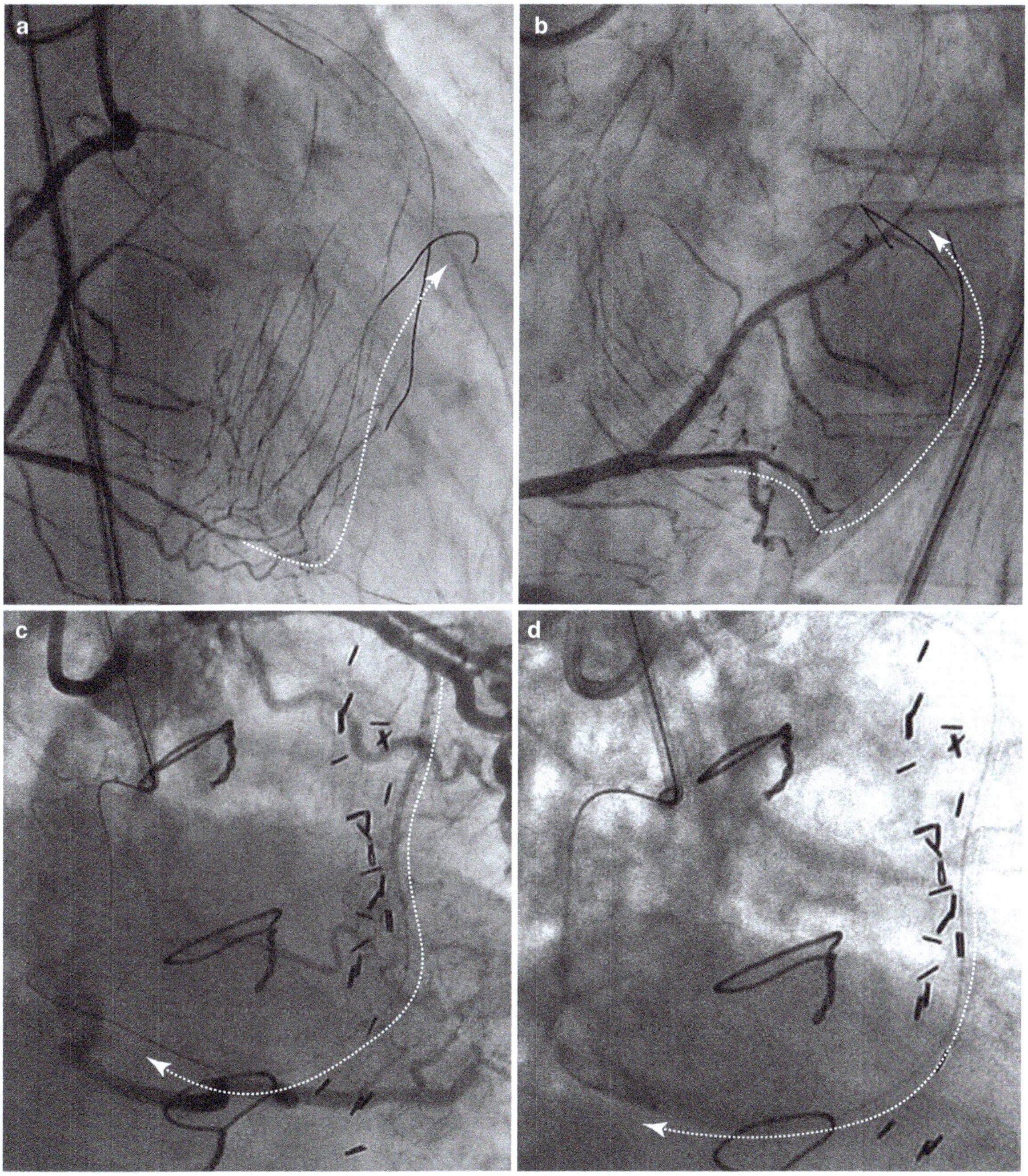

Fig. 1.169 Confirmation of retrograde guidewire crossing by angiography. The guidewire seems to advance toward the septum in the RAO view (**a**), but it shows considerable deviation toward the LCX in the LAO view (**b**). The guidewire appears to have reached the posterior descending artery via a septal branch (**c**), but tip injection demonstrates that it has actually entered a vein running parallel to the artery (**d**)

1.7.10 Advancing a Microcatheter into the Distal True Lumen

After a retrograde guidewire has crossed a collateral channel, you should advance a microcatheter into the true lumen distal to the CTO. A microcatheter can often be advanced easily through a relatively large and less tortuous channel, but frequently will not track a small tortuous channel so well. In the latter situation, the microcatheter will often be easier to advance if it is rotated and pushed simultaneously. However, most microcatheters have a thin shaft and cannot tolerate too much rotation, while the microcatheters with a shaft thick enough to tolerate rotation often fail to penetrate a channel because of their large diameter.

To enable a thin microcatheter to track a collateral channel, you should advance it while alternately performing clockwise and counterclockwise rotation a limited number of times. For example, you can perform three clockwise rotations and then three counterclockwise rotations to reverse the torque back to neutral, after which you can perform an additional three counterclockwise rotations (six counterclockwise rotations in total). This may be followed by six clockwise rotations and then another six counterclockwise rotations and so on. Such rotation is performed to reduce friction, and not for achieving a large screw effect as with a Tornus microcatheter.

If this maneuver does not help the microcatheter to pass through the channel, you may introduce a small-diameter balloon catheter. For this purpose, a small-diameter balloon with a small tip profile and a soft tip is naturally better. Whether the balloon should be inflated to dilate the channel after it has been advanced depends on the risk of cardiac tamponade due to coronary artery perforation following balloon inflation. A ventricular septal branch can be safely dilated by a balloon, but the epicardial part connecting the septal branch with the true lumen distal to the CTO should not be dilated by the edge of the balloon, and the body of the balloon should be used (Fig. 1.170). Dilating an epicardial channel with a balloon is associated with a risk of cardiac tamponade, and forcibly pushing a balloon catheter into the epicardial channel further increases this risk. Rather than attempting to force a large balloon catheter into an epicardial channel, it is safer to pass a balloon catheter with a smaller tip profile through the channel without pushing hard and then inflate the balloon at a low pressure within the channel.

If the balloon catheter fails to cross the collateral channel, you should search for another trackable channel while keeping the guidewire that crossed the first channel in position.

If there is no other trackable channel, you should position the tip of the retrograde guidewire near the distal end of the occlusion as a continuous landmark to assist antegrade wiring. Such a continuous landmark will considerably increase the probability of successful antegrade crossing of the CTO.

If a microcatheter crosses the collateral channel, you should advance the retrograde guidewire and then the microcatheter to near the distal end of the CTO. If there is a side branch near the distal end, it is better to introduce the retrograde guidewire into the side branch. This is because if the retrograde guidewire remains near the distal end of the occlusion, it will often go forward together with the microcatheter when the microcatheter is advanced. This may lead to knuckling of the guidewire tip so that it readily deviates into the subintimal space near the distal cap of the occlusion (Figs. 1.171 & 1.172) and will preclude retrograde intraluminal crossing of the CTO.

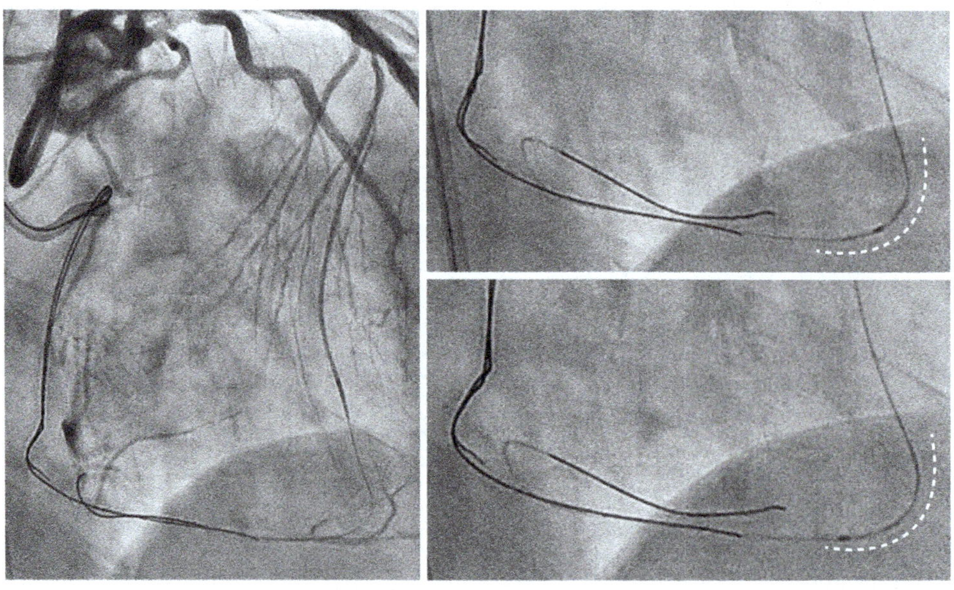

Fig. 1.170 Balloon dilation of a collateral channel that could not be crossed by a microcatheter. When dilating the part of the channel indicated by a dotted line, great care should be taken not to cause perforation as this may lead to pericardial bleeding

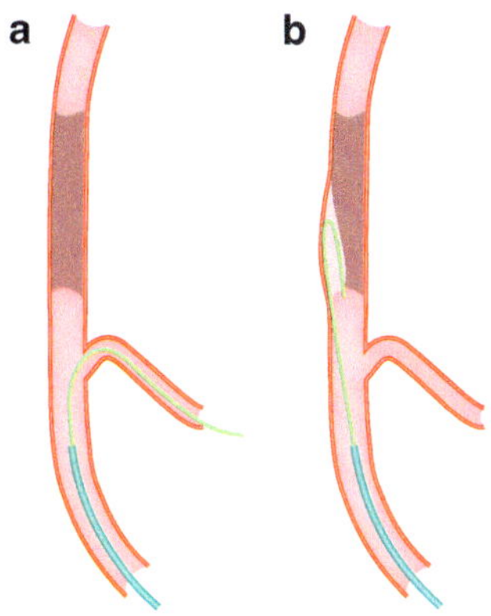

Fig. 1.171 Advancing a retrograde microcatheter. The retrograde guidewire should be introduced into a side branch near the distal end of the occlusion (**a**). If a retrograde microcatheter is advanced without first doing so, the guidewire will deviate into the subintimal space near the distal end of the occlusion (**b**)

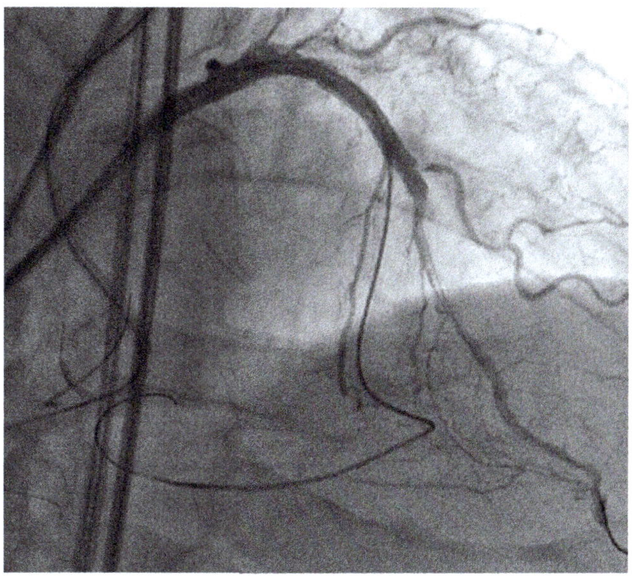

Fig. 1.172 CTO of the distal RCA (Segment #3). A retrograde guidewire that tracked a collateral channel to reach the distal end of the occlusion was introduced into a side branch before advancing a retrograde microcatheter

1.7.11 Selection of (I) Guidewire, (II) CTO Penetration Strategy, and (III) Guidewire Handling Technique

The proximal cap of a CTO is generally harder than the distal cap. As I always start PCI for CTO via the antegrade approach and assess the hardness of the proximal cap before switching to retrograde PCI, I make my first attempt at retrograde crossing with a guidewire that is less stiff than that employed for the antegrade approach. I commonly use a 0.014-inch guidewire with a tip load of about 3.0 g for the retrograde approach and prefer a guidewire that is easier to control with less probability of whipping. Tapered CTO crossing guidewires may also be used, depending on the hardness of the lesion. If it becomes trapped in plaque or the vessel wall, a guidewire from the Gaia series is more likely to be deformed or even fractured than a 0.014-inch guidewire or a Conquest Pro guidewire. Therefore, you should take special care to prevent trapping while retrogradely manipulating such a guidewire. If it becomes impossible to move a retrograde guidewire or advance it further, you should immediately check if it can be pulled back and should then withdraw the wire slightly before advancing it again. It is important to prevent the guidewire from being trapped.

If a retrograde guidewire becomes trapped in the tunica media, you should follow the same procedure that was suggested for a trapped antegrade guidewire, i.e., first advance the tip of the microcatheter toward the point of trapping while pulling the guidewire back slightly, and then rotate the wire alternately clockwise and counterclockwise an identical number of times while continuing to pull it back with minimal force. This maneuver should be performed with patience. If the guidewire can be pulled back into the microcatheter, you should then direct it toward the proximal end of the occlusion from a point just distal to the site of trapping. It is important to be aware of the potential for deformation of the guidewire tip by trapping and withdrawal (rotation). You should withdraw the guidewire from the microcatheter to determine whether its tip has been deformed. If the tip becomes deformed, you should stop using the guidewire and exchange it for a new one (see Sect. 1.9. "Troubleshooting" [page 144]).

1.7.12 Direct Crossing Technique

Since I attempt antegrade PCI for CTO first whenever possible, I rarely perform direct crossing of an occlusion via the retrograde approach. Using the antegrade guidewire as a landmark theoretically makes direct retrograde crossing a subcategory of the kissing wire technique. In fact, manipulation of the guidewire for direct crossing is done in the same way as in the kissing wire technique (see the next subsection).

When antegrade PCI is performed for a bifurcation CTO, the antegrade guidewire may be unable to catch a dimple at the proximal end of the occlusion. In this case, a retrograde guidewire may be able to successfully cross the lesion (direct crossing) if it is manipulated toward the tip of the antegrade wire near the branching point. On the other hand, the antegrade guidewire often starts to cross the occlusion if it is manipulated when the tip of the retrograde guidewire is near the proximal end of the CTO, even if it is in the subintimal space. Thus, PCI is often accomplished successfully by the kissing wire technique or reverse CART (Fig. 1.173).

Some CTOs can only be recanalized by the direct crossing technique. A good example is a CTO at a large coronary ostium where an antegrade guiding catheter cannot catch a

dimple at the proximal end of the occlusion. Only retrograde PCI should be attempted for such a CTO, and if a retrograde guidewire crosses the occlusion, it should be introduced into an antegrade guiding catheter by using a snare (Fig. 1.174). The optimum snaring point may be at the ostium of the target coronary artery or in the innominate artery (Fig. 1.175). To perform snaring, you should use a snare ranging in size from 10 to 15 mm.

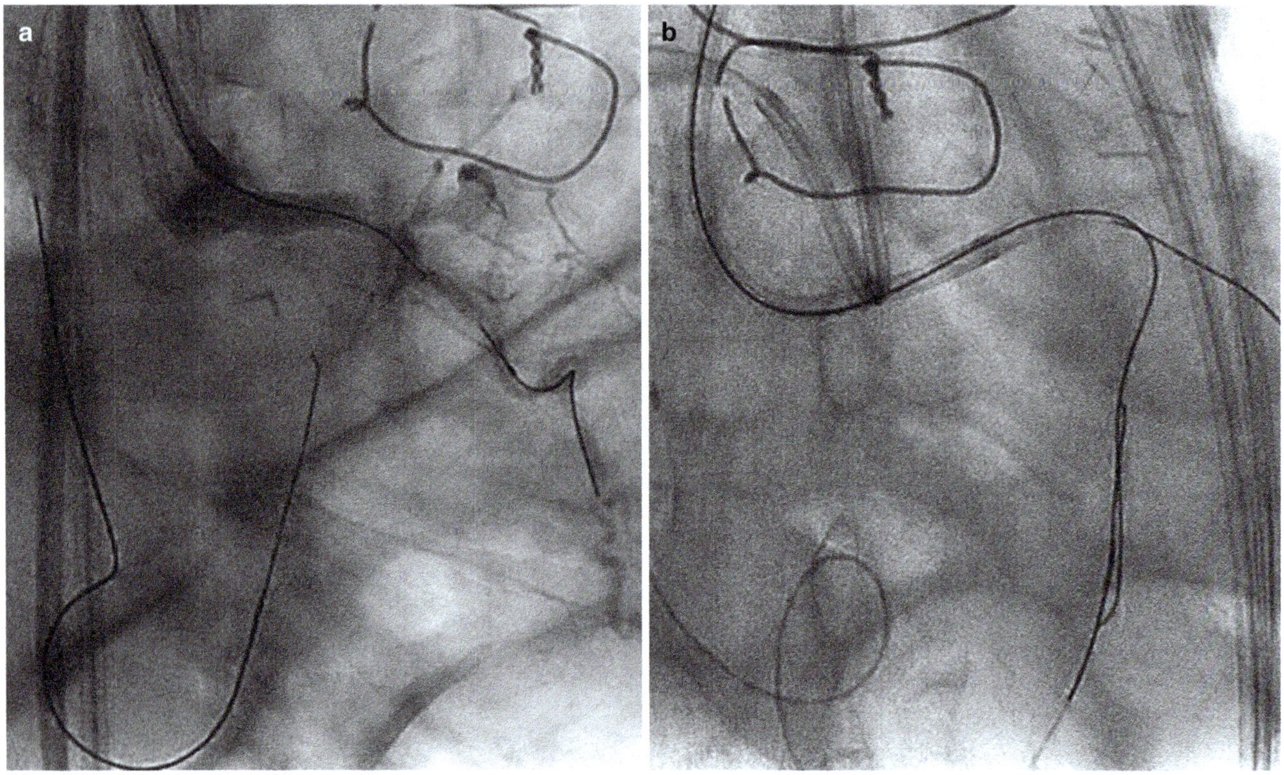

Fig. 1.173 Successful recanalization of a CTO by the kissing wire technique. After failure of antegrade PCI, the strategy was switched to the retrograde approach (**a**). After a retrograde guidewire had almost reached the proximal end of the occlusion, an antegrade guidewire was manipulated again, and the lesion was crossed successfully (**b**)

Fig. 1.174 CTO at the RCA ostium. A retrograde guidewire was captured with a snare and introduced into an antegrade guiding catheter

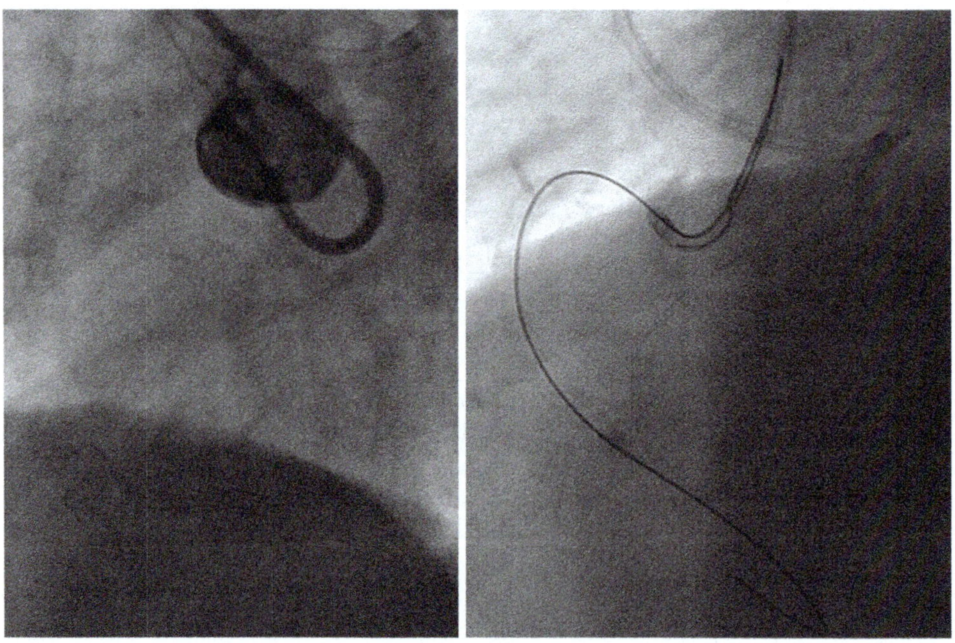

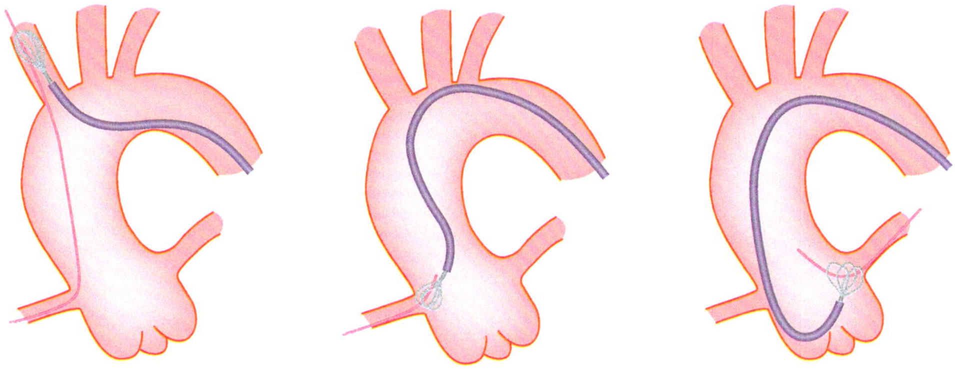

Fig. 1.175 Sites for capturing a retrograde guidewire with a snare

1.7.13 Kissing Wire Technique

I always try to perform antegrade PCI for CTO first, and I only switch to the retrograde approach after failure of this initial attempt. During retrograde PCI, I direct the retrograde guidewire toward the tip of the antegrade guidewire or near the point where the antegrade wire entered the occlusion, which means I am trying to cross the CTO by the kissing wire technique.

For retrograde wiring of a long occlusion, the entry point of an antegrade guidewire alone is not a reliable target. If the antegrade guidewire has gone some distance into the occlusion, its tip is a better target for retrograde wiring. You should not exactly target the tip of the antegrade guidewire, but should advance the retrograde guidewire using little force in parallel with the antegrade wire toward its entry point (even if they are separated by a distance equal to the diameter of the vessel).

If the retrograde guidewire deviates into the subintimal space near the proximal end of the occlusion, you should direct the antegrade guidewire toward the retrograde wire to cross the lesion by the kissing wire technique. PCI can be accomplished successfully when either guidewire crosses the CTO through the proximal or distal true lumen. If you fail to achieve intraluminal crossing with both guidewires, you should try reverse CART. As mentioned in the next subsection, the kissing wire technique brings the antegrade and retrograde guidewires close to each other, which means that reverse CART can be successfully performed by using a small balloon to dilate the space created by either guidewire.

Column 9 Techniques for the Middle and Distal RCA (Segments #2 and 3)

The aim of the kissing wire technique is to cross a CTO through the proximal or distal true lumen with a retrograde or antegrade guidewire by directing one guidewire (that appears to be within the true lumen) toward the other and bringing them into contact. However, it may be difficult to actually bring the two guidewires into contact or even to advance the two wires parallel with each other. A typical example is a CTO in the middle segment (Segment #2) or distal segment (Segment #3) of the RCA that runs along the acute margin of the heart. The RCA runs in the atrioventricular sulcus and has an acute bend at the acute margin of the heart. Its proximal segment runs along the anterior wall of the right ventricle near the tricuspid valve, following a small arc toward the posterior side of the heart. At the acute margin of the heart, the artery suddenly turns to the left and then runs relatively straight toward the crux. Absence of the right ventricular branch and/or atrial branch in this region makes these bends of the RCA more acute and also makes this part of the artery more mobile. Motion of the right atrium and ventricle is opposite during the cardiac cycle, which may amplify movement of the RCA and also lead to unexpected movement.

An attempt to cross a CTO of the RCA (Segments #1 to 3) with an antegrade guidewire often fails because the wire is unable to follow a tortuous part of the artery. When a retrograde guidewire is subsequently manipulated to cross the CTO by using the kissing wire technique, it may also fail to navigate the tortuous region. Although I am an advocate of "non-pushing PCI," you cannot advance a guidewire without pushing it at all. Unless anchored in a side branch, both the antegrade and retrograde guidewires will be directed toward the vertex of a bend when advanced into a tortuous lesion with even minimal force (Fig. 1.176). If the tip of one guidewire becomes trapped in the vessel wall, pull it back a little to reduce the angle of the bend, and then manipulate the other guidewire until it is parallel with the first wire. Then you should be able to advance the second guidewire relatively easily. If neither guidewire is trapped, you should pull one guidewire back a little from its farthest position and then leave it at that site while manipulating the other guidewire.

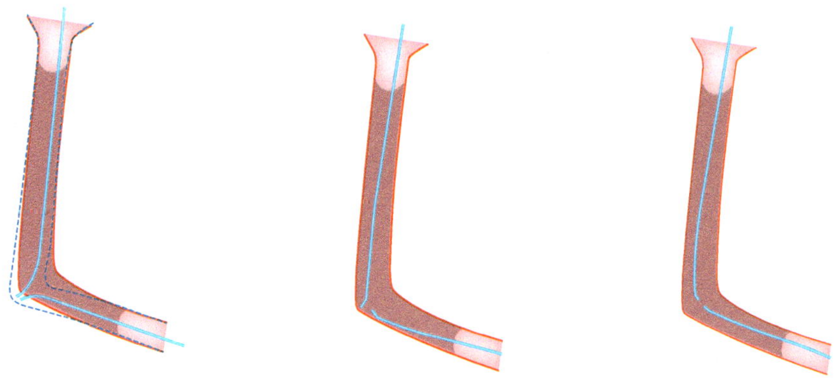

Fig. 1.176 Manipulating guidewires at a bend in the vessel

1.7.14 Reverse CART Technique

The reverse CART technique was originally devised for the situation where both the antegrade and retrograde guidewires have entered a false lumen and are within a common compartment, as shown in Fig. 1.135b. This technique involves enlarging the false lumen and the true lumen near the proximal end of the occlusion by using the antegrade guidewire, puncturing the intima to connect the two lumens, and advancing a retrograde guidewire along the connecting channel. When this technique can be used, the retrograde guidewire can always reach the proximal true lumen.

It should be noted that to successfully accomplish reverse CART, the two guidewires must be within the space created in a common compartment (Fig. 1.177a) and should preferably be close to each other. If the two guidewires are distant from each other, even if they are in a common compartment (Fig. 1.177b), the space created by inflating a small balloon after advancing it over the antegrade guidewire will not be sufficient to accommodate the retrograde guidewire and will need to be enlarged by using a larger balloon (Fig. 1.177c). However, inflation of a larger antegrade balloon is more likely to create a large dissection that evolves toward the distal end of the occlusion (Fig. 1.178).

There are several ways of thinking about how to use the reverse CART technique. Some studies have found comparable mid-term outcomes after placement of a drug-eluting stent (DES) in a false lumen versus the true lumen for recanalization of CTO. Possibly based on this evidence, some interventionalists intentionally advance an antegrade guidewire into the subintimal space from the proximal side of an occlusion if the retrograde guidewire has entered the subintimal space near the proximal end of the occlusion.

In the bare-metal stent (BMS) era, higher rates of restenosis and aneurysm were reported after recanalization of CTO by stenting a false lumen compared with the true lumen. The outcome achieved with DES may be different, and it may be suggested that what will happen after an intervention cannot be predicted without trying it. However, I think we should generally avoid strategies that achieved poor outcomes with BMS when using DES. It is true that we can only determine the eventual outcome of PCI for CTO after long-term follow-up and that a strategy which was ineffective with BMS may have a good outcome when employed with DES. Unfortunately, this means that we can only find the truth after a long time and yet we have to make choices when nobody knows the outcome. Thus, I consider that it is better to avoid strategies achieving a poor outcome with BMS when using DES, at least for the present. When performing PCI for CTO by the reverse CART technique, I always carefully target the true lumen with both the antegrade and retrograde guidewires (kissing wiring), aiming to create a connecting channel between the antegrade and retrograde "true lumens" ("true lumen" reverse CART technique).

Despite such efforts, most attempts at CTO recanalization by the reverse CART technique lead to one of the following outcomes:

1. Both the antegrade and retrograde guidewires enter the subintimal space and miss the true lumen, passing through a common subintimal space on the way to the proximal/distal ends of the occlusion.

2. Both the antegrade and retrograde guidewires eventually enter the subintimal space and miss the true lumen, but pass through the true lumen at some point on the way to the proximal/distal ends of the occlusion. To achieve "true lumen" reverse CART, I always aim to maximize the distance for which the wires are in the true lumen while crossing the occlusion.

After approximating the two guidewires as closely as possible by the kissing wire technique, you should use either wire to advance and inflate a balloon with a diameter corresponding to the distance between the two wires. This will help the two guidewires to enter a common space created by the balloon.

Keeping the antegrade and retrograde guidewires within a common space is an important requirement for successful reverse CART, but it may sometimes be difficult to introduce the retrograde guidewire into the proximal true lumen even if this requirement is met. A typical cause of failure is that the dissection created by balloon inflation extends to the proximal true lumen (Fig. 1.178) and may compress the intimal connection between the false and true lumens soon after ballooning or lead to deformation of the tip curve of the guidewire. Enlargement of the dissection and resultant compression may confine the guidewire within the subintimal space and prevent it from entering the true lumen.

It is also difficult to attempt reverse CART if the antegrade and retrograde guidewires have entered different dissections after being blocked by a hard obstruction in an occlusion (Fig. 1.179). Advancing the retrograde guidewire while leaving the deflated balloon in position to prevent closure of the connecting channel may sometimes be effective in this situation, while withdrawing the deflated balloon to further enlarge the space may also be worth trying. Furthermore, inflating a larger balloon to enlarge the common space and the new connection can help the retrograde guidewire to cross the occlusion into the proximal true lumen. The key to success with reverse CART is to advance the tip of the retrograde guidewire toward the proximal end of the occlusion alongside an antegrade balloon and/or guidewire. If reentry of the retrograde guidewire from the dissection is not achieved despite these efforts, it may be facilitated by IVUS-guided retrograde wiring after confirming the location of the new connection. If this is also ineffective, you should implant a stent under IVUS guidance so that its distal end is within the common space accommodating the two guidewires (Fig. 1.180). The length of the stent should be determined by estimating the distance from the proximal to the distal points by IVUS. If this distance is estimated incorrectly and the stent selected is too short, another stent will also need to be implanted to overlap the first stent within the false lumen. This is a disadvantage of the stent reverse CART technique.

When performing reverse CART, the retrograde guidewire that passes through the occlusion has too high a tip load and too small a tip curve to reenter the proximal true lumen. Therefore, you should advance a retrograde microcatheter into the occlusion until it reaches the tip of the antegrade balloon (or advance the antegrade balloon instead) (Fig. 1.181), and subsequently exchange the retrograde guidewire for a wire with a lower tip load and greater slipperiness. The new guidewire will successfully follow the channel from the false lumen to the true lumen.

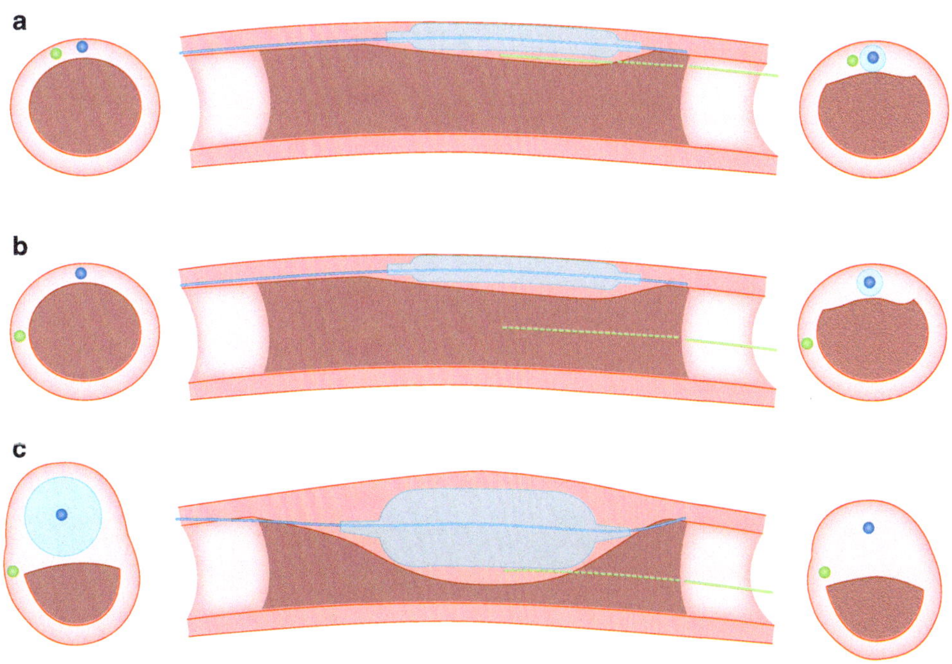

Fig. 1.177 Reverse CART technique. (**a**) If the antegrade and retrograde guidewires are close to each other, inflating even a small antegrade balloon will lead to successful accomplishment of the reverse CART technique. (**b**) If the two guidewires are far apart, even within a common compartment, it is very difficult to accomplish reverse CART by inflating a small antegrade balloon. (**c**) Inflating a larger antegrade balloon will lead to successful accomplishment of reverse CART, but inevitably creates a large dissection

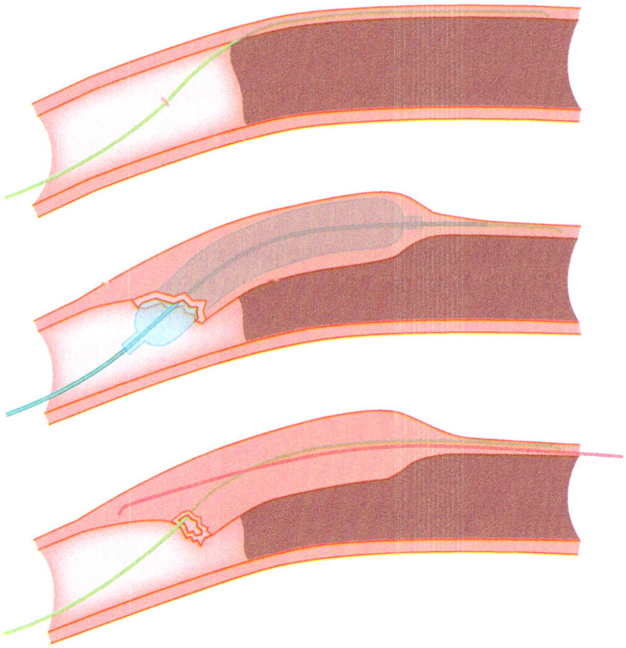

Fig. 1.178 Dissection created by the reverse CART technique. Successful accomplishment of the reverse CART technique requires enlargement of a false lumen, which inevitably creates a dissection of some size. Use of a large balloon will create a large dissection, which can compress or distort the distal true lumen if it extends distally

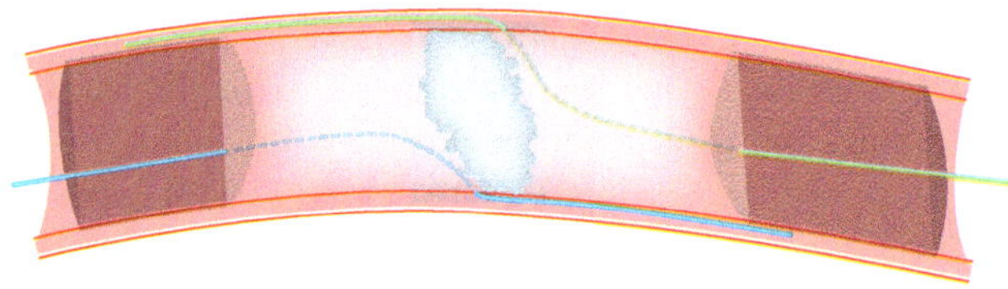

Fig. 1.179 If kissing reverse CART is impossible. If hard plaque in an occlusion blocks the antegrade and retrograde guidewires, causing deviation in different directions, you should search for a more proximal point where the two wires are close to each other to accomplish reverse CART

Fig. 1.180 Stent reverse CART technique. If a large dissection is created and it prevents the retrograde guidewire from passing through a connecting channel created between the false lumen and the true lumen, you should place a stent in the space accommodating both guidewires (as confirmed by IVUS) and then introduce the retrograde guidewire into the stent

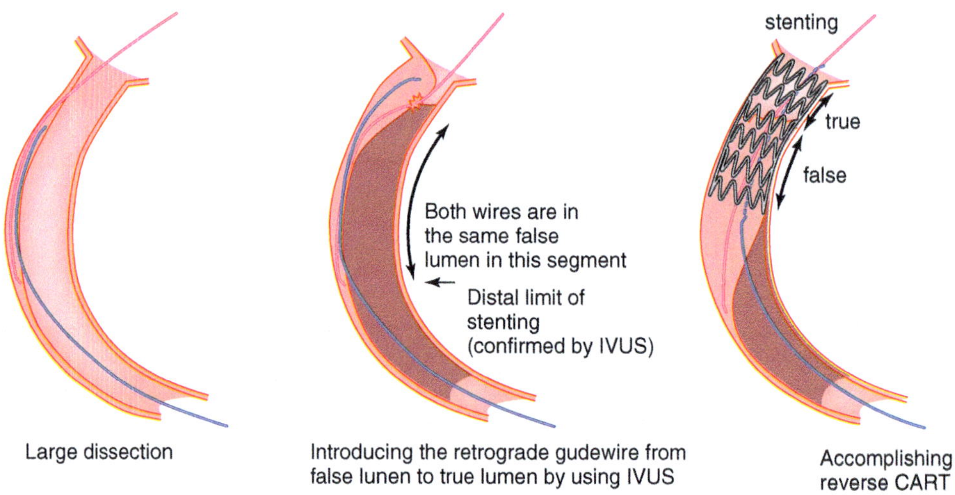

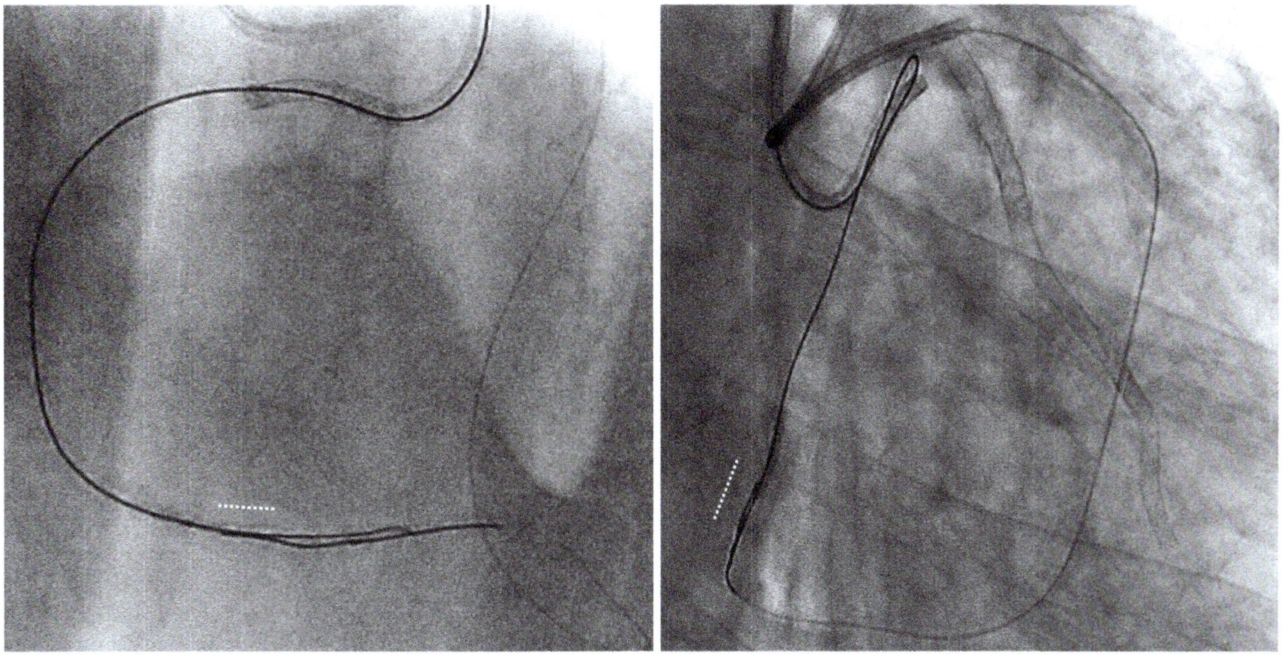

Fig. 1.181 Recanalization of a CTO by reverse CART. Before attempting reverse CART, you should exchange the retrograde guidewire for another with greater slipperiness. Reverse CART can be accomplished if the retrograde guidewire is manipulated in the segment where the two guidewires have been brought into contact (dotted line)

1.7.14.1 Kissing Reverse CART

Even after a previous failed PCI attempt, I always start PCI for CTO via the antegrade approach under appropriate circumstances, and I switch to retrograde PCI after an antegrade guidewire has failed to reach the distal true lumen. There are two patterns for failure of antegrade wiring. First, the antegrade guidewire may fail to reach the distal end of the CTO because advancement within the occlusion becomes impossible or because the wire deviates outside the vessel wall. Second, the antegrade guidewire may reach the distal end of the occlusion, but its tip may be outside the true lumen.

Immediately before starting retrograde PCI, you should perform contralateral CAG to confirm that a collateral channel is available. After a retrograde guidewire and then a retrograde microcatheter have successfully tracked the collateral channel, you can try to cross the CTO retrogradely by using the antegrade guidewire as a landmark (kissing wire technique).

Why should you try the kissing wire technique despite the eventual need to perform reverse CART? Here, let us reconsider the definition of reverse CART. CART is an acronym for controlled antegrade and retrograde subintimal tracking, and it can only be accomplished if both the antegrade and retrograde guidewires are within a common subintimal/subadventitial space (see Fig. 1.135c). Reverse CART is similar to CART, with the only difference between the two techniques being that the subintimal space is enlarged by a balloon introduced antegradely (not retrogradely) when performing reverse CART. As enlargement of the subintimal space is needed anyway, intentionally advancing both guidewires into the subintimal space from both ends of the occlusion saves time. The safest and most efficient way of advancing a guidewire into the subintimal space is to manipulate a knuckled guidewire from the proximal or distal end of the occlusion (Fig. 1.182). However, this will lead to complete subintimal tracking, resulting in subintimal stenting for the full length of the CTO. Although many recent studies have reported no increase in the mid-term risk of adverse events after subintimal stenting with a DES, subintimal stenting clearly had worse outcomes in the BMS era, and no data are available about the long-term outcome of subintimal stenting using DES. In addition, subintimal stenting is incompatible with vascular physiology and not in harmony with nature. Hence, my current PCI strategy for CTO involves implanting a stent in the true lumen whenever possible.

I did not notice that I have never used the original reverse CART technique until it was pointed out by others. In fact, the "reverse CART technique" that I use does not fit the original definition and perhaps should rather be referred to as the "kissing reverse CART technique."

Performance of kissing wiring does not rule out the possibility that both the antegrade and retrograde guidewires have passed through the true lumen in at least part of the CTO. Reverse CART is primarily attempted when the antegrade and retrograde guidewires fail to enter the true lumen at the distal and proximal ends of the occlusion, respectively (Fig. 1.183a). This technique is also used when it becomes impossible to advance one or both of the guidewires within a CTO (Fig. 1.183b).

To accomplish reverse CART, the antegrade and retrograde guidewires have to be in a common compartment that can be enlarged by a balloon. Prior use of the kissing wire technique helps to confirm that the two guidewires are in a common compartment. That is, if the two guidewires can be brought into contact anywhere in an occlusion, the wires are located in the same compartment (Fig. 1.181). Simultaneous imaging in two orthogonal projections makes it easy to alter the direction of a guidewire and advance it toward the other wire and to confirm that the two wires are in contact (Fig. 1.181). Multidirectional imaging or rotational imaging using single plane cineangiography can also facilitate confirmation of contact between the two guidewires, but cannot provide assistance for correcting the guidewire direction in a real-time manner to achieve contact. This is one reason for the importance of being able to perform simultaneous anteroposterior and lateral imaging with biplane cineangiography. If it is confirmed that the two guidewires are in the same compartment, reverse CART can be accomplished. If the shared compartment is the true lumen and not a false, the technique should not be referred to as "controlled antegrade and retrograde subintimal tracking," but as "controlled antegrade and retrograde true lumen tracking."

If the two guidewires are brought into contact with each other in the true lumen, continuing to advance either wire in the same direction may result in crossing the occlusion into the proximal or distal true lumen. We can classify such a method of CTO crossing as direct antegrade or retrograde crossing using the contralateral guidewire as a landmark.

If it proves impossible to bring the two guidewires into contact, it is generally reasonable to conclude that the wires are in different compartments. If one of the guidewires has been advanced along a relatively straight course without an inflection point and the other guidewire takes a spiral course around the former wire, it is reasonable to think that the former wire is in the true lumen and the latter wire is tracking a false lumen (Figs. 1.184 and 1.185).

It may be difficult to bring two guidewires in the same compartment into contact under some circumstances, including the following situations:

1. The two guidewires are within the same subintimal space but are far apart because the vessel has a large diameter (see Fig. 1.177).
2. The two guidewires are inside plaques in the true lumen of a large vessel that has undergone positive remodeling (Fig. 1.186).
3. When the CTO is located in the middle to distal segments of the RCA (Segments #2/3) at the acute margin of the heart (see Fig. 1.176).

Under these circumstances, you should advance the two guidewires with great care by using the kissing wire technique to bring them into contact. Then it is often possible to accomplish reverse CART after inflation of a large balloon. In some cases (e.g., when reattempting PCI), the antegrade subintimal space (dissection) is too large (e.g., with retry) to allow the stabilization of the tips of the two guidewires so that they can be brought into contact (Fig. 1.187).

Thus, I think that you should aim to introduce both guidewires into the true lumen whenever possible when using the kissing wire technique, and you should only try reverse CART if the kissing wire technique fails.

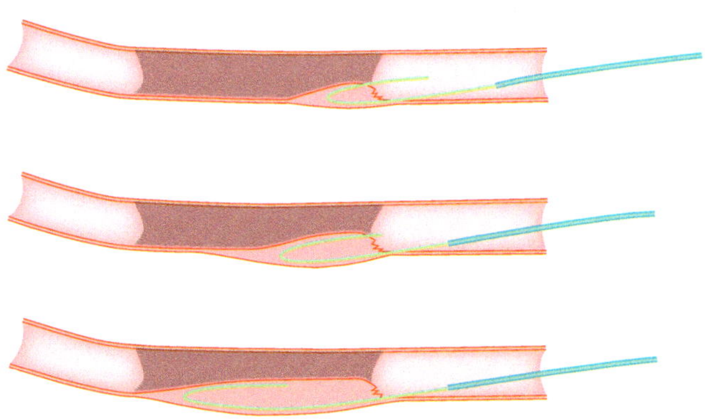

Fig. 1.182 Knuckle wire

a **b**

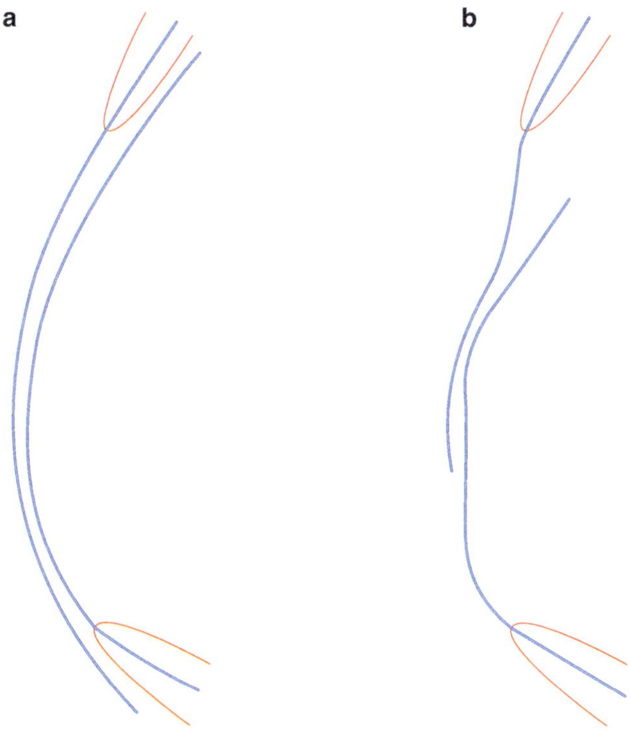

Fig. 1.183 When to switch to the reverse CART technique. (**a**) When a retrograde guidewire fails to enter the true lumen. (**b**) When at least one guidewire is blocked by hard plaque and cannot be advanced any further

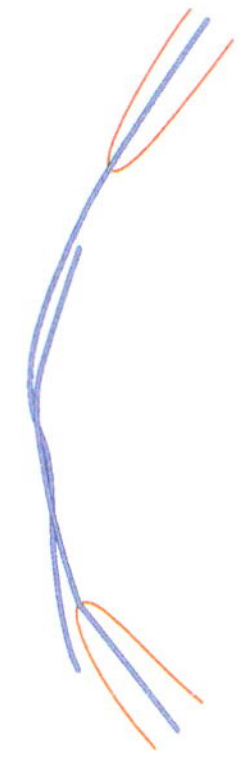

Fig. 1.184 Information from the courses of two guidewires. If one guidewire follows a spiral course and the other follows a relatively straight course, the latter wire is likely to be within the true lumen

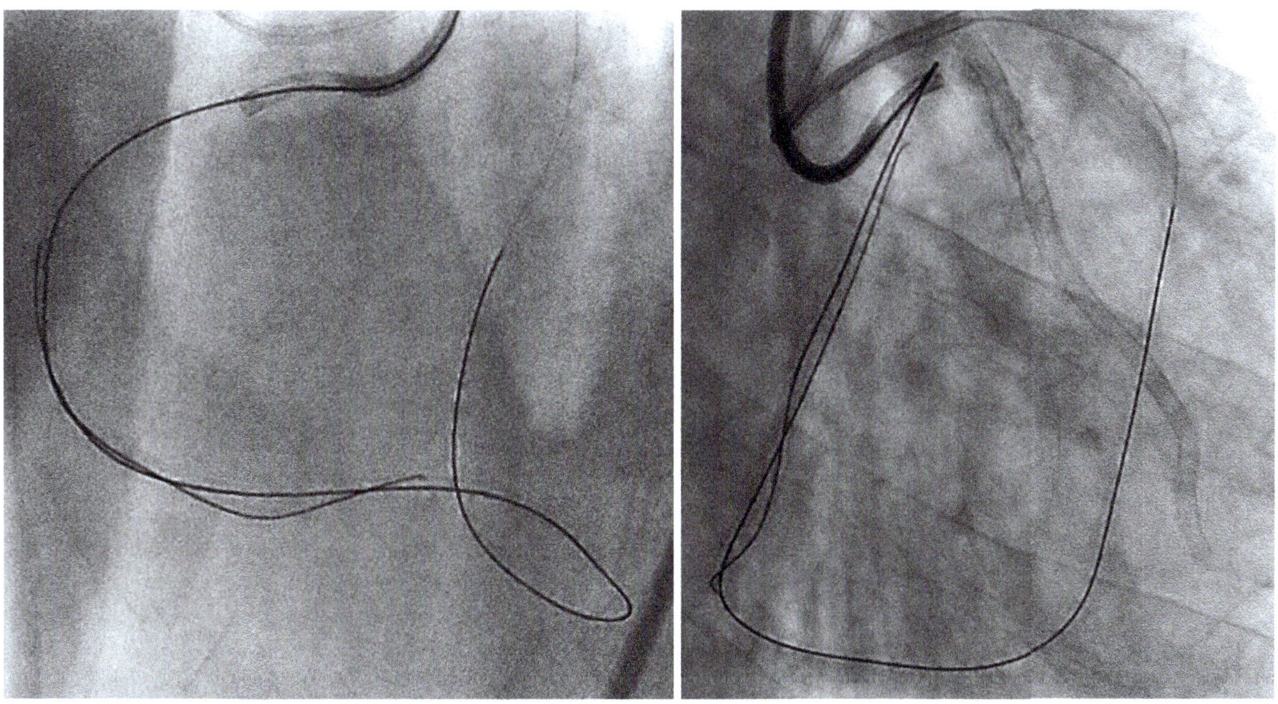

Fig. 1.185 CTO of the distal RCA. In this CTO of the distal RCA, the antegrade guidewire follows a spiral course, and the retrograde guidewire is straight. Therefore, the antegrade guidewire may have entered a false lumen, while the retrograde guidewire has probably tracked the true lumen. To achieve successful recanalization of the lesion, you should advance the retrograde guidewire further with the aim of performing direct retrograde crossing, or you could attempt reverse CART at the proximal part of the occlusion

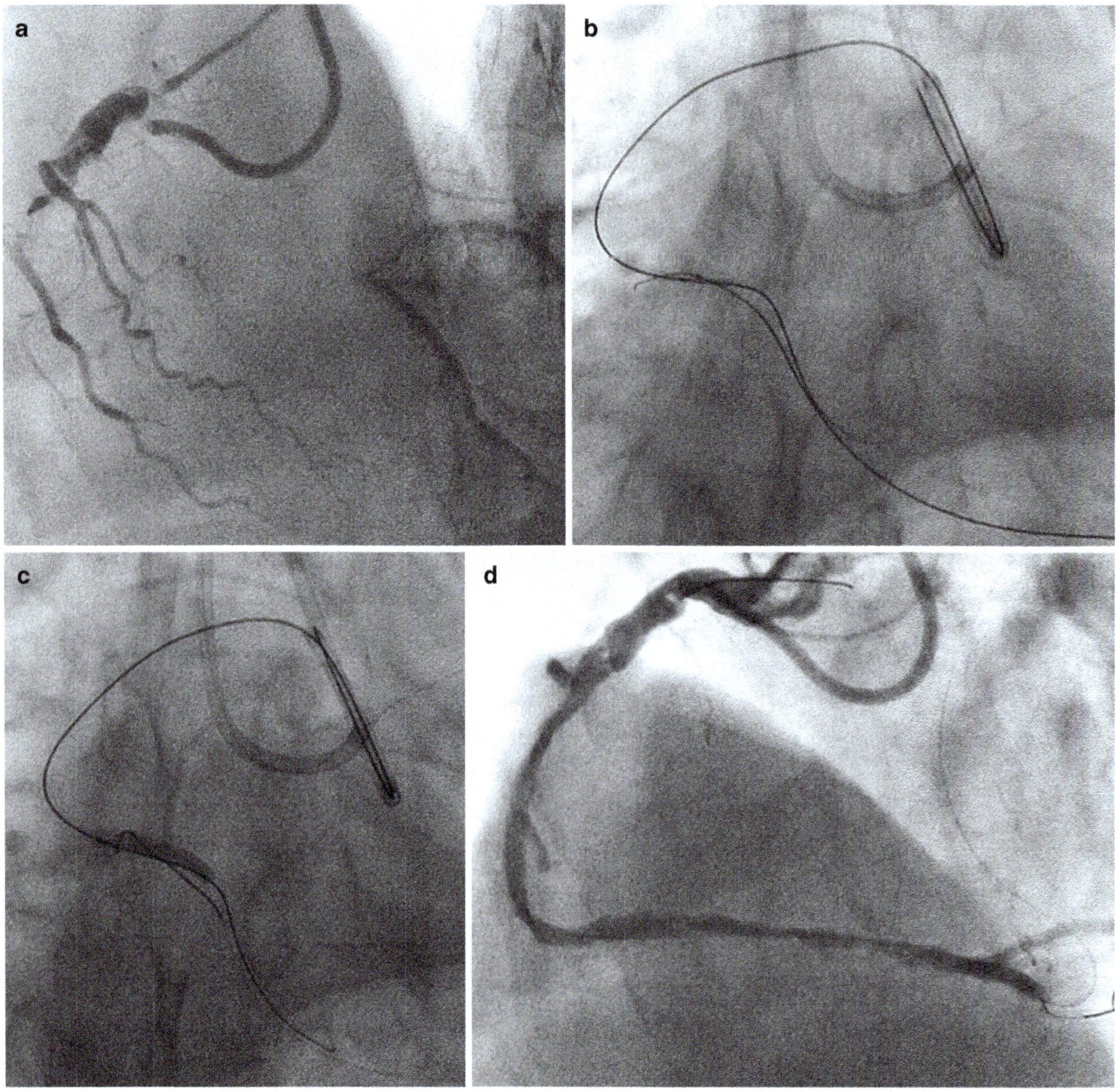

Fig. 1.186 CTO in a large RCA. The RCA has a large diameter proximally and is moderate in size at the distal bifurcation, so the occlusion will also have a large diameter (**a**). Reverse CART failed when it was attempted with a small balloon (**b**), but was accomplished successfully after inflation of a large balloon (**c**). CAG after dilation of the lesion (**d**)

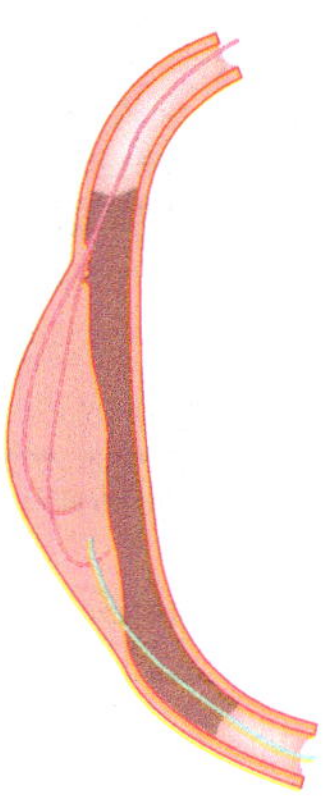

Fig. 1.187 Kissing wire technique in a large dissection. It is difficult to bring the two guidewires into contact when the wires are inside a large dissection

Contemporary Reverse CART Technique

I will discuss the role of antegrade ballooning based on my PCI strategies for CTO that are summarized in Table 1.9. The contemporary reverse CART technique was first advocated by Dr. Osamu Kato around 2013. If the concept described below can be accepted (which is slightly different from the original concept), contemporary reverse CART can be considered an extension of the kissing wire technique.

The contemporary reverse CART technique can be summarized as follows. When an antegrade guidewire fails to reach the distal true lumen or is blocked within an occlusion, a balloon with a small diameter of about 2.0 mm is advanced along the antegrade guidewire and inflated within the occlusion (Fig. 1.188a), while the retrograde guidewire is advanced directly through the occluding tissue toward the

balloon (Fig. 1.188b). Subsequently, the balloon is deflated, and the retrograde guidewire is advanced alongside the balloon until it is introduced into the enlarged proximal space (Fig. 1.188c).

Contemporary reverse CART has the following advantages over classical reverse CART: (1) no enlargement of a distal dissection, (2) the antegrade balloon provides a better landmark when using a retrograde guidewire to connect the antegrade and retrograde spaces, (3) intimal puncture to reach the antegrade balloon can even be done from a different compartment, (4) IVUS guidance is not required, and (5) the procedural time is shorter.

When kissing reverse CART is performed, the antegrade and retrograde guidewires need to be within a common compartment. However, even if the two guidewires are close to each other, they sometimes fail to enter a common space after inflation of an antegrade balloon with a small diameter such as 2.0 or 2.5 mm, as shown in Fig. 1.189. When treating a long CTO, if the antegrade and retrograde guidewires have passed through the same lumen (even if it is a false lumen), a non-stiff retrograde guidewire can often be advanced into the space enlarged by an antegrade balloon; if not, a non-stiff retrograde guidewire often cannot be introduced into the space. On the other hand, it is difficult to advance a stiff CTO crossing guidewire into the space created by the antegrade balloon without IVUS guidance, and it may even be difficult under IVUS guidance. Eventually, you may find it necessary to use a large balloon to enlarge the space created by the antegrade guidewire or else search for another segment where the two guidewires are in the same compartment.

Why would two guidewires that are apparently very close to each other fail to enter a common space? As shown in Fig. 1.190, despite the two guidewires being in the same compartment, the antegrade balloon may be inflated in the opposite direction to that for advancement of the retrograde guidewire, or else the two guidewires may be close to each other but actually within different compartments.

When the two guidewires are in the same compartment or an antegrade balloon is in a false lumen, inflation of the antegrade balloon will occlude the proximal false lumen and allow the retrograde guidewire to be deflected, so you can advance the guidewire toward the balloon (Fig. 1.191).

If a stiff CTO crossing guidewire (a Gaia Second or Conquest Pro 12) can be advanced from the retrograde direction toward an antegrade balloon that has been inflated, the guidewire may enter the space created by the balloon. Biplane cineangiography in two orthogonal projections around the longitudinal axis of thc balloon (thc tip of the retrograde guide wire should be located at the center of the transverse section of the balloon in one projection, and the guidewire tip should be most distant from the balloon in the other) will facilitate successful navigation of the guidewire to the balloon (Fig. 1.192).

While the presence of calcified plaque or any other hard obstruction in an occlusion may have some effect, the ease of accomplishing reverse CART largely depends on the combination of compartments occupied by the antegrade and retrograde guidewires/balloon (Fig. 1.191 & Table 1.10).

I sometimes use contemporary reverse CART as the final step of the kissing wire technique. I particularly prefer this technique when a retrograde microcatheter cannot reach the tip of the antegrade guidewire so that I cannot exchange the retrograde guidewire for another with a lower tip load to accomplish classical reverse CART.

Another situation where contemporary reverse CART may be used is shown in Fig. 1.193. This is one of the settings that will most likely preclude accomplishment of reverse CART. That is, the two guidewires pass through the same compartment (the subintimal space) for only a short distance, with the retrograde guidewire changing direction toward the true lumen immediately after entering the subintimal space and passing through a small channel to the proximal true lumen. As the dissection may sometimes extend to the proximal part of the vessel, even a non-stiff guidewire will be unable to pass through the channel. In this situation, the contemporary reverse CART technique may be effective if it attempted slightly more distally (Fig. 1.193). The retrograde guidewire can be advanced through the subintimal space and enter the connecting channel to the true lumen more proximally, making it easier to abruptly change direction toward the channel.

Retrograde wiring toward an antegrade balloon (plus reverse CART) may be a successful strategy for recanalization of many CTOs. However, it is often difficult to use this technique if the antegrade guidewire is in the true lumen and the retrograde guidewire is in a false lumen. If it is difficult to accomplish reverse CART, you should suspect one of the abovementioned circumstances. Then you should advance a guidewire antegradely as far as possible into the CTO by any method (e.g., using a stiff antegrade guidewire) to try to find a true-true lumen route or you should aim for retrograde reentry into the true lumen within the occlusion by any method (e.g., using a stiff retrograde guidewire) (Fig. 1.194).

Table 1.9 My basic PCI strategies for CTO

Collateral channel status	
Few channels available	There is a trackable channel
– Antegrade true lumen crossing – True lumen crossing by seesaw wiring – Attempt retrograde PCI – IVUS-guided wiring	– Antegrade true lumen crossing – True lumen crossing by the kissing wire technique – Reverse CART technique

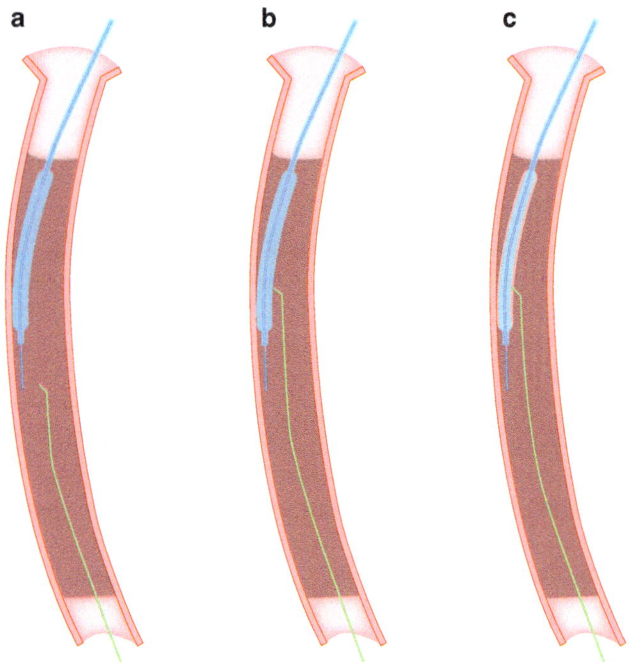

Fig. 1.188 Reverse CART technique. (**a**) The proximal part of the occlusion is dilated by inflating a small antegrade balloon. (**b**) A retrograde guidewire is advanced to bring it into contact with the antegrade balloon. (**c**) The balloon is deflated, and the retrograde guidewire is introduced into the space

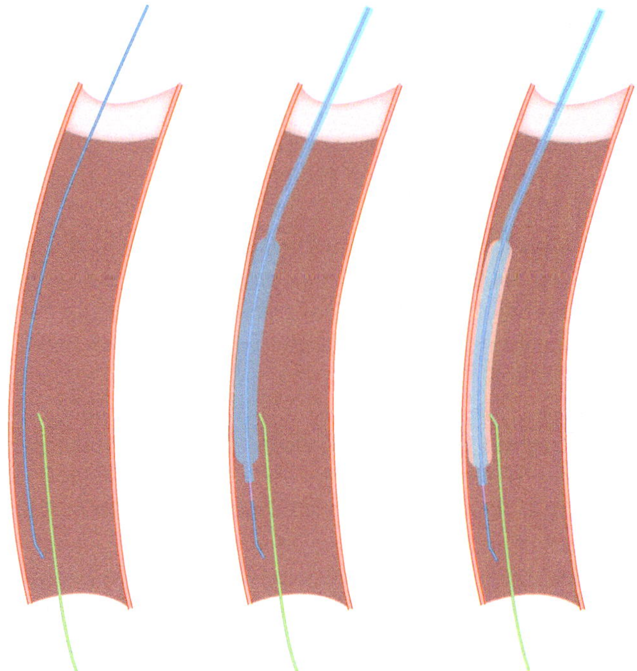

Fig. 1.189 Kissing reverse CART technique. If the antegrade and retrograde guidewires are in the same compartment, reverse CART can be accomplished, since even a non-stiff guidewire can enter the space created by the antegrade balloon

Fig. 1.190 Situations that prevent success with the reverse CART technique. (**a**) Hard plaque in the true lumen blocks the retrograde guidewire and prevents it from reaching the space created by inflation of an antegrade balloon. (**b**) The two guidewires are close to each other, but are in different compartments, making it impossible to accomplish reverse CART

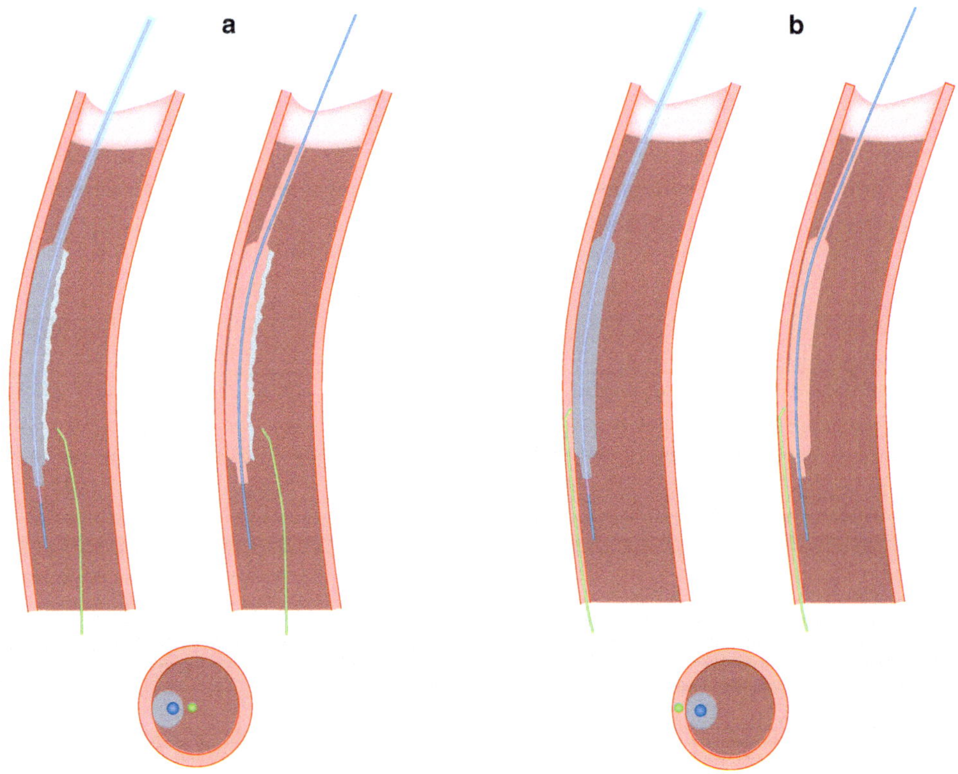

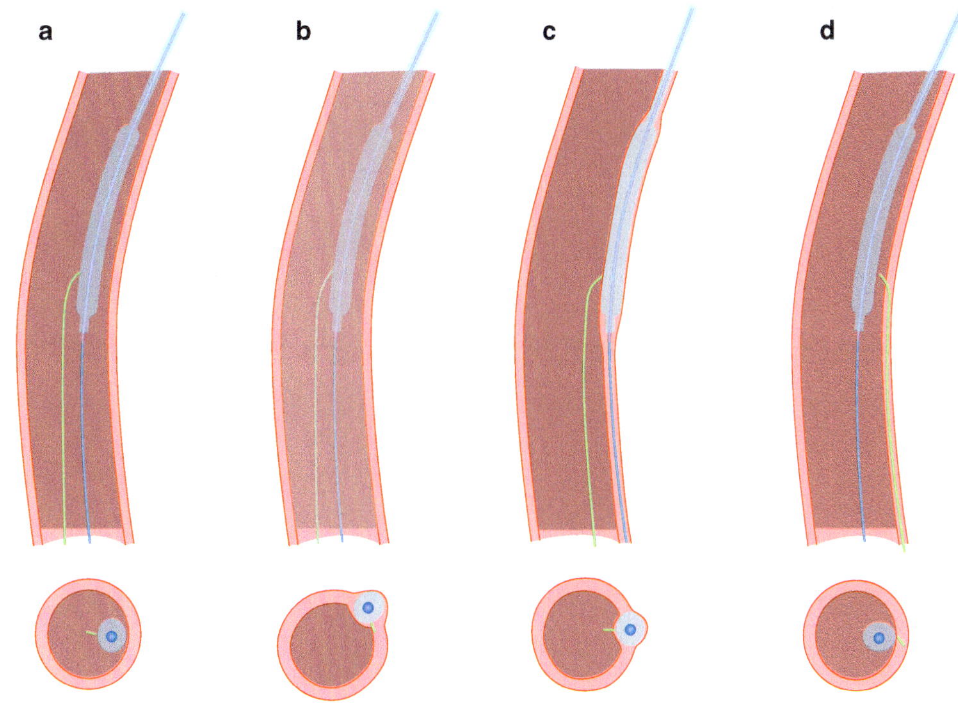

Fig. 1.191 Possible combinations of compartments containing the two guidewires. Reverse CART can be accomplished relatively easily if the two guidewires are in the same compartment (**a** & **b**), or when a retrograde guidewire in the true lumen is manipulated toward a false lumen (**c**). In contrast, it is more difficult to advance a retrograde guidewire from a false lumen toward the true lumen (**d**) because inflating an antegrade balloon has little impact on control of the guidewire, as can be seen from the transverse views of the target vessel

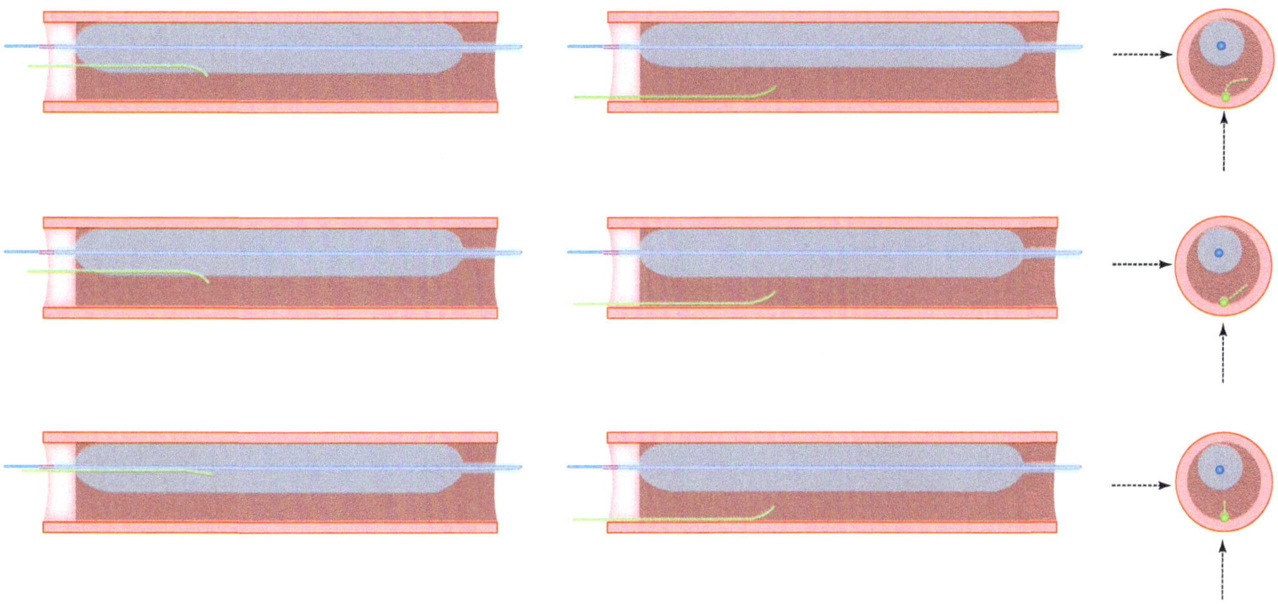

Fig. 1.192 Advancing a crossing guidewire for the reverse CART technique. Inflation of an antegrade balloon should make a retrograde guidewire more deflectable. You should then advance a retrograde crossing guidewire with a higher tip load toward the center of the antegrade balloon in the transverse section (with imaging in two orthogonal projections) so that the wire deflects the balloon and enters the space created by balloon inflation

Table 1.10 Difficulty accomplishing reverse CART depending on the compartments containing the tips of the two guidewires

		Retrograde	
Guidewire		True lumen	Subintimal space
Antegrade	True lumen	+++	+−
	Subintimal space	++	++++

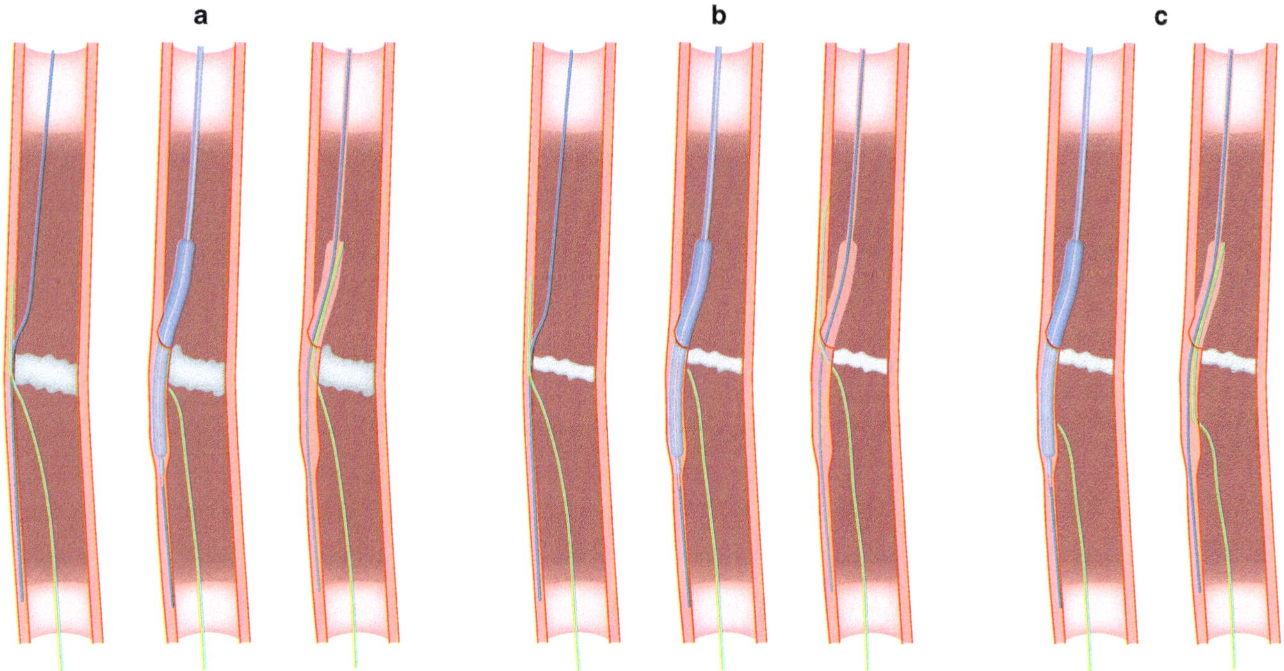

Fig. 1.193 Situations that can preclude success with the reverse CART technique. (**a**) Both guidewires are blocked by hard plaque in the true lumen and undergo deviation into the subintimal space. If the two guidewires are present in a common compartment for only a short distance, it is difficult for the retrograde guidewire to enter a connecting channel to the true lumen. (**b**) Even after reverse CART has been accomplished, the retrograde guidewire may continue to advance through the subintimal space. (**c**) If reverse CART is performed at a slightly more distal site, it becomes easier to alter the direction of the retrograde guidewire

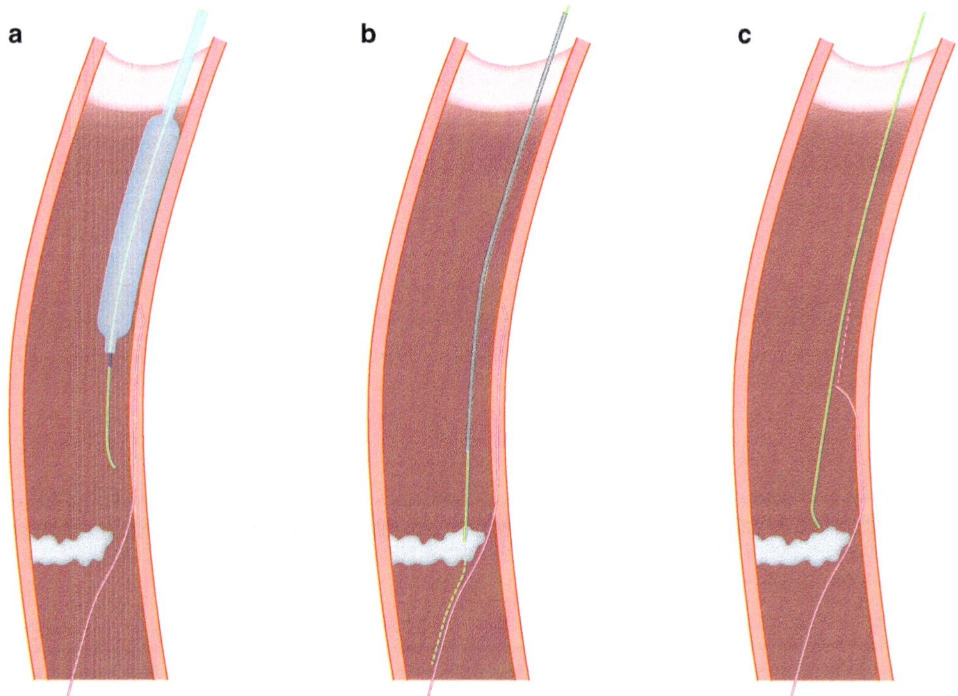

Fig. 1.194 When attempting the reverse CART technique is precluded. (**a**) It is pointless to attempt reverse CART if the antegrade guidewire is in the true lumen and the retrograde guidewire is in the subintimal space. (**b**) You should search for a true-true route by advancing an antegrade guidewire with greater penetrability. (**c**) You should advance a retrograde guidewire with greater penetrability until it comes into contact with the antegrade guidewire

1.7.15 Introducing the Retrograde Guidewire into the Antegrade Guiding Catheter After Crossing the CTO

1.7.15.1 If a Retrograde Microcatheter Crosses the Occlusion Before Introducing the Retrograde Guidewire

After a retrograde guidewire has crossed the CTO, you should advance the retrograde wire further into the coronary artery proximal to the occlusion and introduce it into the antegrade guiding catheter. When performing reverse CART, a retrograde guidewire with a small curve at its tip is better for passing through the connecting channel, while one with a larger tip curve is better for entering the antegrade guiding catheter. Thus, it is often difficult to introduce the retrograde guidewire that has crossed the CTO into the antegrade guiding catheter without changing its tip curve. If you have also been able to cross the occlusion with a retrograde microcatheter, you should withdraw the retrograde guidewire and modify the shape of the curve at its tip. You should then pass the wire through the occlusion again and advance it toward the antegrade guiding catheter. To advance a retrograde microcatheter into the occlusion and reach the proximal true lumen, you often have to push it forward while performing to-and-fro rotation.

To facilitate successful crossing of the occlusion with a retrograde microcatheter, you may consider trapping the retrograde guidewire that has crossed the CTO by inflating a balloon in the artery proximal to the occlusion before advancing the microcatheter. However, I do not use this method because intravascular trapping of the guidewire is unreliable and requires inflation of a balloon compatible in size to the proximal coronary artery at a very high pressure, which may unnecessarily increase the risk of injuring the proximal vessel. To successfully advance a retrograde microcatheter, you should instead push it forward while pulling the retrograde guidewire back. During this procedure, be aware that the retrograde guidewire may be abruptly released by the anchoring balloon and withdrawn completely.

1.7.15.2 If a Retrograde Microcatheter Fails to Cross the CTO

If a retrograde microcatheter fails to cross the occlusion, there is no option but to introduce the retrograde guidewire without changing the size of its tip curve. In this case, you should slightly advance the tip of the antegrade guiding catheter to bring the larger curvature of its tip into contact with the larger curvature of the target coronary artery near its ostium. If you use an anchoring balloon, you should pull it back slightly to allow for optimal positioning of the guiding catheter (Fig. 1.195a). If the antegrade guiding catheter has become slightly wedged into the ostium as it was advanced (based on the pressure waveform), you can often easily introduce the retrograde guidewire into the guiding catheter (Fig. 1.195b).

You should leave the antegrade guidewire and balloon used for reverse CART at the ostium because they make it easier to introduce the retrograde guidewire into the antegrade guiding catheter by helping to keep the guiding catheter coaxial with the ostium of the coronary artery (Fig. 1.196).

It can also be effective to advance a GuideLiner "child" catheter along the antegrade guidewire and introduce the retrograde guidewire into this catheter (Fig. 1.197), because the tip of the GuideLiner catheter can reach the distal edge of a curve in the vessel and because its shaft and the antegrade guidewire ensure the coaxiality with the coronary artery.

Once the retrograde guidewire has entered the antegrade guiding catheter, you should trap the guidewire with a Kusabi or balloon catheter to form a partial loop (Fig. 1.198). Then a retrograde microcatheter can be introduced into the antegrade guiding catheter with a probability of nearly 100%. If the retrograde guidewire shown in Fig. 1.198 is pulled back too strongly relative to the force used to advance the retrograde microcatheter, the guiding catheter may become deeply engaged and may cause dissection at the ostium of the coronary artery. If the ostium of an artery that is being used for the retrograde approach is injured and this results in occlusion, shock may occur. Therefore, you should carefully watch the position of each guiding catheter and the retrograde pressure waveform to avoid deep engagement.

a
b

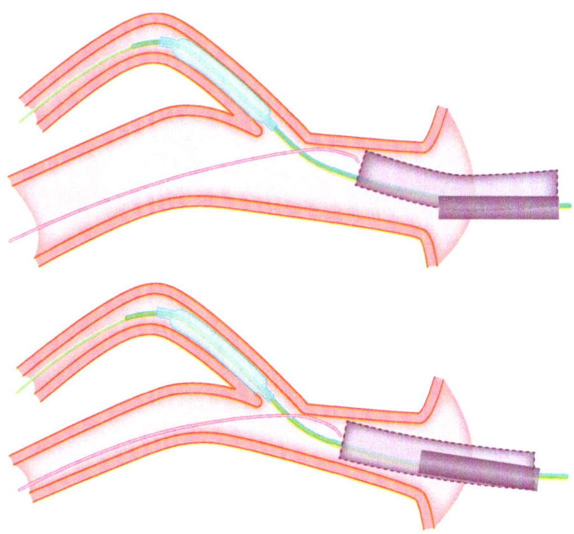

Fig. 1.195 Navigating a retrograde guidewire (1). (**a**) The tip of the guiding catheter should be oriented toward the larger curvature of the artery. If an anchoring balloon is used, the retrograde guidewire should be advanced toward the balloon and introduced into the guiding catheter. (**b**) Advancing the guiding catheter until it has been wedged (as estimated from the pressure waveform) will reduce the gap between the catheter and the vessel wall, making it easier to introduce the retrograde guidewire into the catheter

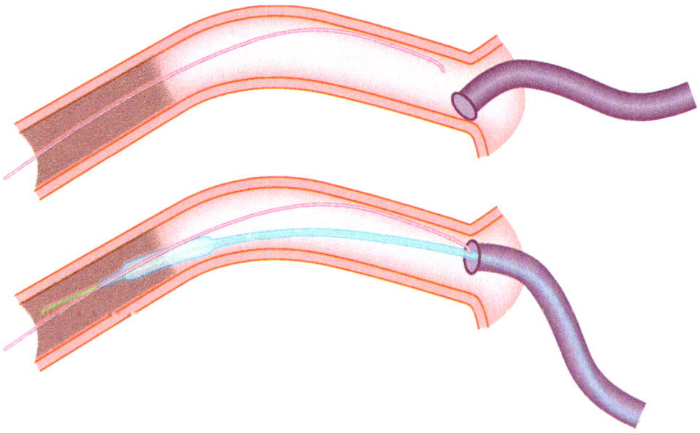

Fig. 1.196 Navigating a retrograde guidewire (2). An antegrade guidewire and antegrade balloon should be left in situ because they make it easier to keep the guiding catheter coaxial with the retrograde guidewire and to introduce the guidewire into the guiding catheter

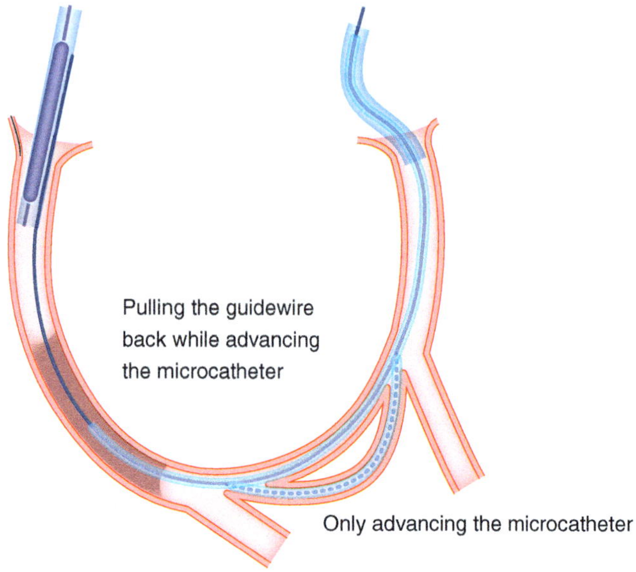

Fig. 1.198 Assisting a retrograde microcatheter to cross the CTO and introducing it into the antegrade guiding catheter. To advance a retrograde microcatheter through an occlusion, there is no alternative but to simply push it forward unless the retrograde guidewire has been trapped. When pushed forward, the retrograde microcatheter trends laterally at a bend of the vessel (dotted line), losing coaxiality with the vessel and stretching that segment. When the microcatheter is in this position, more force is required to push it forward, and there is greater stress on the vessel, increasing the risk of perforation. On the other hand, if the tip of the retrograde guidewire has been trapped, the wire can be pulled back (from the hub of the retrograde guiding catheter) in the opposite direction to that of advancing the microcatheter. If the retrograde guidewire is pulled back while you push the retrograde microcatheter forward, the opposing forces offset each other. As a result, the microcatheter can be kept coaxial with the coronary artery and can be advanced without stretching the vessel while minimizing stress upon it

Fig. 1.197 Navigating a retrograde guidewire (3). If the retrograde guidewire cannot be introduced into the antegrade guiding catheter (**a**), a GuideLiner "child" support catheter should be advanced antegradely to the vertex of a curve of the target vessel (**b**) or to the distal end of the curve (**c**). The retrograde guidewire can then be more easily introduced into the GuideLiner catheter

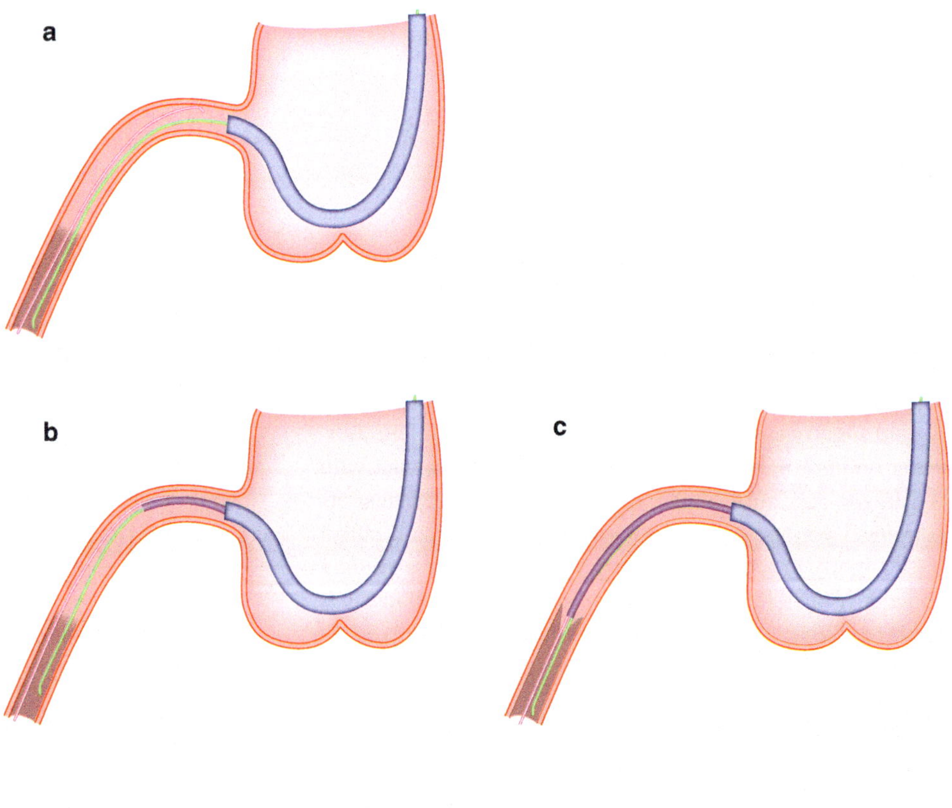

Column 10 Selection and Rationale: Part 2

The reverse CART technique involves enlarging a proximal space by ballooning via the antegrade guidewire. After inflating the balloon, I advance the tip of a retrograde microcatheter to just beyond the tip of the antegrade balloon catheter and exchange the retrograde guidewire for a Runthrough Hypercoat. Although any other 0.014-inch guidewire with a low tip load is a reasonable alternative, I choose the Runthrough Hypercoat because this spring coil guidewire has the optimal slipperiness (not too great) that produces sufficient resistance to signal entry into a proximal false lumen and also helps it to go forward smoothly within an uneven false lumen. I tend to avoid using a polymer-jacketed guidewire because it is too slippery and creates too little resistance when advanced into a false lumen. This may result in the unwitting creation of a new dissection and enlargement of the false lumen toward the proximal side of the lesion.

I rarely try to accomplish reverse CART without exchanging the retrograde CTO crossing guidewire. A guidewire with a stiff tip is absolutely unsuitable for the delicate task of navigating a connecting channel across the intima between the false and true lumens. If the tip of the retrograde microcatheter cannot reach the tip of the antegrade balloon, a retrograde guidewire with a non-stiff tip that has been advanced to replace the CTO crossing guidewire may also not be able to reach the antegrade balloon. In such cases, it is sometimes unavoidable to use a CTO crossing guidewire as the retrograde wire for reverse CART.

1.7.15.3 If the Retrograde Guidewire Fails to Enter the Antegrade Guiding Catheter

It may be impossible to introduce the retrograde guidewire into the antegrade guiding catheter in some circumstances, e.g., if the CTO is located at the ostium of a coronary artery and does not have a dimple in which an antegrade guiding catheter can be engaged, or if the CTO is in a vessel with a large diameter ostium and it is difficult to maintain coaxiality of the antegrade guiding catheter. In such cases, capturing the tip of the guidewire with a snare (e.g., a Gooseneck snare, Ensnare, or Soutenir NV) is an effective measure (see Figs. 1.174 and 1.175).

After you have captured the tip of the retrograde guidewire, it is pulled into the antegrade guiding catheter. After introduction of the retrograde wire into the guiding catheter, you should trap the guidewire at its interlocked site with a Kusabi or balloon catheter to facilitate advancement of the retrograde microcatheter (Fig. 1.199).

If the retrograde guidewire has a non-stiff tip, it can be retracted into the retrograde microcatheter within the antegrade guiding catheter even if the tip is bent by snaring. In contrast, a retrograde guidewire with a stiff shaft near the tip (e.g., a Conquest Pro) cannot be retracted into the retrograde microcatheter as its tip cannot be completely straightened after it is bent (Fig. 1.200). When using a CTO crossing guidewire with a stiff shaft near the tip, you should employ a snare with adequate stiffness and keep the snare locked while introducing the retrograde microcatheter into the antegrade guiding catheter. You should take appropriate measures to prevent unintentional de-snaring, including trapping the site of interlocking with the snare by using a balloon.

After a retrograde microcatheter has been sufficiently introduced into the antegrade guiding catheter and the retrograde guidewire is no longer necessary, you should withdraw the snare together with the guidewire. While the hard proximal part of the guidewire passes through the microcatheter during withdrawal, this procedure only takes a short time and rarely causes injury to the collateral channel.

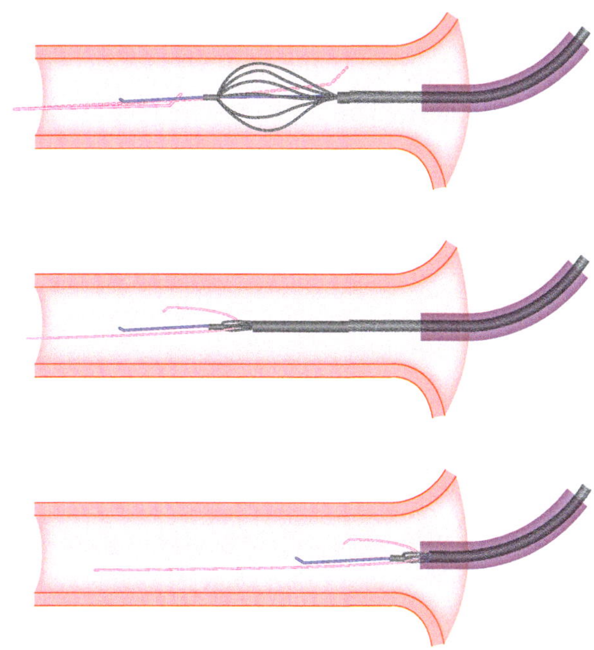

Fig. 1.199 Navigating a retrograde guidewire. If a retrograde guidewire cannot be introduced into the antegrade guiding catheter, a snare should be advanced antegradely (**a**) to capture the retrograde guidewire (**b**). After it is subsequently introduced into the guiding catheter, the guidewire should be trapped, and then a retrograde microcatheter should be advanced (**c**)

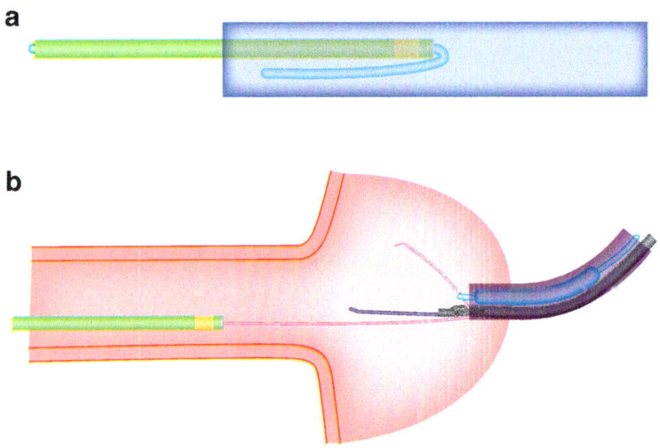

Fig. 1.200 Navigating a retrograde microcatheter. (**a**) If the retrograde guidewire has a non-stiff tip, it should be captured by a snare and then introduced into the antegrade guiding catheter. Subsequently, a retrograde microcatheter should also be introduced into the guiding catheter. (**b**) A retrograde guidewire with a stiff shaft near the tip cannot be retracted into the antegrade guiding catheter because its shaft cannot be completely folded over by a snare. Therefore, such a guidewire should be captured by the snare, and then a retrograde microcatheter should be advanced. The retrograde guidewire can be trapped by a balloon to prevent de-snaring

1.7.16 Introducing the Retrograde Microcatheter into the Antegrade Guiding Catheter

If a retrograde guidewire has successfully been introduced into the antegrade guiding catheter, it is not difficult to subsequently introduce a retrograde microcatheter into the antegrade catheter. First, you should attempt to advance a retrograde microcatheter by pushing it forward. If you become unable to advance the microcatheter, you should trap the retrograde guidewire in the antegrade guiding catheter by using a balloon and pull the wire back while simultaneously pushing the microcatheter forward. An important tip is to disengage the antegrade guiding catheter while advancing the retrograde microcatheter, because advancement of the microcatheter may cause deep engagement of the guiding catheter, potentially injuring the ostium of the target artery.

If the antegrade guiding catheter is 7 Fr in size, the trapping balloon can be 2.0 mm or more in diameter. Although I inflate a 2.25-mm or 2.5-mm balloon at 10 atm, it should be noted that a balloon ranging from 2.0 mm to 3.0 mm or larger usually needs to be inflated at 14 atm. A small balloon must be inflated at a high pressure to trap a 0.014-inch guidewire as there is a small gap between the balloon and the inner surface of the catheter. A large balloon forms wrinkles when inflated. If the wrinkles are parallel with the longitudinal axis of the guidewire, the guidewire may slide into one and slip through the balloon unless it is inflated at a sufficiently high pressure.

When using the rendezvous technique explained in the next subsection, a retrograde microcatheter must be advanced into the antegrade guiding catheter far beyond its optimal position. This is because deflating the trapping balloon will disengage the antegrade guiding catheter and reversal of the shrunken coronary segment proximal to the CTO will pull back the retrograde microcatheter. An RG-3 wire can be used if the retrograde microcatheter even slightly enters the antegrade guiding catheter after withdrawal of the retrograde guidewire.

1.7.17 Switching to the Antegrade Approach

After the retrograde microcatheter has been introduced into the antegrade guiding catheter, you should advance the antegrade guidewire through the CTO to facilitate antegrade delivery of devices to complete PCI. For this purpose, I use either of the following techniques. The rendezvous technique is suitable in most cases (>95%), and I only use the externalization method if the rendezvous technique seems inappropriate.

1.7.17.1 Rendezvous Technique

The rendezvous technique involves placing the tip of the retrograde microcatheter at the vertex of the curve of the antegrade guiding catheter (Fig. 1.201) and pulling the retrograde guidewire back to 2 to 3 cm from the tip of the microcatheter. Without extruding the antegrade guidewire, you should then advance an antegrade microcatheter and bring its tip into contact with the tip of the retrograde microcatheter. If you then advance the antegrade guidewire slightly, its tip will readily enter the retrograde microcatheter. Whether the antegrade guidewire has successfully entered the retrograde microcatheter can be determined by checking if the antegrade guidewire deviates from the radiolucent marker of the retrograde microcatheter and/or if it retains its tip curve when it comes out of the antegrade microcatheter. Final confirmation is obtained when the antegrade guidewire is blocked by the tip of the retrograde guidewire.

The tips of the two microcatheters must not be brought into contact with each other vigorously because doing this will deform the tip of the antegrade guidewire (Fig. 1.202), precluding successful introduction of the antegrade guidewire into the retrograde microcatheter. Making gentle contact between the two guidewires is important for achieving success with the rendezvous technique.

This technique utilizes the very simple phenomenon that all devices advance along the larger curvature of each bend within a guiding catheter. You might wonder if the distance between the tip hole of a microcatheter and the wall of the guiding catheter on the larger curvature varies with the thickness of the microcatheter wall at its tip. However, in actual practice an antegrade guidewire can readily enter a retrograde microcatheter whatever combination of antegrade and retrograde microcatheters is used, even if they are very different with respect to size or wall thickness.

Next, I will discuss the circumstances where it is difficult for an antegrade guidewire to enter the retrograde microcatheter and effective countermeasures.

It can be difficult for an antegrade guidewire to enter the retrograde microcatheter in the following situations:

1. If the tips of the antegrade and retrograde microcatheters cannot be brought into contact with each other within the antegrade guiding catheter, which may be due to the following factors:
   - Inappropriate rendezvous point: The optimal position of the two microcatheters is with their tips on the larger curvature of a bend in the guiding catheter. If either microcatheter cannot reach the larger curvature (Fig. 1.203a) or the tips of the two microcatheters are at an acute angle to each other (Fig. 1.203b), the antegrade guidewire may not be able to enter the retrograde microcatheter.
     - Severe deformation of a microcatheter tip (Fig. 1.204a): Even if the tip of a microcatheter is severely deformed, advancing both an antegrade and a retrograde guidewire toward the tip of the catheter will usually straighten it and bring the tip into contact with the tip of the other microcatheter. Advancing a retrograde guidewire to 1.5 to 2.0 cm from the tip of a deformed microcatheter should be able to straighten it (Fig. 1.204b & c).
   - Isolation by a guidewire or device within the guiding catheter (Fig. 1.205): If a guidewire or device has divided the lumen of the guiding catheter into two compartments and if the two microcatheters pass through different compartments, their tips cannot come into contact with each other (Fig. 1.205a). In this situation, you should withdraw the antegrade microcatheter through the O-ring and confirm its original position. Inserting the antegrade microcatheter again on the opposite side (Fig. 1.206) may be a good solution to this problem.

     If the two microcatheters are in the same compartment within the guiding catheter, a guidewire or other device in the guiding catheter will tend to act as a guide that helps the microcatheters meet each other (Fig. 1.205b).

     If there is more than one guidewire in the guiding catheter and if the two microcatheters are in different internal compartments created by at least one guidewire, "rendezvous" cannot be accomplished. Therefore, you should withdraw and reinsert one of the microcatheters. If this also fails to bring the tips of the two microcatheters into contact with each other, you should switch to the externalization strategy.
2. If the tip curve of the antegrade guidewire is too acute to maintain coaxiality with the retrograde microcatheter at the rendezvous point (Fig. 1.207a).

This problem occurs with a Sion guidewire that has a small curve at its tip and when a guidewire designed for retrograde channel tracking is used as an antegrade guidewire. The antegrade guidewire should be withdrawn and the tip curve should be stretched with a fine (25-G) dull needle. If you are planning to employ a guidewire with a small curve at its tip for retrograde collateral channel tracking when performing the rendezvous technique, you should enlarge the tip curve before use (Fig. 1.207b).

Once an antegrade guidewire has entered the retrograde microcatheter, you should immediately pull the retrograde guidewire back into the retrograde guiding catheter and then advance the antegrade guidewire into the retrograde catheter. Subsequently, you should inflate a balloon between the antegrade guiding catheter and antegrade guidewire to trap the antegrade guidewire and slowly withdraw the retrograde microcatheter until it is near the entrance of the collateral channel. During this procedure, you should take care to prevent injury to the coronary ostium by the retrograde guiding catheter. Trapping the antegrade guidewire allows you to reliably and definitely disengage the retrograde guiding catheter and thus safely withdraw the retrograde microcatheter.

You should then also withdraw the antegrade microcatheter.

Next, you should advance an angioplasty balloon to near the trapping balloon and deflate the latter balloon, with the aim of bringing trapped air near to the proximal segment of the artery to reduce the time needed for deaeration.

The externalization technique discussed in the next subsection has the advantage of permitting continuous use of a guidewire loop involving the heart if PCI is continued with a 300-cm guidewire. Only the antegrade guidewire is left in situ with the rendezvous technique, so some interventionalists may be concerned about loss of the guidewire loop, but I have no such concern for the reasons described below. Actually, I have not had any difficulty in accomplishing PCI for CTO with this technique.

At this stage, a retrograde guidewire and a retrograde microcatheter have already crossed the CTO through the antegrade guiding catheter. Therefore, any device that is advanced antegradely can almost always cross the occlusion without such a guidewire loop.

If a loop should become necessary, you can easily create a loop by trapping the antegrade guidewire within the retrograde guiding catheter. When doing so, you should always keep in mind the fact that the 0.014-inch antegrade guidewire is directly in contact with the coronary artery wall in the segment between the tip of the antegrade device and the tip of the retrograde guiding catheter. This means that the antegrade guidewire can cause coronary perforation if you apply too much force.

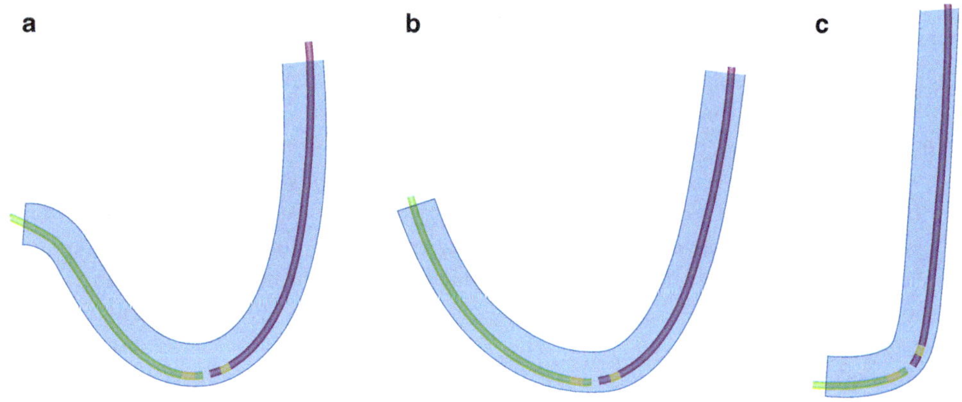

Fig. 1.201 Optimal position of the "rendezvous" point. The rendezvous technique should be performed at the vertex of the bend in the guiding catheters (**a**, **b**, **c** are different catheters)

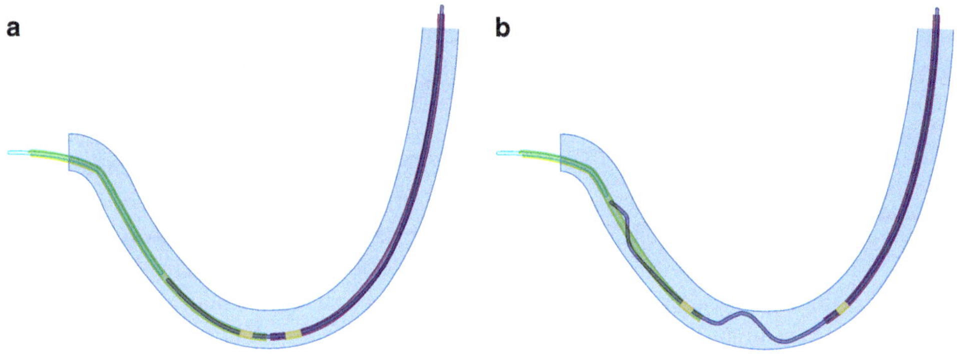

Fig. 1.202 Advancing a guidewire for the rendezvous technique. (**a**) Advance a guidewire while keeping gentle contact between the two microcatheters. (**b**) Pushing the guidewire forward too hard may deform its tip, preventing entry into the retrograde microcatheter

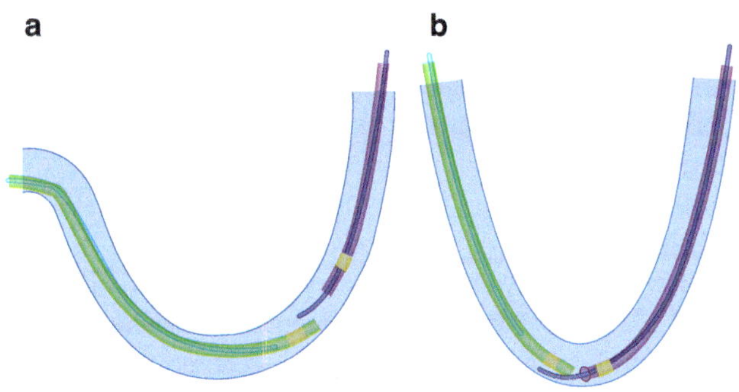

Fig. 1.203 Major impediments to achieving "rendezvous." (**a**) The tips of the two microcatheters are not at the vertex of the bend in the guiding catheter. (**b**) The two microcatheters are at an acute angle to each other, leaving a gap between their tips even after they come into contact

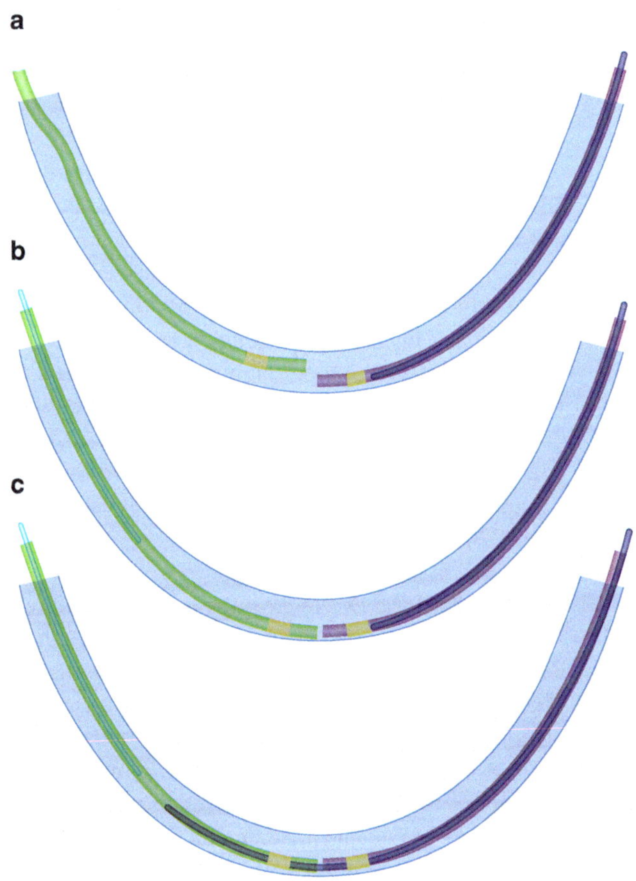

Fig. 1.204 Impediment to achieving "rendezvous" and the solution. (**a**) The retrograde microcatheter is deformed and is not oriented toward the larger curvature of the bend in the guiding catheter. (**b** & **c**) Advancing a retrograde guidewire to near the tip can straighten the microcatheter

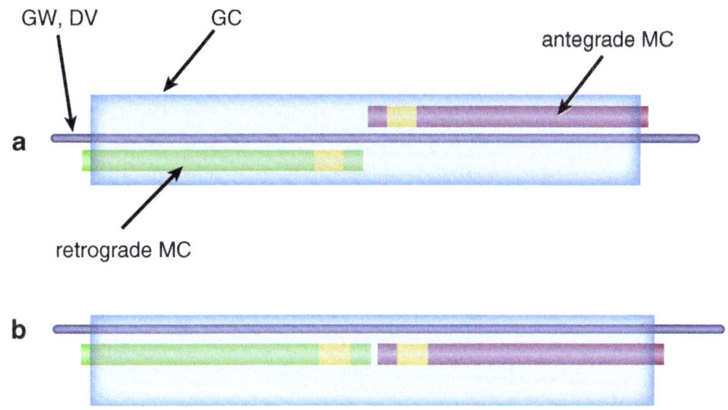

Fig. 1.205 Potential positions of the two microcatheters inside a guiding catheter that also contains a guidewire (GW) or other device (DV) introduced antegradely. (**a**) If the antegrade and retrograde microcatheters (MC) are in different compartments of the guiding catheter created by the GW (or DV), their tips cannot meet each other, preventing "rendezvous." (**b**) On the other hand, if the antegrade and retrograde MCs are in the same compartment created by the GW (or DV), the GW (or DV) will act as a guide that helps the tips of the two MCs meet

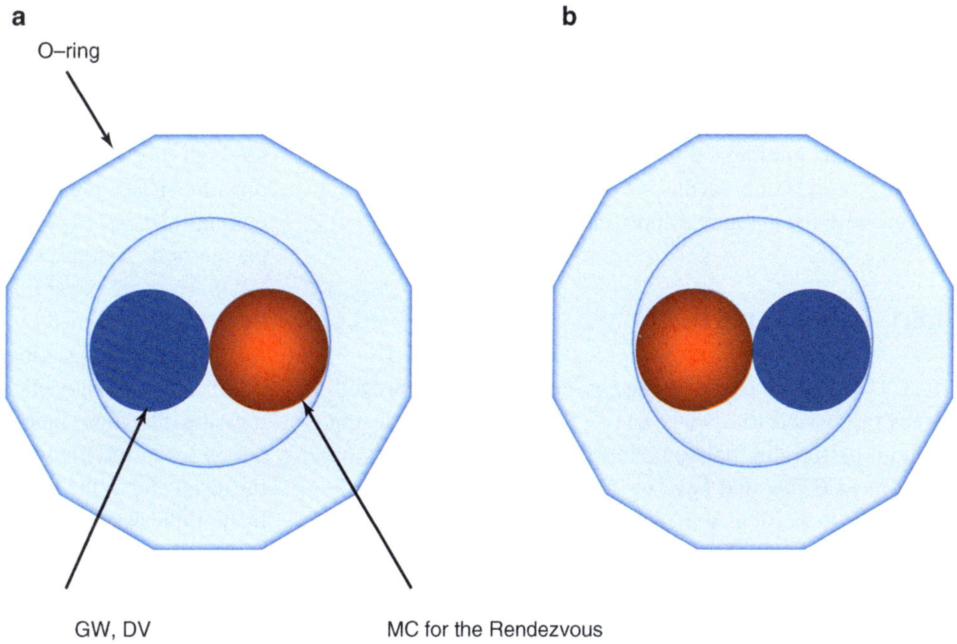

Fig. 1.206 Position of the antegrade microcatheter relative to an antegrade guidewire (or device) seen from the Y-connector. If the antegrade microcatheter (MC) is on the opposite side relative to an antegrade guidewire (GW) or device (DV) when you attempt to use the rendezvous technique (**a**), you should confirm the position of the MC relative to the GW/DV (on the right side in this example) at the Y-connector and then completely withdraw the MC. Then you reintroduce the MC on the opposite (left) side (**b**)

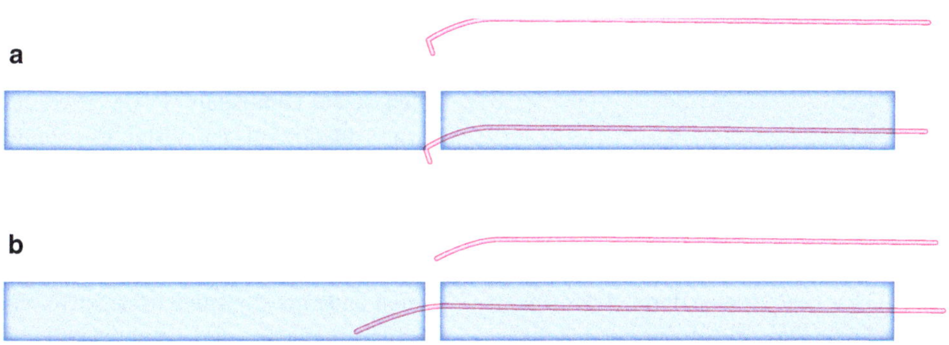

Fig. 1.207 Further major impediments to achieving "rendezvous." (**a**) A guidewire with an acute curve at its tip for collateral channel tracking should not be used as the antegrade guidewire, since it may not be able to enter the retrograde microcatheter. (**b**) The guidewire should be reshaped with a less acute tip angle before it is used as an antegrade "rendezvous" guidewire

1.7.17.2 Externalization Using an RG-3 Wire

Externalization using an RG-3® wire is most commonly performed to revisit the antegrade approach. This technique is very simple, since it just involves advancing the RG-3 wire after withdrawing the retrograde guidewire. After completely withdrawing all balloons and other devices from the antegrade guiding catheter, you should carefully push the RG-3 wire forward without needing CAG confirmation. Once the tip of the wire has reached the radiolucent part near the hub of the Y-connector attached to the antegrade guiding catheter,

you should disconnect the Y-connector and pull the tip of the RG-3 wire out of the O-ring by using an inserter.

While leaving the wire in this way, you could advance a balloon and/or other device from its soft tip to accomplish PCI. However, I always trap the RG-3 wire with a balloon and advance a microcatheter antegradely to exchange the wire for a 0.014-inch guidewire. As mentioned above, I do not think that it is difficult to advance a device antegradely without a guidewire loop. If the microcatheter is unable to reach the distal end of the CTO even using a guidewire loop, it needs to be exchanged for a Tornus catheter. After the catheter has crossed the lesion, you should consider using a Rotablator.

1.8 Antegrade Approach Revisited

After a retrograde guidewire has crossed the CTO through the antegrade guiding catheter, PCI is accomplished by performing a series of procedures from ballooning to stenting as is done with the antegrade approach.

1.8.1 Balloon Inflation

If a CTO has been easily crossed by the antegrade approach, it may be possible to advance an IVUS catheter into the lesion without performing balloon dilation, but it is difficult to do so in most CTOs that have been crossed by the retrograde approach. In particular, if reverse CART has been accomplished via the false lumen, the false lumen has a remaining blind distal end. To prevent distal enlargement of this false lumen, you need to create a channel leading to the distal true lumen as soon as possible. Ballooning is considered successful if you can use a 1.0- to 1.5-mm balloon to create such a channel, in order to reduce the pressure in the false lumen and permit advancement of an IVUS catheter.

1.8.2 IVUS

You should introduce an IVUS catheter into the space enlarged by the balloon for the following purposes: (1) to determine how the CTO has been crossed (through the true or false lumen), (2) to estimate the external and internal diameters of the target vessel proximal and distal to the occlusion, (3) to estimate the luminal diameter and the characteristics of plaques at the occlusion, (4) to characterize plaques in the entire target vessel, (5) to assess side branches at the occlusion, and (6) to assess a bifurcation distal to the occlusion.

1. Mode of guidewire crossing lumen: You should determine the extent to which the CTO has been crossed through the true and false lumens. Even if the lesion has been crossed through a false lumen, the standard procedure is to dilate the lumen and place one or more stents. However, if the false lumen is long, you may reattempt tracking the true lumen in parallel under IVUS guidance (see 1.8.3 "Retry for Tracking the True Lumen").

   If the proximal part of a previously stented CTO cannot be crossed through the true lumen, the first antegrade guidewire may not be able to pass through the stent. Also in this case, you may reattempt tracking the true lumen through the stent from the proximal true lumen under IVUS guidance.
2. Diameter of the target vessel proximal and distal to the occlusion: If there is no plaque in the proximal or distal stent landing zone, you should dilate these parts of the vessel using a balloon compatible with the external vessel diameter in these zones. For post-dilatation, I use a balloon at least 0.25 mm smaller than the external vessel diameter estimated by IVUS. To obtain sufficient dilation, I inflate the high-pressure balloon at an average of its rated burst pressure (RBP) plus 4 to 6 atm. Inflating a balloon of the optimal size at 14–16 atm may effectively dilate hard, plaque-rich lesions such as CTOs, as indicated by IVUS. Even so, better dilation of such lesions (as indicated by IVUS) is obtained by inflating a high-pressure balloon that is a quarter size smaller to its RBP plus 4–6 atm. To avoid creating a dissection at the edge of the stent by high-pressure dilatation, I increase the pressure more slowly as I get closer to the final target pressure. If there is plaque at the distal end of the stent or the vessel may be over-dilated by high-pressure dilatation, I perform high-pressure dilatation by placing the distal end of the balloon 2–3 mm proximal to the distal end of the stent and dilate the vessel at the edge of the stent by inflating a balloon at 14–16 atm.

   The coronary artery lumen distal to a CTO often shows negative remodeling (shrinkage). In this case, you should administer intracoronary nitrate before performing IVUS, although this treatment cannot promptly dilate the remodeled vessel completely. IVUS after stenting often confirms dilation of the distal true lumen. If a marked vasodilatory response of the distal true lumen occurs, you should dilate the vessel with a balloon of the optimal size.
3. Luminal diameter and characteristics of plaques at the occlusion: The occluded segment of a coronary artery often undergoes positive or negative remodeling. In particular, if plaques are scattered through the remodeled part of a long occlusion, you must not overlook calcified plaques or plaques showing attenuation because their presence influences the technique to be used in the next step. A CTO with severe calcification that has been crossed through the true lumen is a good indication for using a Rotablator or scoring balloon, while the presence of plaques with attenuation may require protection of the coronary artery distal to the CTO, depending on the properties and volume of the plaque in question.

4. Plaques in the entire target vessel: The presence/properties of plaques in the entire target vessel, as well as at the occlusion, influence selection of the subsequent PCI strategy.

   When treating a CTO that has been crossed through the true lumen, the important considerations are the same as those when treating a non-occluded lesion and should include (1) the need for rotablation, (2) the need for a Lacrosse NSE balloon, (3) the preference for a high-pressure balloon, (4) the need to protect the distal coronary artery, (5) the need to protect any side branch, (6) the need for bifurcation stenting, (7) the need for ostial stenting, and (8) the optimal size of each device.
5. Side branch at the CTO: If there is a large side branch at the occluded segment, you should attempt to isolate the branch by using a Crusade catheter or under IVUS guidance, provided that the IVUS catheter has been introduced into the true lumen, the ostium of the side branch is not severely calcified, and the side branch is visible on IVUS (Fig. 1.208). If the side branch cannot be isolated and if there is a collateral channel leading to the branch, you should also perform retrograde PCI for the occluded side branch. You should introduce a retrograde guidewire into the antegrade guiding catheter to eventually accomplish stenting of the bifurcation lesion.
6. Bifurcation distal to the CTO: If the vessel undergoes bifurcation at the distal end of the occlusion, even an antegrade guidewire in the true lumen of the main vessel (or side branch) may not easily enter the distal lumen of the side branch (or main vessel) (Fig. 1.209). If a guidewire that was tracking in the subintimal space or in plaque distal to the branching point has gone into the true lumen, the intima of the main vessel (or side branch) may close the ostium of the side branch (or main vessel), precluding isolation of the side branch by antegrade wiring.

Under such circumstances, you should take the following measures:

- Dilate the occluded vessel with a scoring balloon (e.g., a Lacrosse NSE balloon) to make longitudinal cracks in the intima of the main vessel (or side branch). Such cracks may possibly extend to the intima of the side branch (or main vessel), facilitating side branch isolation through a Crusade catheter.
- Manipulate a CTO stiff guidewire through a Crusade catheter to penetrate the plaque and enter the side branch (or main vessel) (Fig. 1.210).
- Approach the side branch retrogradely via any collateral channel that is available (Fig. 1.211).
- Use the reverse wire technique (Fig. 1.212).

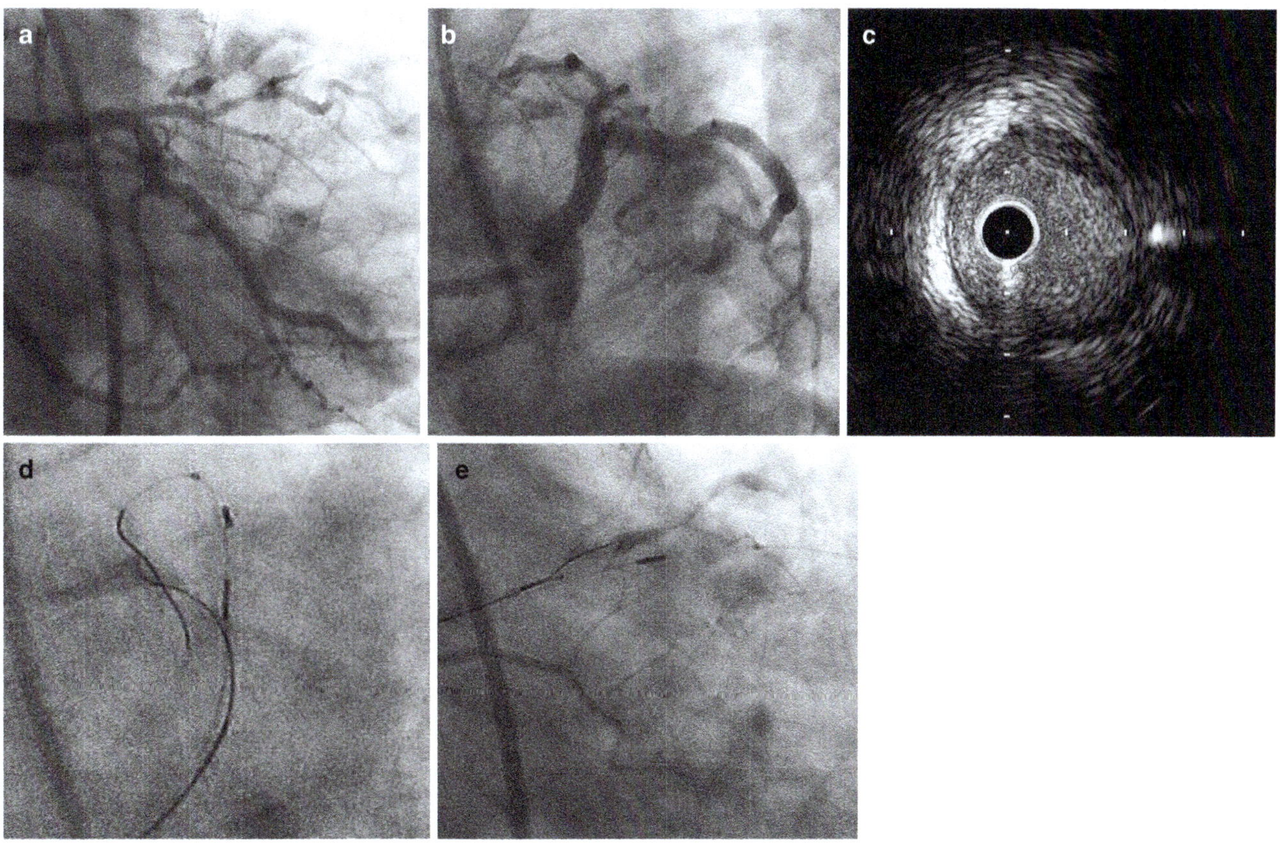

Fig. 1.208 CTO of the proximal LAD. It was difficult to identify the ostium of the side branch on CAG (**a**, **b**). An IVUS catheter was advanced to the side branch to identify its ostium (**c**), leading to successful wiring of the branch (**d**, **e**)

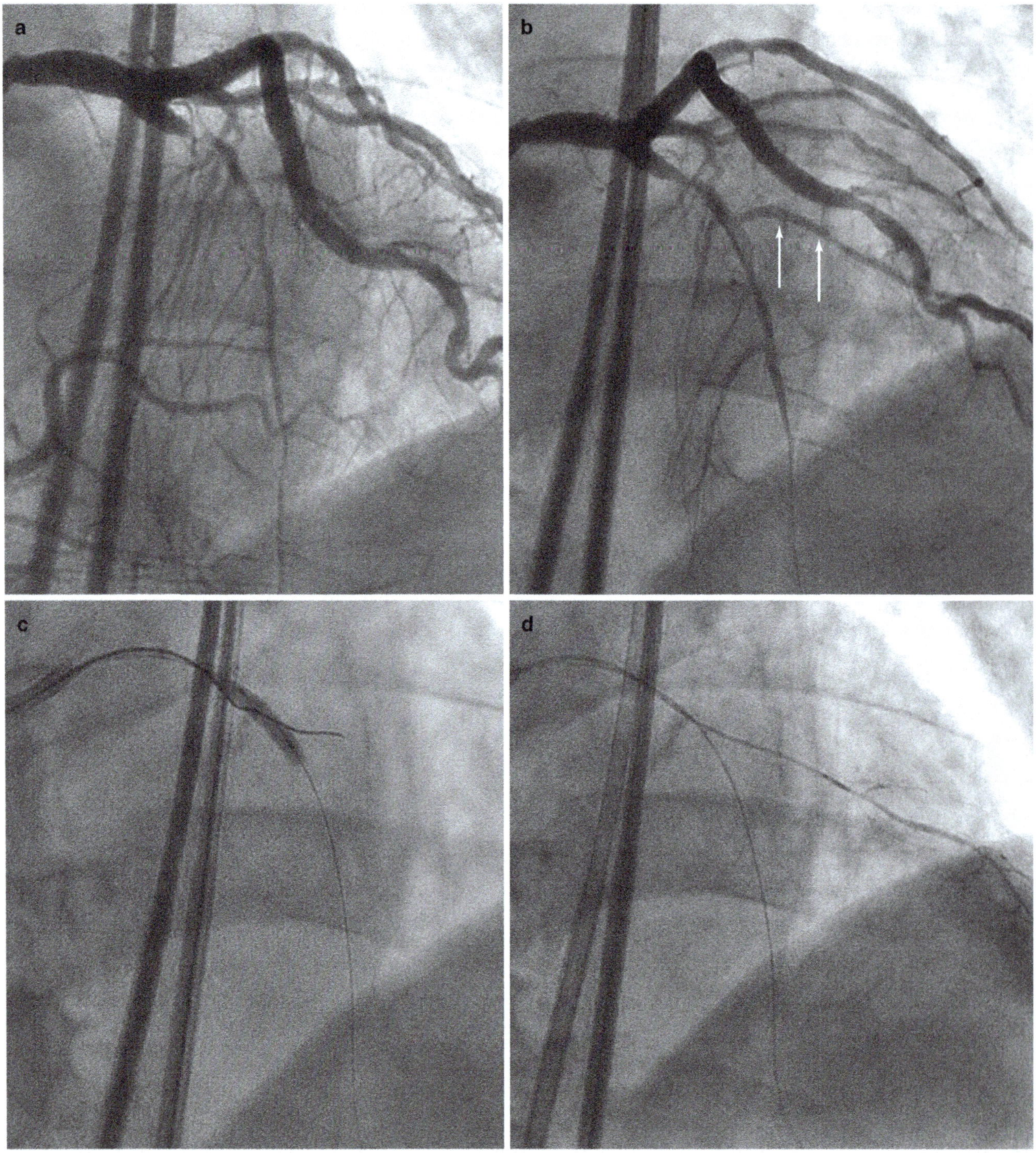

Fig. 1.209 Short CTO of the LAD (**a**). A guidewire has crossed the CTO through a subintimal space and enlarged it, so a stent implanted in the lumen may occlude the side branch indicated by arrows (**b**). Dilation of the main trunk by a Lacrosse NSE balloon (**c**) resulted in successful entry into the side branch (**d**)

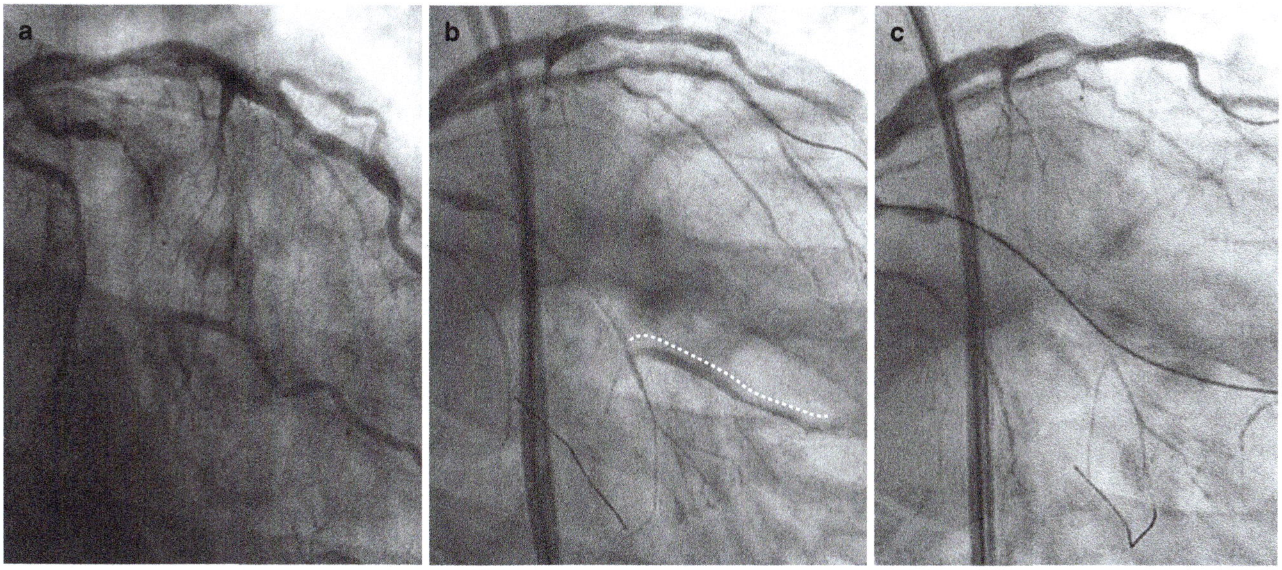

Fig. 1.210 CTO of the LCX (**a**). After a Gaia First guidewire had successfully crossed the CTO, the ostium of the side branch indicated by a white dotted line was closed by plaque, and it was difficult to pass a guidewire (**b**). A Gaia Second guidewire penetrated the plaque obstructing the entry to the side branch (**c**)

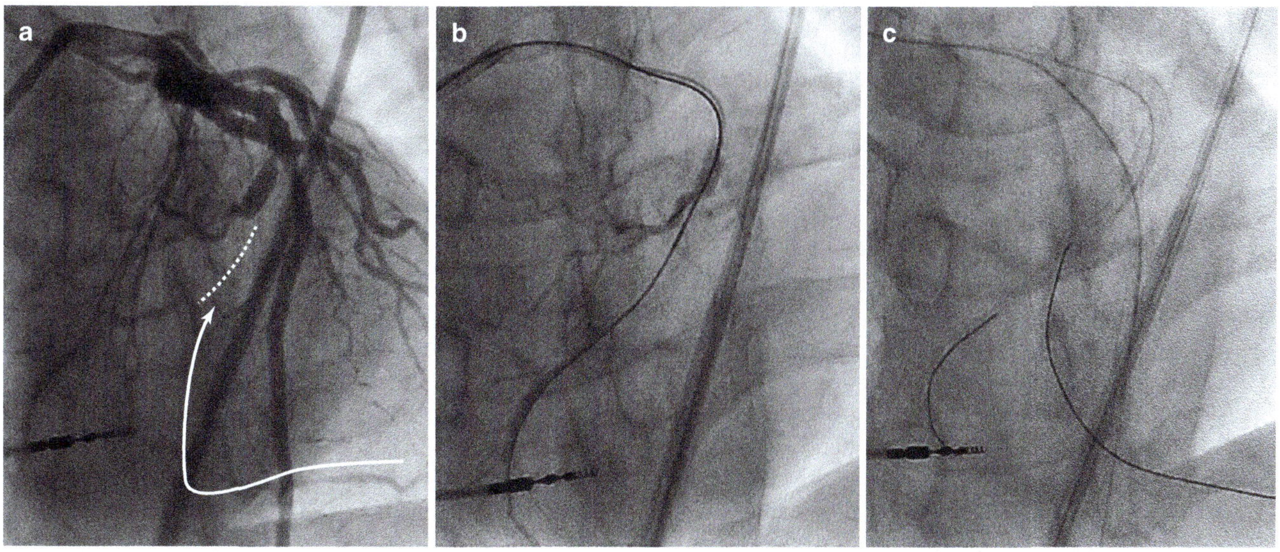

Fig. 1.211 CTO of the LCX (**a**). After failure to advance an antegrade guidewire into a side branch, retrograde tracking of a collateral channel from the LAD led to successful wiring of the side branch (**b** & **c**)

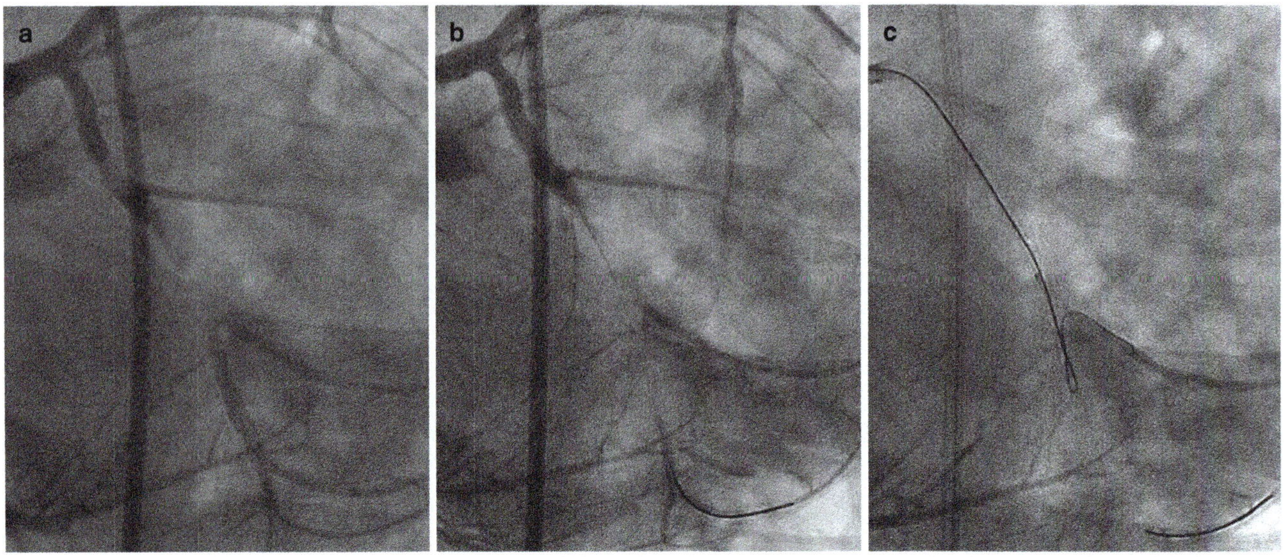

Fig. 1.212 CTO of the LCX (**a**). After a guidewire crossed the CTO (**b**), the reverse wire technique was used for isolation and wiring of the side branch (**c**)

1.8.3 Retry for Tracking the True Lumen

While keeping an IVUS catheter on a guidewire without a stiff tip, you should use a CTO stiff guidewire with a tip load equal or higher than that of the Gaia Second. Before IVUS-guided wiring, you should position the IVUS catheter so that the transducer is between the true and false lumens. When a guidewire is advanced into the false lumen previously enlarged by a balloon, it always goes along the larger curvature at a bend in the vessel. Since the true lumen must be on the smaller curvature of the bend, you should orient the tip of the crossing guidewire medially at the bend and use IVUS to confirm that the tip is oriented toward the true lumen. Then you should slightly advance the guidewire and use IVUS to confirm that the tip is moving toward the true lumen. After the guidewire enters the true lumen, you should also advance the IVUS catheter to monitor the course of the wire and confirm that it is inside the true lumen. After confirming this point, you should advance the guidewire slightly further to explore the correct direction and also advance the IVUS catheter to confirm the position of the guidewire tip. This method of tracking the true lumen is the same as the technique for antegrade IVUS-guided wiring of the false lumen, with the important difference that there is no risk of further enlarging the false lumen since its internal pressure has been reduced by creation and dilation of a channel connecting it to the distal true lumen. Tracking the true lumen across the entire route from entrance to exit of the occlusion can also be monitored by IVUS.

However, the initial subintimal tracking process often takes considerable time, which then limits the radiation exposure and time available for further interventions. In patients with RCA occlusion, an attempt to achieve true lumen tracking is usually only made for CTOs in Segments #1–3 if a long false lumen has previously been tracked within a relatively short time.

After a guidewire enters the true lumen of a side branch at an occlusion, you may be unable to advance another guidewire into the true lumen of the main vessel by the parallel wire technique. If the main vessel cannot be approached retrogradely in this situation, tracking the true lumen under IVUS guidance is the only remaining way to cross the CTO to the distal true lumen (see Fig. 1.128).

1.8.4 From Pre-dilatation to Stenting and Post-dilatation

When performing the steps from pre-dilatation onward, several factors influence the PCI strategy and determine the optimum devices to use, as well as the optimum balloon type, size, and inflation pressure.

Such factors may include the following: (1) whether the CTO was crossed through the true or false lumen, (2) the length of subintimal tracking if the lesion was partly crossed via each lumen, (3) whether the occlusion is tapered or not, (4) calcification of the lesion, (5) the presence of plaque with attenuation, (6) negative remodeling of the occluded vessel, and (7) whether the occlusion involves a bifurcation.

1. If the CTO was crossed through the true lumen, the factors from ③ onward should be considered. If the CTO was crossed through a false lumen, the only option is a simple PCI strategy consisting of balloon angioplasty and stenting, although additional care is needed for an occlusion involving a bifurcation.
2. If the CTO was crossed through both lumens with subintimal tracking for a very short distance, you can apply the same strategy as that employed after tracking the true lumen through the entire occlusion. However, you should limit the size of a Rotablator burr to 1.5 mm, and the inflation pressure of a Lacrosse NSE balloon in the false lumen should be limited to 4–6 atm.
3. A tapered CTO can be treated in the same manner as a non-occluded lesion. Briefly, the entire lesion should be pre-dilated with a balloon of compatible size to the diameter of the distal true lumen where a stent will be implanted. Then the proximal part of the occlusion should be additionally pre-dilated with a high-pressure balloon or scoring balloon of compatible size to the proximal vessel.
4. If the lesion shows calcification severe enough to prevent the entry of a balloon catheter or has extensive circumferential calcification, rotablation is often chosen. A lesion that is less severely calcified should be dilated with a scoring balloon (e.g., a Lacrosse NSE balloon), while a lesion that is mainly affected by fibrosis should be pre-dilated with a high-pressure balloon.
5. If there are extensive plaques showing attenuation, a filter device should be placed to protect the vessel distal to the occlusion.

   It is often difficult for the Filtrap (filter) to pass through an occlusion if it has only been dilated by a small balloon. If so, an aspiration catheter should be used to assist delivery to the distal segment.

   If it is hard to advance the aspiration catheter through the occlusion, a microcatheter with a large lumen should be used together with a Parachute (filter) guidewire.
6. In patients with CTO, the occluded segment or the artery distal to the occlusion often shows negative remodeling. If the distal segment has undergone marked shrinkage, it should be dilated by inflating a balloon 0.5 mm larger than the vessel diameter at a low pressure such as 2 atm.

   If negative remodeling is only partial, the vessel should be dilated by slowly inflating a balloon of compatible size to the diameter of the vessel proximal and distal to the remodeled region. I increase the balloon inflation pressure at the rate of 1 atm per second once the pressure has reached 4 atm because rapid inflation of a balloon to dilate the vessel is generally more likely to cause dissection.
7. If there is a branch vessel just proximal to the CTO: Myocardial infarction resulting from occlusion of a side branch proximal to the CTO should be prevented whenever possible. If occlusion of a side branch might result in infarction, the branch should be protected from occlusion with a guidewire even if it is small. If balloon angioplasty or stenting of the CTO will cause stenosis of the side branch, the kissing balloon inflation (KBI) should be adopted.

   A relatively large side branch should be treated by stenting plus the KBI to dilate the main vessel proximal to the branch. If the proximal segment has a large diameter so that the struts of the implanted stent cannot approximate the vessel wall, the proximal optimization technique (POT) should be performed followed by the KBI (refer to Chap. 2. "Stenting of Bifurcation Lesions").
8. If there is a branch vessel just distal to the CTO: Typically, this scenario is encountered when the distal RCA bifurcates to form the posterior descending branch and the atrioventricular branch, when a diagonal branch originates from the LAD, and when the posterolateral branch (Segment #14) arises from the distal LCX (Segment #13). If a guidewire crossed through the true lumen of the CTO at the branching point, stenting should be done by the KBI, or culotte stenting should be performed.

   If a guidewire crossed through the subintimal space at the branching point and if provisional T-stenting of the main trunk may prevent guidewire entry into the side branch, modified T-stenting may be performed.
9. If a guidewire involving a bifurcation crossed through the subintimal space, provisional T-stenting is also difficult, so modified T-stenting should be performed.
10. A CTO of the LAD ostium is usually treated by implanting stents through the entire LMT and the proximal LAD using the POT and KBI. If the LMT branches into three vessels, the POT should be used with triple KBI.

Column 11 Distal Protection

If attenuated plaques are extensively distributed within the CTO, the distal coronary artery should be protected against occlusion by plaque debris from the CTO. Among several protection methods, I choose the Filtrap filter. It is very difficult to advance a Filtrap filter past a long CTO along a bare wire. To facilitate delivery of the filter, you should pre-dilate the occlusion with a small balloon around 1.5 mm in diameter and advance an aspiration catheter beyond the occlusion.

Even if there is temporary "no flow" after balloon inflation before delivering a Filtrap filter, I think that blood flow through the affected vessel often recovers slowly during the next procedure. Lipids trapped by the 100-μm pores of the filter may become fragmented, and small lipid fragments may pass through the filter into the distal vessel. Even so, ST elevation is unlikely to occur after placement of a Filtrap filter because the capillary walls are permeable to many small lipid fragments.

A Parachute filter guidewire can be passed through a microcatheter with a larger diameter. However, this guidewire has a net with relatively large mesh, so it is suitable for trapping large thrombi but not for trapping small lipid particles.

1.9 Troubleshooting

1.9.1 Guidewire Entrapment

If a guidewire has a tip load equal to or greater than that of a Gaia Second guidewire, its tip often becomes trapped and difficult to withdraw from the CTO, especially after reaching an obstruction. The tip of the guidewire may sometimes be trapped inside severe calcification, but it is usually trapped after the wire enters the tunica media and is advanced through this layer for some distance.

Sometimes the guidewire enters the tunica media and advances through it, going forward relatively smoothly along the adventitia. In this case, the guidewire can be withdrawn slightly, but may then become trapped so that it cannot be withdrawn further. CTO guidewires have a small curve at the tip, and this may prevent withdrawal of the wire.

A tightly trapped guidewire is difficult to withdraw, so you should always check whether the tip is free or not by pulling the wire back slightly if it stops advancing. If it is not trapped, you can advance the wire again while exploring to find the right direction. If advancement of the guidewire is blocked in a certain direction, you should never attempt to force it forward in that direction, but should check whether the guidewire can be withdrawn. If you cannot find a route through the CTO without the guidewire becoming trapped, you should suspect that it has been blocked by a hard obstruction within the true lumen and has deviated into the subintimal space. Therefore, you should exchange the guidewire for another with a higher tip load.

In this way, you can generally avoid tight entrapment of a guidewire. Despite these precautions, it may sometimes be difficult to withdraw the guidewire. If this happens, never attempt to forcibly pull the guidewire back or rotate it excessively in the same direction, because this may lead to fracture of the core of the wire.

If entrapment occurs, the best option is to perform 6 to 8 to-and-fro rotations of the guidewire while pulling back slightly. You may also need to wait patiently for spontaneous release of a trapped guidewire after administration of a coronary vasodilator such as a nitrate.

If the guidewire becomes trapped, you should advance the microcatheter while pulling the wire back slightly. Then the microcatheter will often enter the occlusion and reach the site where the wire is trapped. Advancing the microcatheter to the trapping point in this way provides optimal support for the guidewire, allowing secure to-and-fro rotation of the wire.

However, the proximal fibrous cap of a CTO may sometimes be hard enough to prevent penetration or advancement of the microcatheter. In this situation, you will also have to pull the microcatheter back while performing to-and-fro rotation, but you must not pull strongly in order to avoid fracture of the wire core. The tip of the guidewire is prone to deformation, so the frequency and angle of rotation should be reduced to prevent unnecessary deformation. Even if the guidewire cannot be withdrawn despite these efforts, never pull it back forcibly or rotate it excessively in the same direction.

1.9.1.1 If a Trapped Guidewire Cannot Be Withdrawn

If a guidewire cannot be withdrawn after trying the above-mentioned maneuvers for several minutes, it may be a good

idea to wait for reversal of vasospasm of smooth muscle caused by the wire. You should advance another guidewire by the same approach or the contralateral approach, aiming to achieve direct crossing of the CTO while simultaneously making preparations for bailout. If the guidewire remains trapped for a long time, you should attempt the following bailout procedure:

If an antegrade guidewire has been trapped, one of the most likely solutions is to advance another guidewire by the parallel wire technique and enlarge the space where the first wire is trapped by inflating a balloon (Fig. 1.213).

Crossing the occlusion with a retrograde guidewire and then enlarging an adjacent space with an antegrade balloon is an acceptable variation of the above method (Fig. 1.214). In some cases, you may attempt the reverse CART technique and use the antegrade guidewire for ballooning (Fig. 1.215).

Entrapment of a retrograde guidewire is a more serious problem because it is very difficult to recover a guidewire if its core is ruptured and the spring coil is stretched. A guidewire is often trapped after its advancement has been blocked by an obstruction. If advancement of a retrograde guidewire is blocked, you should attempt to pull it back slightly as soon as possible. If the guidewire cannot be withdrawn at all, you should continue to pull back slightly while performing to-and-fro rotation until it moves. If you still cannot free the wire even after administration of a nitrate, you should advance another guidewire antegradely toward the distal true lumen by the kissing wire or parallel wire technique until it is distal to the entrapment point. Even if the antegrade guidewire cannot reach the distal true lumen, if you can enlarge a space near the entrapment point by advancing a balloon over the antegrade wire, you should be able to withdraw the trapped retrograde guidewire and accomplish reverse CART.

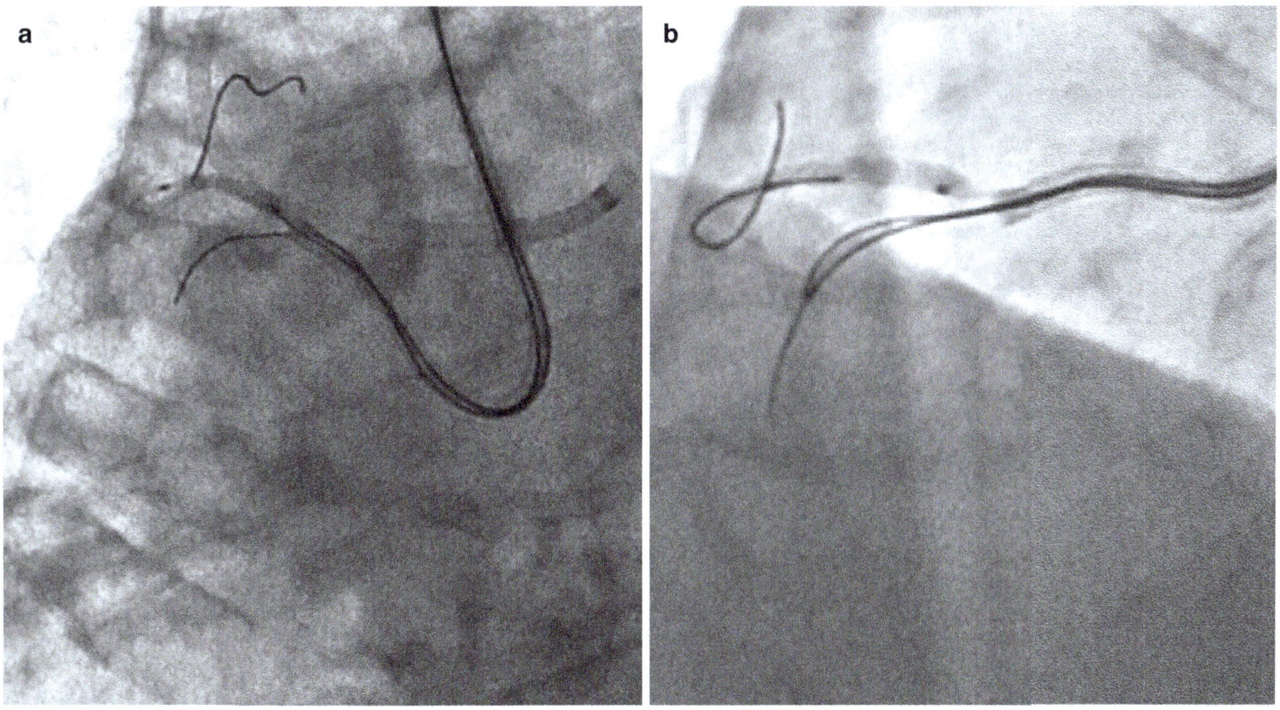

Fig. 1.213 Guidewire entrapment. In a patient with CTO of the proximal RCA (**a**), direct antegrade crossing of the occlusion was attempted with a Gaia Second guidewire using the anchor balloon technique because the guiding catheter provided poor backup. However, the guidewire tip became trapped and its core fractured, leaving the spring coil in the occlusion (**b**). To recover this part of the fractured wire, a Conquest Pro guidewire was advanced along the first guidewire, and then a balloon catheter was also advanced to that point. After a space was created by inflating the balloon, the spring coil was successfully recovered using a snare

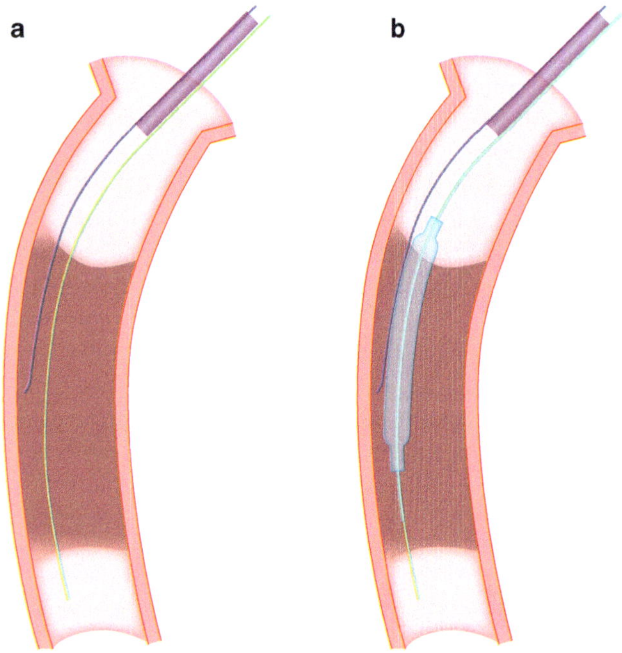

Fig. 1.214 Solution for guidewire entrapment. (**a**) Cross the occlusion with a retrograde guidewire. (**b**) After you achieve access for a balloon, advance a balloon to near the point of entrapment, and inflate it to enlarge the space. This may help to free the tip of the guidewire and permit its withdrawal

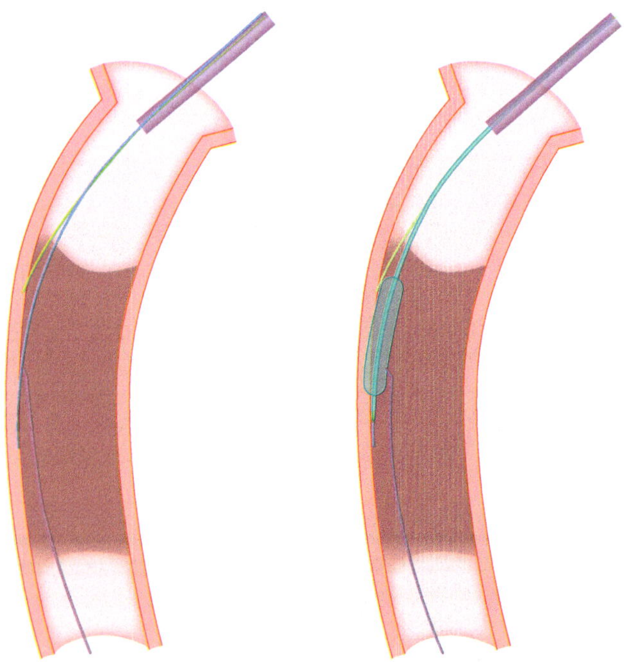

Fig. 1.215 Solution for guidewire entrapment. Perform the reverse CART technique, and inflate a balloon at the point of entrapment. This may help to free the tip of the guidewire and permit its withdrawal

1.9.1.2 If the Guidewire Core Is Fractured and the Spring Coil Is Stretched

With regard to the products made by Asahi Intecc, guidewires in the Miracle series are unlikely to become trapped because the diameter of the tip is the same as that of the shaft (0.014″), providing a large torque, and because the tightly wound spring coil allows these wires to tolerate rotation even in the muscular layer or in calcified plaque.

Gaia and Conquest Pro guidewires are more likely to become trapped because they have a tapered tip (0.009″ to 0.011″) and thus a smaller torque. In particular, fracture of the core of the wire is likely to occur if Gaia guidewires are rotated repeatedly because the tip shaft is not stiff and the spring coil is not wound tightly. While wires in the Conquest Pro series are also susceptible to trapping, fracture of the core is less likely because these guidewires have a stiff core and tightly wound spring coil.

If the core of a guidewire is fractured, the guidewire can be pulled back with almost no resistance by applying a slight force that is sufficient to stretch the spring coil. Never completely withdraw a guidewire, even if it can be pulled back easily. If the proximal part of the stretched spring coil snaps and remains inside the guiding catheter, it is difficult to recover this part of the guidewire with a snare.

1.9.1.3 Recovering a Spring Coil Connected to the Proximal Guidewire Shaft

If possible, you should enlarge the space around the trapped tip of the guidewire by inflating a balloon introduced along another guidewire (Fig. 1.216a & b). If you cannot advance another guidewire or inflate a balloon, you should advance a snare along the spring coil as far as possible before attempting to capture the spring coil with the snare and withdraw it (Fig. 1.216c). If a GuideLiner catheter is advanced along the stretched spring coil to near the proximal end of the occlusion, it will provide good support to the distal portion of the spring coil and facilitate its recovery.

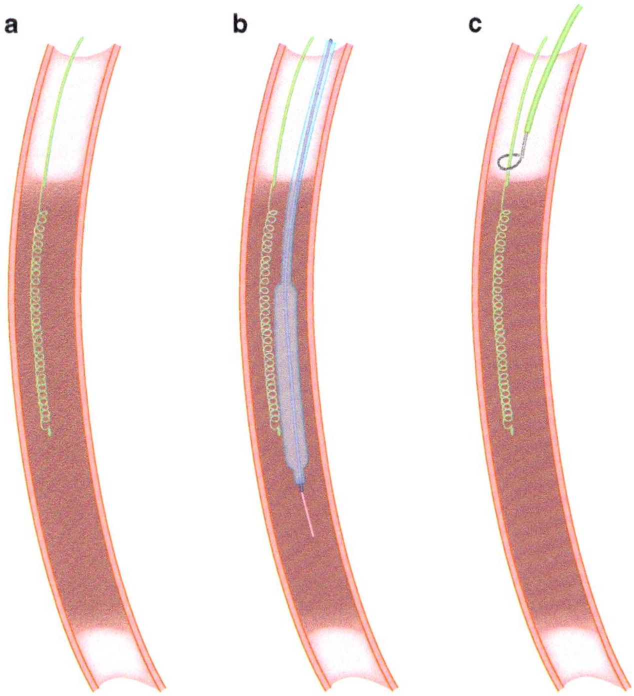

Fig. 1.216 Recovering a guidewire after rupture of the core (**a**). (**b**) Advance a balloon along another guidewire and inflate it. (**c**) Advance a snare as far as possible to capture the ruptured guidewire and withdraw it

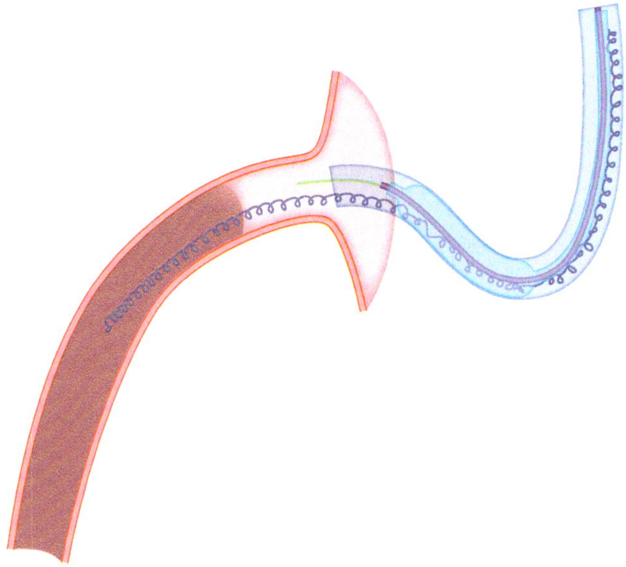

Fig. 1.217 Recovering a guidewire after rupture of the core and fracture of the shaft. It is difficult to capture the damaged guidewire with a snare inside the guiding catheter. Therefore, you should inflate a balloon to anchor the spring coil within the guiding catheter and then withdraw the guidewire together with the whole PCI system

1.9.1.4 If the Proximal Part of the Spring Coil Has Become Separated from the Guidewire Shaft

In this situation, a guidewire cannot be used to advance a snare. The separated spring coil (due to its fineness, softness, and winding shape) contacts the wall of the guiding catheter over a large area, so attempts to capture the spring coil with a snare inside the guiding catheter often fail as the snare just pushes the coil aside and cannot be advanced beyond its proximal end. However, you can advance a guidewire or a small balloon through the guiding catheter beyond the spring coil. Therefore, you should be able to inflate a balloon about 2.5 mm in diameter near the tip of the guiding catheter at a pressure of not less than 10 atm and then withdraw the guidewire together with the guiding catheter (Fig. 1.217).

1.9.1.5 If a Stretched Spring Coil Has Escaped from the Guiding Catheter

While confirming the position of the proximal end of the spring coil by fluoroscopy, you should advance a large (15 mm) snare from the guiding catheter and catch the proximal end of the coil with the loop of the snare (Fig. 1.218). After capturing the coil with the snare, you should advance the guiding catheter to the ostium of the coronary artery. As mentioned above, you should then inflate a balloon inside the guiding catheter near the coronary ostium and withdraw the spring coil together with the guiding catheter.

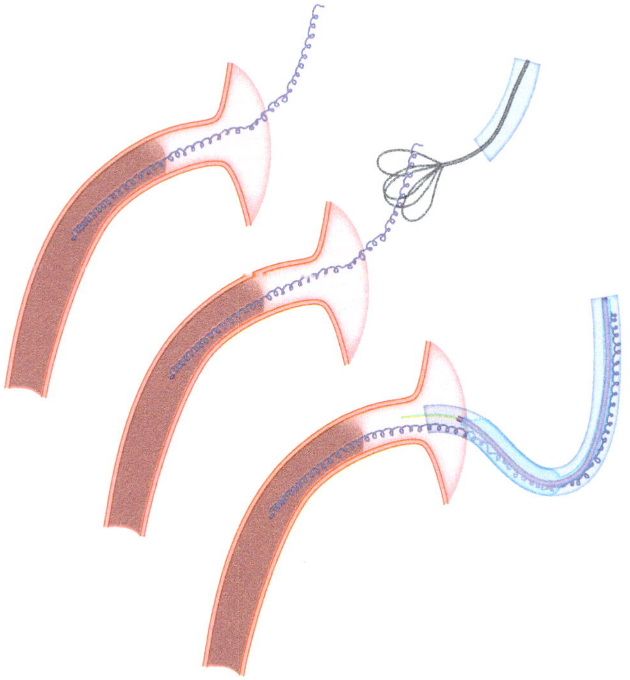

Fig. 1.218 Recovering a spring coil that has escaped from the guiding catheter. While confirming the position of the proximal end of the spring coil, capture it with a large snare and pull it into the guiding catheter. Inflate a balloon within the guiding catheter to anchor the coil and then withdraw it together with the PCI system

1.9.2 Perforation by the Guidewire

Coronary artery perforation by the guidewire tip most commonly occurs with CTO crossing guidewires. To prevent this complication, you should take the following precautions when performing PCI for CTO:

1. Once an antegrade guidewire has crossed the CTO, do not advance it much further.
2. Do not vibrate a balloon while advancing it.
3. Once a microcatheter has crossed the CTO, immediately exchange the guidewire for a non-tapered spring coil guidewire with a lower tip load and moderate slipperiness.
4. After inflating a crossing balloon, promptly exchange the balloon catheter for a microcatheter, and also exchange the guidewire for another wire (using a Kusabi catheter rather than an extension wire for the safety).

Use a non-tapered spring coil guidewire in the main vessel. While advancing the guidewire beyond a branching point in the proximal segment, you should carefully monitor the position of its tip as the guidewire may go too far or deviate into a side branch and cause perforation of the smaller vessel. If the guidewire causes perforation despite these precautions, you should take the following measures to achieve hemostasis:

1. Administer protamine intravenously to neutralize about half of the antithrombin effect of heparin (if 10,000 units of heparin was administered, the initial dose of protamine should be 50 mg [10,000 ÷ 200]). If the activated clotting time (ACT) becomes about 120 to 150 seconds, further doses of protamine are not required.
2. If hemorrhage originates from a small side branch, place a balloon of a size compatible with the diameter of the distal coronary artery segment in the main vessel across the branching point, and inflate it at 2–4 atm (Figs. 1.219a & 1.220). Confirm the absence of antegrade hemorrhage, and keep the balloon inflated for 5–10 minutes.
3. If the main vessel has been perforated directly, place a balloon in the lumen at the site of hemorrhage, and inflate it at a low pressure for a long period as explained above (Figs. 1.219b, 1.220, & 1.221).
4. During balloon inflation, flush the guiding catheter and the dilated coronary artery with heparinized saline every 1–2 minutes to prevent thrombus formation.
5. Hemostasis can usually be achieved by measures (2) or (3). If hemostasis cannot be obtained with these measures, repeat prolonged balloon inflation. If hemostasis is still not achieved, but blood loss is decreasing, repeat prolonged balloon inflation again. To prevent thrombus formation, continue to perform measure (4) without fail until hemostasis is achieved.
6. In rare cases, even prolonged balloon inflation will fail to obtain hemostasis, and delivery of a hemostatic plug through a microcatheter will be required. The following can serve as a hemostatic plug: (1) a blood clot formed by arterial puncture, (2) subcutaneous fat, (3) hemostatic material such as Spongel, and (4) a coil. To deliver a blood clot or a block of subcutaneous fat into the bleeding vessel, inject it by using saline mixed with an equal volume of contrast medium. Both a blood clot and subcutaneous fat will float in an equal mixture of saline and contrast medium. Inject the hemostatic plug floating in saline/contrast medium into a microcatheter through a syringe with the hub kept upward, and stop injection when the bleeding vessel can be imaged for a distance of several millimeters. Withdraw the microcatheter until its tip reaches the site where sufficient backflow of blood is detected, and slowly perform tip injection to confirm hemostasis. If tip injection is too rapid, it may push the hemostatic plug away and lead to recurrent bleeding, whereas uncontrolled hemorrhage may be missed if the microcatheter reduces the distal perfusion pressure and tip injection is too slow. Final CAG should be performed via the guiding catheter after placing the tip of the guidewire in the side branch or in the proximal segment and after pulling the microcatheter back sufficiently.

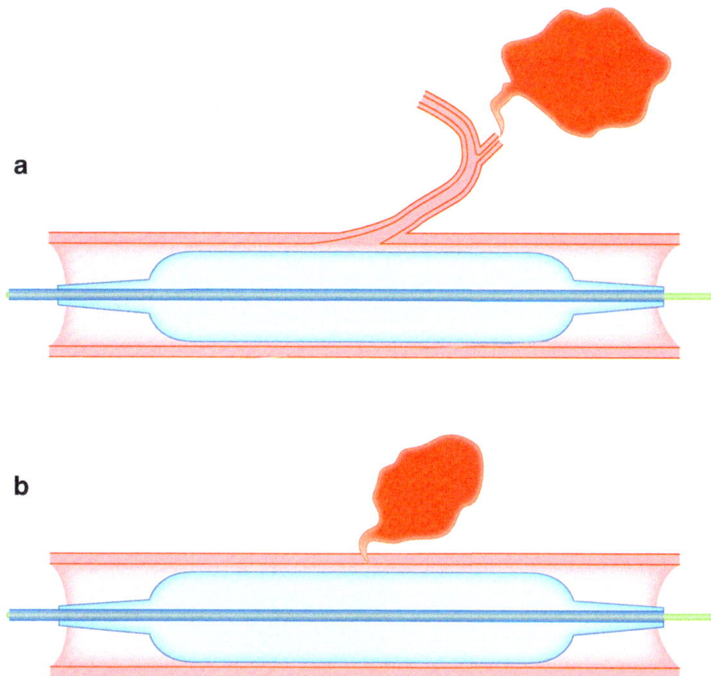

Fig. 1.219 Coronary artery perforation by a guidewire. (**a**) To control hemorrhage from a side branch, place a balloon in the main vessel across the branching point, and inflate it at a low pressure. (**b**) To control hemorrhage from the main vessel, place a balloon in the vessel at the site of hemorrhage, and inflate it at a low pressure

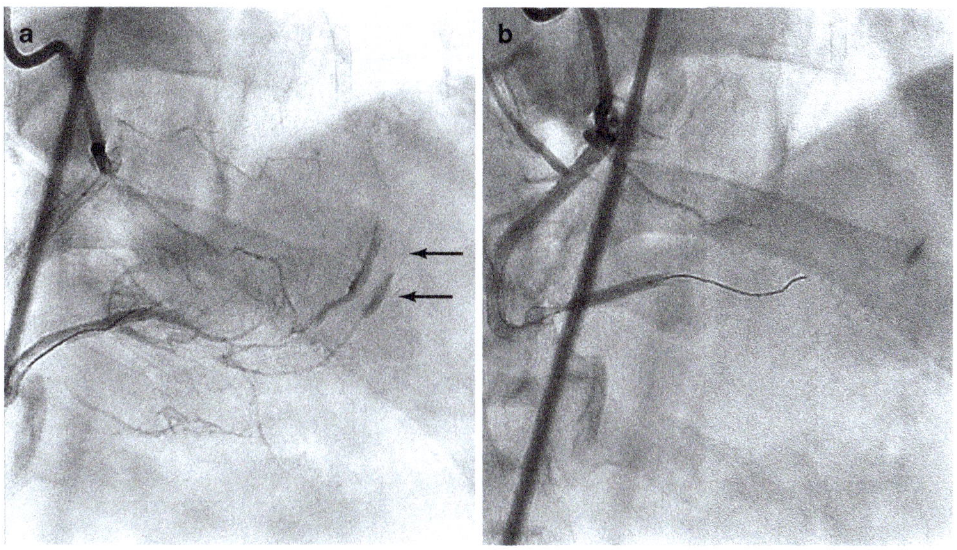

Fig. 1.220 Hemorrhage from the distal coronary artery segment (**a**). Place a balloon in the proximal segment, and inflate it at a low pressure. Confirm that the distal segment is not visualized during balloon inflation (**b**)

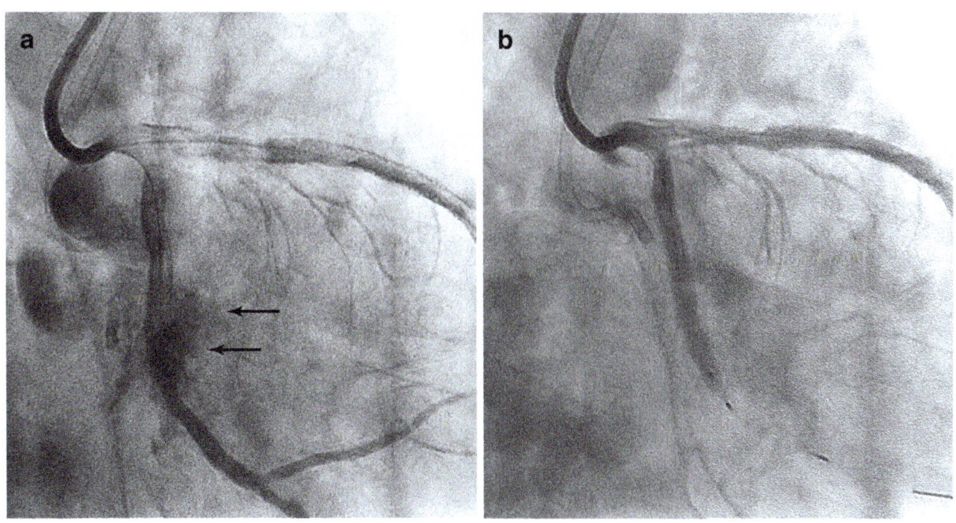

Fig. 1.221 Hemorrhage after stenting a CTO of the LCX (**a**). Hemostasis was achieved by inflating a balloon in the lesion at a low pressure (**b**)

1.9.3 Perforation or Laceration of a Retrograde Collateral Channel

Perforation or laceration of a septal channel is not so serious. Even if it leads to intramyocardial bleeding, blood will flow into the ventricle and rarely creates a large hematoma in the myocardium. However, if there is a hematoma showing progressive enlargement and poor clearance of contrast medium, you should take measures to secure hemostasis. If bleeding into the ventricle does not occur, the perforation is probably large, so a coil is more reliable for stopping the bleeding than a blood clot or a block of subcutaneous fat (Fig. 1.222). After successful hemostasis, similar measures should be taken from the contralateral side (Fig. 1.223).

If there is intramyocardial bleeding, it is difficult to estimate the size of the connection between the artery and the cardiac chamber. In this case, coil embolization should basically not be performed (Fig. 1.224) because the connection may be too large to retain a coil that is delivered as a hemostatic plug.

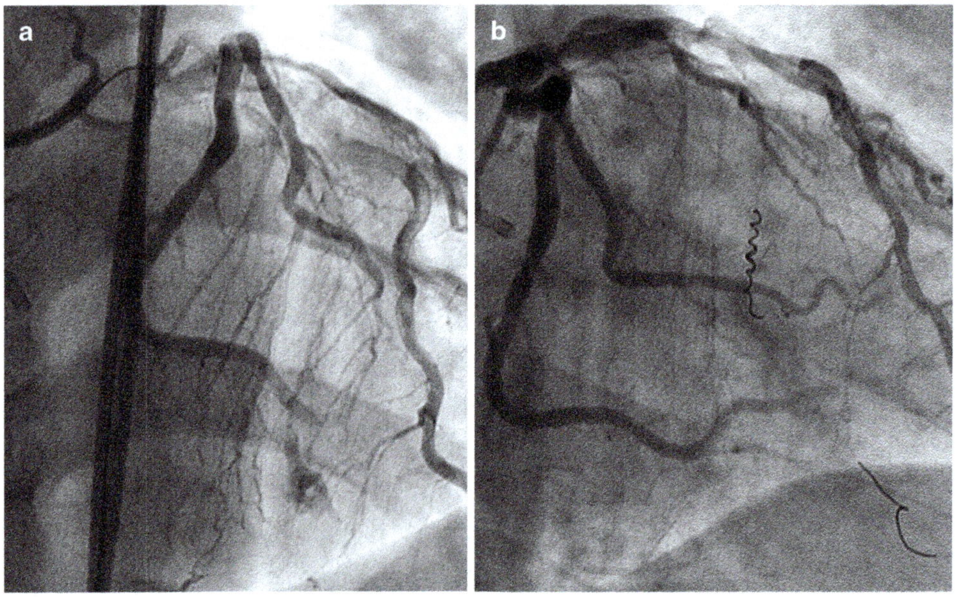

Fig. 1.222 Septal channel perforation caused by inflating a balloon after a microcatheter failed to cross the channel (**a**). The hematoma was enlarging and showed poor washout of contrast medium, so a coil was implanted to achieve hemostasis (**b**)

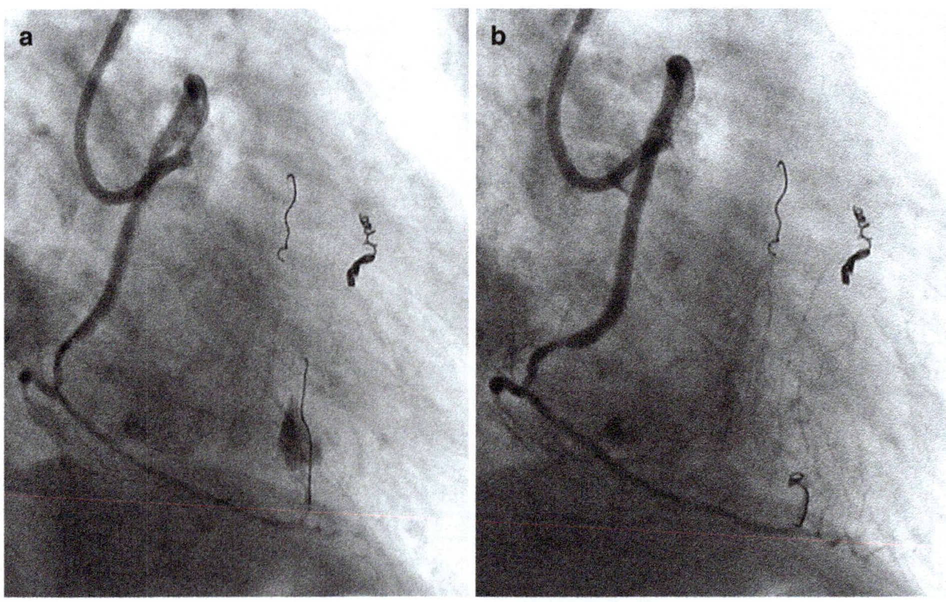

Fig. 1.223 Septal channel perforation caused by inflation of a balloon after a microcatheter failed to cross the channel retrogradely from the LAD in a patient with CTO of the RCA. The hematoma was enlarging and showed poor washout of contrast medium, so a coil was implanted from the LAD. Angiography of the RCA showed bleeding (**a**), so a coil was also implanted from the RCA to consolidate hemostasis (**b**)

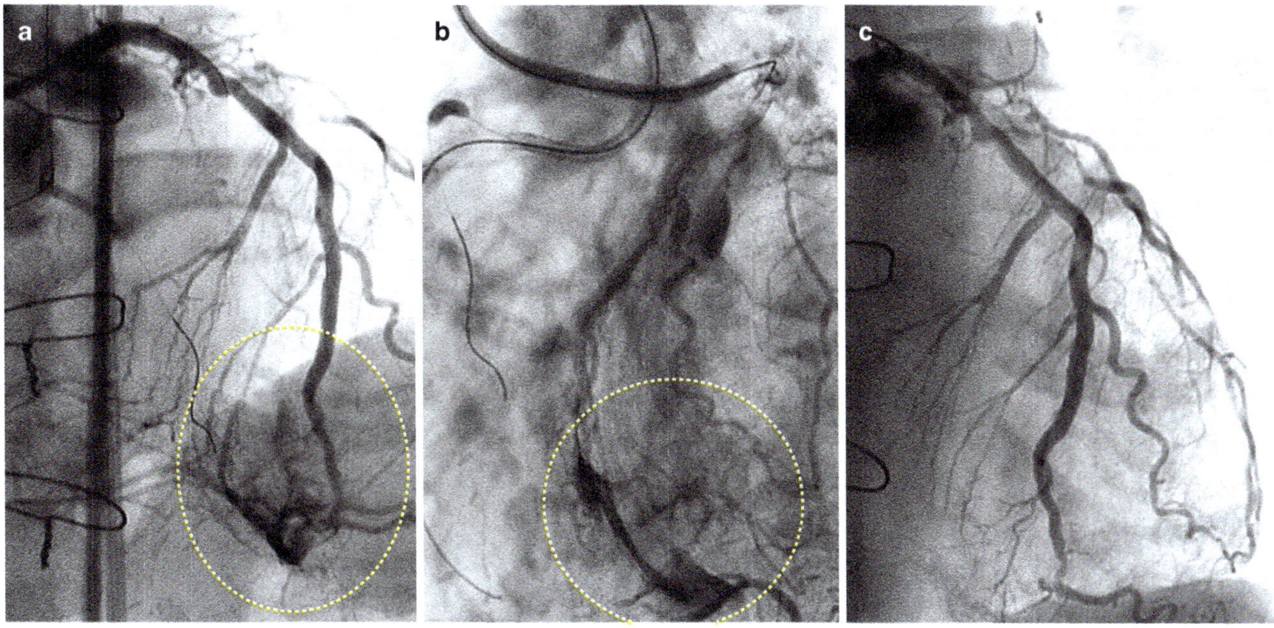

Fig. 1.224 Connection to the right ventricle created by a guidewire during retrograde tracking of a septal channel from the LAD in a patient with CTO of the RCA (**a** & **b**). The patient was followed up without any specific treatment. After 3 months, CAG confirmed disappearance of the connection to the ventricle (**c**)

1.9.4 Uncontrollable Bleeding: Management of Coronary Perforation

Typical cases are presented below (Figs. 1.225 & 1.226).

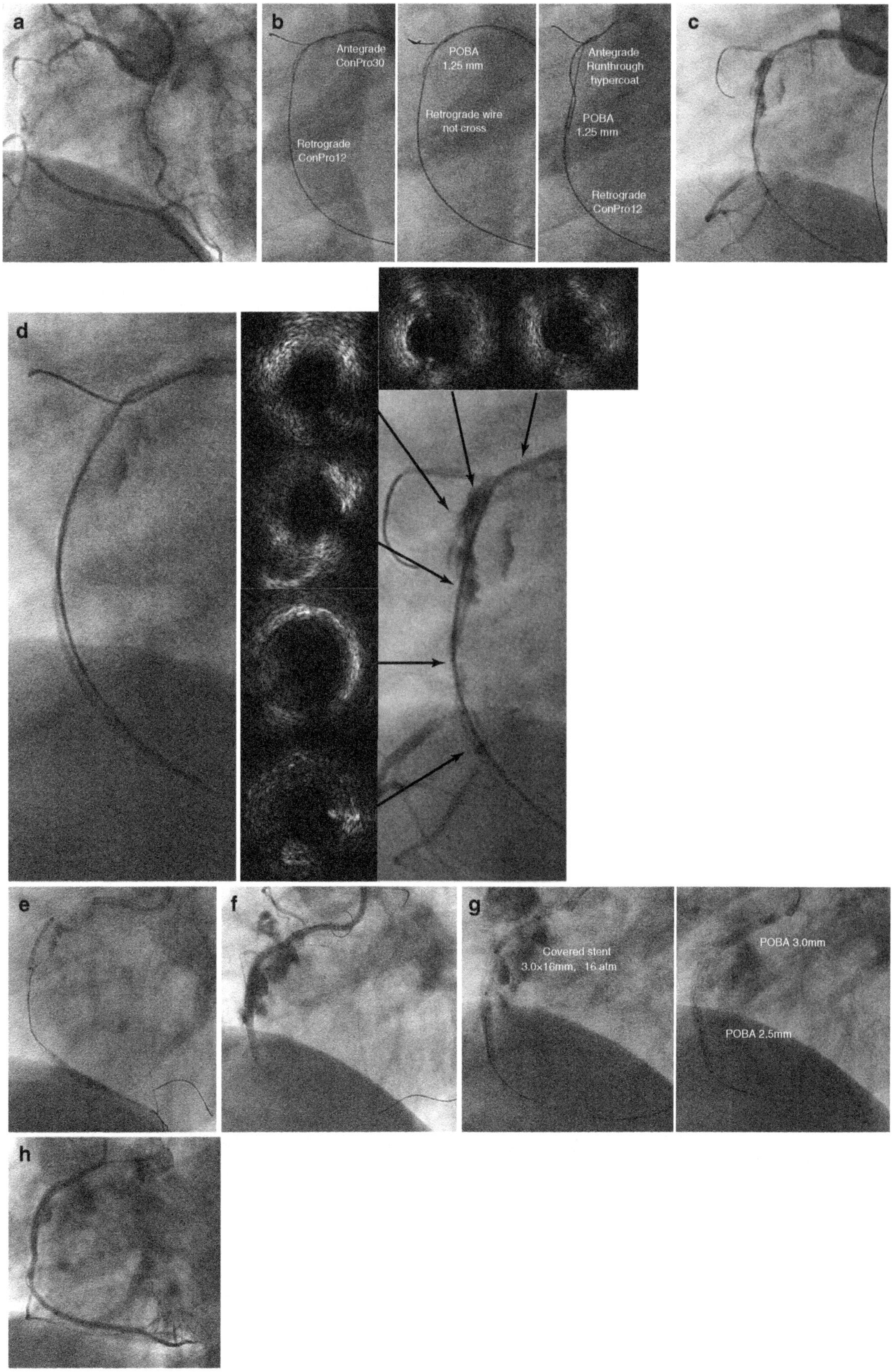
a
b
Antegrade
ConPro30
Retrograde
ConPro12
POBA
1.25 mm
Retrograde wire
not cross
Antegrade
Runthrough
hypercoat
POBA
1.25 mm
Retrograde
ConPro12
c
d
e
f
g
Covered stent
3.0×16mm, 16 atm
POBA 3.0mm
POBA 2.5mm
h

Fig. 1.225 Bleeding during PCI for CTO of the RCA (1) (**a**). (**b**) The retrograde guidewire was parallel with the antegrade guidewire in the proximal true lumen and followed the same route when manipulated repeatedly. It reached a site of resistance, and the tip was deflected when the guidewire was pushed further, indicating that the tip was in the subintimal space. Since reverse CART could not be accomplished, CART was attempted, and antegrade crossing of the CTO was successful. Subsequent CAG showed coronary artery perforation (**c**), and IVUS confirmed that the antegrade guidewire was outside the vessel wall (**d**). After the antegrade guidewire was anchored with a retrograde balloon, a covered stent was delivered and implanted (**e**). To control persistent hemorrhage (**f**), another covered stent was implanted, and prolonged plain old balloon angioplasty (POBA) was performed from both directions. Simultaneously, protamine was injected intravenously (**g**). Hemostasis was achieved and the CTO was successfully recanalized (**h**)

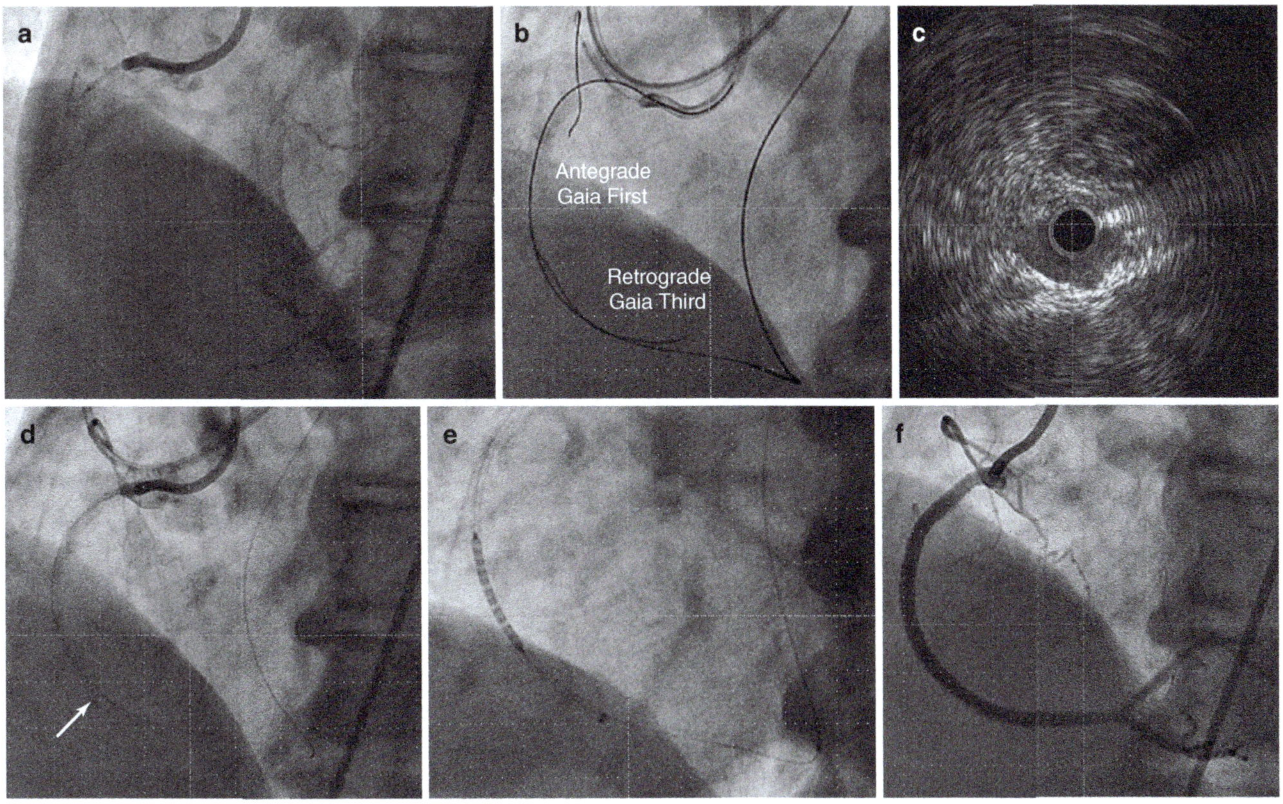

Fig. 1.226 Bleeding during PCI for CTO of the RCA (2) (**a**). (Images generously provided by Dr. Ryohei Yoshikawa, Sanda City Hospital) After reverse CART appeared to be successful (**b**), externalization was done, and the lesion was dilated with a 2.00-mm balloon. However, IVUS showed that the guidewire ran outside the vessel wall in the segment where subintimal tracking occurred (**c**). CAG revealed coronary artery perforation (arrow) (**d**). A GuideLiner catheter was advanced, and a covered stent was delivered through the catheter at the site of bleeding (**e**). The GuideLiner catheter not only facilitates smooth delivery of a difficult stent (e.g., a covered stent) but also has a physical hemostatic effect and helps identify the site of bleeding by tip injection. In this case, hemostasis was achieved by placing a covered stent at the bleeding point. Then PCI was completed successfully by implanting DES at the proximal and distal stenotic lesions (**f**)

2 Stenting of Bifurcation Lesions

With regard to stenting of bifurcation lesions, the choice between one and two stents, the need for kissing balloon inflation (KBI) following implantation of a single stent, and the optimal two-stent technique have been controversial issues. Some recent studies have provided evidence that the proximal optimization technique (POT) is useful for bifurcation stenting, while other reports have suggested the importance of understanding the relationship between the diameters of the two distal vessels and that of the proximal vessel when performing PCI for bifurcation lesions. Various dedicated bifurcation stents and balloons have been developed. The usefulness of bioresorbable vascular scaffold (BVS) systems when performing PCI for bifurcation lesions has also been suggested.

This chapter reviews several stenting strategies and techniques that can be used for bifurcation lesions. Although there is no evidence to support the superiority of these strategies/techniques over others, there also seem to be no data to justify the solutions to the previous controversies.

For example, the controversy over the choice between one and two stents appears to have been resolved with the conclusion that a single stent is better, but is this really correct? The angiographic and clinical outcomes after bifurcation stenting using general-purpose stents may be influenced by several factors, including (1) the stent design, (2) the stenting technique (provisional T-stenting, culotte stenting, crush stenting, etc.), (3) the details of stent implantation (point of stent wire crossing, use of the Crusade, timing of proximal optimization, kissing balloon inflation [KBI], etc.), (4) the extent of jailing or stent malapposition, and (5) unfavorable stent deformation.

Some stents are not designed for bifurcation stenting, while others are only compatible with certain stenting techniques. If a stent with an unsuitable design is selected, it may be impossible to prevent jailing or malapposition when it is used for a bifurcation lesion. KBI may not sufficiently expand the proximal part of some stents. The stenting technique has an influence on the risk of jailing, stent malapposition, and stent deformation. The outcome of single versus double stenting of bifurcation lesions should be compared after optimization of all these factors, but it is doubtful that previous studies comparing one versus two stents achieved optimization of other factors. If any of these factors is undergoing clinical evolution, at least the best-available current combination of stenting techniques and stent implantation methods should be employed when comparing single and double stenting. However, none of the previous studies comparing one or two stents employed a standardized (optimized) stenting protocol with regard to stent design and the details of stent implantation.

This chapter describes the evolving state-of-the-art procedures for bifurcation stenting using general-purpose stents and reviews the rationale for current practice.

K. Mitsudo, *Non-Pushing PCI Techniques*, https://doi.org/10.1007/978-981-15-7043-8_2

Column 12 Stent Design and Stenting Technique

The design of a stent often limits the choices of stenting techniques and the details of stent implantation. That is, stents with a certain design can only be implanted by using certain techniques in certain situations.

Some interventionalists formerly used a Cypher stent to treat left main trunk (LMT) bifurcation lesions. The average diameter of the LAD ostium is 3.5 mm, and it may sometimes be larger than 4 mm. After expansion by KBI, the strut cells of the Cypher stent open up to <3.5 mm (Fig. 2.1a). Although balloon inflation in the side branch (SB) appears to cause wider opening of the strut cells on imaging (which is two-dimensional), KBI has to produce three-dimensional stent expansion, leading to insufficient strut cell opening for access to the SB when the reference diameter is ≥3.5 mm at the ostium. This inevitably results in jailing and stent malapposition. When culotte stenting is performed by placing a stent from the LMT to the LCX after stenting from the LMT to the LAD, the main branch (LAD) ostium is jailed instead of the SB (LCX) ostium (Fig. 2.1b). A stenting technique that results in jailing of the main branch (MB) is absolutely undesirable. Performing treatment on the basis that you do not know what is possible until you try it is not good science or medicine.

In order to perform culotte stenting of an LMT bifurcation lesion, we need stents that are designed to prevent jailing of the LAD after LCX stenting and KBI. If such stents are not available, research should focus on developing something suitable. In fact, an appropriate stent has already been developed in Japan (Fig. 2.2). This stent can be expanded up to 6 mm and has made a significant contribution to stenting of LMT bifurcation lesions, as well as other lesions in large coronary arteries.

If protecting the SB is not considered important along with the risk of SB jailing or plaque shift, it may be felt that crossover stenting (placing a stent in the MB across the SB) with or without POT is sufficient. If a Cypher stent (6-link BX Velocity stent) is used for bifurcation stenting, it would be better to omit KBI, because this stent is likely to show suboptimal expansion with jailing of the SB and because KBI leads to unnecessary stress on the SB. In contrast, using a 2-link stent that permits optimal dilatation of both MB and SB will probably result in a satisfactory outcome after KBI. If it is combined with an optimal stenting technique and optimal stent implantation, a 2-link stent can make a two-stent strategy practicable. If stenting techniques are adopted on the basis of minimizing the risk of jailing (discussed later), culotte stenting will often be superior to crossover stenting.

When SB rewiring is done after stent implantation in the MB, I have proposed that the wire should cross the strut through the most distal cell at the SB ostium since around the time when the Wiktor stent was introduced. This proposal is based on the assumption that bifurcation stenting will always be performed by using coil or ring stents with 0 to 2 links (Wiktor, AVE Microstent, GFX, S-6, S-7, Endeavor [Driver], and Nobori [S-Stent]), and not with stents that have a larger number of links.

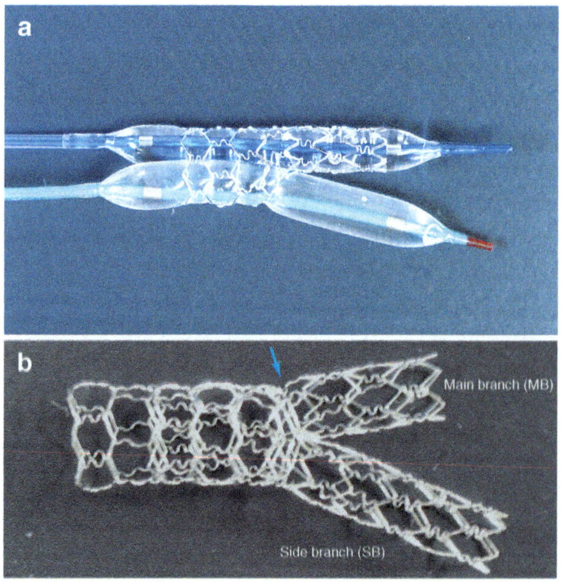

Fig. 2.1 A BX Velocity stent (Cypher stent platform) after expansion by inflation of two 3.0-mm kissing balloons. (**a**) The stent in the SB has not expanded to 3.0 mm, with an indentation at the carina. Inflation of two 3.5-mm kissing balloons also failed to sufficiently expand a 3.5-mm stent in the SB, which had the same design as the 3.0-mm stent. (**b**) Culotte stenting with these stents leads to jailing of the MB (arrow)

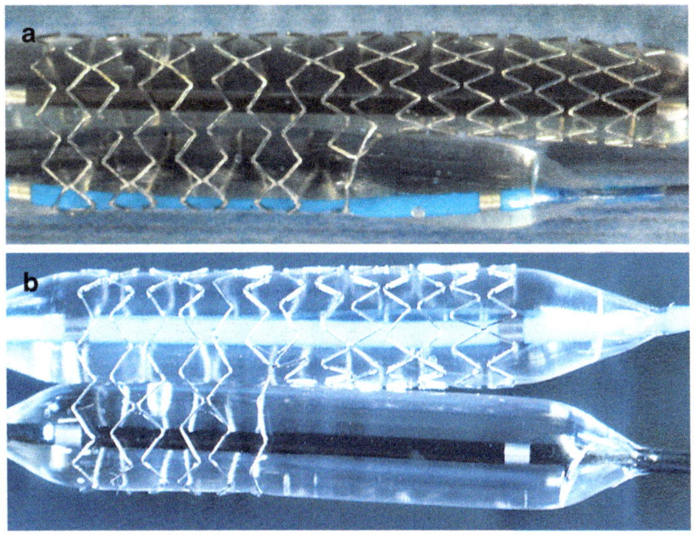

Fig. 2.2 Nobori stent. (**a**) A 3.5-mm Nobori stent expanded with two 3.5-mm kissing balloons inflated at their nominal pressure. (**b**) A Nobori stent expanded to an estimated proximal diameter of 5.8 mm with two 4.0-mm kissing balloons, leaving no indentations

Next, I will discuss the implications of the MB stent wire crossing through the most distal cell of a Cypher stent at the SB ostium. Figure 2.3a, b shows diagrams of the structure of 2-link Driver and 6-link BX Velocity stents on the same scale. The blue circles have a diameter of 3.5 mm. In the case of the Cypher stent, a wire crossing through the most distal cell as indicated by one red dot within the circle would cause minimal SB jailing, whereas a wire crossing through the most distal cell as indicated by the other red dot within the circle would aggravate SB jailing. There is no other route for the wire that minimizes the risk of SB jailing. With the Driver stent, if the wire crosses through the cell as indicated by either red dot, it will only cause minimal SB jailing, even if jailing cannot be completely avoided. Figure 2.4a–e shows structural diagrams of currently available stents on almost the same scale. By moving the blue circle over the view of each stent, it is possible to estimate the extent of SB jailing when the wire crosses through different cells.

The crush stenting technique (Fig. 2.5a) was developed with introduction of the Cypher stent. Regarding this technique, many interventionalists have suggested the risk of the wire crossing a non-apposed stent through a cell distal to the carina. In addition, crush stenting leads to three layers of struts overlapping in part of the proximal MB and limits subsequent strategies if treatment of restenosis is required. Also, this technique has never been used with BMS. Due to its closed cell design, the Cypher stent is crushed parallel to the MB wall. On the other hand, a 2-link stent is crushed in an oblique direction to the MB wall, which may prevent introduction of a guidewire into the SB across the stent. Moreover, overlapping of three strut layers impairs conformability of the stent. At best, the crush stenting technique is only useful for placing Cypher stents at bifurcation lesions.

What about the V-stenting (simultaneous kissing stenting [SKS]) technique (Fig. 2.5b)? Considering its principle, SKS will cause stent malapposition and is far from the ideal method for bifurcation stenting (mentioned later). This technique is also only practicable with multi-link stents that have a closed cell design. When it is used with stents that have no links or a few links, the overlapping stent struts will interlock with each other, and this will gradually reduce the diameters of stents expanded simultaneously.

The strategy for bifurcation stenting can only be optimized when a stenting technique is chosen that is compatible with the stent design and when stent implantation is as sophisticated as possible. The feasibility of adopting a particular stenting strategy also depends on lesion anatomy. Therefore, we should not compare the outcomes achieved with one versus two stents or classify individual techniques as good or bad strategies without considering the various technical aspects of bifurcation stenting.

Comprehensive evidence can only be obtained by comparison of all possible combinations of stent design and stenting techniques, but performing such comparisons is not practical. Therefore, we need to devise optimal stenting strategies on the basis of theoretical principles, as well as the results of bench tests and stent expansion experiments using models.

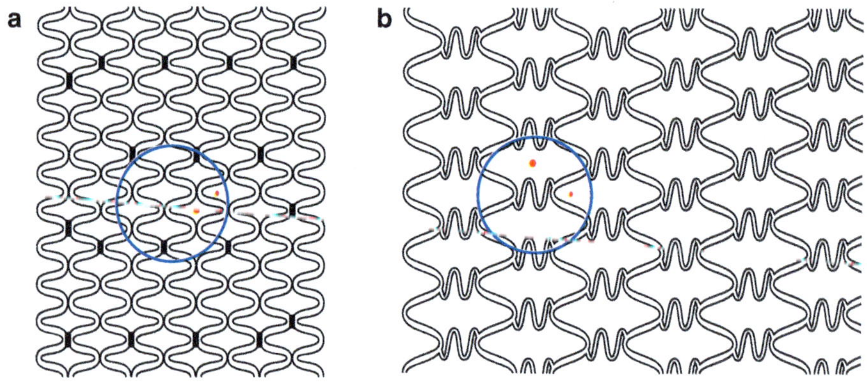

Fig. 2.3 Structural diagrams of 2-link and 6-link stents. (**a**) Driver stent. (**b**) Cypher (BX Velocity) stent

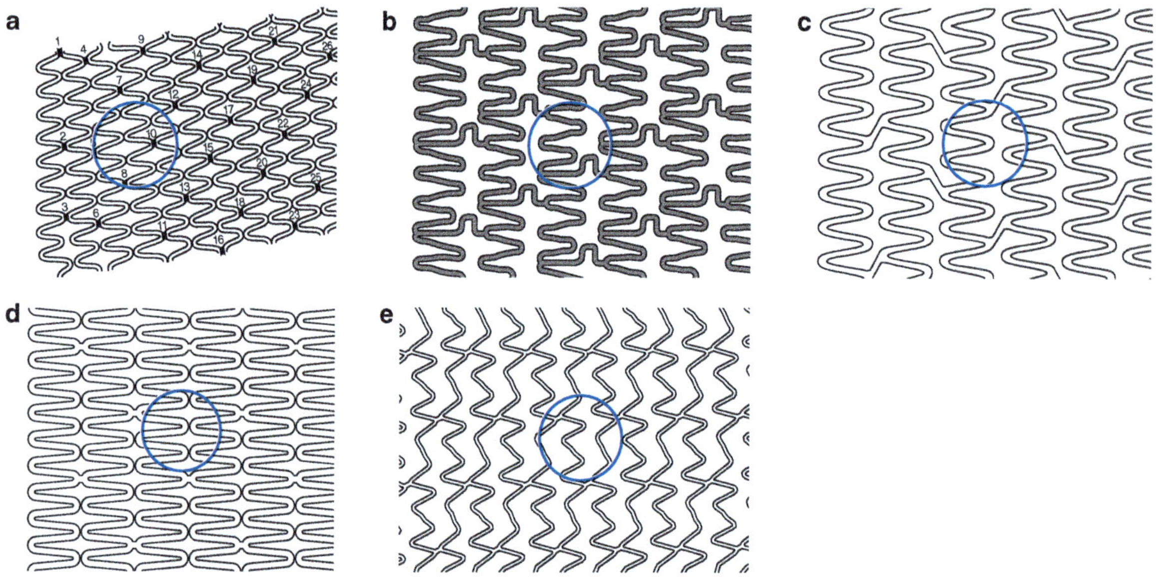

Fig. 2.4 Structural diagrams of currently available stents. (**a**) Resolute Integrity stent. (**b**) Xience Prime stent. (**c**) PROMUS Element stent. (**d**) Nobori stent. (**e**) Ultimaster stent

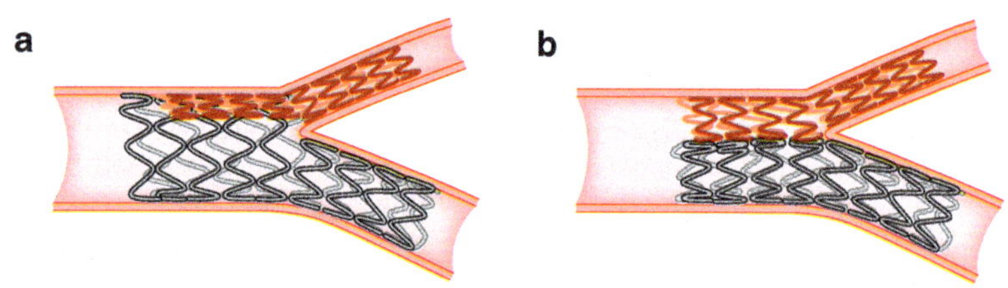

Fig. 2.5 Stenting techniques. (**a**) Crush stenting. (**b**) V-stenting or simultaneous kissing stenting (SKS)

2.1 Dedicated Bifurcation Stents

Various dedicated bifurcation stents have been developed and can be classified into several categories. Many of them can be used to achieve satisfactory outcomes if the stent is positioned optimally so that its carina fits into the SB ostium. However, it is often challenging, and sometimes nearly impossible, to achieve optimal positioning of a dedicated bifurcation stent (Fig. 2.6). The greatest limitation of dedicated bifurcation stents is probably the fixed distance between the proximal edge and carina. The stent may be too short for full coverage of the proximal MB

including its ostium, which will then require implantation of an additional stent for this purpose. Alternatively, the stent may be too long to allow the proximal edge to remain within the MB lumen, precluding its use.

Various difficulties may be encountered during bifurcation stenting with a dedicated stent. If a stent mounted on two balloons becomes blocked by an obstacle in the lumen during delivery, it is often difficult to withdraw the stent into the guiding catheter and reattempt advancement. This is because mounting the stent on two balloons makes it very bulky and liable to become stuck, deformed, or lost during withdrawal into the guiding catheter. Another significant limitation of a dedicated bifurcation stent is that repositioning the stent to improve access to the SB may be impossible after initial failure to place it in the optimal position (Fig. 2.7). SB rewiring through a strut cell far from the carina may be required, resulting in loss of the original advantage of the dedicated stent (Fig. 2.8).

Thus, the dedicated bifurcation stents developed so far have various limitations, including little flexibility of indications, complexity of the stenting procedure, and difficulty in correcting the stent position/direction. These limitations have prevented their extensive use in PCI.

Next, I will consider the designs of several of the dedicated bifurcation stents that are currently available. Many dedicated stents have been developed, all of which have embodied interesting concepts. However, further assessment is needed to determine whether any of these dedicated stents is sufficiently useful for performing optimal bifurcation stenting.

Figure 2.9 shows the dedicated bifurcation stent developed by Advanced Stent Technologies. Although this stent has an extendable petal that is a very interesting idea, the design raises important questions such as whether its carina can always reach the vascular carina between the MB and the SB and whether the center of the petal can be positioned precisely at the center of the SB lumen (Fig. 2.7). In addition, this stent may show poor conformability with the SB at its origin.

Figure 2.10 displays Abbott's dedicated bifurcation stent. It has a simple design and is intended for simultaneous stent implantation and KBI. This attractive stent mimics a general-purpose stent suitable for provisional stenting that has been applied to a bifurcation lesion. However, it also has limitations, including difficulty in achieving optimal positioning and proper alignment of the carina (i.e., the distance from the vessel carina and orientation relative to the SB). Also, the position of this stent cannot be corrected. If the stent is positioned wrongly, SB rewiring has to be performed through a different strut cell, followed by KBI, resulting in loss of the original functionality of a dedicated stent (Fig. 2.8).

Figure 2.11 illustrates the dedicated stent system developed by Advanced Bifurcation Systems. This system is designed to deliver a stent to the SB first so as to automatically achieve optimal alignment. Although it is interesting, this stent does not appear to conserve dynamic conformability with the SB origin and thus may not ensure optimal alignment if guidewire entanglement occurs.

Figure 2.12 illustrates the Y stent developed by Medtronic, which joins two Driver stents into a "Y" shape. If it can be implanted at a bifurcation lesion without deformation, its design appears to ensure optimal bifurcation stenting. However, optimizing the carinal position and alignment remain challenging with this stent, while inability to correct suboptimal carinal position and alignment is another limitation.

The Tryton stent is displayed in Fig. 2.13. This stent is based on a unique concept and may be practical, with the stent being composed of three zones (Fig. 2.13a). The distal zone (SB zone) is implanted in the SB, while the proximal zone for the MB (MB zone) consists of a wedding band and a triple linkage to the middle zone, which is referred to as the transit zone. Two types of stent delivery balloon are available, a stepped balloon and a straight balloon. The Tryton stent can be implanted by a "simplified" culotte stenting technique, which involves implanting the SB stent, inserting the SB guidewire into the MB, implanting the MB stent, reinserting the guidewire into the SB, and final KBI (Fig. 2.13b). However, it cannot be used for provisional stenting. Also, the transit zone has very little radial strength, so it may not be able to provide an adequate scaffold at the carina.

The STENTYS stent is shown in Fig. 2.14. It has a unique self-expanding mesh linked by small interconnections between the struts, which can be disconnected by KBI. This structure will ensure almost optimal bifurcation stenting plus KBI if the SB take-off angle from the proximal MB is medium to small. If the SB take-off angle is large, conformability of this stent is insufficient to ensure excellent apposition in the SB and possibly in the MB on the contralateral side. Also, its self-expanding nature prevents correction of malapposition by KBI.

The AXXESS stent is displayed in Fig. 2.15. It is a self-expanding stent designed to treat bifurcation lesions of the LMT or other large coronary arteries. Although they cannot be seen in this figure, the stent has one and three markers at the proximal and distal edges, respectively, for optimizing its position. As its distal end expands into an elliptical bell, the strut edge becomes orthogonal to the longitudinal axis of each branch. This results in little or no overlap between it and the stent implanted in one branch and also minimizes jailing of the other branch. The bell at the distal end of the stent can expand to a diameter as large as 8–12 mm. This allows conformity to a bifurcation with a large SB take-off angle, but possibly not to a distal LMT bifurcation with a large SB take-off angle versus the LMT. In addition, if the proximal LMT has a large diameter (either anatomically or due to progressive dilatation after CTO), the distal end of this self-expanding stent will open to a smaller extent, and stent malapposition will occur at the lateral wall of the branch, especially the LCX because of its extreme take-off angle. A similar phenomenon may occur when the SB take-off angle becomes progressively larger year after year.

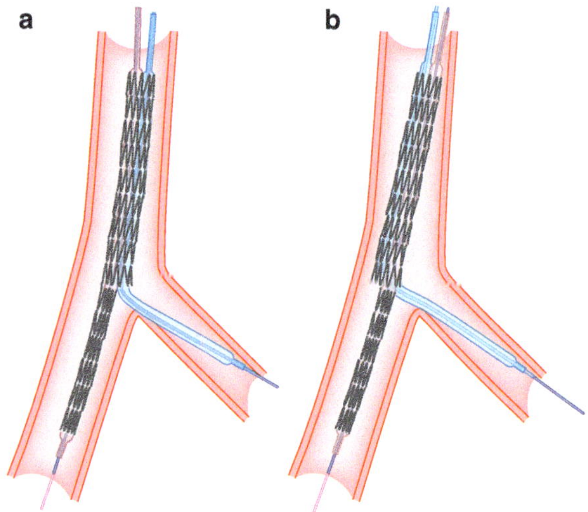

Fig. 2.6 Positioning a dedicated bifurcation stent. A dedicated stent positioned optimally for access to the SB (**a**) and a stent with the carina positioned on the opposite side (**b**)

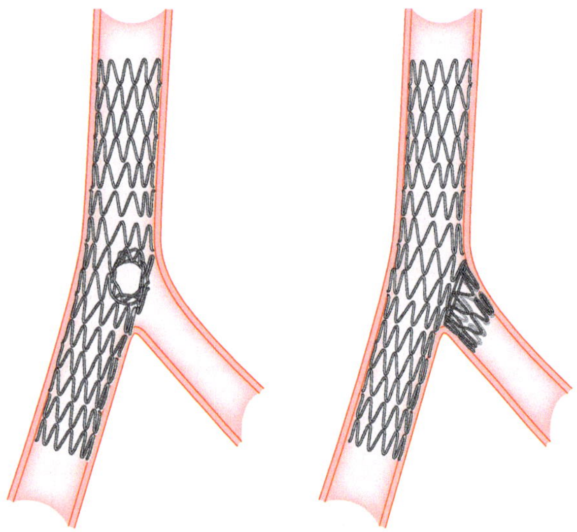

Fig. 2.7 Failure to optimally position a dedicated stent. It may be impossible to place the center of the petal of a dedicated stent exactly at the center of the SB lumen, as shown on the left

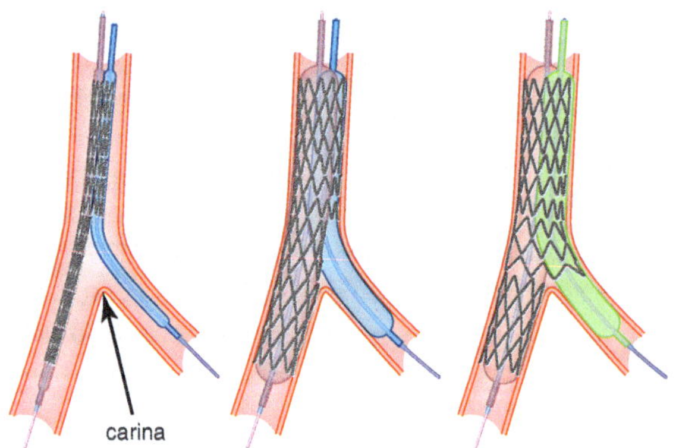

Fig. 2.8 Incorrect deployment of a dedicated stent proximal to the carina. It is necessary to reinsert a guidewire/balloon into the SB through a cell closer to the carina and perform KBI again

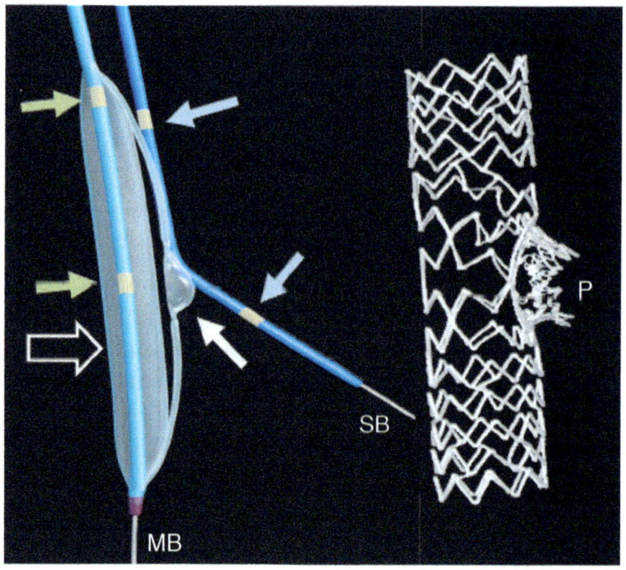

Fig. 2.9 Boston Scientific Petal stent. The stent is mounted on the dedicated stent delivery system shown on the left. Inflation of the spherical balloon at the SB ostium extends the petal obliquely into the SB. Subsequently, KBI is done to optimally reshape and align the petal

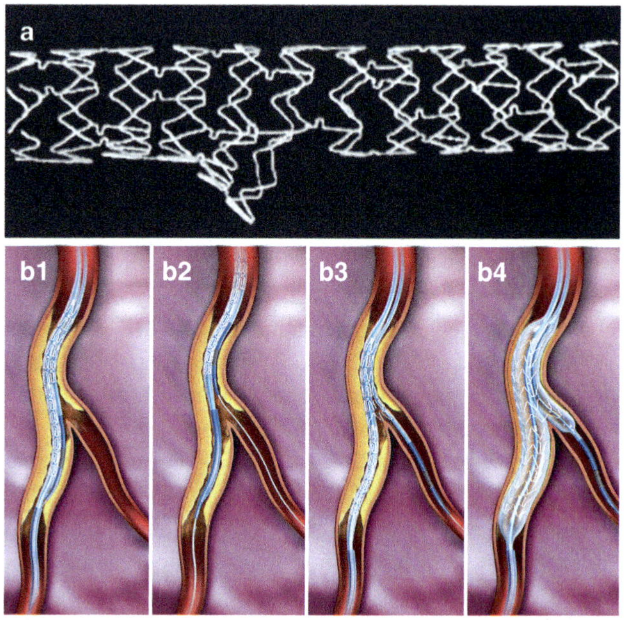

Fig. 2.10 Abbott Xience SBA stent (**a**). This dedicated stent is suitable for provisional stenting, which is simply accomplished by simultaneous stent implantation and KBI. The stent delivery system mounts a single stent on two balloons and accommodates the SB guidewire near the tip (**b1**). The stenting procedure includes the following steps: advancing the stent until the SB balloon is just beyond the carina, releasing the SB guidewire tip and withdrawing the wire, pulling the entire system back slightly, advancing the guidewire with a reshaped tip into the SB (**b2**), advancing the stent until its carina meets the vascular carina (**b3**), and performing local KBI (**b4**)

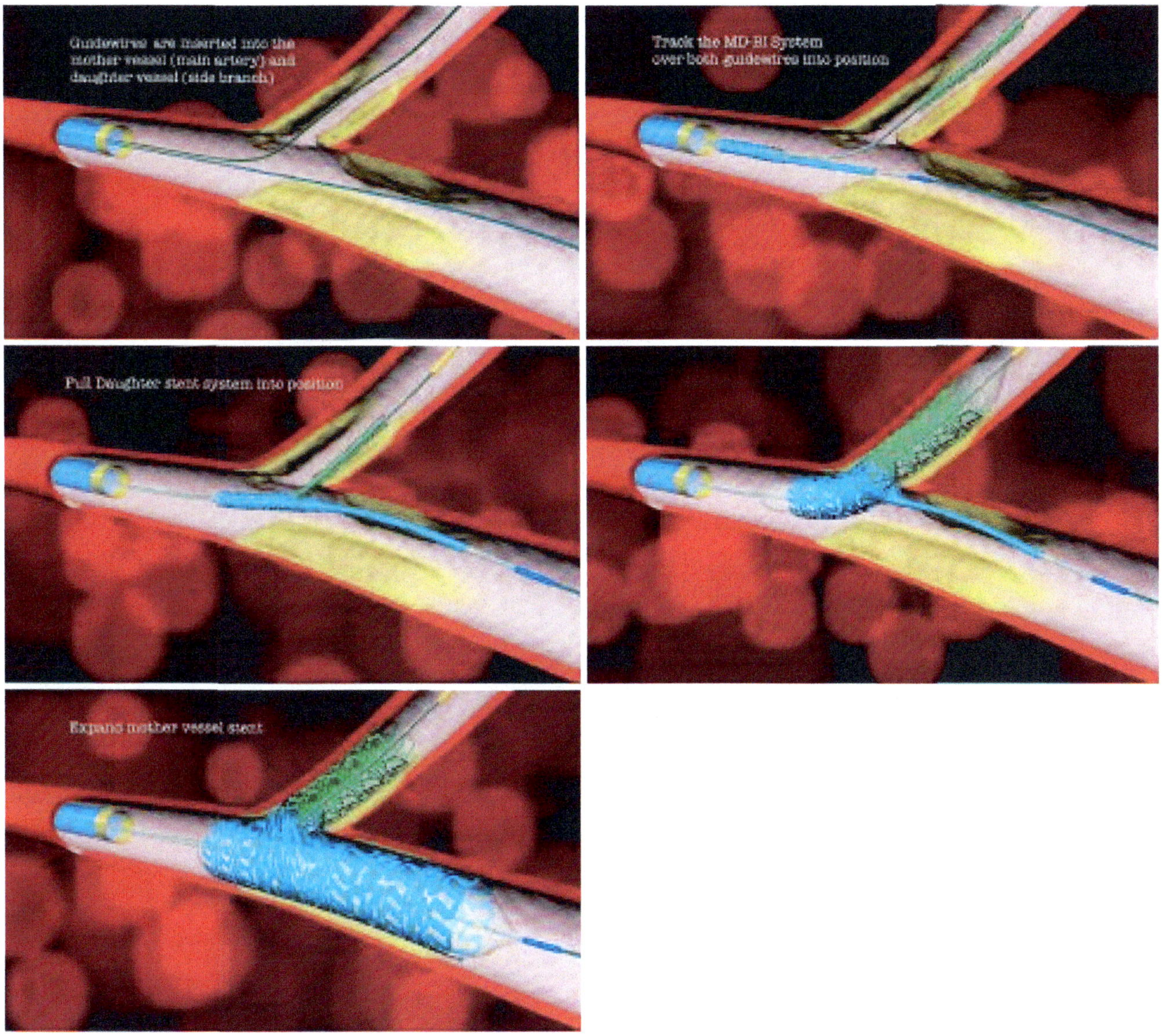

Fig. 2.11 Advanced Bifurcation Systems stent

Fig. 2.12 Medtronic Y stent

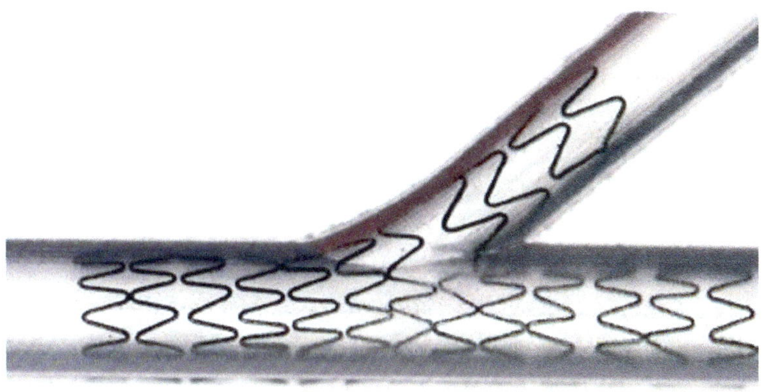

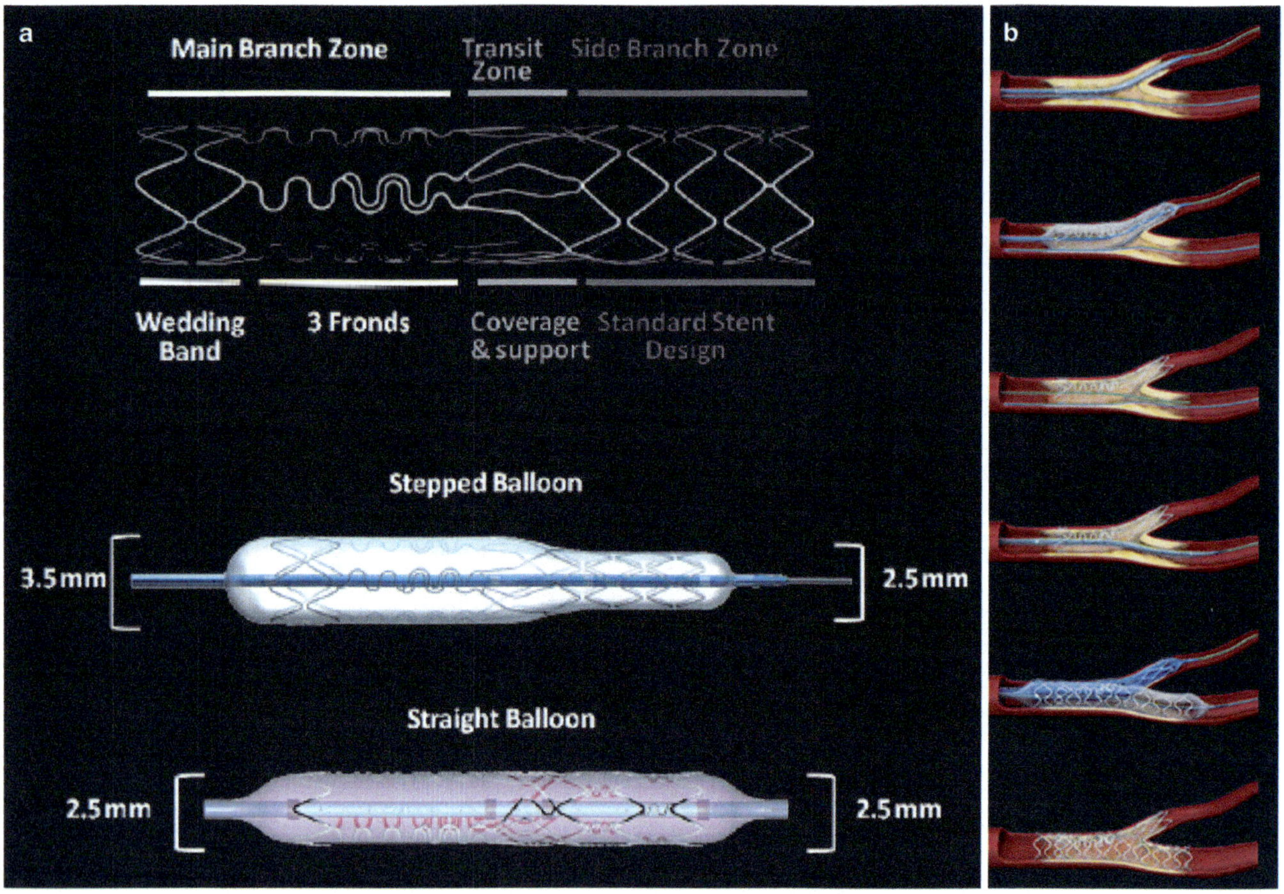

Fig. 2.13 Tryton stent (**a**, **b**)

Fig. 2.14 STENTYS stent

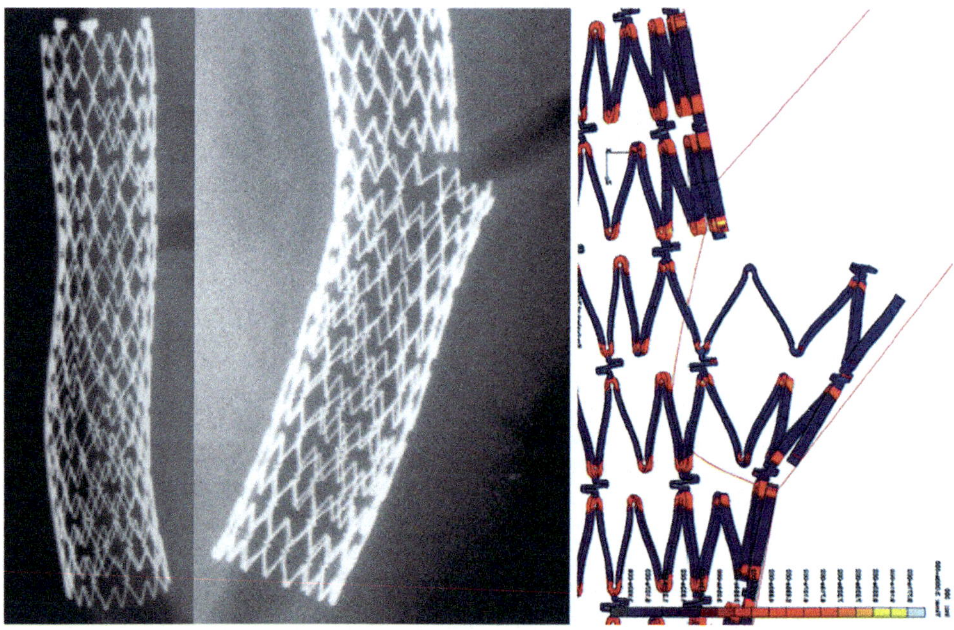

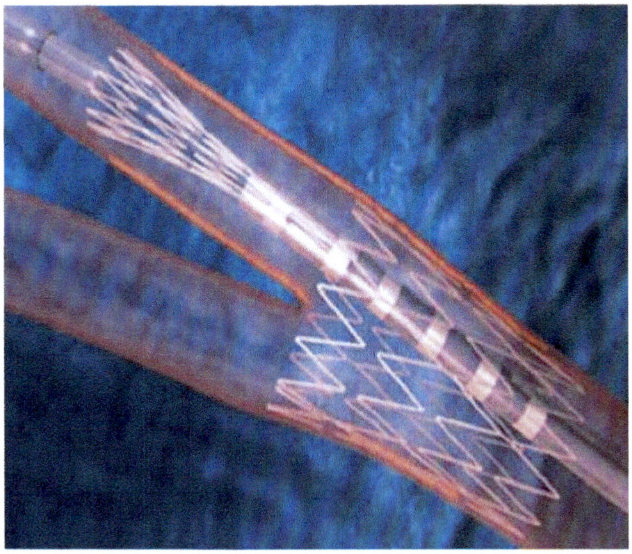

Fig. 2.15 AXXESS stent

2.2 Optimizing General-Purpose Stents for Bifurcation Lesions

As shown in Fig. 2.16, the ideal bifurcation stent should achieve excellent apposition of a single layer of struts over the entire vessel wall at the bifurcation without causing SB or MB jailing. A general-purpose stent that can provide the ideal bifurcation scaffold needs to meet the following requirements:

1. High flexibility (conformability): Bifurcation lesions are often tortuous (Fig. 2.17), and many side branches have a steep take-off angle (Fig. 2.18). Hence, a stent for bifurcation lesions requires high conformability. Highly conformable stents usually have little edge effect. In general, stents with fewer links are more conformable.
2. No risk of SB jailing after optimal KBI: The optimal stent for a bifurcation lesion can dilate the lesion correctly without causing SB jailing if optimal KBI is performed, which is defined as inflation of appropriately sized kissing balloons at the optimal pressure that does not injure the proximal MB after SB (re)wiring through the most distal cell near the carina.
3. Minimum risk of malapposition: The optimal stent for bifurcation lesions must have high overall conformability as well as being easily deployed by balloon inflation. Ease of stent expansion is influenced by the design as well as the material used to make it.

   To achieve optimal apposition in a bifurcation lesion, a stent with fewer links and with more and longer crowns is preferred. In addition, a stent made of a material with higher plasticity (e.g., stainless steel or platinum-chromium alloy) is better able to undergo plastic deformation when implanted at a complicated bifurcation lesion and thus achieve optimal apposition. A stent made of cobalt-chromium alloy, which has lower plasticity (i.e., higher elasticity), may be slightly inferior with respect to fine plastic deformation at bifurcation lesions.

   However, a stent with higher elasticity can undergo greater distortion before reaching the limit of elasticity, which makes the occurrence of fracture (especially acute fracture) or dynamic deformation less likely. Thus, the balance between elasticity and plasticity of the stent material leads to significant trade-offs for stent performance.
4. Little or no risk of fracture: Stents with no risk of fracture have long been awaited, but no such stent has been developed so far. I consider that stent fractures can be classified as "good" or "bad." It would be ideal to completely prevent stent fractures, but this is impossible. Therefore, stents should be designed so that any fracture is likely to be a good fracture.
5. Drug-eluting: Unlike metal stents, BVS cannot be used extensively for bifurcation lesions at present because performing KBI leads to collapse of the scaffold. DES will remain the standard type of stent for bifurcation lesions, at least for a while.
6. Polymer-free: A polymer coating may peel off after KBI or culotte stenting. The peeling polymer can lead to thrombosis, even if it is bioresorbable, and there is less drug release from the part of the stent where the coating has been lost. Therefore, a polymer-free DES is preferable for bifurcation stenting.
7. Proximal edge structure compatible with the aorto-ostial anatomy: The aortic ostium, whether normal or occluded/stenosed, can usually be dilated to its original diameter, although its anatomy may prevent this. When treating an LMT bifurcation lesion, it is often necessary to dilate the bifurcation through the LMT ostium. Since the ostium can be as large as 6 mm in diameter, a stent for an LMT bifurcation lesion has to be expandable to a large diameter. On the other hand, the part of the stent implanted outside the ostium may be deformed by a guiding catheter or other device. To prevent such stent deformation that could impair the system integrity, the stent must have two links within 2–3 mm of the proximal edge. Two links are both necessary and sufficient for preserving stent conformability and preventing deformation, while three or more links are not required.

A stent that meets all of requirements (1) through (4) above should have no links, but it is virtually impossible to implant a no-link stent without marked deformation. Hence, the ideal stent for bifurcation lesions should have links that can prevent excessive deformation during implantation and lose these links as soon as possible after implantation.

If all of the stent links facing the SB ostium can be fractured during KBI, there is no risk of SB jailing. Thus, I would like to discuss the concept of a stent with temporary (easily fractured) links later.

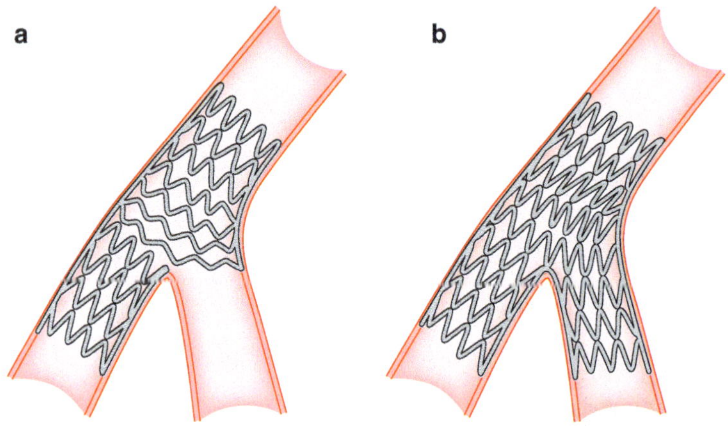

Fig. 2.16 Optimal bifurcation stents. Whether bifurcation stenting is performed by the MB crossover technique (**a**) or the MB/SB full coverage technique (**b**), the optimal stenting strategy must meet the following requirements: (1) complete coverage, (2) complete apposition, (3) complete expansion, and (4) optimal stent design

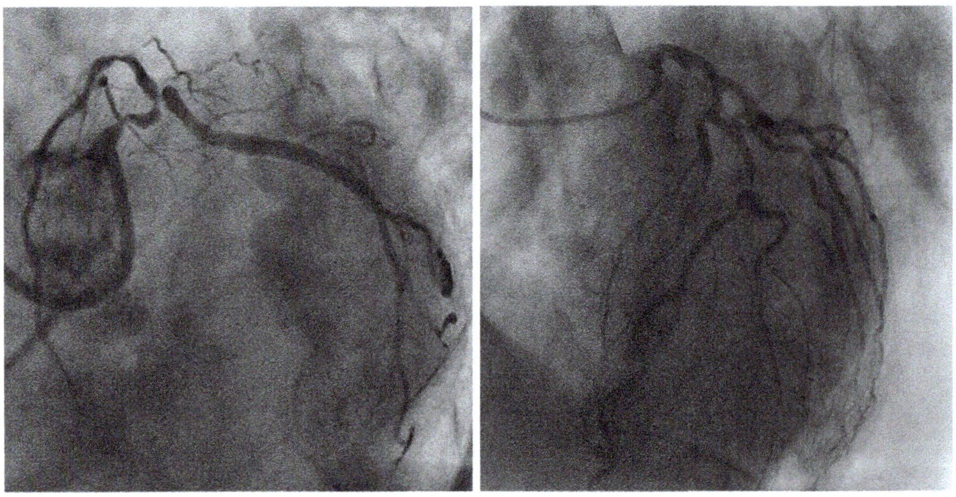

Fig. 2.17 A tortuous bifurcation lesion

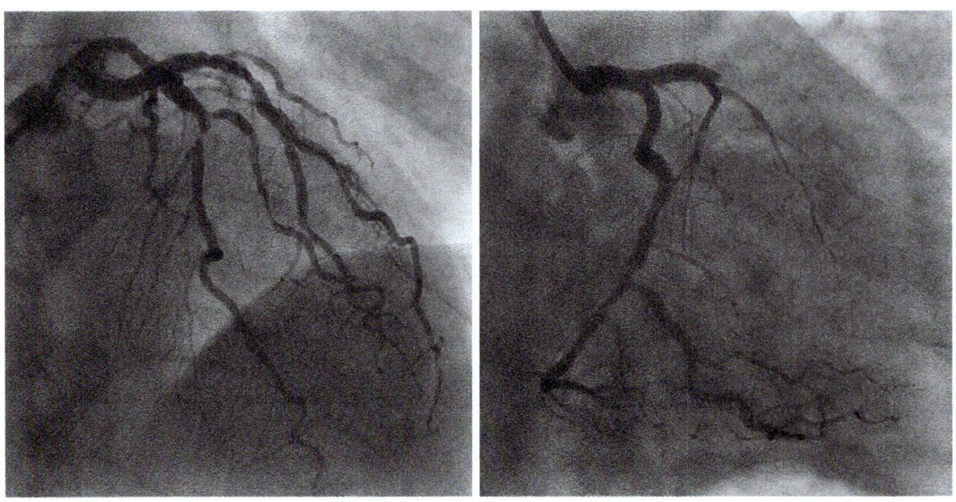

Fig. 2.18 A bifurcation lesion with extreme SB angulation

Column 13 Good Versus Bad Fracture

[Bad fracture]

1. When one of the links is fractured in a stent with low conformability (e.g., a multi-link stent), both edges of the stent will become more mobile, and this will cause static or dynamic edge effects (Fig. 2.19).
2. When the long link in a stent is fractured, the stumps of the link may cause stimulation of the intima or malapposition can occur at the fractured link.

3. A stent with at least one link can be fractured at a strut rather than at a link (Fig. 2.20). If strut fracture occurs, the stumps of the strut will stimulate the intima. In addition, the fractured strut loses its radial strength due to loss of continuity of the supporting arch. Thus, the fractured strut can easily be deformed by vascular recoil, narrowing the lumen that was previously expanded by balloon inflation of the stent. This mechanism may be involved in some cases of in-stent occlusion (restenosis) at a fractured strut.

[Good fracture]

When can stent fracture be considered good? A good fracture can occur if a stent is designed with fracturable short links between the strut peaks and valleys (Fig. 2.21). If fracture occurs at a short link, it is unlikely that the stumps of the fractured link will stimulate the intima or that the strut will lose radial strength. These outcomes are even more unlikely if the stent has few links and high conformability.

I have long sought for a stent that can undergo good fracture. The Driver stent initially appeared to be suitable, but it was found that fracture occurred at the struts and not at the links. However, I have found that the Nobori stent (particularly the 3.5-mm stent) is more likely to be fractured at a link than at a strut. This may account for the low restenosis rate after implanting a Nobori stent, although this type of stent is liable to fracture if used at the RCA ostium. A modified Nobori stent that is much more likely to undergo fracture at a link than a strut is needed. Moreover, a stent with no links or one designed with disappearing links could provide a good solution to the problem of stent fracture.

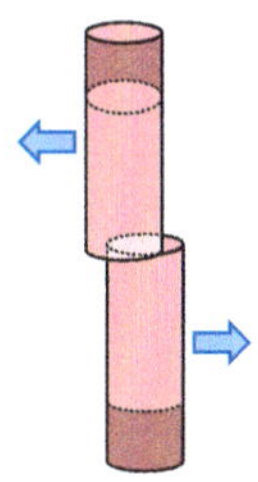

Fig. 2.19 Bad fracture. The parts of the stent proximal and distal to the fracture have shifted horizontally in opposite directions

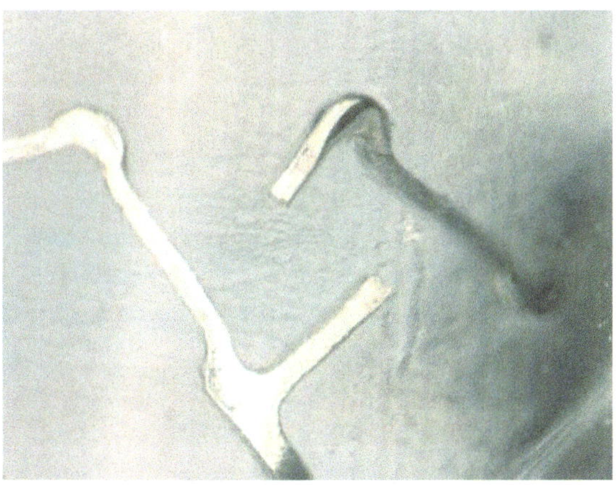

Fig. 2.20 Another example of bad fracture. The stent strut has been fractured

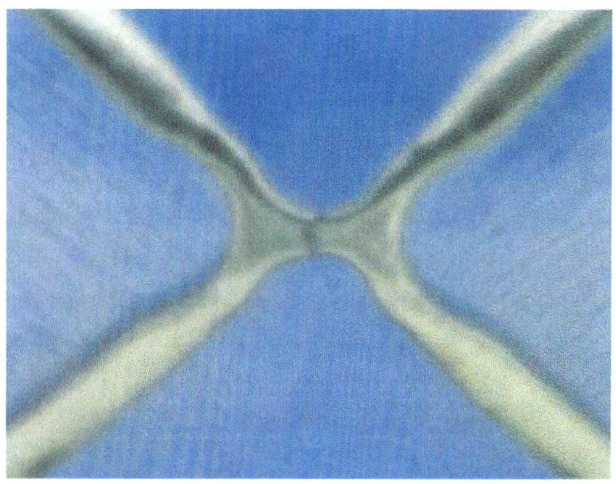

Fig. 2.21 Good fracture. The stent has fractured at a short link

[Stent "recoil"]

I often feel that something is wrong when I hear someone referring to stent deformation by external force as stent recoil. This is because recoil means spontaneous movement of an object to return to its original shape. Thus, stent recoil describes the tendency of a stent that has been expanded by a balloon to shrink slightly due to its inherent elasticity after deflation of the balloon. Partial luminal loss after balloon deflation when implanting a balloon-expanded stent cannot be referred to as stent recoil because this phenomenon arises from recoil of both the vessel and the stent. A stent will show minimal deformation if it is implanted in a soft lesion, but severe deformation will occur after implantation in a hard lesion that has not been prepared sufficiently.

In the POBA era, sudden luminal loss at the end of intervention was referred to as acute recoil, while late lumen loss attributable to restenosis was called chronic recoil. Analogous with vascular luminal loss, narrowing of the stent lumen may therefore have also been referred to as recoil. While "recoil" may reasonably be used to describe luminal loss due to spontaneous narrowing of the target vessel after POBA, should it be used to describe narrowing of the stent lumen? It is clear that stent luminal loss is largely due to deformation caused by external forces, rather than spontaneous motion of the stent. In particular, chronic stent deformation (late stent luminal loss) is never due to stent recoil. If the term "stent recoil" is used to describe stent deformation, it does not accurately express the essence of this phenomenon. It may lead to classification of some stents as prone to "recoil" and possibly to an inappropriate focus on stent-related factors when investigating the mechanism of stent deformation. The vascular factors potentially involved in stent lumen loss should also be considered, in order to elucidate the mechanism applying external force to the stent and to devise countermeasures. In this sense, I think that we should pay careful attention to use of the term "recoil."

2.2.1 Temporary Link Stents

2.2.1.1 Concept of the "Temporary Link Stent"

I use the term "temporary link stent" to describe a stent with intact link(s) until it is expanded in a vessel, after which the link(s) are fractured or lost because of vascular movements or with the passage of time. A link facing the SB ostium can be easily fractured by application of horizontal force during KBI, and the stumps of the link will not stimulate the vessel. After loss of the links, it is desirable that the stent does not break up into rings and that continuity of the struts is maintained.

2.2.1.2 Classification of Temporary Link Stents

1. Bioresorbable link stent: The links of the stent are made of a bioresorbable (drug-eluting) polymer and disappear from several months to about 1 year after implantation.
2. Separable link stent: The links are made of metal but are designed to be easily disconnected by KBI and by vessel movements. If the stent is fractured at a link, the stumps of the link do not stimulate the vessel, so it can be intentionally fractured at a link to ensure high conformability while preventing vascular injury.

A stent with disconnectable links (Fig. 2.22) has been developed, but it has not been marketed in Japan so far.

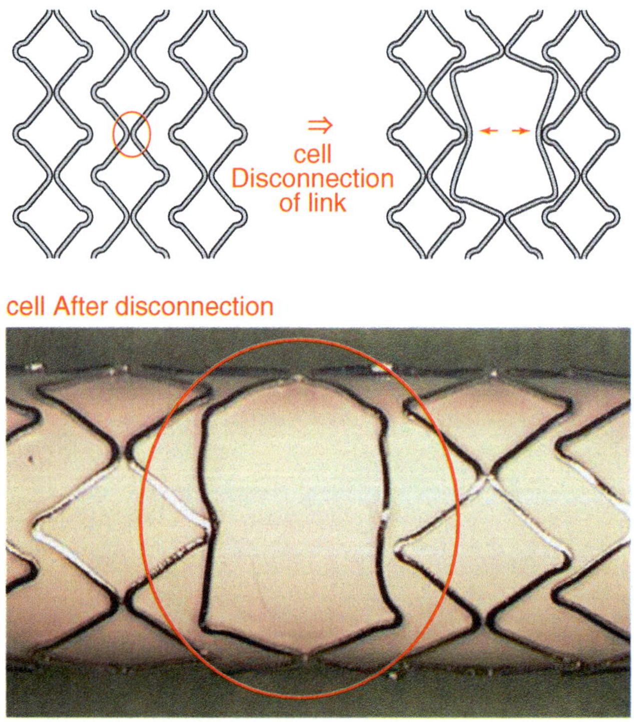

Fig. 2.22 A stent with disconnectable links. Balloon inflation in the SB disconnects a link, producing a larger cell and resolving SB jailing

2.2.1.3 Helical Coil Stents

Loss of links in a temporary link stent means that the individual strut rings are independent of each other in the vessel lumen and malapposition may allow movement or shift of the stent struts. To preserve the integrity of a stent after loss of all links, it has to have a helical coil structure. Helical coil stents have very high conformability. Even if overlapped, such stents rarely become rigid and are unlikely to undergo strut fracture.

However, if a helical coil stent deployed in an aorto-ostial lesion is not optimally apposed (even temporarily), longitudinal deformation can readily occur, and the stent may sometimes be extruded into the aorta. If used for an aorto-ostial lesion, a helical coil stent should have several proximal struts with a durable 2-link pattern.

2.2.1.4 Optimal Design of a Stent for Use with KBI

The optimal stent for deployment with KBI should be designed as follows:

1. It should permit sufficient enlargement of a strut cell for side branch access.
2. It should have few links (Figs. 2.23 and 2.24) to permit sufficient enlargement of a cell while causing less vascular damage near the SB ostium and to minimize the risk of SB jailing or stent malapposition.
3. It should have disconnectable links (refer to Fig. 2.21).
4. It should provide an adequate scaffold for SB shoulder support (Fig. 2.24b).
5. Its struts should be uniformly expandable in every direction by KBI.

A laser-cut stent, polished and bordered, generally has struts that are square in the cross-sectional view. A strut with a square cross section can be bent easily by application of force in a direction parallel to a side of the square, but not in a direction that is at an angle to the side. Such a strut is most difficult to bend at an angle of 45 degrees to the side of the square.

A strut with a rectangular cross section can easily be bent by application of force in the direction of the shorter side, but not in other directions, especially the direction of the longer side. A filamentous strut with a round cross section can be bent in every direction by application of identical force (Fig. 2.25).

In principle, a stent with cylindrical struts is considered to be best able to fit into the two branches. On the other hand, cylindrical struts have a smaller contact area with the vessel wall and are prone to excessive deformation when contacted by a balloon. Thus, designing a stent with cylindrical struts involves a trade-off between these two characteristics, although the actual clinical performance of stents with different strut shapes for bifurcation stenting is uncertain.

At least, it can be said that a stent with rectangular struts is not suitable for bifurcation stenting. A stent with cylindrical struts is the best option, while a stent with rectangular struts (chamfered squares in cross section) is second best.

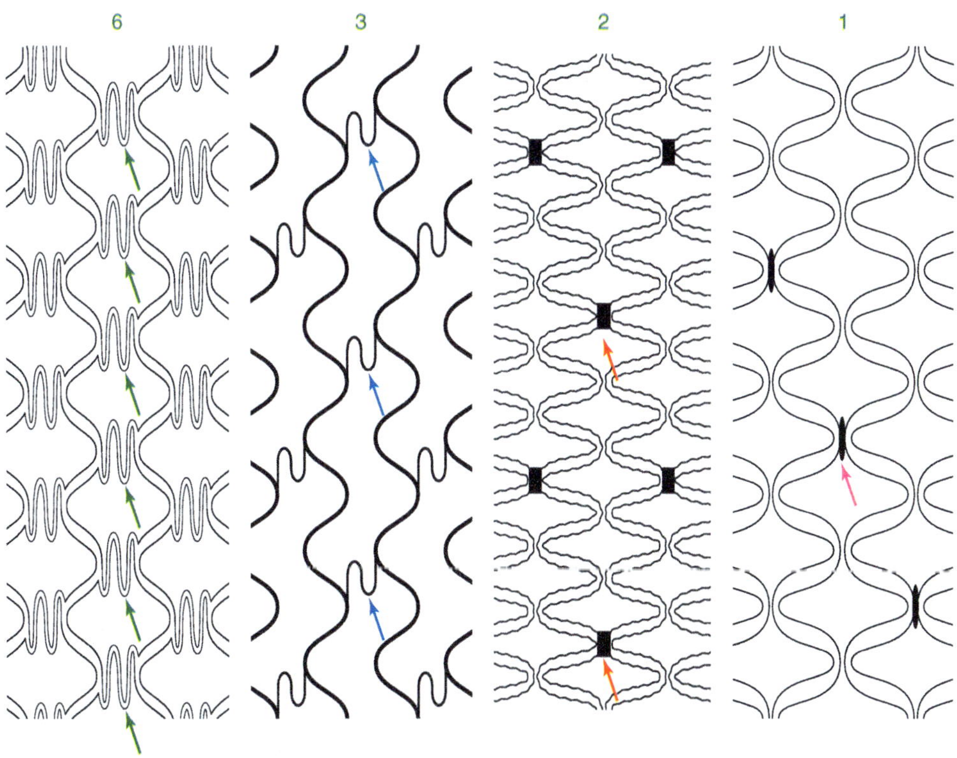

Fig. 2.23 Design of 6-, 3-, 2-, and 1-link stents. A stent with fewer links is less likely to cause link-induced SB jailing

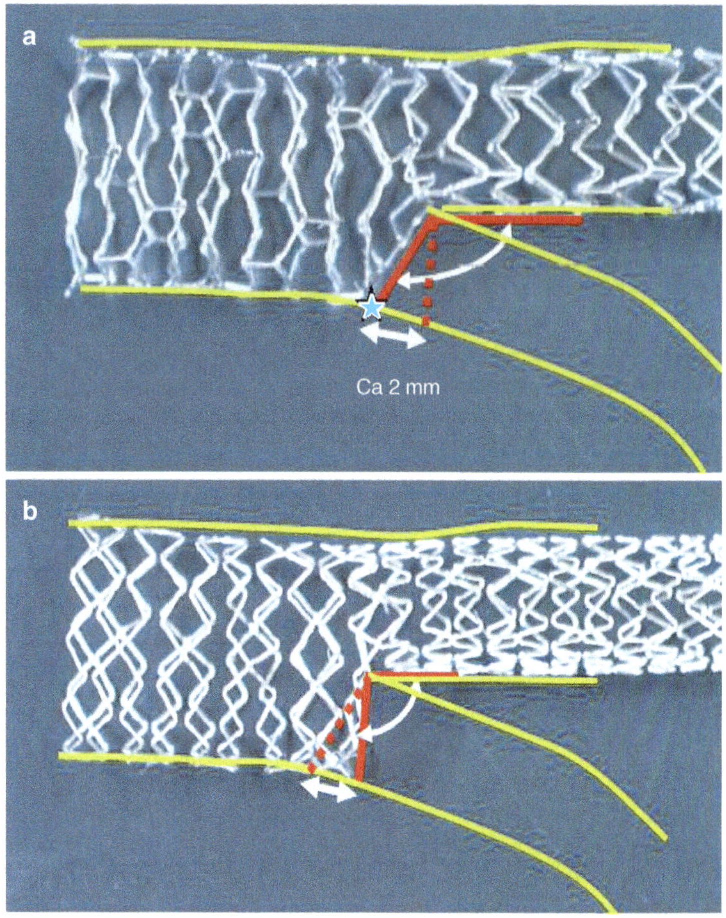

Fig. 2.24 Stents expanded by KBI ex vivo. (**a**) Expanding a 3-link stent results in enlargement of a strut cell at the SB ostium to an elliptical hole about 3 mm in diameter with no zigzag strut. Hence, the lateral border of the hole (★) is proximal to the stent carina, with the average distance being about 2 mm or slightly more. (**b**) Expanding a 2-link stent results in enlargement of a strut cell at the SB ostium to about 3 mm in diameter while retaining the zigzag structure of the struts. This allows the stent to provide a more adequate scaffold for the SB shoulder (arrow) compared with a 3-link stent

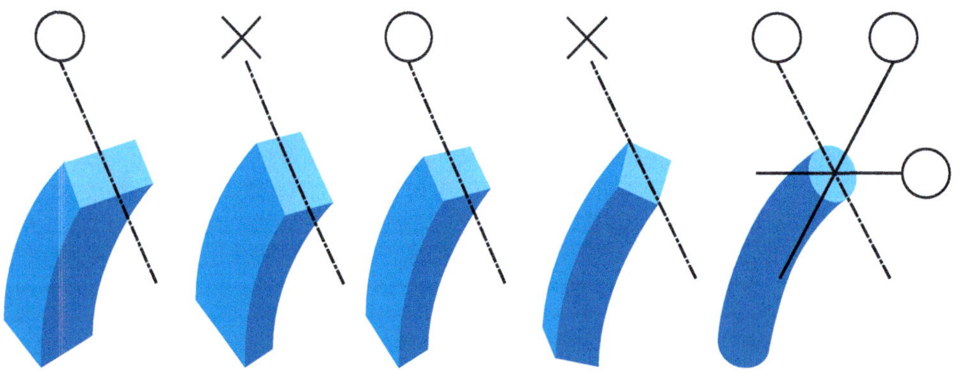

Fig. 2.25 Cross-sectional views of stent struts. A strut with a rectangular cross section can easily be bent if force is applied in the direction of the shorter side, but not in the direction of the longer side. A strut with a square cross section can be bent more easily if force is applied in a direction parallel with its sides, but not in a direction at 45 degrees to a side. A cylindrical strut can be bent in any direction by the same force

2.3 Optimal Stenting Techniques for Bifurcation Lesions

2.3.1 Need for KBI Pre-dilatation and Practical Approach

Although many interventionalists question the use of KBI for pre-dilatation, I often perform this technique for pre-dilatation of a bifurcation lesion with plaques around the carina (including the SB ostium), provided the diameter of the proximal MB is significantly larger than that of the distal MB. The objectives of performing KBI in this situation are (1) to assess the responsiveness of the proximal MB to balloon angioplasty (Figs. 2.26 and 2.27) to reduce the risk of plaque shift after stent implantation and the risk of occlusion/severe stenosis of the SB ostium by carina shift during alternating balloon inflation (Fig. 2.27). For pre-dilatation, I first perform KBI at a pressure of only 6–8 atm.

If such low-pressure KBI cannot dilate the lesion sufficiently, I perform alternating balloon inflation at escalating pressures until sufficient dilatation of the SB ostium and the distal MB is achieved. I then repeat low-pressure (about 10 atm) KBI and check if there is any residual indentation.

Even if alternating balloon inflation seems to have removed all indentations in the MB and SB balloons and to have sufficiently dilated both branches, one or more indentations may reappear in the body of either or both balloons during KBI. Such pre-dilatation failure typically occurs in patients who have an LAD-diagonal branch (Dg) ostial lesion with hard plaque at the shoulder of the branch. In such lesions, alternating balloon inflation often causes carina shift (Fig. 2.28) that obscures balloon indentations, so that it appears that the SB ostium has been dilated sufficiently. For optimal preparation of these lesions, I have often used a scoring balloon in recent years. The Lacrosse NSE is my favorite scoring balloon. In general, I combine scoring balloon angioplasty and POBA as required to prepare bifurcation lesions according to the size of the MB/SB and the pattern of stenosis (Fig. 2.29). IVUS guidance is absolutely required for optimizing the combination of these angioplasty procedures.

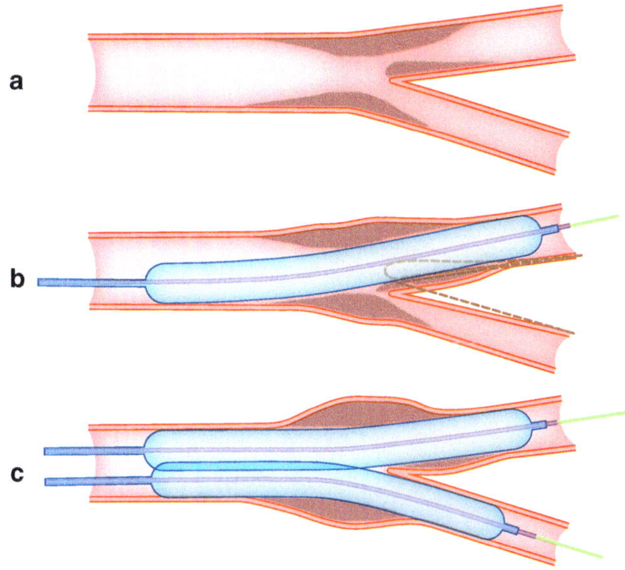

Fig. 2.26 Need for KBI in pre-dilatation. At a bifurcation stenosis (**a**), alternating balloon inflation appears to have sufficiently dilated the MB and the SB since there are no indentations when the balloon is inflated in either branch (**b**). However, alternating inflation has actually caused carina shift and deformation of the SB shoulder, resulting in transient elimination of indentations in the body of the SB balloon so that it appears as if the SB ostium has been sufficiently dilated (**b**). During KBI, one or more indentations may reappear in the SB balloon, but such indentations can be eliminated by raising the KBI pressure to 8 atm. As a result, both the MB and SB can be dilated sufficiently as optimal preparation for stenting with KBI (**c**)

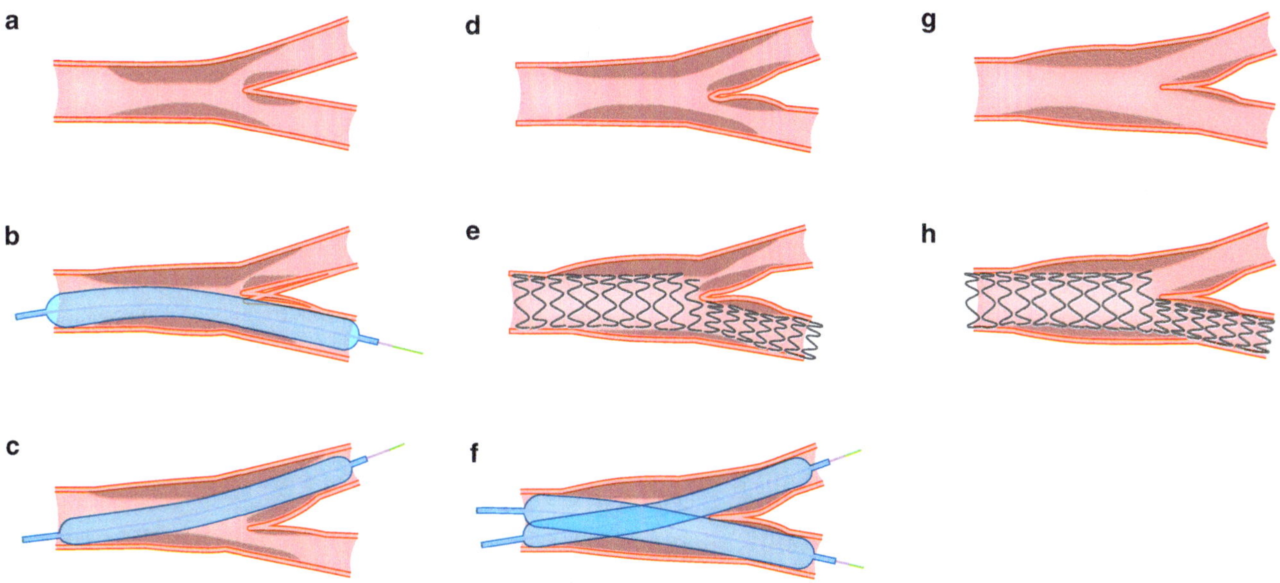

Fig. 2.27 Need for KBI in pre-dilatation of true bifurcation lesions. If pre-dilatation of a bifurcation lesion (**a**) is performed by alternating balloon inflation, the carina shifts toward the SB after inflation of the MB balloon (**b**) and then shifts back toward the MB after inflation of the SB balloon (**c**). After balloon deflation, it is found that only minimal dilatation of the lesion has been achieved (**d**). Following minimal pre-dilatation of a bifurcation lesion, placing a stent in the MB can cause plaque shift that leads to severe stenosis or occlusion of the SB (**e**). With pre-dilatation by KBI (**f**), the lesion will be optimally dilated (**g**), minimizing the risk of SB occlusion (**h**)

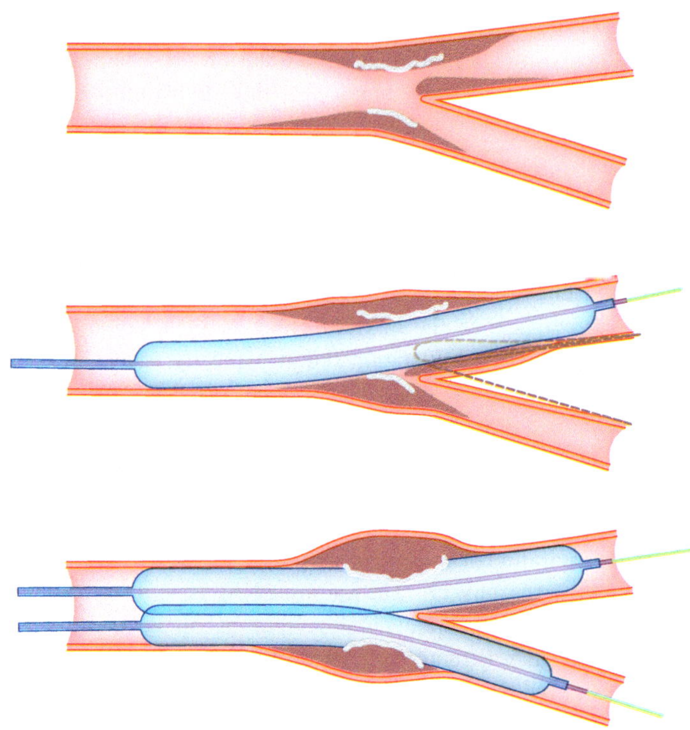

Fig. 2.28 Bifurcation lesion with calcified plaque. In a bifurcation lesion with calcified plaque (**a**), alternating balloon inflation appears to have sufficiently dilated both the MB and SB, since there are no indentations when the balloon is inflated in either branch (**b**). However, alternating balloon inflation has caused carina shift and deformation of the SB shoulder, which have transiently eliminated the indentations in the body of the SB balloon so that the SB ostium seems to have been dilated sufficiently (**b**). During KBI, one or more indentations may reappear in the body of the balloon (**c**). In this setting, it is uncertain whether such indentations can be eliminated by raising the KBI pressure. Since high-pressure KBI is associated with a significant risk of dissection or perforation, performing KBI with two scoring balloons (e.g., a Lacrosse NSE) at a low pressure is better

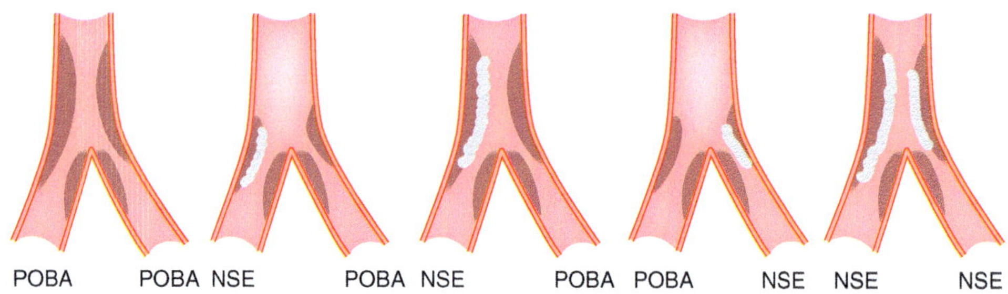

Fig. 2.29 Optimal selection of scoring balloon angioplasty or POBA according to the severity of stenosis and calcification

Bifurcation lesions should be adequately prepared by appropriate use of a scoring balloon (e.g., a Lacrosse NSE) as required. The scoring balloon should usually be one-quarter size smaller than the diameter of the target vessel

2.3.2 KBI for Post-dilatation

Even if the side branch is protected with a guidewire, KBI may not need to be performed for pre-dilatation or post-dilatation in the following situations: (1) if the SB has a relatively small diameter (<2.0 mm) and only perfuses a small territory (Fig. 2.30), (2) if the proximal MB has a similar diameter to the distal MB, (3) if there is little plaque at the ostium of the SB, (4) if coronary angiography shows no significant stenosis at the SB ostium after stenting or POT of a LAD-Dg bifurcation lesion, and (5) if SB blood flow does not decrease after removal of the SB guidewire or after high-pressure balloon inflation in the SB.

Except in these situations, stenting should generally be followed by KBI. If the proximal MB has a large diameter, POT should be performed before final KBI. The reasons for this recommendation are as follows: (1) POT alone cannot achieve sufficient dilation of a bifurcation, including the carina (accurate POT is possible for an LAD-Dg ostial lesion that can be viewed en face on angiograms, but not for an LM-LAD-LCX lesion that is difficult or sometimes impossible to view en face). (2) An attempt to perform POT along the carina without knowing its true position may lead to over-dilatation and injure the proximal segment of the distal MB. (3) A balloon employed for POT, even if it reaches the carina, cannot be used to evenly dilate the proximal MB if plaques show maldistribution in this segment. (4) Considering that the proximal MB originally has an elliptical lumen, POT should be combined with KBI to dilate the proximal MB to an ellipse and thus achieve complete stent apposition (Fig. 2.31).

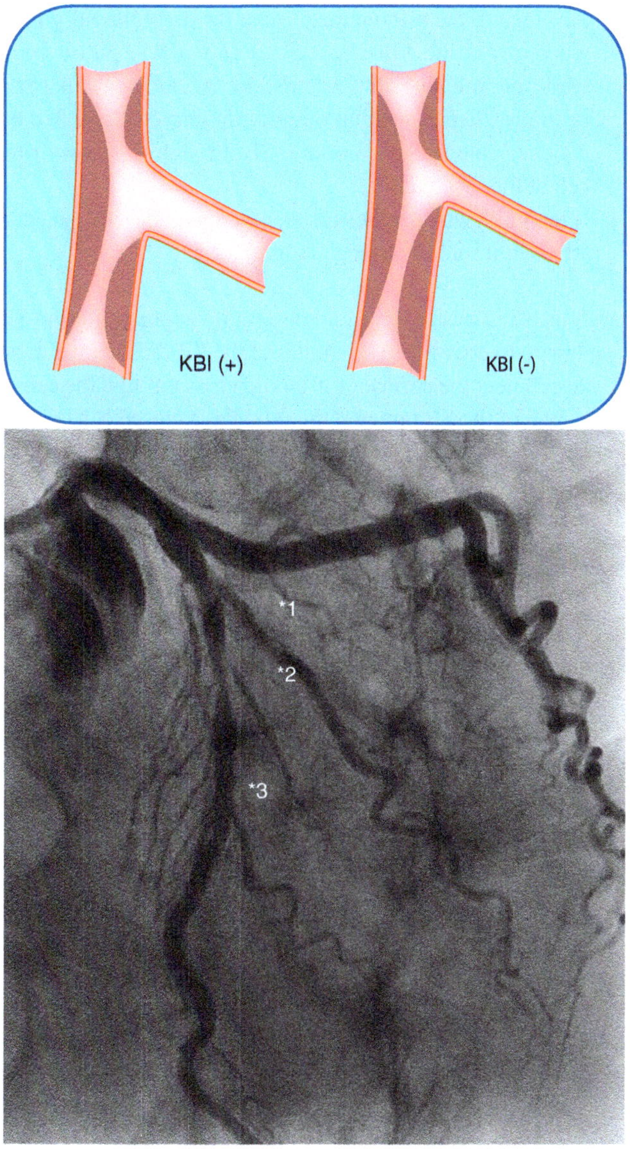

Fig. 2.30 A situation where KBI may not be required. In a bifurcation with a small SB <2 mm in diameter (*1, *2), only guidewire protection is adequate without addition of KBI if there is no decrease of blood flow through the SB after stenting (+ post-dilatation). However, KBI should be considered if the SB is larger and perfuses a large territory (*3)

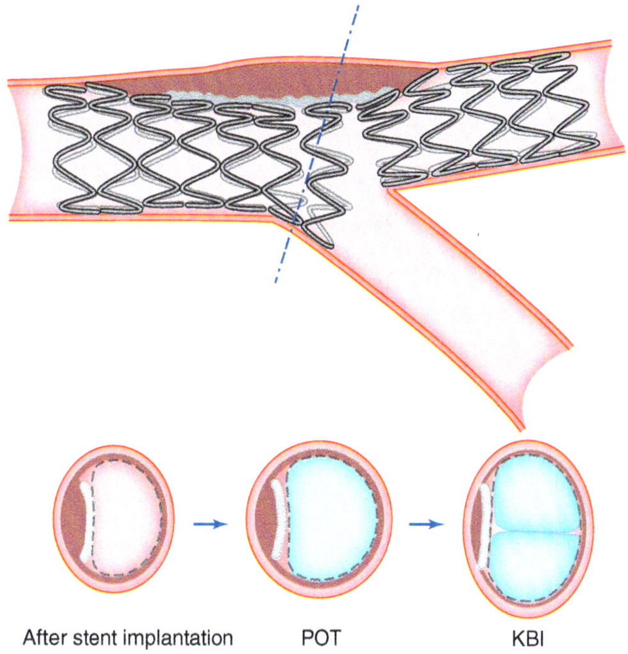

Fig. 2.31 Achieving complete stent apposition. Since the proximal MB has an elliptical lumen, POT combined with KBI should be used to dilate the proximal MB to an ellipse and thus achieve complete stent apposition

Column 14 Selection of the Balloon Type and Inflation Pressure

Here, I will explain my ideas about how to select the ideal type of balloon (including stent) and the ideal balloon size, as well as how to determine the balloon inflation pressure. These points are also applicable to PCI for non-bifurcation lesions.

For pre-dilatation, you should basically choose a slightly undersized balloon that can be inflated to the desired diameter at its rated burst pressure plus 4 atm. You should steadily pre-dilate the lesion to adequately prepare it for stenting while preventing stent edge dissection due to over-dilatation of the lesion. If the lesion is severely calcified and is not dilated sufficiently by POBA (even after rotablation), you should perform scoring balloon or cutting balloon angioplasty, since this is the best way to completely avoid suboptimal dilatation after stenting. The Lacrosse NSE balloon for this purpose should be one-quarter size smaller than the diameter of the target vessel, so that it can be inflated to the optimal size at its RBP plus 4 atm. The balloon inflation pressure should generally be escalated to the RBP plus 4 atm.

The optimal balloon size depends on the situation. To determine the optimal size, you should assess the risk/benefit ratio by considering the vessel diameter (external elastic membrane), inner diameter, and plaque eccentricity (particularly calcified plaques).

2.3.3 Basic Procedures for Stenting with KBI

2.3.3.1 SB Rewiring

There are three key points to keep in mind when recrossing a guidewire into the SB again across the MB stent.

Dual Lumen Catheter (Crusade Catheter)

The Crusade catheter is used for SB (MB) wiring. If SB wiring is performed before stent implantation, the bare wire technique can generally be employed. If SB wiring is found to be difficult after MB wiring or if MB wiring is difficult after SB wiring (intentionally done before MB wiring), you should advance a Crusade catheter over the first guidewire. If you are treating a bifurcation lesion distal to a long CIO, you should also use the Crusade catheter for SB wiring.

I always use a Crusade catheter for SB wiring after MB stenting. Although some interventionalists may criticize the overuse of limited medical resources, employing the Crusade catheter ensures wire crossing through the optimal cell of the stent, thus reducing the risk of SB jailing and difficulty implanting a stent in the SB. It also alleviates possible problems related to future SB intervention.

The Crusade catheter is also advantageous for SB wiring after ostial dissection or occlusion of the SB. If a Crusade is not used (bare wire technique), SB wiring will be difficult because the guidewire tip tends to become stuck on the proximal stent struts. Attempts at SB wiring by using a single guidewire with its original tip shape tend to fail and may rather enlarge the dissection. If you use a Crusade catheter, SB wiring can be retried many times by advancing the guidewire from the tip of the catheter, and there is no stress on the wire from the proximal part of the stent. The Crusade also facilitates SB rewiring by using the same guidewire after modifying the tip shape or with a different guidewire. Thus, the Crusade catheter is useful for SB rewiring in most occlusions with most types of dissection.

Overall, use of the Crusade catheter improves the quality of PCI and eventually reduces the impact on medical resources.

Using a Crusade Catheter (SB Wiring After Stenting)

1. You should insert an SB guidewire into the over-the-wire (OTW) lumen of the Crusade catheter (but do not allow the tip to protrude from the catheter) and advance the Crusade along the MB guidewire in the stent (Fig. 2.32a).
2. Advance the tip of the SB guidewire through a side hole at the tip of the OTW lumen to reliably place the guidewire tip distal to the SB ostium in the stent (Fig. 2.32b).
3. While keeping the two guidewires in place, you should pull the Crusade catheter back so that its tip is 1–2 cm proximal to the bifurcation. Orient the tip of the SB guidewire toward the SB (Fig. 2.32c) and slowly pull it back while maintaining this orientation. A guidewire that has been pre-shaped with an optimal tip curve (Fig. 2.32d★) is better able to cross into the SB through the most distal cell at the bifurcation.
4. If the guidewire crosses the stent to reach the SB, you can advance it into the branch (Fig. 2.32e).

If the stent has an open cell design, it is optimal for the SB guidewire to cross the MB stent into the SB through the most distal cell near the carina, or it should cross through the cell at the center of the SB lumen if the stent has a closed cell design.

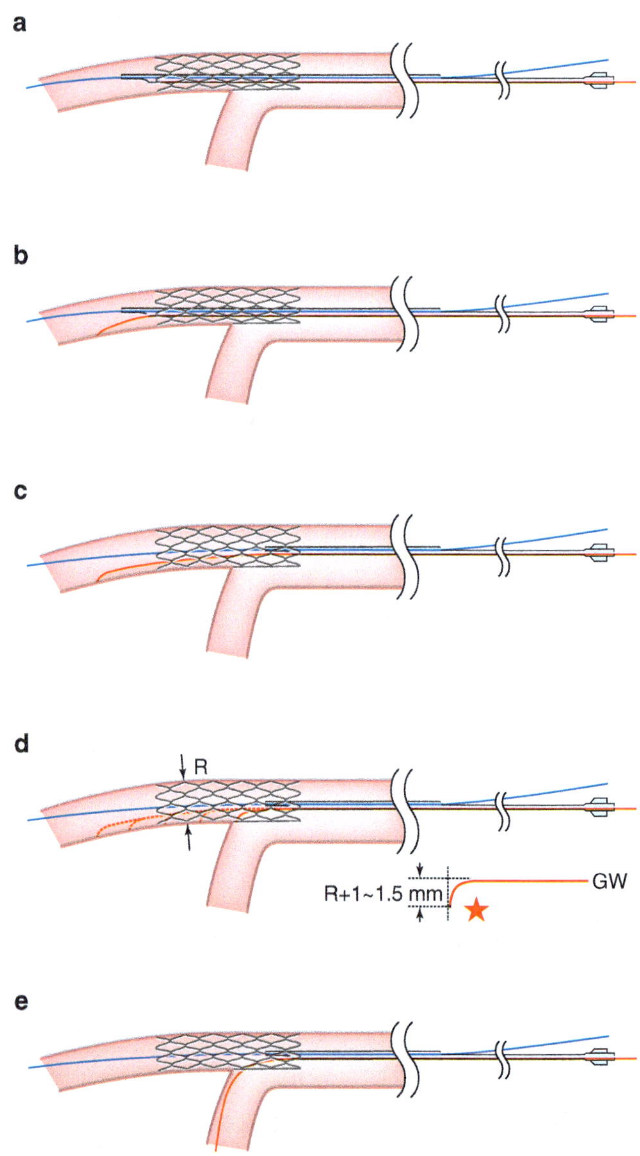

Fig. 2.32 Using the Crusade catheter (**a**–**e**)

Removing the Crusade Catheter

1. Trapping technique (Fig. 2.33)

While maintaining the two guidewires in position, withdraw the Crusade catheter into the guiding catheter. Introduce a Kusabi® trapping balloon or a large-diameter (2.0 to 2.5 mm) balloon catheter directly into the guiding catheter. Inflate the balloon at about 10 atm to trap the two guidewires and pull them back together with the balloon catheter. Never fail to remove the air trapped in the guiding catheter after deflating the balloon. This is the safest and most reliable method for removing the Crusade.

2. Nanto's technique (Fig. 2.34)

This technique involves fixing the guidewire in the monorail lumen and removing the Crusade catheter while advancing the guidewire in the OTW lumen. It is safer to use an inflation device (indeflator) to advance the guidewire. I prefer this technique because it is quicker than the trapping technique.

1. First, you fix the guidewire in the monorail lumen of the Crusade catheter. While checking the position of the tip of the guidewire in the OTW lumen by cineangiography, pull the hub of the Crusade catheter back to the proximal end of the OTW guidewire.
2. Monitor the pressure waveform and confirm that the catheter is not wedged in the vessel. If the catheter becomes wedged, air may be aspirated, or air that unexpectedly enters the vessel from an inflation device may not be let out, possibly leading to air embolization.
3. Completely remove air from the inflation device and confirm that the wire passes through the center of the inflation device connector and is not caught by the connector. Then connect the inflation device to the Crusade catheter.
4. Apply pressure on the OTW lumen of the catheter by using the inflation device.
5. In reaction to the advancing OTW guidewire, the Crusade catheter will move back through the guiding catheter. To prevent unexpected air embolization, keep the O-ring of the Y-connector open.
6. You must continue to hold the guidewire in the monorail lumen with your left hand or the guidewire will come out spontaneously. Place your right hand lightly on the Crusade catheter to support it.
7. When removing the Crusade catheter, the exit port of its monorail lumen will get stuck on your left hand. While continuing to apply pressure on the OTW lumen, move your left hand to a more proximal part of the monorail lumen guidewire. Then slowly withdraw the Crusade catheter while monitoring the position of the OTW lumen guidewire by cineangiography to confirm that it is still in place. When the exit port of its monorail lumen gets stuck on your left hand again, stop removing the catheter and repeat the above procedure. As is done during removal of monorail (rapid exchange) devices, you continue to apply pressure on the OTW lumen and to hold the Crusade catheter.
8. When the tip of the Crusade catheter exits the Y-connector, you reduce the pressure on the OTW lumen to atmospheric pressure. Carefully hold and fix the guidewires in both lumens near the O-ring and remove the Crusade catheter.
9. If a jailed guidewire remains after SB rewiring, it must be the third guidewire (not the two guidewires you are holding). Remove the jailed guidewire as soon as possible after removing the Crusade catheter (after the wire is confirmed to be jailed).

3. Extension wire technique

This technique involves fixing the guidewire in the monorail lumen, fixing the guidewire extended by an extension wire or guidewire, and removing the Crusade catheter.

I do not use this technique because of the complexity of the procedures required to simultaneously fix the two guidewires.

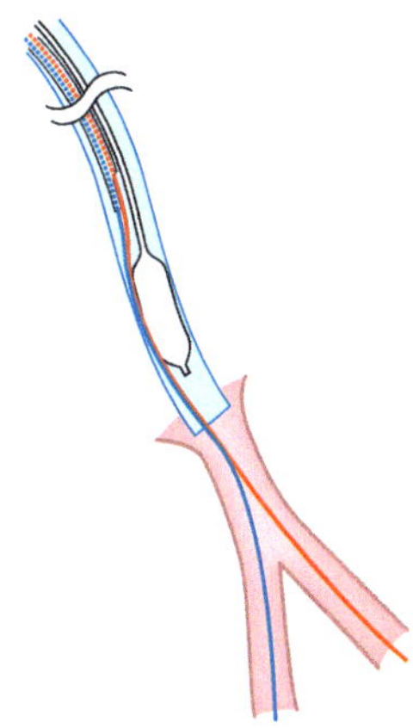

Fig. 2.33 Trapping technique. This technique requires a Kusabi trapping balloon or a large-diameter (2.0–2.5 mm) balloon

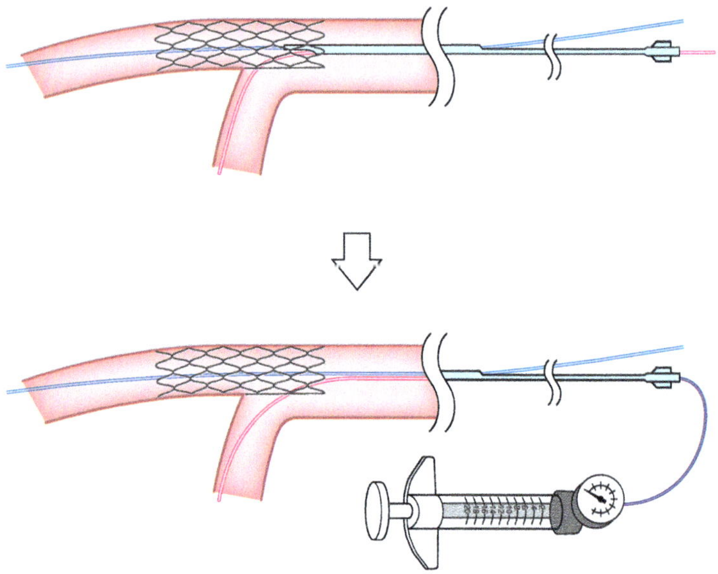

Fig. 2.34 Nanto's technique

Column 15 Preventing Guidewire Entanglement and Countermeasures

[Crusade catheter]

Using a Crusade catheter to facilitate SB wiring also contributes to preventing guidewire entanglement. A Crusade catheter allows delivery of a guidewire within its OTW lumen beyond the carina, which is associated with a much lower risk of guidewire entanglement compared with the bare wire method.

[Organizing guidewires]

Organizing the guidewires is also important to prevent entanglement. I recommend organizing your guidewires in the order of the directions in which they are viewed by fluoroscopy. Two kissing balloons are difficult to withdraw individually because the other may also be withdrawn spontaneously while removing one balloon. However, simultaneous withdrawal of two kissing balloons may disturb the organization of your guidewires. Therefore, I recommend reorganizing the two guidewires by separating their proximal parts while keeping the topological relationship at the O-ring. The same applies to wiring with the assistance of a Crusade. You should put the proximal parts of the two guidewires in the correct order while keeping their topological relationship at the O-ring, and cover them with wet gauze for stabilization.

[Countermeasures for entanglement]

1. Case 1

The first device (e.g., balloon and stent) to be delivered into the MB may not go beyond the bifurcation due to guidewire entanglement. In this case, you should pull the device back to the hub and advance it again, which often allows you to successfully deliver the device into the MB. If this maneuver fails, retract the guidewire into the device and then push it gently forward while slightly pressing the device into the bifurcation. The device will often become disentangled, permitting it to advance beyond the bifurcation.

2. Case 2

A previously inflated balloon may become entangled due to poor rewrapping of the balloon or twisting of the shaft. Therefore, I recommend selecting a balloon that rewraps well with a shaft that is strong near the exit port. A balloon that has become entangled should be exchanged for a new one, which can often be delivered smoothly

3. Blocking of the second device by the guidewire exit port of the first device

The guidewire exit port of a device that has already been advanced into the guiding catheter may block advancement of a second device. In such a situation, you should pull the latter device back to the hub and then advance it again. This maneuver often allows the device to be delivered successfully. If it fails, you should withdraw both devices and then readvance them simultaneously.

2.3.3.2 Optimal Projections

The optimal projection for visualizing each coronary bifurcation should permit en face observation of the plane in which both the MB and SB lie (Fig. 2.35). However, it is not always easy to find the specific projection for each situation, and interventionalists can sometimes be mistaken about the optimal projections for visualizing bifurcations.

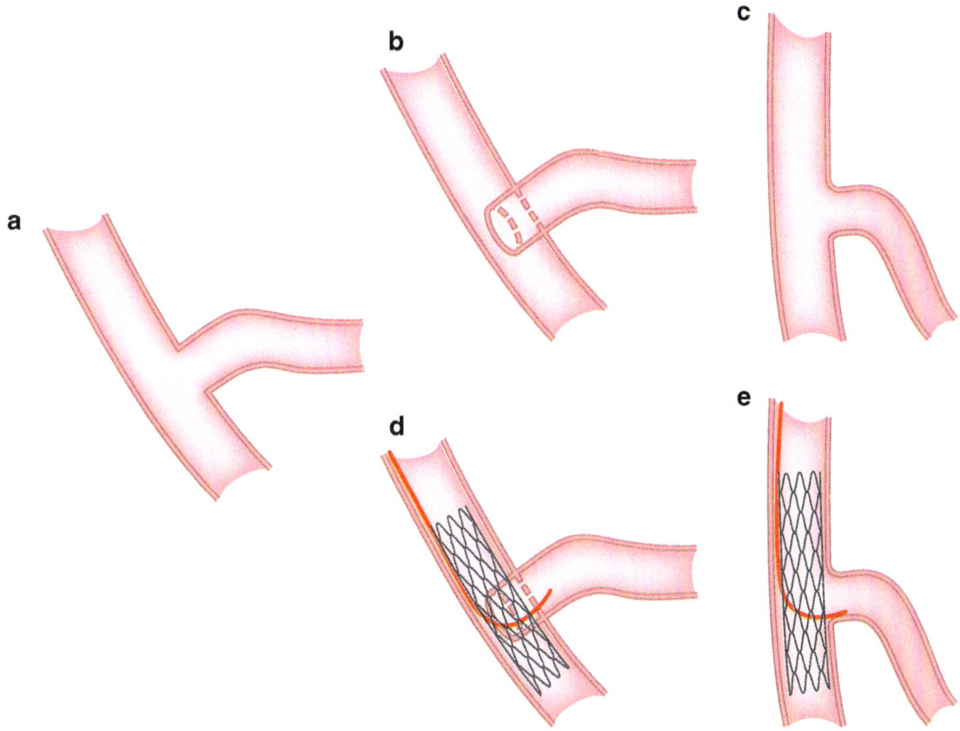

Fig. 2.35 Optimal projections. CAG guidance (**a**) using a projection that deviates considerably from that perpendicular to the plane of the MB and SB (**b** or **d**) will only allow successful wiring of the MB or SB by chance, since it is impossible to assess whether the wire has come into contact with the carina. Conversely, CAG in a projection perpendicular to the plane of the two branches (**c** or **e**) facilitates SB wiring and assessment of whether the guidewire has contacted the carina

Examples of Wrong Projections

The most frequently chosen wrong projection is use of the RAO cranial projection for separating the Dg from the proximal LAD. The RAO is relatively parallel to the plane of the proximal LAD and the Dg, so the two vessels overlap in most parts when viewed in this projection. The cranial projection is good for separating the Dg from the mid-distal LAD, but not for visualizing the LAD-Dg bifurcation. According to standard practice, the LAO cranial projection is optimal for separating the Dg from the proximal LAD. Figure 2.36 shows typical CAGs explaining this point. It is easy to understand that the longest view of the LAD is obtained in the cranial projection as this artery runs leftward and anteriorly. The Dg is located posterior to the LAD and runs caudally in the LL cranial projection, while it is on the left of the LAD in the AP cranial view. The LAO projection is excellent for visualizing a bifurcation with leftward and posterior SB angulation. As the longitudinal axis of the LAD is oriented anteriorly, marked cranial angulation is better. The LAO cranial projection separates the Dg from the LAD very well (Fig. 2.36c). If the LAD takes extremely anterior course, even greater cranial angulation may be needed to achieve good separation from the LCX, but such a projection imposes stricter radiographic conditions. Some interventionalists prefer the RAO cranial projection, probably because this projection had better radiographic conditions and provides clearer images than the LAO view. However, the RAO cranial projection is not optimal for visualizing the LAD-Dg bifurcation.

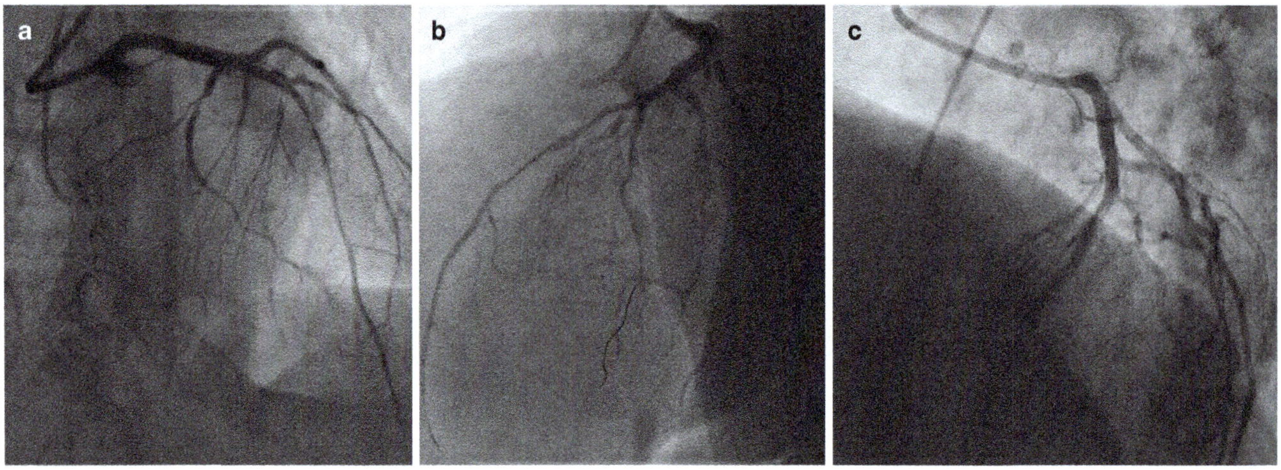

Fig. 2.36 Optimal projection for separating the Dg from the LAD. (**a**) AP cranial view. (**b**) AP/LL view. (**c**) LAO cranial view. The LAO cranial projection is optimal for separating the Dg from the LAD

Typical Projections Allowing En Face Observation of Various Coronary Bifurcations (Table 2.1)

The projections presented in the table often allow the SB to be separated from the MB at individual bifurcations and should be tried first. If the recommended projection is not appropriate, you will generally need to adjust the fluoroscopy angle to optimize it.

The bifurcation of LMT to form the LAD and the LCX is a special case. At other coronary bifurcations, the two branches run in the same plane on the surface of the ventricle for some distance, so it is relatively easy to identify the plane encompassing both branches and find a projection perpendicular to that plane. However, both the LAD and the LCX immediately change directions at the LMT bifurcation, with the former running to the left, anteriorly and caudally, while the latter runs posteriorly. The LM bifurcation offers a point of deflection for both branches. In other words, there is no plane which encompasses even the proximal segments of both the LAD and LCX. It is hard to find the optimal projection for visualizing the LMT bifurcation by reviewing various images of the proximal LAD/LCX, so you have to estimate the take-off angle of each branch. This is sometimes difficult and requires many fine adjustments.

Table 2.1 Projections allowing en face observation of different coronary bifurcations

Coronary bifurcation	Projection perpendicular to the bifurcation plane	Ancillary projection for biplane cineangiography
LAD and LCX	LAO + CA(spider)	AP(RAO) + CA
LAD and Dg(Prox)	LAO + CR	AP + CR(RAO + CR)
LAD and Dg(M ~ Dist)	LAO ~ AP + CR	
LAD and Sept	RAO + CR	
LCX and PL (Prox)	RAO + CA	LAO + CA
LCX and PL (M)	RAO	
LCX and PL (Dist)	RAO + CR	
4-AV and 4-PD	LAO + CR	AP + CR

Rules for Fine Adjustment of Fluoroscopy Angles

1. If the standard Spider view cannot separate the LCX from the LAD, a more steeply angled LAO projection is needed. In a view with more caudal angulation, the LMT-LAD often becomes "elevated" and easier to distinguish from the LCX (Fig. 2.37).
2. When performing biplane coronary angiography of a bifurcation, exploration along a line that is assumed to connect the two branches can lead to identification of the optimal fluoroscopy angle. The two projections do not necessarily need to be orthogonal to each other.

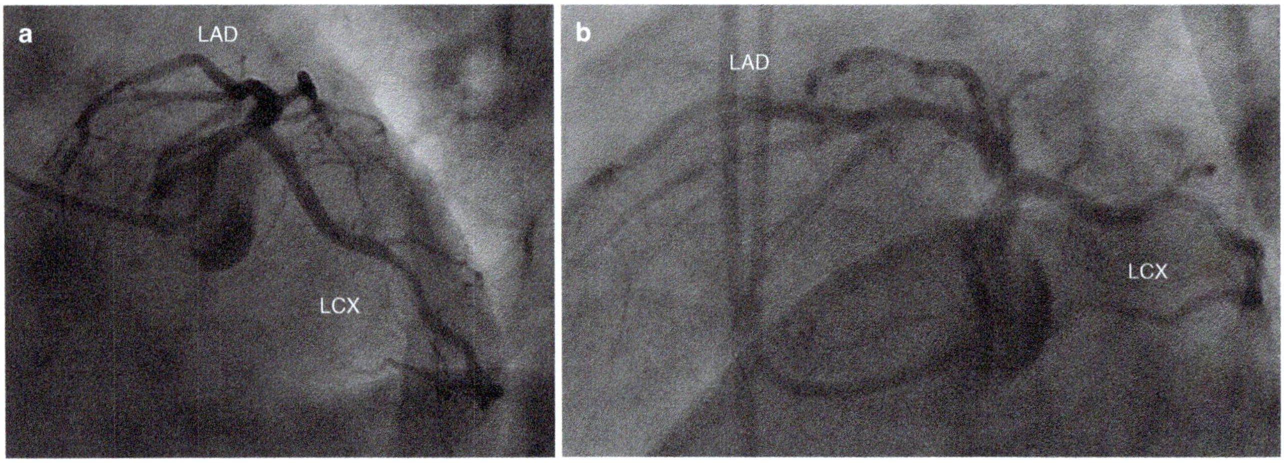

Fig. 2.37 Adjusting the Spider view. (**a**) LAO 44.3° and caudal 17°. In this shallow Spider view, there is poor separation of the LAD from the LCX (occluded). (**b**) LAO 89.6° and caudal 37.2°. In this steeper Spider view, the LAD shows good separation from the LCX

Reliable Method of Finding the Optimal Projection for En Face Observation of a Specific Bifurcation

The optimal projection may be determined in an empirical manner, as described above. However, if you have no idea which projection will allow en face observation of the bifurcation, the following procedure can be followed to reliably identify the correct projection. First, you should find the projection that provides the longest view (red line) of the bifurcation (deep green) and the longitudinal axis of the MB (green) (Fig. 2.38). Then you should rotate the detector at 90 degrees around the line projected on the surface of the fluoroscope. The longest view of the longitudinal axis of the MB will be provided by the new projection, since the MB is being viewed in a projection orthogonal to the plane of the vessel (Fig. 2.39). Subsequently, you should rotate the detector around the axis to find a plane in which the branching angle is maximal, i.e., a projection in which the bifurcation can be viewed en face (Fig. 2.40). The optimal projection is not always required for simple wiring before stenting. However, if the optimal projection is found in this way after wiring the two branches, coronary angiography will not be required. If SB wiring is difficult, you may leave the guidewire in the MB and inject small test doses of contrast medium while seeking the optimal projection that displays the maximal branching angle.

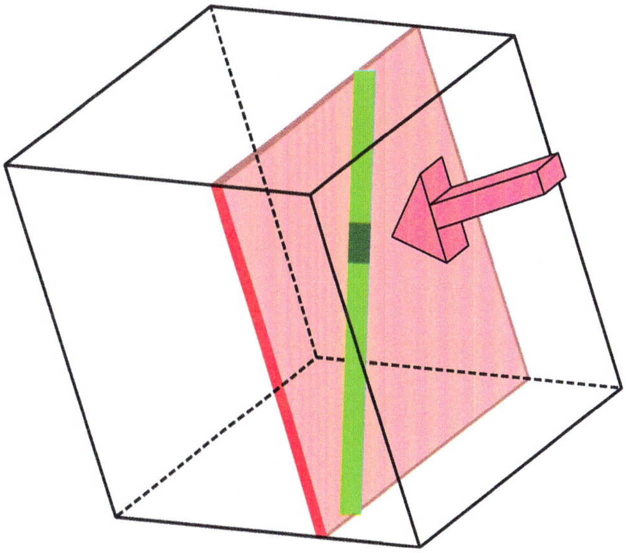

Fig. 2.39 Visualizing the longitudinal axis of the MB: 2. The longest view of the longitudinal axis of the MB is obtained when the ROI is seen in a projection orthogonal to the plane encompassing the axis

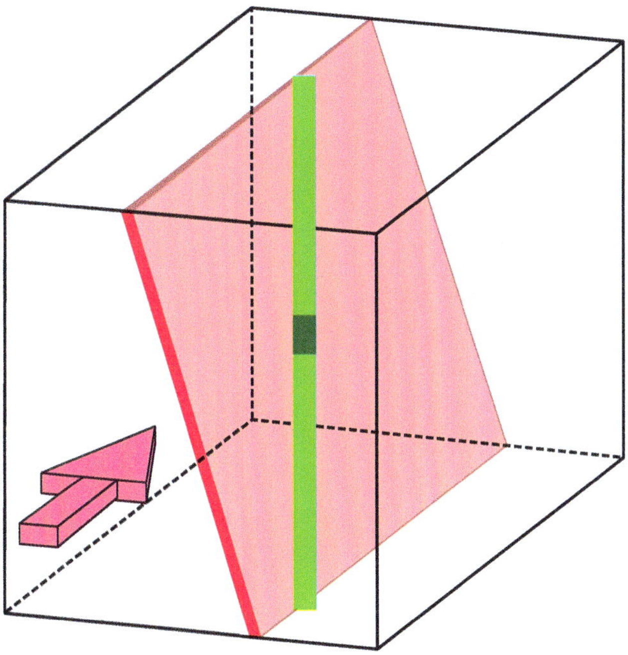

Fig. 2.38 Visualizing the longitudinal axis of the MB: 1. The green line represents the axis of the ROI (dark green). This axis is viewed as the thick red line on the anterior detector. To visualize the true axis, you rotate the detector 90 degrees around the projected axis

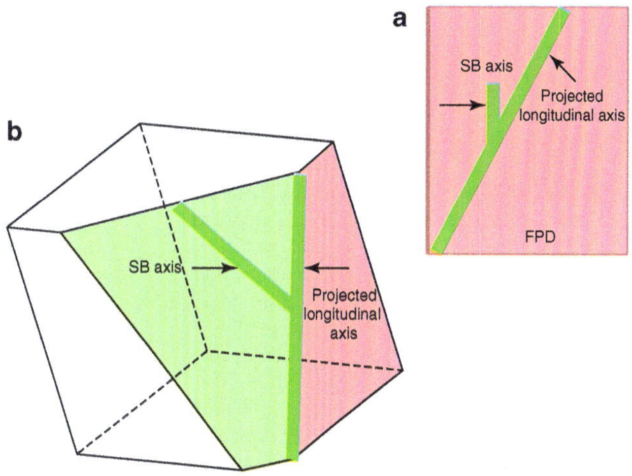

Fig. 2.40 Finding a projection that allows en face observation of the bifurcation plane after identifying the optimal projection for visualizing the longitudinal axis of the MB. Assuming that the SB is viewed on the fluoroscopy detector (FPD) as shown in (**a**), while the actual branching pattern is shown in (**b**), a projection that is en face to the green plane will be optimal. You should seek the green plane with the maximal branching angle by rotating the red plane clockwise or anticlockwise around the longitudinal axis projected on the detector. Several test doses of contrast medium may be injected during this step

2.3.4 SB Wiring

Shaping the Tip Curve of the SB Guidewire

If POT has not been performed, the tip of the guidewire for the SB should be bent to an angle of 90° relative to its shaft, and the curve should have a radius about 1.0 mm longer than the diameter of the distal MB (Fig. 2.41a).

If POT has been performed, the tip of the SB guidewire should be bent to slightly less than 90° relative to its shaft, and the curve should have a radius about 1.0 mm longer than the diameter of the proximal MB (Fig. 2.41b).

You should aim for the guidewire to cross the stent through the most distal cell at the SB ostium so that the wire comes into contact with the carina (Fig. 2.42). This minimizes the risk of jailing.

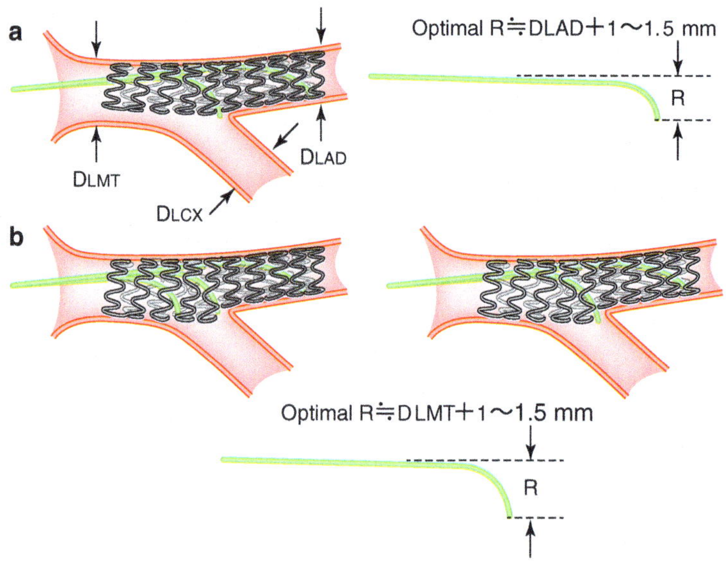

Fig. 2.41 Shape of the tip curve for the SB guidewire. (**a**) Without POT: Optimal radius ≈ D_{LAD} + 1 to 1.5 mm. (**b**) With POT: Optimal radius ≈ D_{LMT} + 1 to 1.5 mm. D_{LAD} diameter of the LAD; D_{LMT} Diameter of the LMT

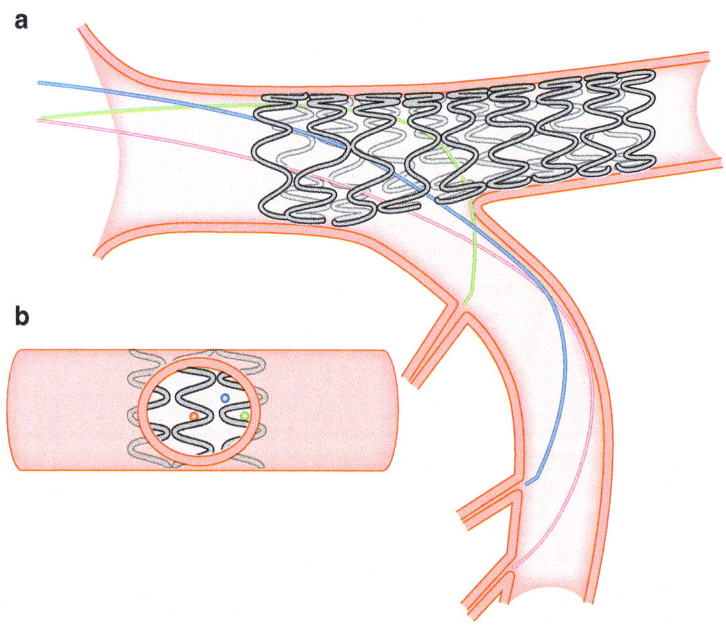

Fig. 2.42 Point of stent wire crossing. (**a**) Diagram of a bifurcation in a projection perpendicular to the plane encompassing both the MB and SB. (**b**) Diagram of the SB ostium in a projection parallel to the axis of the SB. The blue line and the blue dot indicate the optimal route of the wire and the optimal point of stent crossing, respectively. If the SB guidewire follows the route indicated by the green line, KBI will cause injury to the distal MB and the SB at the time of dilatation. If the SB guidewire follows the route indicated by the red line, KBI will result in SB jailing. A guidewire following the red or blue route can move about 1.2–2.5 mm within the stent cell when pushed forward or pulled back slightly. In contrast, a guidewire following the green route can only move less than 1 mm and will feel stuck (although guidewire maneuverability also depends on the stent type and strut configuration)

Confirmation of Wire Crossing Through the Most Distal Cell at the SB Ostium

If the SB guidewire comes into contact with the carina when advanced slightly in a projection that allows en face observation of the bifurcation, it can be considered to have crossed the stent through the most distal cell at the SB ostium (Fig. 2.43). Although the shaft of the guidewire crossing into the SB is not always biased toward the carina, its tip is often biased toward the larger curvature of the SB when the radiopaque marker passes the SB ostium. If coronary angiography is performed at this time and shows the tip of the guidewire in contact with the carina, it confirms that the wire has crossed the stent into the SB through the most distal cell. Alternatively, the SB guidewire can be anchored at a very small branch or dimple and then pushed slightly to bias it toward the carina. If coronary angiography subsequently shows that the guidewire is in contact with the carina (Fig. 2.44), this confirms that the wire has crossed the stent through the most distal cell.

Thus, if the SB guidewire comes into contact with the carina when pushed toward the larger curvature, it is reasonable to consider that the wire has crossed the stent into the SB through the most distal cell at the SB ostium. Conversely, if the guidewire does not come into contact with the carina, the stent has jailed the SB, possibly to a significant extent (Fig. 2.42). For accurate radiographic assessment of SB wiring, coronary angiography must be performed in the optimal projection (as discussed above).

1. If the SB guidewire does not come into contact with the carina when it is advanced appropriately, you should remove the guidewire and make another attempt to cross the stent through the most distal cell.
2. If the SB guidewire crosses the stent through a cell that is actually distal to the SB ostium, KBI may induce carinal injury by the most distal strut (Fig. 2.42). Whether or not the cell is distal to the SB ostium can be roughly assessed from guidewire mobility within the cell. If the SB guidewire moves forward and back at least about 1.2 mm within a cell at the SB ostium and is in contact with the carina, you can assume that the wire has safely crossed the stent. In contrast, a virtually immobile SB guidewire has probably crossed the stent through a cell distal to the SB ostium (Fig. 2.42).

If the SB guidewire crosses the stent through a cell distal to the SB ostium, it may cause dissection at the carina. In such rare cases, culotte stenting may be indicated.

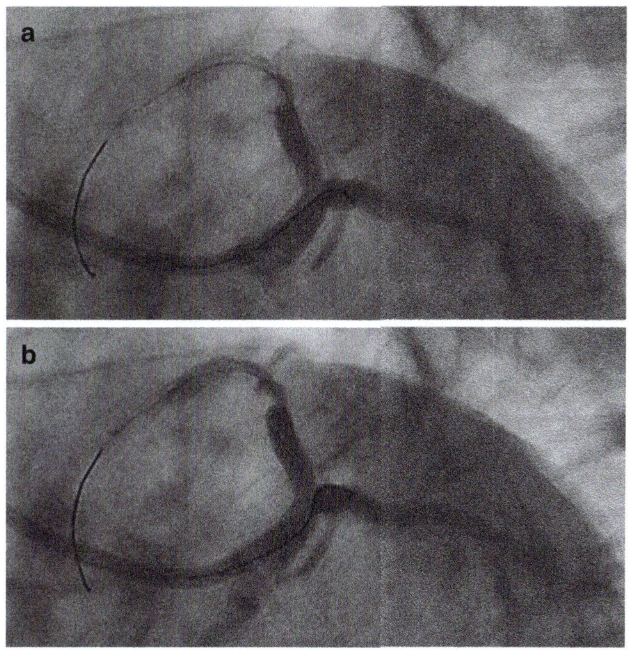

Fig. 2.43 Confirmation of crossing the stent into the SB. A guidewire is advanced with its bias toward the larger curvature of the SB immediately after entering the branch. If the guidewire does not come into contact with the carina (**a**), you should reattempt crossing the stent by the optimal route that brings the wire into contact with the carina (**b**)

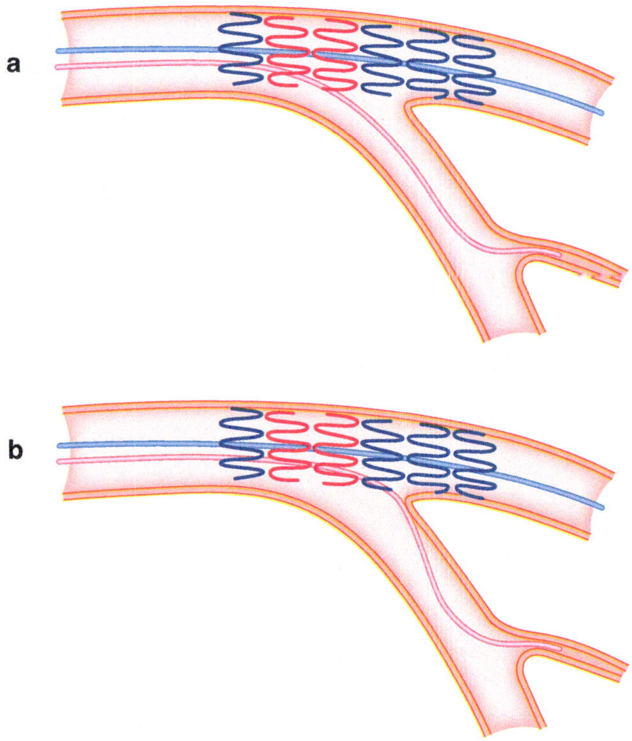

Fig. 2.44 Confirmation of wire crossing through the most distal cell at the SB ostium. If an SB guidewire is anchored in a very small branch (**a**) and then pushed forward (**b**), its proximal portion will be deflected toward the larger curvature of the vessel. If the deflected guidewire comes into contact with the carina, you may assume that the guidewire has crossed the stent into the SB through the most distal cell at the branch. If this does not happen, the guidewire has probably not crossed the stent through the most distal cell. Therefore, you should reattempt crossing the stent through a more distal cell

Factors That Prevent the Wire Crossing Through the Most Distal Cell

1. Plaque shift or dissection (not carinal shift) caused by MB stenting that leads to SB ostial stenosis (Fig. 2.45a).
2. Severe tortuosity of the target vessel.
3. Using a suboptimal fluoroscopy projection that misleadingly suggests a guidewire has crossed the stent through the most distal cell at the SB when it has actually crossed through a more proximal cell. This is often a problem in LMT bifurcation stenting (Fig. 2.45b).

If the SB perfuses a large territory or has a diameter ≥ 3.0 mm, you should perform IVUS after KBI to check whether the SB guidewire crossed the stent through the most distal cell at the SB. If necessary, you should reattempt to cross the stent into the SB through the most distal cell.

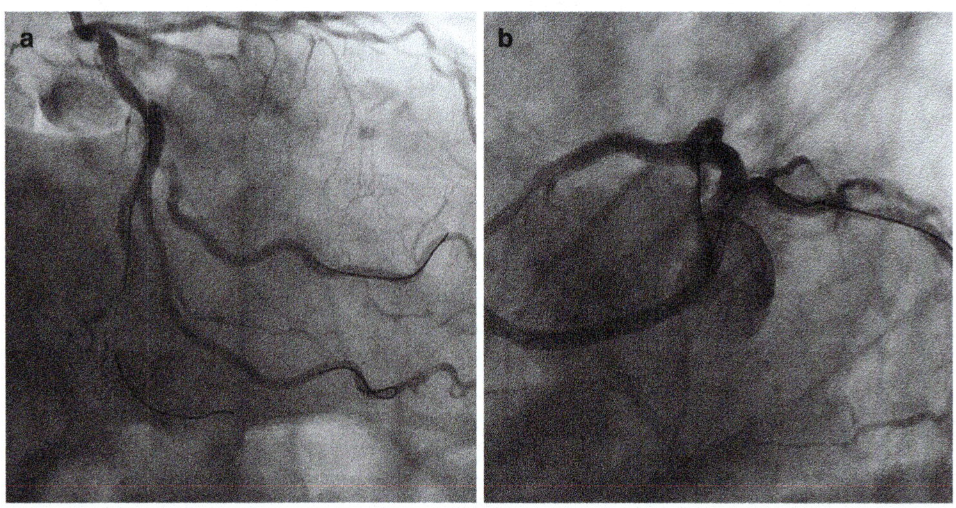

Fig. 2.45 Failure to cross the stent through the most distal cell at the SB. (**a**) After stenting the central vessel, dissection occurred in the left vessel and interfered with wiring it. The right vessel was very tortuous and also difficult to rewire. (**b**) The SB guidewire appeared to have crossed the stent into the SB through the most distal cell on coronary angiography, but IVUS showed it crossing the stent through a central cell. Using a suboptimal CAG projection led to this error

Removing a Jailed Guidewire

I limit the stent balloon inflation pressure to 14 atm so as to prevent failure to remove the jailed wire. I also limit the inflation pressure for POT (mentioned later) to 14 atm. A jailed guidewire should be removed after first withdrawing the Crusade catheter. Removing the jailed guidewire is usually easy, even after withdrawal of the Crusade catheter, although there is some resistance. If a jailed bare wire proves difficult to remove, you should advance a balloon catheter over the wire and position the balloon near the proximal edge of the stent (Fig. 2.46). The balloon may facilitate removal of the guidewire by reducing friction between the wire and the wall of the proximal MB and by helping the jailed part of the guidewire to become more coaxial with its proximal part.

With the aid of a balloon, you can usually remove a jailed guidewire without too much difficulty, but you may sometimes encounter great resistance. In this case, you should pull the guidewire back strongly without pushing the balloon in. By doing so, you can usually remove the guidewire without deforming the stent. However, when using a PROMUS Element stent, the proximal edge of the stent may be deformed by the tip of a balloon catheter advanced along the jailed guidewire. Some stent deformation patterns prevent introduction of a balloon into the MB stent. When removing a jailed guidewire, you should take care not to cause such stent deformation. To overcome this potential problem, I recommend introducing a balloon into the MB stent before removing the jailed guidewire (Fig. 2.46). Even if the MB stent becomes deformed, the previously introduced kissing balloon can still be inflated to achieve optimal stent apposition. Since balloons are absolutely required for subsequent KBI, introducing a balloon into the MB stent does not complicate the procedure; the only difference is whether the balloon is introduced before or after removal of the jailed guidewire.

a

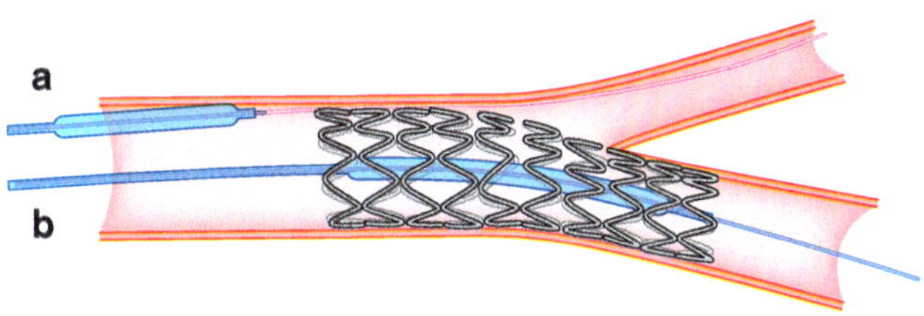

b

Fig. 2.46 Removing a jailed guidewire trapped by a stent. A balloon is advanced over the jailed guidewire (**a**) until it is close to the proximal end of the stent to facilitate removal of the guidewire. When the guidewire is pulled back, the balloon may be pushed into the stent and deform it. To avoid problems due to stent deformation, a balloon can be introduced into the MB stent (**b**) before removing the jailed guidewire. Even if the stent becomes deformed, the previously introduced balloon can still be inflated to achieve optimal stent apposition

Kissing Balloon Inflation (KBI)

To discuss the optimal size of the kissing balloons and the optimal inflation pressures for bifurcation stenting, let us consider the equations that can be used to predict the diameters of the MB and side branch(es) and to calculate the dilated diameter of the proximal MB after KBI.

Before performing KBI for bifurcation stenting, I have used the following equation to calculate the dilated diameter of the proximal MB after ballooning since around the mid-1990s:

1. Area conservation equation (Fig. 2.47)

$$r_p^2 = r_{d1}^2 + r_{d2}^2 + r_{d3}^2 + r_{d4}^2 + \cdots + r_{dn}^2,$$

where r_p is the diameter of the parent vessel and r_{dn} is the diameter of the *n*th daughter vessel.

This equation was not intended to accurately predict the diameter of one (parent) vessel from the known diameters of two (daughter) vessels. Instead, it shows that performing KBI for a bifurcation lesion always dilates the proximal MB to a diameter that can be calculated from the sum of the cross-sectional areas of the two balloons used. Neither this equation nor Murray's law (presented below) can accurately predict the actual diameter of a blood vessel in the body because the vessel may have undergone positive or negative remodeling and because vessel size does not change in precise units of 0.25 millimeters. I reiterate that KBI actually dilates the proximal MB to a diameter that can be calculated from the sum of the cross-sectional areas of the two balloons used. Therefore, if the proximal MB has a smaller diameter than the calculated diameter, you should inflate the kissing balloons at a low pressure or use undersized balloons for the MB and SB in order to prevent dissection of the proximal MB. On the other hand, if the proximal MB has a diameter equal to or larger than the calculated diameter, KBI may be performed at a relatively high pressure. The primary aim of using this equation is to raise awareness of the need to make such adjustments to the size of the kissing balloons and the balloon inflation pressure. It should be noted that Murray's law (presented below) is quite useless for this purpose. Indeed, this law is used to predict the normal diameter of each occluded vessel at a bifurcation CTO. Even in that case, the area conservation equation is needed to confirm whether the proximal MB can be safely dilated by kissing balloons of a size compatible with the predicted vessel diameters.

Needless to say, the optimal size of the balloon for POT should not be based on the theoretical (calculated) diameter of the proximal MB, but on the diameter observed by IVUS or optical coherence tomography (OCT). At a trifurcation, it is also easy to adjust the inflation pressures for triple KBI by

comparing the observed diameter of the proximal MB with its predicted diameter after dilatation calculated from the diameters of the three distal vessels measured by IVUS. If the observed diameter is greater than the predicted diameter, the inflation pressure should be about 10 atm. If the observed value is smaller than the predicted value, the kissing balloons should be inflated at a low pressure of about 6 atm.

For example, let us assume that triple KBI is planned for a trifurcation lesion involving the LAD, the high lateral branch (HL), and the LCX. If IVUS shows that the diameters of the three branches are 3.0, 2.5, and 2.5 mm, respectively, the dilated LMT diameter triple KBI can be calculated as follows:

$$\sqrt{3^2 + 2.5^2 + 2.5^2} = \sqrt{9 + 6.25 + 6.25} = \sqrt{21.5} \approx 4.64.$$

Assuming that the LMT diameter is measured as 4.7 mm by IVUS, POT may be performed by inflating a 4.5-mm balloon at a high pressure (14–20 atm), and triple KBI can be performed at standard pressure (8–10 atm). On the other hand, if the LMT diameter is 4.4 mm, POT should be performed by inflating a 4.5 mm balloon at a lower pressure (≤10 atm), and triple KBI should be done by inflating 2.25 mm balloons in the HL and LCX and a 3.0 mm balloon in the LAD at the standard pressure (8–10 atm) ($\sqrt{2.25^2 + 2.25^2 + 3^2} = \sqrt{19.13} \approx 4.4$). If the three kissing balloons are 3, 2.5, and 2.5 mm in diameter, respectively, balloon inflation should be done at a low pressure of about 6 atm.

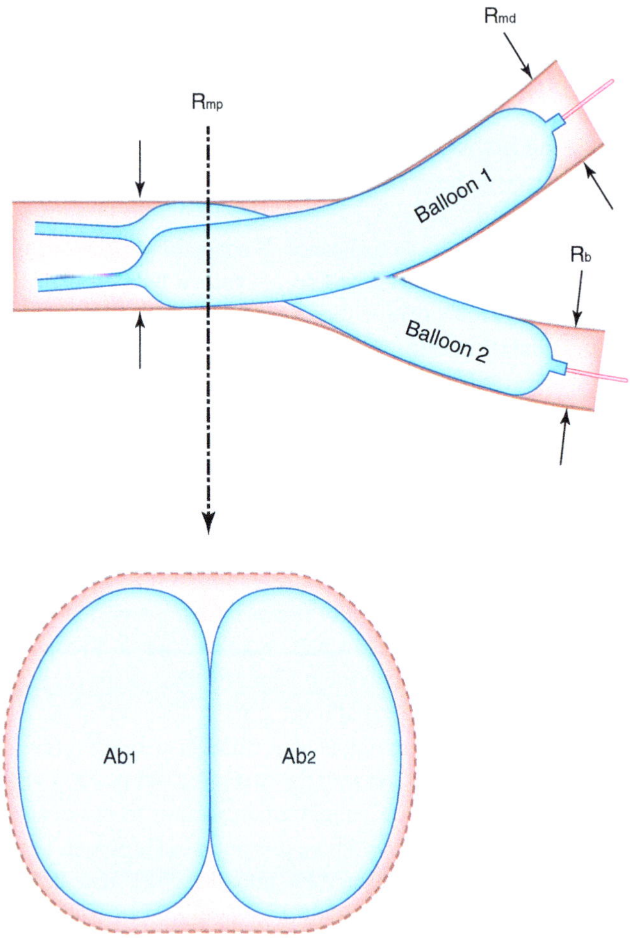

Fig. 2.47 Area conservation equation: $R_{mp}^2 = R_{md}^2 + R_b^2$. R_{mp} diameter of the proximal main vessel; R_{dn} diameter of the *n*th daughter branch. $R_p^2 = R_{d1}^2 + R_{d2}^2$; R_{md} diameter of the distal main vessel; R_b diameter of the side branch. Ab1 Area of balloon1. Ab2 Area of balloon2

2. Murray's law (Table 2.2)

Murray's law describes the diameters of a bifurcated tube with a certain rheological friction coefficient that is used to model a bifurcated human vessel. The equation is:

$$r_{\mathrm{p}}^{(7/3)} = r_{\mathrm{d1}}^{(7/3)} + r_{\mathrm{d2}}^{(7/3)} + r_{\mathrm{d3}}^{(7/3)} + r_{\mathrm{d4}}^{(7/3)} + \cdots + r_{\mathrm{dn}}^{(7/3)}.$$

where r_{p} is the diameter of the parent vessel and r_{dn} is the diameter of the nth daughter vessel.

If there are only two daughter vessels, the equation can be simplified as follows:

$$r_{\mathrm{mp}} = 0.67\left(r_{\mathrm{md}} + r_{\mathrm{b}}\right).$$

where r_{mp} is the diameter of the proximal MB, r_{md} is the diameter of the distal MB, and r_{b} is the diameter of the SB.

However, I measure the diameters of the individual vessels by IVUS and OCT to determine the size of each balloon for POT and KBI, and I never used this formula to estimate them.

Murray's law is also impracticable for triple KBI because it requires complicated calculations. It is quite doubtful that such theoretical values can be useful for bifurcation stenting. The actual size of a patient's vessel is not always rheologically optimal and often tends to be suboptimal due to vascular remodeling and plaque deposition. Despite these reservations, I will discuss the use of this formula for predicting vessel size at a bifurcation before KBI.

According to Table 2.2, a vessel branching into two daughter vessels of equal diameter (3.5 mm) is predicted to have a diameter of 4.7 mm immediately upstream of the bifurcation ($4.7^{(7/3)} = 37.00 \approx 37.20$).

KBI with two 3.5-mm balloons can be predicted to dilate the proximal MB to a diameter of 5.0 mm as follows:

$$\sqrt{3.5^2 + 3.5^2} = \sqrt{24.50} \approx \sqrt{25.0} = 5.0\ (\mathrm{mm}).$$

Even if the diameter of the proximal MB is observed to be 4.7 mm, the same as that predicted by Murray's law, should KBI be performed using two 3.5-mm balloons?

Based on the area conservation equation, it would be recommended to gradually inflate the two kissing balloons at a low pressure or to downsize one balloon to 3.25 mm in order to prevent injury to the proximal MB. This is why I recommend using the area conservation equation to predict the dilated diameter of the proximal MB, rather than using a formula that just predicts the size of the MB at a bifurcation.

Table 2.2 Predicted size of the main vessel according to Murray's law

f_{as}	2.25	2.5	2.75	3.0	3.25	3.5	3.75	4.0	4.5
	6.63	8.43	10.60	12.98	15.65	18.60	21.85	25.40	33.43
2.25	13.26	15.11	17.23	19.61	22.28	25.23	28.48	32.03	40.06
2.5		16.96	19.08	21.46	24.13	27.08	30.33	33.88	41.91
2.75			21.20	23.58	26.25	29.20	32.45	36.00	44.03
3.0				25.96	28.63	31.58	34.83	38.38	46.41
3.25					31.30	34.25	37.50	41.05	49.03
3.5						37.20	40.05	44.00	52.03
3.75							43.70	47.25	55.28
4.0								50.80	58.83
4.5									68.86
5.0	42.75								
5.5	53.40								
6.0	65.42								

Delivery of Kissing Balloons

1. As kissing balloons, use a high-pressure balloon for the MB and a balloon with a small soft tip for the SB. For reasons of medical economy, the balloons that were employed for pre-dilatation are generally reused.
2. In principle, the balloon for the MB is delivered first and then the balloon for the SB. This is because the MB stent may be deformed during delivery of the SB balloon, and such deformation may preclude subsequent delivery of the MB balloon. Another reason is that the MB balloon can be used to assist delivery of the SB balloon. While introducing a balloon into the stent, you should take care to prevent unnecessary deformation of the stent struts by the tip of the balloon or its irregular surface. This is particularly important for 2-link stents that are prone to deformation, such as the PROMUS Element and Nobori stents.
3. If the MB balloon cannot be delivered, you should clarify whether this is because the balloon tip is being blocked by the edge of the stent or because of excessive friction between the shoulder or body of the balloon and the stent. You can easily distinguish between these two causes. If the distal balloon marker is several millimeters from the stent edge, the first cause is more likely, while if the balloon marker is very close to the stent edge, the tip of the balloon must have entered the stent and the second cause is more likely.

(1) Blocking of the Balloon Tip by the Stent Edge

To deliver a balloon into a stent, you should push the balloon very gently and advance it very slowly. If the proximal edge of the stent is in the proximal part of an ostium or at a vessel angle, the tip of a kissing balloon or a post-dilatation balloon may be blocked by the stent edge so that the balloon cannot be advanced with minimal force. However, an attempt to forcibly advance the balloon can easily lead to stent deformation. This risk is particularly high when the stent shows suboptimal apposition in a proximal MB with a large diameter (before POT or KBI). If the balloon is advanced rapidly, it can deform the stent immediately on coming into contact with it. Stent deformation induced by the balloon may be mild, such as slight disturbance of the stent strut configuration. However, the balloon can elevate one or more stent struts, which may further inhibit balloon delivery and could possibly result in catastrophic stent deformation. Continued attempts to advance the balloon may also cause similar severe deformation of the stent. To successfully deliver a blocked balloon into the stent without deforming the stent struts, you can use any of the following procedures:

1. Pull the balloon back to straighten the balloon shaft and then push it in slightly. Never continue to push it strongly into the stent.
2. Change the orientation of the guiding catheter to separate the balloon tip from the stent.
3. Pull the balloon back a little (to straighten the guidewire) and then immediately push it forward slightly.
4. Use the buddy wire technique (Fig. 2.48a).
5. Use the buddy balloon technique (Fig. 2.48b).
6. If even the buddy balloon technique is ineffective, keep the buddy balloon in place and exchange the kissing balloon for a new low-profile balloon.

(2) Friction Between the Shoulder or Body of the Balloon and the Stent

If the balloon has been used for pre-dilatation, you should withdraw it into the guiding catheter and inflate it at about 10 atm inside the catheter. Then immediately deflate the balloon and advance it into the stent again. If this procedure fails to deliver the balloon, you should completely remove the balloon and rewrap it. If the rewrapped balloon still cannot be delivered, you should try the buddy wire technique (Fig. 2.48a). After failure of this technique, you should use the buddy balloon technique (Fig. 2.48b). The buddy balloon technique rarely fails, but if it does, you should exchange the balloon for a new low-profile balloon.

4. If the SB balloon cannot be delivered, never try to push it into the stent forcibly either. When advancing a balloon across the stent into the SB, take great care as it often causes severe strut deformation if it becomes stuck. This is particularly the case with a stent having few (or no) links, which is prone to marked deformation. Use a balloon with a small soft tip for the SB. Considering the possible need for rewrapping, choose a balloon that is easy to rewrap. Anchoring is not recommended, or rather is contraindicated, for delivering a balloon into a stent with 0 to 2 links. Anchoring reinforces backup of the balloon and allows it to be pushed too strongly, inducing stent deformation.
5. If the tip of the SB balloon is blocked by a stent strut (the distal balloon marker is far from the stent carina), you should inflate the MB balloon to a high pressure. This will achieve better stent deployment and apposition, facilitating delivery of the balloon into the SB. If this method fails, check whether the balloon tip has become frayed (see (8)).

6. If the tip of the SB balloon has crossed the stent struts, but its shoulder is blocked, you should inflate the two balloons at a low pressure (about 6 atm) by using the hugging balloon technique. After deflating them, gently advance the SB balloon (Fig. 2.49), and it will often cross the stent struts. Several inflation/deflation cycles of the two hugging balloons may allow gradual advancement of the SB balloon.
7. Repeated dilatation of the proximal MB by a large-diameter balloon (POT) using the MB guidewire can facilitate delivery of the SB balloon.
8. If the tip of the SB balloon cannot cross the stent struts, withdraw the balloon and check whether its tip has become frayed (Fig. 2.50). Fraying is often too small to identify by visual inspection. Continued use of a balloon with a frayed tip will worsen the fraying. Forcibly pushing such a balloon forward will cause its tip to spread open, further exacerbating the difficulty in achieving smooth advancement and increasing the risk of stent deformation (one reason that anchoring the balloon is contraindicated in bifurcation lesions). If fraying is identified, never reuse the balloon without cutting off the frayed tip (about 0.3 mm) by using sharp scissors. This markedly improves deliverability of the balloon, although it removes part of the tapered tip, which suggests that fraying of the balloon catheter tip poses a major impediment to delivery across a stent. Although cutting off the tip of a device is not officially recommended, I often do this to avoid using a new balloon catheter for reasons of medical economy.

   A balloon catheter may become frayed at its tip while crossing stent struts, as well as when it is advanced through a CTO. As shown in Fig. 2.50, I cut the balloon catheter tip at right angles, not obliquely to the shaft, for the reason explained in Fig. 2.51. Although it might seem that a balloon catheter with an obliquely cut tip will be easier to advance, the resulting angle at the tip is usually oriented toward the larger curvature of the guidewire during advancement of the catheter (Fig. 2.51a). Due to lack of support from the contralateral side, the leading edge of the cut tip tends to lift away from the guidewire, so the angled tip is more likely to get stuck on a stent strut and subsequently become more severely frayed. Theoretically, a balloon catheter with an obliquely cut tip can easily cross a stent if it is advanced gently and is pulled back slightly and rotated at about 180 degrees before attempting readvancement after getting stuck (Fig. 2.51b). However, it is uncertain whether a balloon catheter that has become stuck can actually be rotated appropriately in practice.

   Although the tip of a rotatable balloon catheter may be cut off obliquely, balloon catheters are generally difficult to rotate. Therefore, I always cut off the tip of the balloon catheter at right angles to its shaft.
9. If the balloon catheter still cannot cross the stent struts after its frayed tip has been cut off, exchange it for a new one.
10. If the new balloon catheter also cannot cross the stent, it is highly probable that the guidewire has not passed through an appropriate cell. While keeping the guidewire in place, try SB rewiring with a second guidewire along a new route with the aid of a Crusade catheter. Then advance a balloon catheter along the second guidewire that has crossed the stent through a different cell to deliver it into the SB. If the first guidewire actually crossed the stent through an appropriate cell and the second guidewire has passed through the same cell (although this cannot be verified by coronary angiography), the buddy wire technique may be effective. Therefore, slowly advance the balloon catheter along the second guidewire. This technique may be more effective if the first guidewire is pushed in slightly. If the buddy wire technique also fails (although it is rare), the last possibility is to deliver the smallest-diameter balloon into the SB. After dilating the cell by inflating the balloon, it should be exchanged for a larger balloon.

In summary, when delivering a balloon into the SB, never push the balloon forward forcibly so as to prevent stent strut deformation and never use the anchor technique.

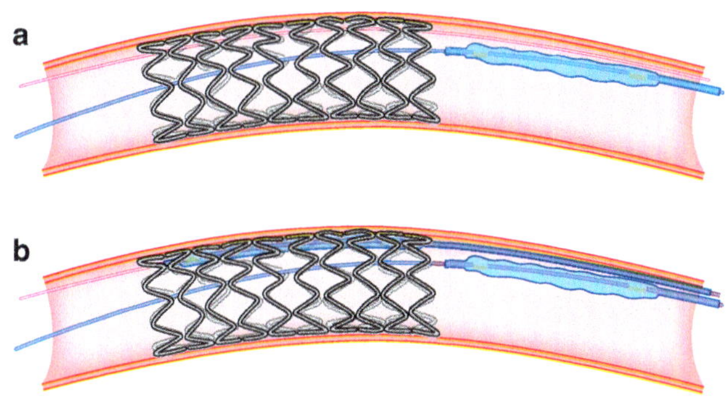

Fig. 2.48 Buddy wire technique (**a**) and buddy balloon technique (**b**). (**a**) Introduction of a new guidewire changes the environment for the balloon tip and/or reduces friction between the balloon and the stent struts. (**b**) If the buddy wire technique fails, advance a new balloon with good deliverability over the buddy wire. This facilitates delivery of the second balloon

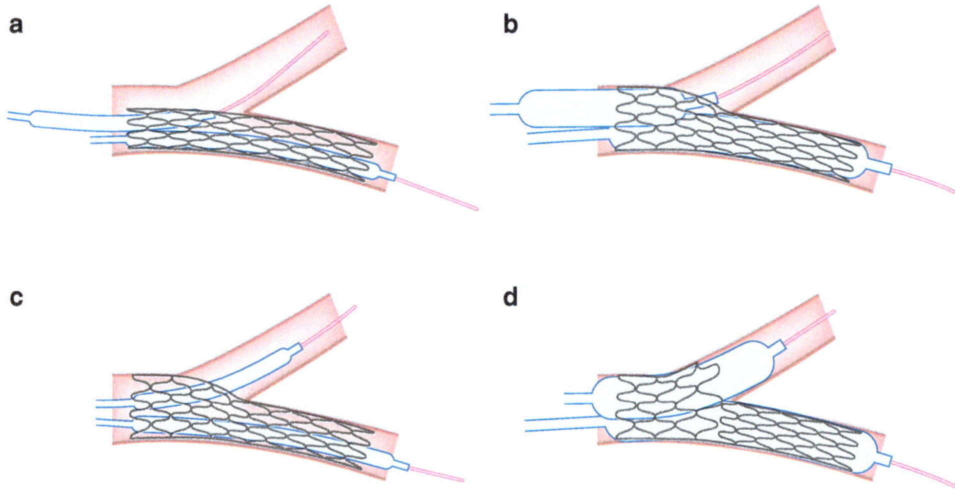

Fig. 2.49 Handling an SB balloon that has failed to cross the MB stent (hugging balloon technique). (**a**) The SB balloon cannot cross the MB stent. (**b**) SB and MB balloons are inflated at about 6 atm using the hugging balloon technique. Ensure that the proximal marker of the MB balloon is located at the proximal edge of the stent, because dissection may occur in the proximal MB if the two balloons overlap outside the stent. (**c**) After both balloons are deflated, the SB balloon can often readily cross the stent into the SB. (**d**) Performing KBI

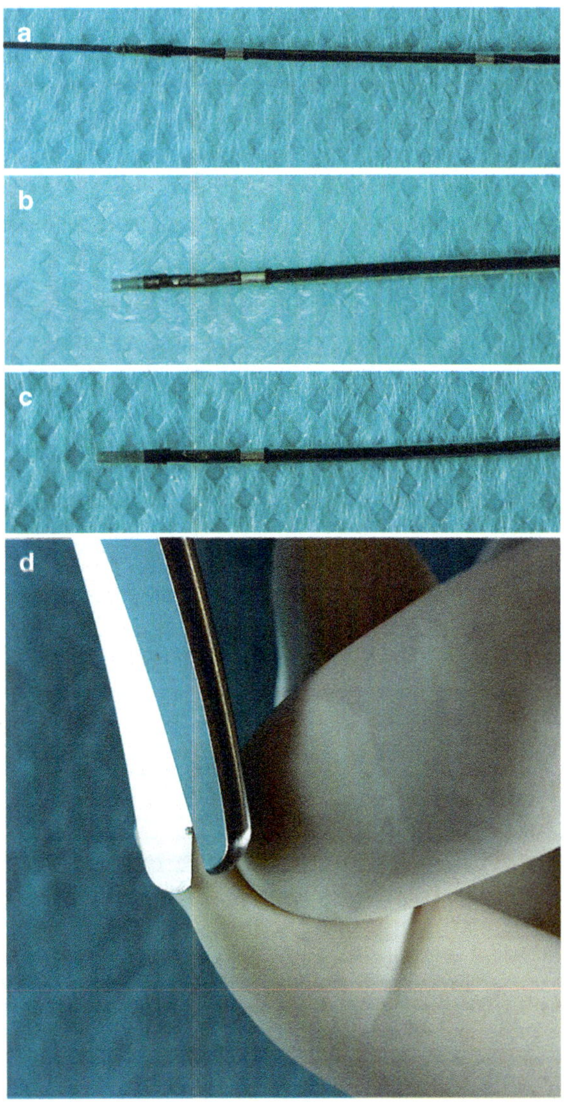

Fig. 2.50 Countermeasures for a frayed balloon tip. (**a**) The tip of a balloon catheter has become frayed and deformed. (**b**) The frayed tip (about 0.3 mm) has been cut off a balloon catheter, so it has lost its tapered end compared with an intact catheter (**c**). (**c**) The tip end of a new balloon catheter that has been chamfered modestly. (**d**) Using Cooper scissors to cut off the tip of a balloon catheter

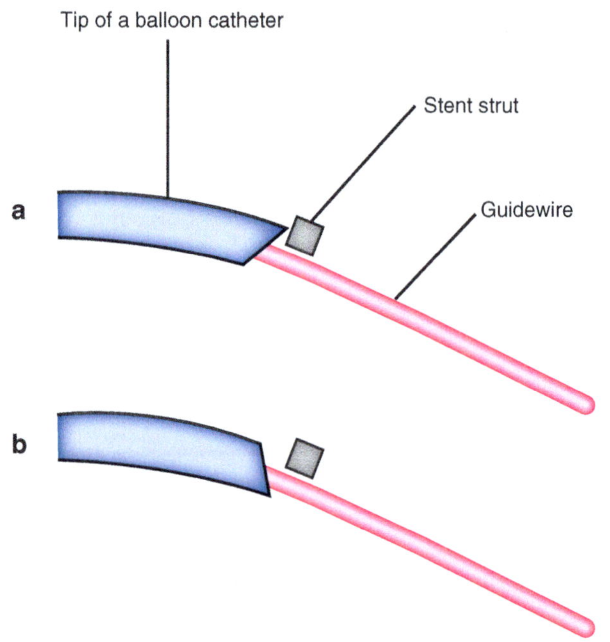

Fig. 2.51 Balloon catheter with the tip cut obliquely. If the angle at the balloon tip is oriented toward the lateral side (larger curvature) of the guidewire during advancement of the balloon, the leading edge is more likely to get stuck on a stent strut and become severely frayed (**a**). A balloon catheter with an obliquely cut tip should be advanced gently. If it becomes stuck, it should be pulled back slightly and rotated about 180 degrees before attempting readvancement (**b**). In practice, a balloon catheter often cannot be rotated appropriately

Column 16 Balloon Rewrapping

To reduce resistance to the irregular surface of a rewrapped balloon, you should minimize irregularity by using the protective sheath to cover the balloon as follows. Insert the stylet introducer for the sheath into the balloon catheter from its tip under negative pressure, and slide the sheath over the balloon from the tip to reduce its profile. Rotate the sheath while sliding it over the balloon to prevent balloon deformation and to facilitate coverage with the sheath

Column 17 Importance of the Correct Fluoroscopy Angle

When confirming the position of the tip of the SB balloon, it is important to use a projection that allows en face observation of the bifurcation. For example, the LAD-Dg bifurcation must be viewed in the LAO cranial projection, and not in the RAO cranial projection. As shown in Fig. 2.52, the distal marker of the balloon appears to be well past the carina in the LAO cranial view but is only just beyond the carina in the RAO cranial view. It is very important to decide whether or not the balloon tip has passed the carina because this determines the subsequent procedures.

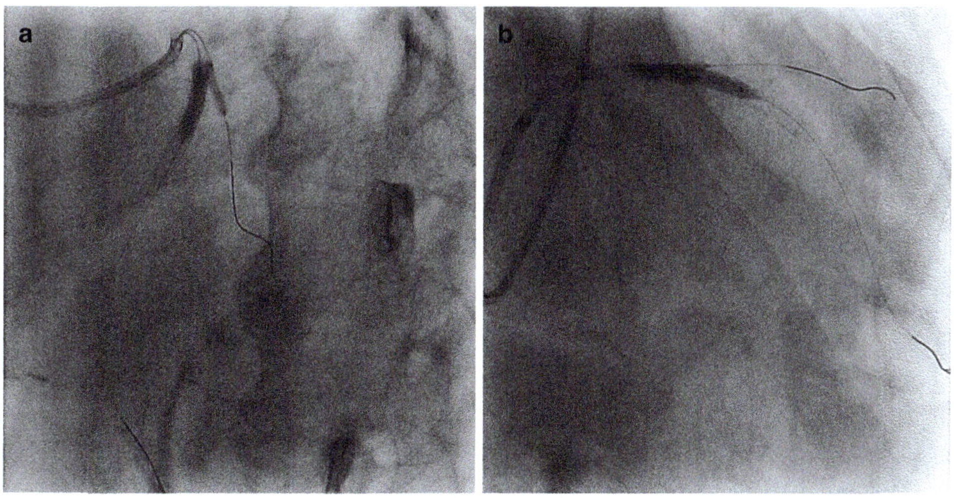

Fig. 2.52 Views obtained in different projections. The distal marker of the balloon appears to be well past the carina in the LAO cranial view (**a**) but is only just beyond the carina in the RAO cranial view (**b**)

Balloon Inflation

1. Initially inflate the kissing balloons at a relatively low pressure of about 8 to 10 atm to expand the stent into a shape compatible with the bifurcation (Fig. 2.53).
2. If the proximal MB has not been dilated with a large-diameter balloon (POT), the proximal ends of the two kissing balloons must be positioned at or proximal to the proximal edge of the MB stent, and the two balloons must not overlap beyond the proximal edge of the stent (Fig. 2.54). If the proximal ends of the two kissing balloons are distal to the proximal edge of the stent, inflation will lead to suboptimal expansion and malapposition of the proximal part of the stent (Fig. 2.54e). Also, the balloon surfaces will become irregular after inflation and deflation, so a balloon may get stuck in the proximal part of the stent and deform it during subsequent withdrawal of the two balloons.
3. After KBI, only inflate the SB balloon at a sufficient pressure to dilate the SB ostium.
4. Perform final KBI at a relatively low pressure.

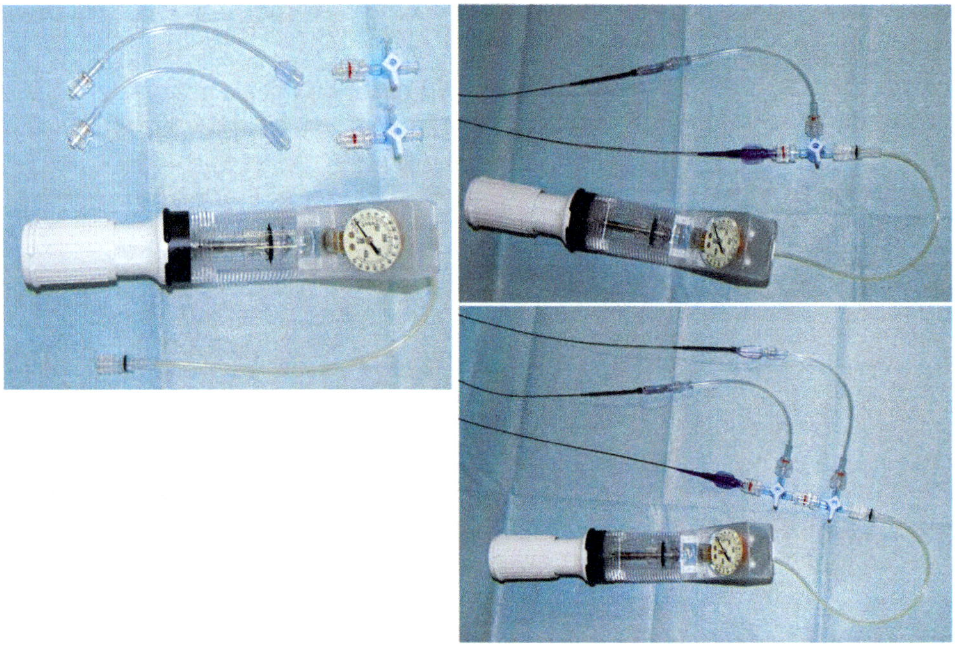

Fig. 2.53 Kissing balloon inflation using a male-male connector. Use of a male-male connector with KBI permits synchronous inflation and deflation of multiple (2–3) balloons at equal pressures. This is a cost- and labor-saving procedure, since the interventionalist can operate the indeflator without an assistant.

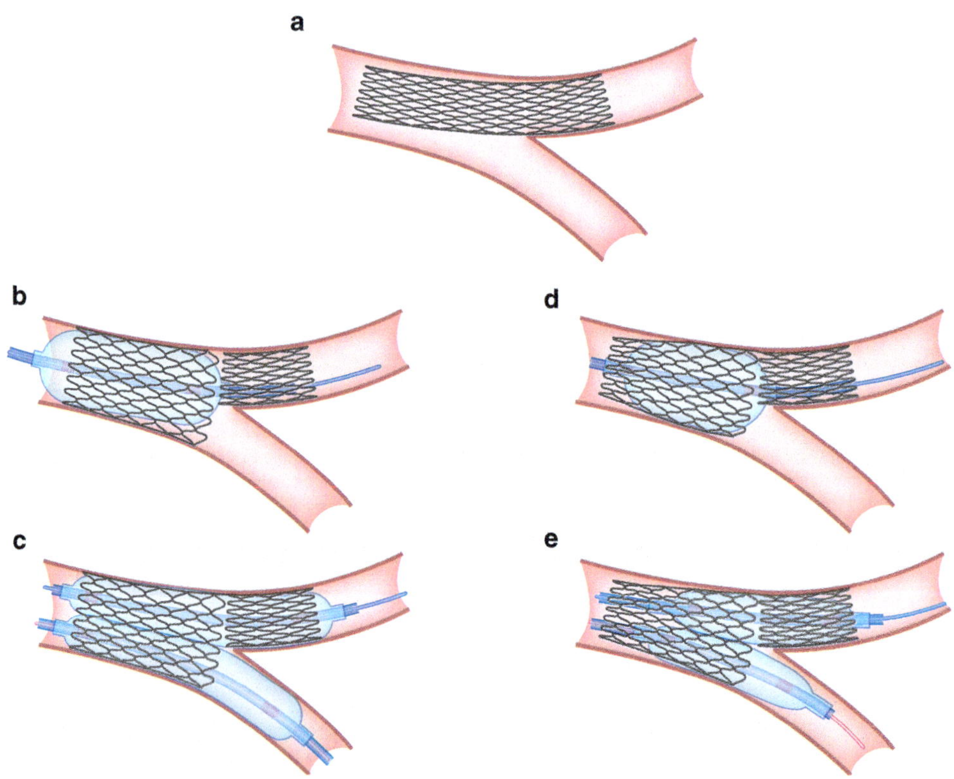

Fig. 2.54 Dilating a bifurcation and the proximal MB. When performing POT (**a**), the proximal end of the balloon must be proximal to the proximal edge of the stent (**b**). After optimal POT, KBI could be performed adequately (**c**). If the proximal part of the stent undergoes suboptimal expansion (**d** or **e**), one or both balloons may get stuck on malapposed stent struts and deform the stent during withdrawal after inflation and deflation. If a short balloon cannot sufficiently expand the distal part of the stent and cannot be advanced into the stent, it should be withdrawn and rewrapped before attempting readvancement

Proximal Optimization Technique

The proximal optimization technique (POT) refers to dilating the proximal MB by inflating an optimally sized balloon in a stent placed from the proximal MB to the distal MB or the SB (Fig. 2.55).

The diameter of the proximal MB may be too large compared with the diameters of the distal MB and SB to achieve optimal stent apposition in the proximal MB by only inflating a stent delivery balloon. In such cases, you should inflate a balloon of the optimal size for the proximal MB only in this segment (POT), and then perform SB rewiring before KBI. Performing POT will prevent deformation of the proximal part of the stent by KBI. Ensure that the stent is positioned to cover more than 6 mm of the proximal MB. To minimize damage to the MB segment proximal to the proximal edge of the stent, the balloon should only be inflated within the stent and should not overlap the stent into the proximal MB. Therefore, it is better for the stent in the proximal MB to be longer than the shortest balloon currently available.

It is not always easy to achieve optimal positioning of the balloon for POT. If a balloon with a tapered tip is used, it can over-dilate and injure the ostium of the distal MB. A sandbag-shaped balloon with a less tapered tip should be used and positioned so that its distal marker is just proximal to the carina (Fig. 2.56). Even if slight stent malapposition occurs near the carina, subsequent KBI can optimize apposition at this site (which originally had an elliptical lumen).

a
b
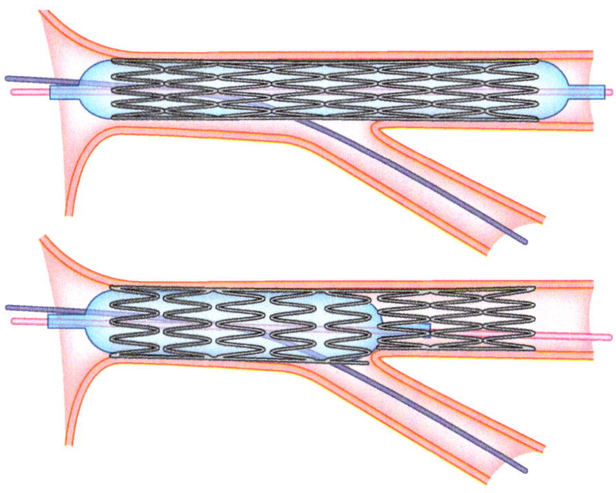

Fig. 2.55 Proximal optimization technique (POT). (**a**) A stent placed in the MB may not show optimal apposition in the proximal MB if the diameter of the vessel is too large. (**b**) Subsequent inflation of a balloon with the correct size for the proximal MB only in this segment can achieve optimal stent expansion and apposition. If the patient has a non-ostial lesion, the balloon should be inflated to a diameter compatible with the stent landing zone in the proximal MB, while it should be inflated to the diameter of the proximal MB for an ostial lesion. If there is a jailed guidewire, the inflation pressure should not exceed 14 atm, in principle

a
b
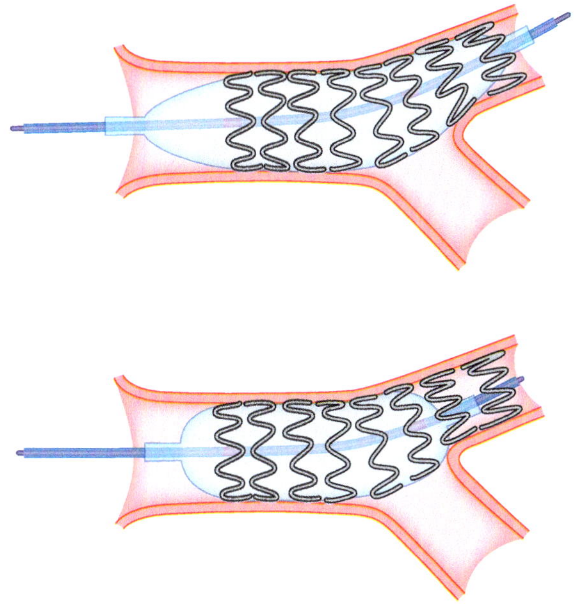

Fig. 2.56 Balloons suitable for POT. (**a**) A balloon with a tapered tip can injure the ostium of the distal MB because its tip may enter this segment. (**b**) A sandbag-shaped balloon with a less tapered tip is suitable for POT

Column 18 Necessity of Performing POT and KBI

When bifurcation stenting using POT is performed according to the following procedure, there may seem to be no need for KBI.

1. Implant a stent compatible with the diameter of the distal MB using the MB crossover technique.
2. Perform POT.
3. Perform SB wiring.
4. Dilate only the SB ostium.

However, I object to this procedure for the following reasons:

- While better mid-term outcomes have been reported for some stents (e.g., Cypher) without KBI than with KBI, this does not mean that KBI should be absolutely avoided even with such stents.
- KBI should be performed proactively if the stent design permits culotte or provisional stenting to salvage a compromised SB after KBI and if the long-term outcome of PCI will be better than without KBI
- When employing KBI, the optimal stent needs to be selected and placed as sophisticatedly as possible in order to safely accomplish optimal bifurcation stenting.

The disadvantages of not using KBI should also be considered, since bifurcation stenting without KBI theoretically has the following disadvantages:

- Performing POT does not ensure optimal stent apposition at the carina and does not completely eliminate SB jailing. If the POT balloon impinges on the distal MB, performing POT can cause carina shift toward the SB and injury of the distal MB. The outcome of stenting plus POT alone is markedly different from that of optimal bifurcation stenting.
- Can these issues be overcome without performing KBI by only dilating the SB, i.e., by opening a cell for SB access with a very short balloon? Even if inflating a very short balloon can achieve optimal dilatation of the SB ostium, the contralateral stent struts at the carina will be drawn toward the SB, just as when the SB is dilated by a long balloon (Fig. 2.57). Optimal stent apposition cannot be achieved without dilating the ostium of the distal MB.
- The risk of complications associated with KBI can be minimized by using a 2-link stent, by wiring the SB through the most distal cell at the carina, and by optimizing the sizes of the kissing balloons and their inflation pressures.

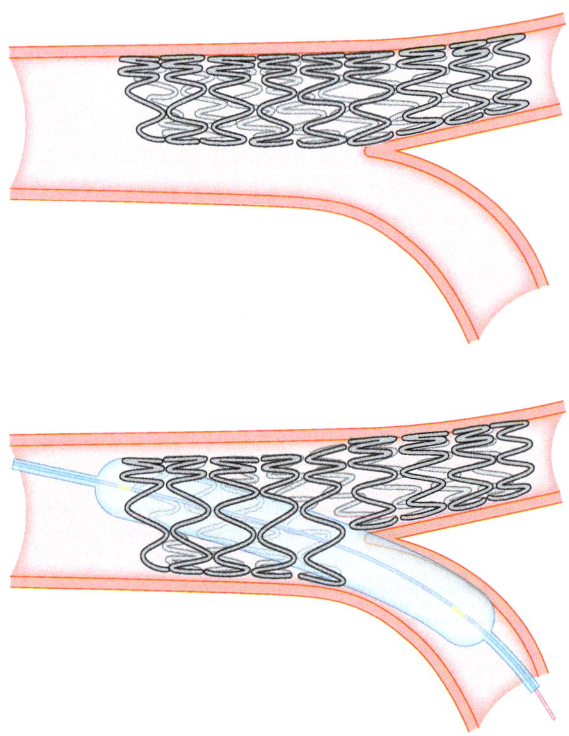

Fig. 2.57 Dilating only the SB with a balloon after stent implantation. This procedure results in malapposition of the contralateral stent struts

Confirmation of Jailing and SB Rewiring

1. IVUS

IVUS is the best method to check for jailing after KBI. You should advance an IVUS catheter into the MB and estimate the extent of stent jailing from the edge of the carina. If it is within 1 mm, jailing may be considered acceptable. If it exceeds 1.5 mm, you should always perform SB rewiring.

2. SB rewiring using a Crusade catheter
   - Crusade catheter advanced over the MB guidewire (Fig. 2.58)

You should advance a Crusade catheter over the MB guidewire while maintaining the SB guidewire as a landmark. To ensure that the probing guidewire goes through a cell just distal to the landmark guidewire, you should pull the landmark wire back slightly and bring it into contact with the proximal rim of the cell after placing its radiolucent part at the SB ostium. Then you should pull the probing guidewire back very gently and stop. If the probing guidewire is distal to the landmark guidewire and if the two wires are not in contact with each other, it is highly probable that the probing guidewire has crossed the stent through a cell at least one strut more distal to that of the landmark guidewire.

   - Crusade catheter advanced over the SB guidewire (Fig. 2.59)

You should advance a Crusade catheter over the SB guidewire (landmark) while keeping the probing guidewire within the catheter. After confirming smooth entry of the Crusade into the SB, you should withdraw it so that the side hole is in the proximal MB and then advance the probing guidewire into the distal MB. Subsequently, you should pull the guidewire back while orienting its tip toward the SB and try to insert it into the SB through a more distal cell. When the guidewire just enters the SB, you should advance the Crusade a little. If the probing guidewire has crossed the stent through a different cell from that of the landmark guidewire, there will be at least one strut between the tip of the Crusade and the probing guidewire delivered through its side hole, and this will prevent advancement of the catheter beyond the carina. If the Crusade catheter does not go beyond the carina, the probing guidewire may be considered to have crossed the stent through a cell at least one strut more distal to that of the landmark guidewire. If the probing guidewire has crossed the stent through the same cell as the landmark guidewire, the Crusade will readily go beyond the carina.

3. Final KBI

If SB rewiring through the most distal cell is considered to be highly probable, you should perform final KBI with balloons chosen as described above using the abovementioned technique.

4. IVUS

Then you should repeat IVUS to confirm that the extent of jailing is acceptable (≤1 mm).

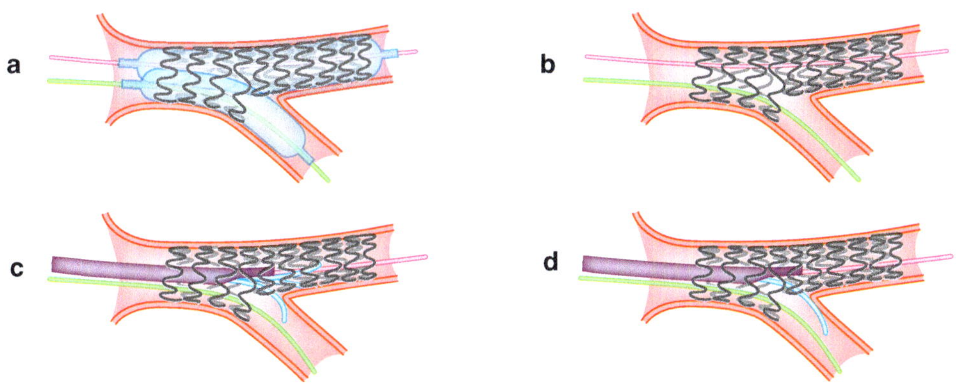

Fig. 2.58 SB rewiring using the Crusade microcatheter (advanced over the MB guidewire). (**a**) Kissing balloon technique for suboptimal side branch rewiring. (**b**) Side branch wire is in the more proximal cell (**c**) Advance a Crusade catheter over the MB guidewire to the distal MB and pull the probing guidewire back together with the catheter. (**d**) If the probing guidewire is distal to the landmark guidewire and if the two wires are not in contact with each other, it is highly probable that the probing guidewire has crossed the stent through a more distal cell

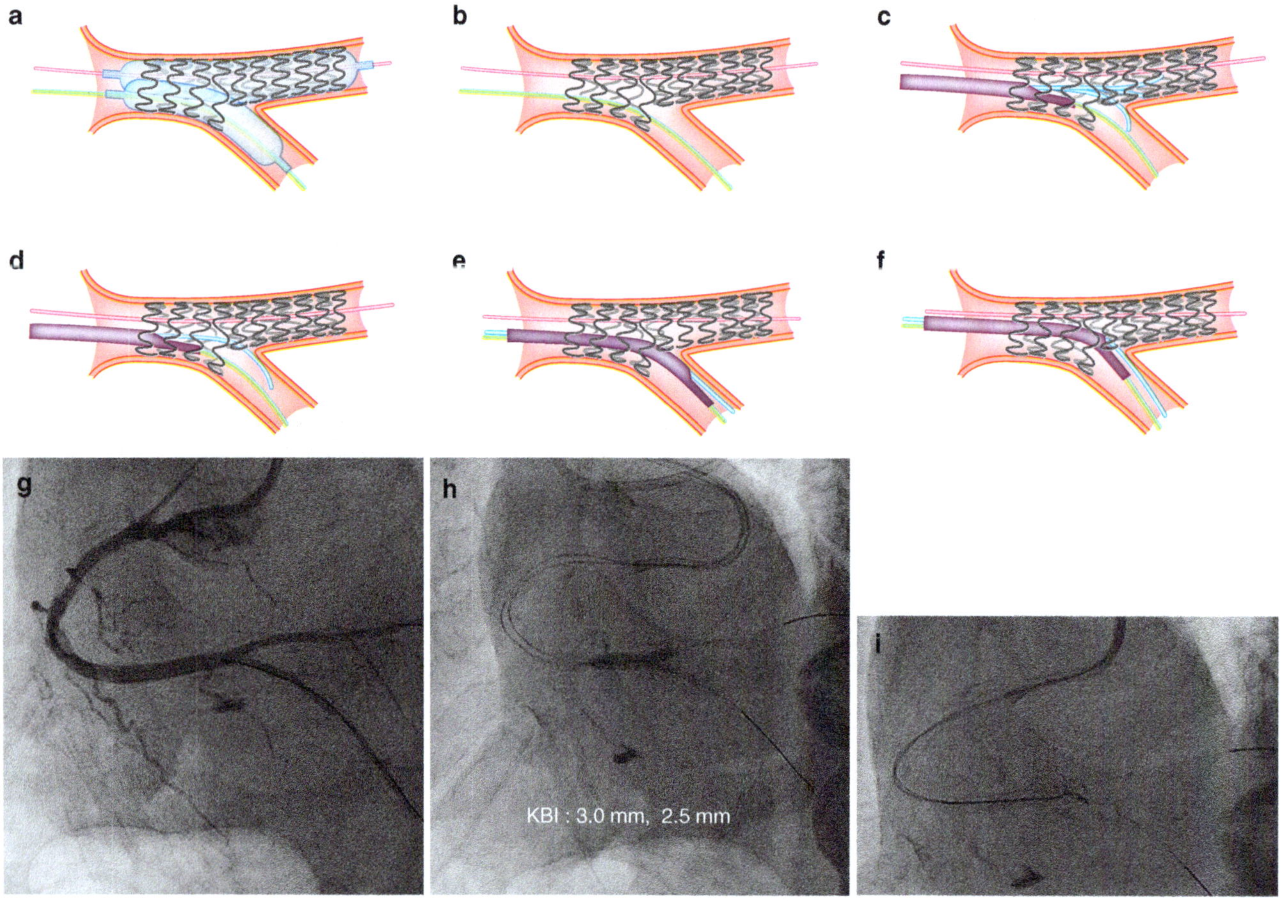

Fig. 2.59 SB rewiring using the Crusade microcatheter (advanced over the SB guidewire). (**a**) Kissing balloon technique for suboptimal side branch rewiring. (**b**) Side branch wire is in the more proximal cell. If the probing and landmark guidewires have crossed the stent through different cells (**c**, **d**), the Crusade catheter will never go beyond the carina (**f**). If the two guidewires have crossed the stent through the same cell, the Crusade will readily go beyond the carina (**e**). (**g**) SB rewiring after placing a stent from Segment 3 to Segment 4 in the RCA. (**h**) KBI. (**i**) To overcome severe jailing, SB rewiring is done with the aid of a Crusade catheter advanced over the SB guidewire

2.4 Ideal Double Stenting of Bifurcation Lesions

The controversy over the choice between single and double stenting is generally relevant to bifurcation lesions, for which both strategies appear to achieve equally good short-term outcomes. It is true that only double stenting can achieve favorable short-term results in some bifurcation lesions. What is the ideal double stenting method for bifurcation lesions? To achieve ideal double stenting for a bifurcation lesion, what stent design, wiring strategy, device strategy, and dilatation/deployment strategy should be used?

Section 2.2 of this chapter provides diagrams of the ideal scaffold for bifurcation lesions which also involve the SB (see Fig. 2.60 [p. XX]). Figure 2.60a depicts a single stent, as we cannot rule out the possibility that one stent may be optimal for bifurcation lesions. Although the figure legend does not specify whether this bifurcation scaffold can be constructed with one or two stents, at least two stents are needed currently, and two-stent or three-stent methods have been proposed for handling bifurcation lesions. Here, I will discuss how closely these methods correspond to the ideal method.

2.4.1 Comments on Various Two-Stent Methods

The key to procedural success with provisional T-stenting, modified T-stenting, mini-crush stenting, or sleeve stenting is to accurately position the SB stent without its struts entering the MB and without a gap between the two stents. One of the problems with all of these stenting techniques is creation of a gap between the stents, particularly at the shoulder of the SB. When performing provisional T-stenting, you can minimize the risk of creating such a gap by placing the SB stent

exactly from the SB ostium while maintaining the option to switch to culotte stenting if the proximal edge of the stent protrudes into the MB. With provisional or modified T-stenting, half of each strut ring in the proximal part of the SB stent loses the support of the vessel wall, which may reduce the radial strength of the stent (Fig. 2.60).

If provisional T-stenting is performed at a large (≥2.75 mm) bifurcation with a small SB take-off angle, some struts of the SB stent will show malapposition and fail to contribute to the radial strength of the stent (Fig. 2.61a). If both the MB and SB are small, the distal struts of the SB stent will protrude into the MB lumen more prominently relative to the MB diameter (Fig. 2.61b). If the branching angle is larger, protrusion of SB stent struts into the MB lumen becomes less prominent (Fig. 2.61c).

When the sleeve technique is used (Fig. 2.62), even if the distal struts of the SB stent protruding into the MB lumen are pressing on the MB wall, the struts oblique to the MB stent may lose radial strength because the SB stent cannot show optimal apposition to the walls of the SB while maintaining its original zigzag structure (Fig. 2.62b). At the ostium of the SB, it is highly probable that the struts of the SB stent have been distorted (Fig. 2.62c). This is particularly likely if there is a calcified lesion at the ostium of the SB.

With the V-stenting (SKS) technique, each stent will always have insufficient radial strength in the proximal MB. The principle of this technique also prevents optimal stent apposition (Fig. 2.63).

Culotte stenting (Fig. 2.64) is a relatively simple technique, which involves two cycles of stenting with KBI. However, interventionalists often seem to think that this technique is complicated and thus avoid it. Although the two stents overlap in the proximal MB, proper deployment of optimally designed stents will achieve complete stent apposition and adequate radial strength while avoiding MB/SB jailing. Therefore, culotte stenting is a near-optimal strategy for bifurcation stenting.

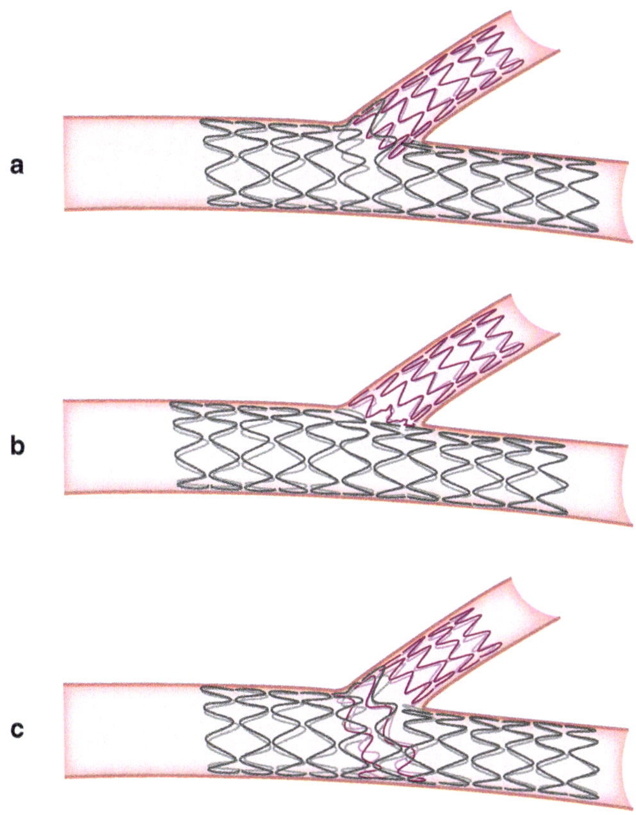

Fig. 2.60 Provisional T-stenting (**a**), modified T-stenting (**b**), and culotte stenting (**c**). With provisional or modified T-stenting, the stent may lose radial strength on the contralateral side

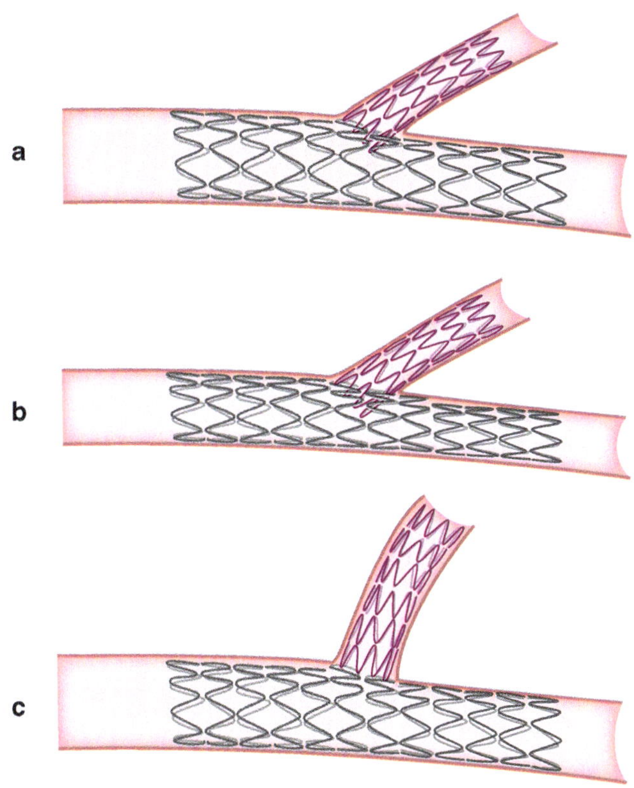

Fig. 2.61 Various T-stenting patterns. (**a**) If the bifurcation has a small SB take-off angle, the SB stent struts protruding into the MB lumen are unable to contribute to the radial strength of the stent. (**b**) If the bifurcation has a small MB and small SB, struts from the SB stent will protrude into the MB lumen more prominently relative to the MB diameter. (**c**) If the bifurcation has a large SB take-off angle, protrusion of SB stent struts into the MB lumen becomes less prominent

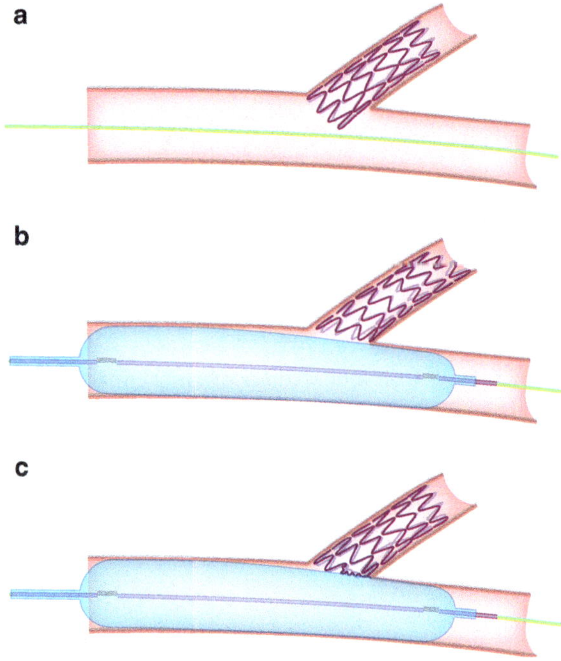

Fig. 2.62 Sleeve stenting. (**a**) Side branch stent is protruded to main vessel. After the stent is returned to the SB, it is unlikely to preserve its zigzag strut structure (**b**) and is likely to have been distorted (**c**)

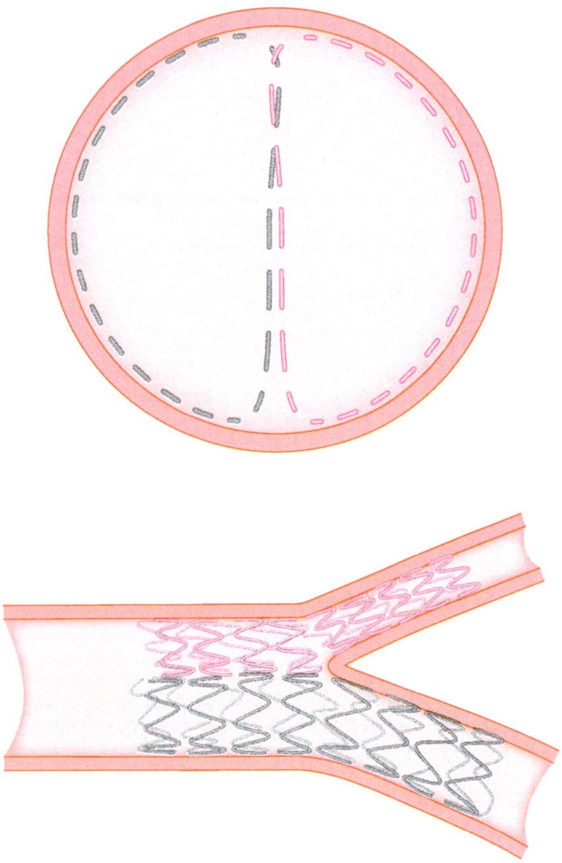

Fig. 2.63 V-stenting. The radial strength of each stent is very low as it depends on the strength of the contralateral stent struts.

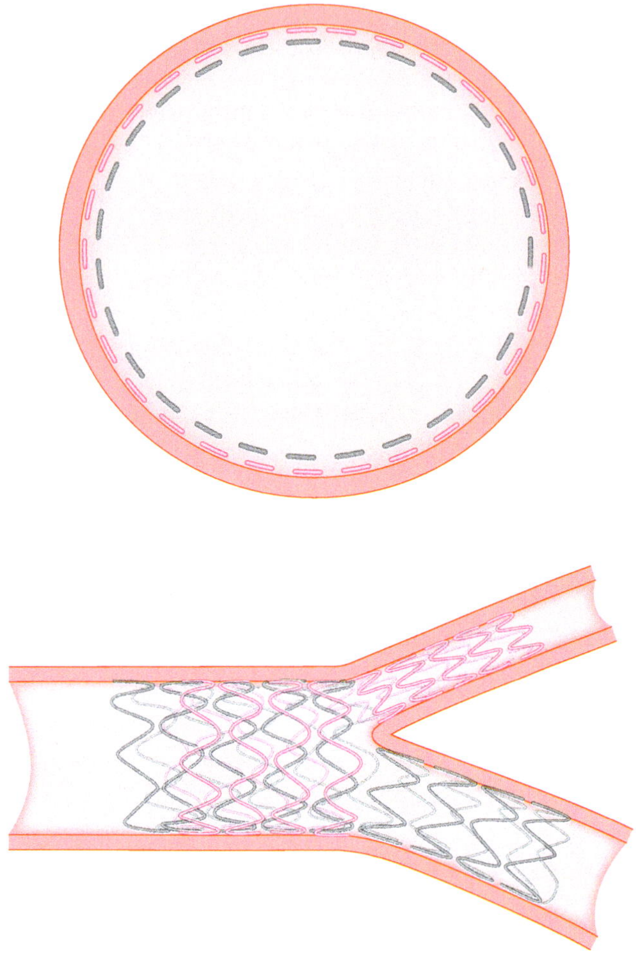

Fig. 2.64 Culotte stenting. Culotte stenting allows complete stent apposition and preserves high radial strength of both stents.

2.4.2 Culotte (Y) Stenting

2.4.2.1 Indications for Culotte Stenting

1. A true bifurcation lesion where stenting with KBI has caused SB dissection with a risk of occlusion or restenosis or significant SB stenosis due to plaque or carina shift.
2. A bifurcation lesion with an extreme SB take-off angulation that is likely to prevent SB stenting after MB stenting. In this setting, upfront culotte stenting should be planned so that SB stenting precedes MB stenting.
3. A bifurcation lesion where pre-dilatation has caused severe SB dissection that is likely to prevent SB wiring after MB stenting in provisional stenting. In this case, SB stenting should precede MB stenting, with the intention of performing culotte stenting.

2.4.2.2 Practical Approach to Culotte Stenting

1. Perform MB stenting with KBI as described above. If SB wiring through the most distal cell has not been confirmed, assess the extent of jailing by IVUS. If jailing exceeds about 1.0 mm, try SB rewiring through a cell that is at least one strut more distal. Perform KBI and then check stent apposition by IVUS.
2. Place a stent in the SB. Note that stent size should be compatible with the SB diameter at the ostium, e.g., if the SB diameter at the ostium exceeds 4.0 mm, a 3.5-mm stent should be placed and expanded by balloon inflation at low pressure.
3. Overlap the two stents in the proximal MB for a distance of about 3 to 5 mm. If SB stenting is done before MB stenting, place the proximal edge of the SB stent 3 to 5 mm proximal to the carina. Cover the entire proximal MB with the MB stent (Fig. 2.65).
4. Advance the SB stent slowly and with great care so as to prevent its distal edge from hitting the MB stent. If the distal edge of the SB stent contacts the MB stent during rapid advancement, the struts at the edge will be distorted and damaged, so that it may become impossible to advance the stent into the SB. It is important to advance the stent into the SB slowly and gently, and you should never attempt to push the stent in if it is blocked even slightly.
5. There are several ways of advancing an SB stent that has been blocked by struts of the MB stent.
   (a) When stenting the proximal MB (e.g., LMT), withdrawal and advancement of the guiding catheter should be repeated until its tip is as coaxial with the SB ostium as possible.
   (b) Slightly press the stent into the struts to deflect the stent delivery balloon a little, withdraw the balloon catheter to straighten the deflected part, and then immediately push it in again (Fig. 2.66).
   (c) Insert another guidewire (buddy wire) to advance the stent gently. If delivery of the stent is still not achieved even after these procedures, advance the stent while pushing the buddy wire forward after confirming the safety of pushing in a wire with a prolapsed tip.
   (d) Advance a buddy balloon along the buddy wire to push in the stent with minimal force. Alternatively, advance the buddy balloon first and then gently push in the stent.
6. It may become difficult to advance the stent or even to withdraw it, if deformation occurs during any of the abovementioned steps. There is a temptation to push harder with the intention of advancing the stent "just a little further," but even a slight increase of force can easily deform the stent, so you must not push a stent in. By using the abovementioned procedures, you can almost always deliver a stent. If all of these procedures fail, you can try the mother/child guiding technique. This technique involves introducing a child catheter into the affected coronary artery by using an anchor balloon previously introduced via the catheter and inflated at a low pressure. You should advance the child catheter very gently while pulling the anchor balloon back to prevent coronary artery injury and stent deformation by the catheter tip. The stent can be delivered successfully if the catheter is advanced so that its tip is just distal to the carina.
7. After placing a stent in the SB, perform KBI by the same method as that for initial stenting with KBI. For in-stent dilation, use an optimally sized (not oversized) semi-compliant balloon inflated to a relatively high pressure. If necessary, perform final KBI with noncompliant balloons inflated to a relatively high pressure.

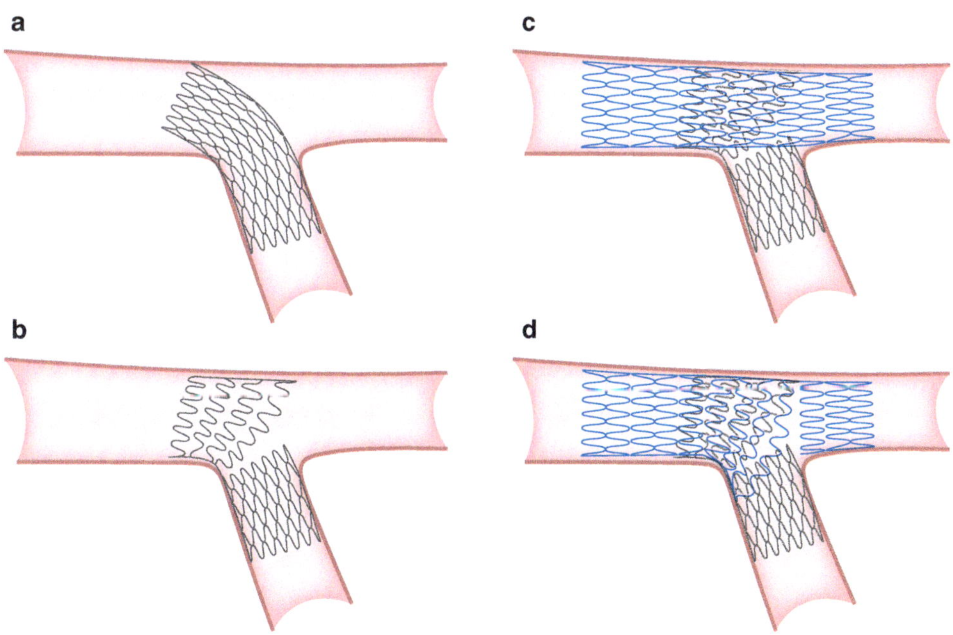

Fig. 2.65 Stent implantation for culotte (Y) stenting. (**a**) Place a stent in the SB. Limit the protrusion of struts into the MB to about 3 mm. (**b**) After KBI. (**c**) Place a stent in the SB. (**d**) After KBI

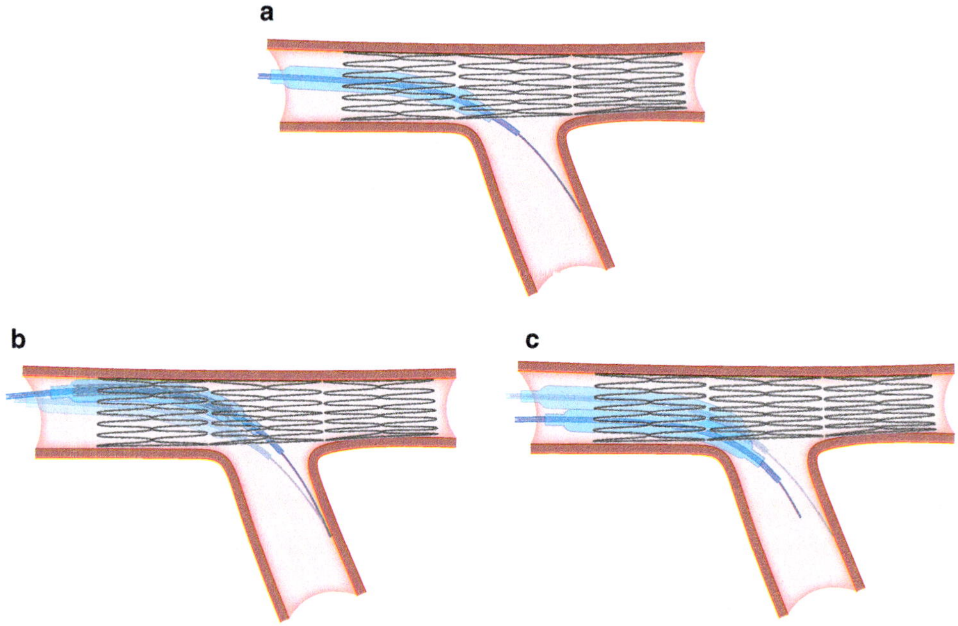

Fig. 2.66 Measures to take if the balloon tip is blocked by stent struts (**a**). (**b**) Never forcibly push the stent delivery balloon (SDB) catheter, but slightly press the stent into the struts to deflect the tip of the SDB a little. (**c**) Pull the catheter back slightly to straighten the tip of the SDB and promptly push it in a little way. This may allow smooth stent delivery into the SB

3 Stenting of RCA Ostial Lesions

PCI of RCA ostial lesions has long posed a challenge for interventional cardiologists for the following two reasons: (1) the RCA ostium is too rigid to be dilated successfully and is likely to show severe recoil, resulting in a high restenosis rate, and (2) stent fracture and restenosis occur frequently at the region several millimeters from the ostium.

The high rigidity and recoil of the RCA ostium have been attributed to the sphincter-like arrangement of myofilaments in the aorto-ostial smooth muscle, while prominent movement of the aorto-ostial junction has been suggested to contribute to the high frequency of stent fracture and restenosis after stenting at this site.

3.1 Radial Force

When a vessel is poorly dilatable and likely to recoil after stenting, how strong does the resistance of the stent to radial force (i.e., its radial stiffness) need to be in order to support the vessel wall and prevent "stent recoil" (actually vascular recoil)?

Before discussing this question, it is important to confirm how strong a stent can be. Although this depends on the definition of radial force and the method of measuring it, let us assume a stent is implanted in a silicone tube immersed in water and consider what will happen if the water pressure is increased. With an increase of the external pressure, the stent will change shape and its diameter will gradually decrease. When the pressure reaches a certain level, the stent will abruptly collapse. This is referred to as the buckling point (radial strength). If the water pressure at the buckling point is defined as the radial strength of the stent, resistance to a radial force of about 2 atm (2000 hPa) may be regarded as adequate. If so, a stent with "adequate" radial strength would show "recoil" due to vascular compression at a pressure greater than 3 atm. If it was implanted in a lesion that was pre-dilated at 16 atm or could only be post-dilated at ≥22 atm, the stent might be compressed at ≥3 atm after post-dilatation.

When IVUS is performed after stent implantation, it shows adequate dilation of many lesions, and follow-up angiography rarely shows stent lumen loss. This means that compression of the stent (due to recoil of the vascular wall) is often no more than moderate. Nevertheless, compression of about 3 atm may readily be applied to the stent in the presence of severe fibrosis or calcification of the vascular wall. In fact, vascular recoil often occurs at the RCA ostium even after pre- and post-dilatation at an adequate pressure for eliminating balloon indentations.

In such situations, the vessel may be regarded as having a recoil force of about 2 to 3 atm. Recoil of such a vessel may be preventable by placing a stent with adequate resistance to compression. However, a vessel with rubberlike recoil after being dilated by balloon inflation at high pressure (without the balloon popping out) will probably compress the stent with a force much larger than its radial strength. A stent with low to medium radial strength cannot be an adequate scaffold for such a vessel. Unfortunately, all attempts to strengthen the scaffold (e.g., by using a stent with a larger radial strength or overlaying two stents) and prevent restenosis at the RCA ostium have failed, as was theoretically predicted before these attempts. Hence, the consensus has been reached that strengthening the scaffold is useless for lesions with a hardness exceeding a certain threshold, while adequate lesion preparation to attenuate the recoil force of the vessel is much more practical.

3.2 Lesion Preparation

Therefore, we need to consider how a hard lesion should be prepared to attenuate vascular recoil and to make the vessel wall redundant like that at a soft lesion. Although the same principles apply to hard non-ostial lesions, the situation at the RCA ostium is special.

Some calcified lesions can be successfully debulked by rotablation, cutting balloon angioplasty, or directional coronary atherectomy (DCA). However, the DCA system is

K. Mitsudo, *Non-Pushing PCI Techniques*, https://doi.org/10.1007/978-981-15-7043-8_3

unsuitable for lesions at the RCA ostium, which displays extreme angulation and tortuosity, and thus is not a universal PCI device.

The best method of lesion preparation currently available involves combined use of a Rotablator to debulk a calcified lesion and a cutting or scoring balloon to create cracks in a calcified or hard fibrosed lesion, as well as a pressure-resistant balloon inflated at high pressure (Fig. 3.1). Performing these procedures effectively and safely is the major key to success with lesion preparation. Whenever possible, high-pressure inflation should be performed to dilate the lesion to the normal vessel diameter in order to attenuate vascular recoil and reduce the relative plaque burden. Expanding a stent to a large diameter after implantation in a softened lesion is also effective for increasing its resistance (even slightly). Before performing high-pressure balloon inflation, you should assess the severity and distribution of calcification by IVUS to determine the optimal balloon expansion diameter from the viewpoint of safety.

Rotablation for debulking should be performed with a burr up to 2.25 mm in size, which is the maximum size that can be used through an 8-Fr guiding catheter. In principle, the Lacrosse NSE balloon selected for this procedure should be one size smaller than the normal diameter of the target vessel. If the RCA ostium has a diameter ≥ 4.5 mm, a 4.0-mm Lacrosse NSE balloon has to be selected since this is the maximum available diameter. If the calcified plaque is eccentric with little or no plaque on the opposite side, a smaller Lacrosse NSE balloon should be used. If the calcified plaque has an abrupt (not tapered) edge, the lesion should be dilated with a Lacrosse NSE balloon of equal length to the calcified segment plus about 0.5 mm, regardless of the vessel diameter. If IVUS shows that scoring balloon angioplasty has created cracks in the calcified lesion, the vessel should then be dilated gradually to its normal diameter by high-pressure balloon inflation. If the calcified lesion has not cracked and dissection has occurred on the opposite side, the vessel must not be dilated using a large balloon. The only option in this case is to implant a stent that is compatible in size with the internal diameter of the distal part of the RCA Segment 1.

High-pressure inflation should be performed with a balloon that has an RBP of at least 20 atm, and a balloon that can be inflated to the target diameter at its RBP plus 4 atm should be chosen. For both pre- and post-dilation, the balloon should be inflated at gradually escalating pressures until it reaches the target diameter. If balloon inflation is rapid, it is more likely to cause dissection or perforation, so I always inflate the balloon very slowly. For example, assuming that the final inflation pressure is 26 atm, I escalate the pressure to 10 atm relatively quickly (within 2 or 3 s), after which I take about 1.5 times longer to reach 20 atm and increase the pressure at 2 atm per second thereafter.

When implanting a stent in a tapered ostium, the balloon and even the stent may slide out of the ostium if balloon inflation is too rapid. Gradual inflation of the balloon can avoid most of these problems.

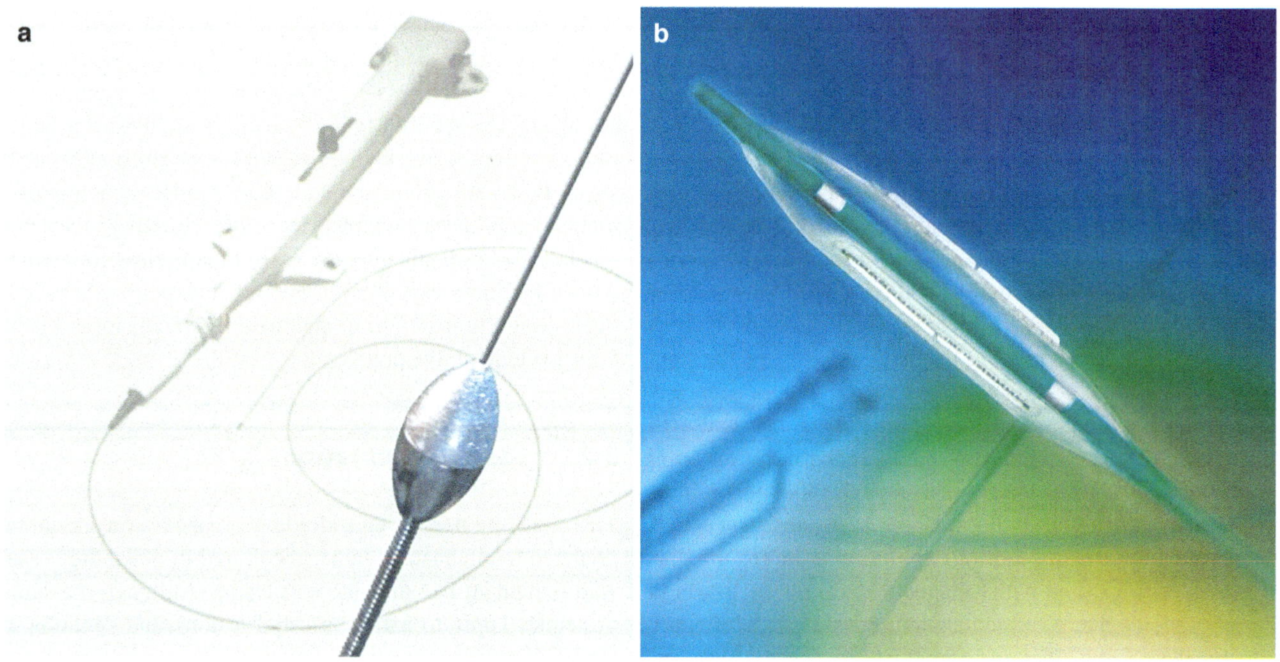

Fig. 3.1 Devices for lesion preparation. (**a**) Rotablator (Boston Scientific Corp.). (**b**) Flextome cutting balloon (Boston Scientific Corp.). (**c**) Lacrosse NSE ALPHA (Goodman/Nipro)

c

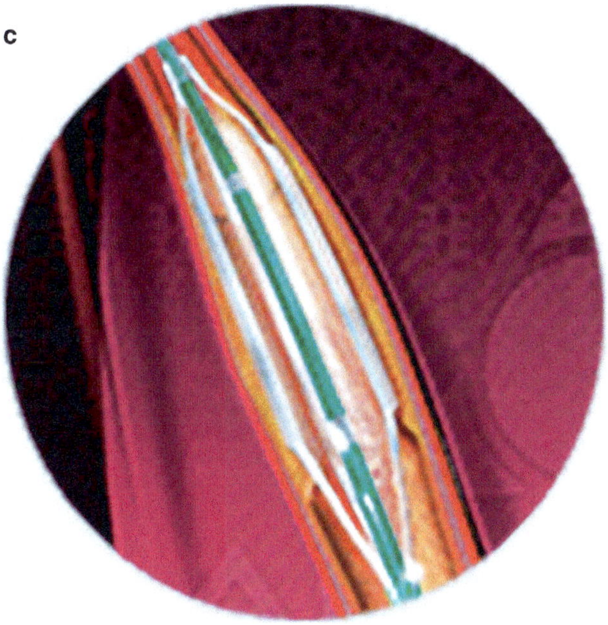

Fig. 3.1 (continued)

3.3 Stents

For the reasons mentioned above, the stent should be expanded to the ostial diameter to prevent deformation and to achieve complete apposition at the ostium. At the RCA ostium, a stent may have to be expanded to a diameter of 5 to 6 mm, so an adequately expandable stent should be chosen for an aorto-ostial lesion.

Another problem with RCA ostial stenting is a high frequency of stent fracture and restenosis at a site several millimeters from the ostium. The effect of aortic movement on a stent in the RCA ostium may account for these events. The most common pattern is that repetitive bending causes stent fracture, which leads restenosis. Therefore, a type of stent should be selected with which progression of stenosis is less likely, even after fracture.

3.3.1 Optimal Stent Design for RCA Ostial Lesions

The optimal stent for RCA ostial lesions should meet the following requirements: (1) a larger radial strength (less important); (2) 0 to 2 links; (3) likely to be fractured at a link rather than at a strut; (4) no stimulation of the vessel wall by the stumps of a fractured link; and (5) expandable to a large diameter to fit the RCA ostium (most important).

I will discuss various hypotheses about RCA ostial stenting with the Nobori 3.5-mm Japanese Version (JV) stent, which has achieved favorable outcomes when used for RCA ostial lesions.

3.3.1.1 Expansion to a Large Diameter

The Nobori 3.5-mm JV stent is designed to be expanded to a maximum diameter of 6.0 mm so as to ensure complete apposition in large coronary arteries (e.g., the LMT and the RCA ostium). For the stent to expand to a diameter of 6.0 mm, the full length of the crowns covering the circumference has to be about 19 mm (6π). In addition, each strut should become linear after stent deployment, but this is practically impossible. The engineers who developed the Nobori stent concluded that to allow a 10-crown stent to expand to a diameter of 6.0 mm with a crown height of 1.26 mm, each strut had to be 25.2 mm long (1.26×20). If the number of crowns was increased to 12, the height of each crown could be reduced to 1.05 mm. However, the stent struts would overlap when a 12-crown stent is mounted on a balloon, so the number of crowns in the stent was set at 10.

The Nobori 3.5-mm JV stent is the only stent that can be expanded to a diameter ≥ 5.5 mm.

3.3.1.2 High Conformability

It is necessary to reduce the number of links in a stent in order to increase its conformability. A stent composed of rings interconnected by link(s) must have at least one link. A 1-link stent shows high conformability, but its proximal rim can easily be rolled up if this type of stent is extruded from the ostium (Fig. 3.2).

A 2-link stent has a well-balanced design, since two links maintain the integrity of the stent but do not impair conformability.

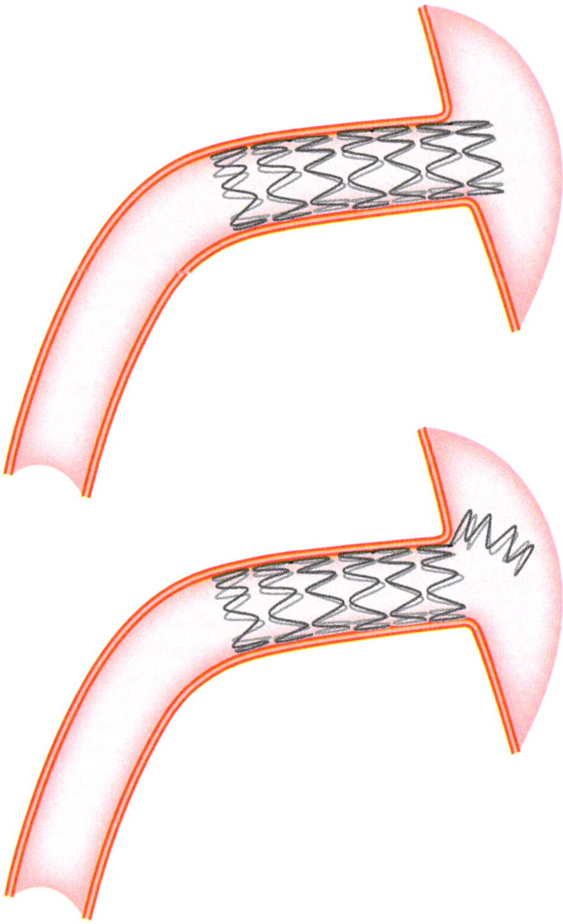

Fig. 3.2 Disadvantages of a 1-link stent. If a 1-link stent is extruded from the ostium, its proximal rim can easily be rolled up

3.3.1.3 Likely to Fracture at a Link

Some 2-link stents are composed of struts in which the peaks and valleys are interconnected directly or by a short link. In the Driver stent era, it was thought that when such a 2-link stent fractured at a link, the stumps of the link would not cause significant stimulation or injury of the vessel wall and that these stents would reduce the risk of in-stent restenosis and thrombosis. However, it was found that the Driver stent was actually much more likely to undergo fracture at a strut than at a link. The currently available helical coil integrity stent retains its integrity even after fracture, and this stent is equally likely to be fractured at a strut or at a link (Fig. 3.3a).

The PROMUS Element stent is also resistant to fracture, but fracture exclusively occurs at a strut (Fig. 3.3b).

What happen if a stent is fractured at a strut? At a minimum, the fractured ring will lose its structural strength and malfunction. Part of the strength may be retained if the stumps of the fractured strut support each other or are supported by the vessel wall, but such support will probably be lost over time.

In contrast to the above stents, the Nobori 3.5-mm JV stent predominantly undergoes fracture at a link (Fig. 3.3c). Even after a link has fractured, the stent maintains its original strut configuration and does not lose strength.

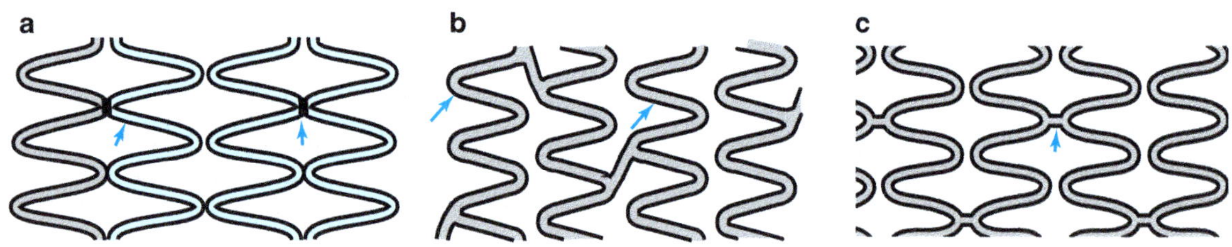

Fig. 3.3 Designs of 2-link stents. (**a**) The Integrity stent is equally likely to fracture at a link or a strut. (**b**) The PROMUS Element stent only fractures at a strut. (**c**) The Nobori stent predominantly fractures at a link

3.3.2 Effect of Stent Fracture on the Vessel

A native coronary artery is normally subjected to three types of stress, which are (1) tensile or compressive stress, (2) bending stress, and (3) torsional stress (Fig. 3.4). After a stent is implanted in an artery, it will also be affected by these stresses if it shows complete apposition to the vessel wall and is integrated with it. Many studies have examined the changes of stents after implantation and have demonstrated that different stents exhibit differing behaviors. However, few studies have addressed long-term interactions between the movement of a fractured stent and the stented coronary artery.

A stent implanted in a coronary artery is primarily subject to recurrent bending stress. If the stent is fractured, apposition becomes incomplete so that shear stress arises at the edges in addition to bending stress (Fig. 3.5). I have often seen the proximal and distal parts of a fractured Cypher stent shift horizontally in opposite directions. This stent shift applies shear stress to the coronary artery. While considerable shear stress may be generated by the Cypher stent due to its very low conformability, some level of shear stress may also arise after fracture of a 2-link stent with high conformability. I think that shear stress is the underlying cause of in-stent restenosis or progression of stenosis at a site of stent fracture associated with deformation, because bending stress alone is unlikely to deform a stent.

It is certain that loss of strength of a strut at the stent edge due to strut fracture has an important role in the development of in-stent restenosis. However, even after strut fracture, bending stress alone is insufficient to deform the stent in the radial direction (Fig. 3.6). Unlike stent fracture, stent deformation is not attributable to metal fatigue. Continuous application of external stress to a stent may cause the stent to be deformed (luminal loss) to some extent by overcoming its radial stiffness.

However, this mechanism is unlikely to explain the progression of stenosis when there is no preexisting stenosis. To clearly explain progression of stenosis, we need to introduce the concept of stent edge deformation by shear stress and the concept of metal yield (elastic limit) that helps to maintain the deformed shape. If the stent loses radial stiffness at its edge due to strut fracture, resistance to shear stress applied to the edge is decreased, allowing stent deformation to occur at the edge. Shear stress is not applied continuously, but only during a certain phase of the cardiac cycle, and is nullified in the other phases. Accordingly, stent deformation only occurs during that phase. If the deformation remains within the elastic limit of the metal used to make the stent, deformation will be transient and the stent will subsequently return to its original shape. If deformation exceeds the elastic limit (yield point) of the stent material, the stent will not return to its original shape during the other phases of the cardiac cycle. If the resulting stent deformation increases shear stress, deformation will progressively become more severe until shear stress is no longer strong enough to deform the stent further.

If a stent maintains its radial strength, intimal proliferation (even if aggressive) is limited to the stented site. I have never heard of endothelial cell growth into the lumen causing stent deformity or in-stent restenosis. It is more reasonable to hypothesize that stent deformation is caused by stress from the vessel wall and that intimal proliferation occurs after or in parallel with stent deformation.

The concepts of shear stress and metal yield combined with stent fracture seem to provide a better explanation of how clinical events occur. This discussion can also suggest the optimal design of a stent for treating RCA ostial lesions and how a new stent should be designed for this special anatomical region.

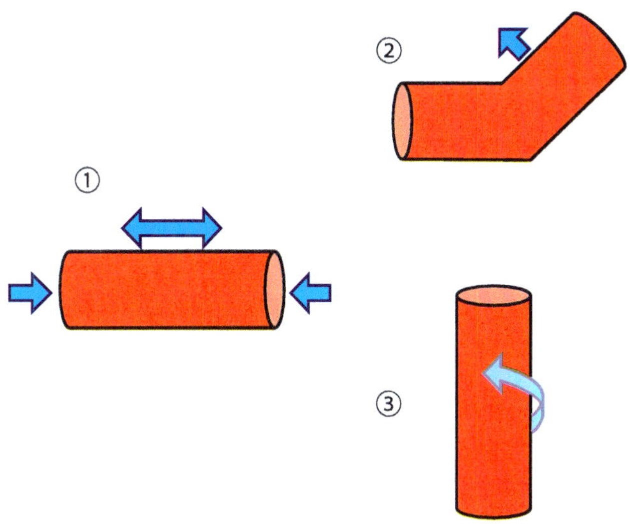

Fig. 3.4 Stresses acting on the coronary arteries. Movement of the myocardium induces three types of stress on the coronary arteries: (1) tensile or compressive stress, (2) bending stress, and (3) torsional stress

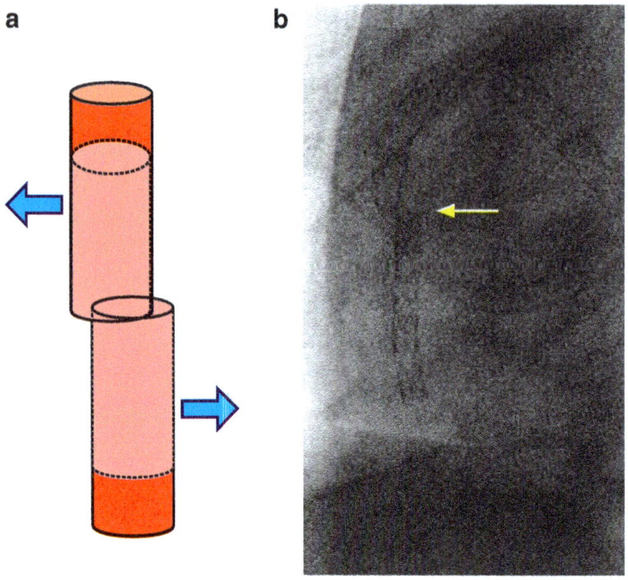

Fig. 3.5 Movement of a fractured stent. (**a**) A fractured stent is also affected by shear stress. (**b**) After fracture of a Cypher stent, the two parts of the stent shift horizontally in opposite directions at the fracture site

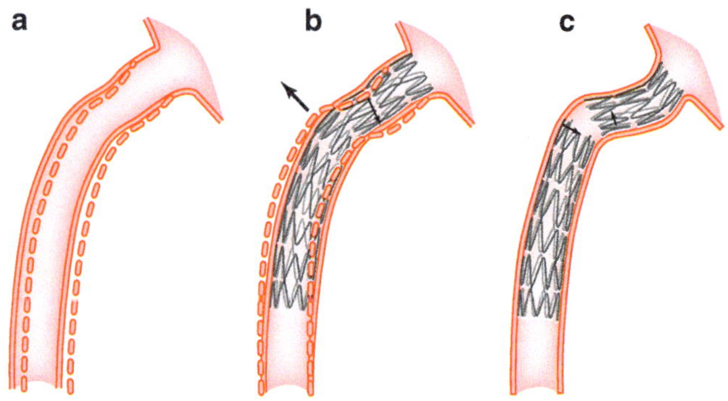

Fig. 3.6 Mechanisms of stent fracture. (**a**) Bending stress is the main stress applied to a native coronary artery. (**b**) After stenting, the coronary artery becomes more rigid and is also affected by shear stress. (**c**) The two parts of a fractured stent separate from each other due to transmission of stress from the vessel

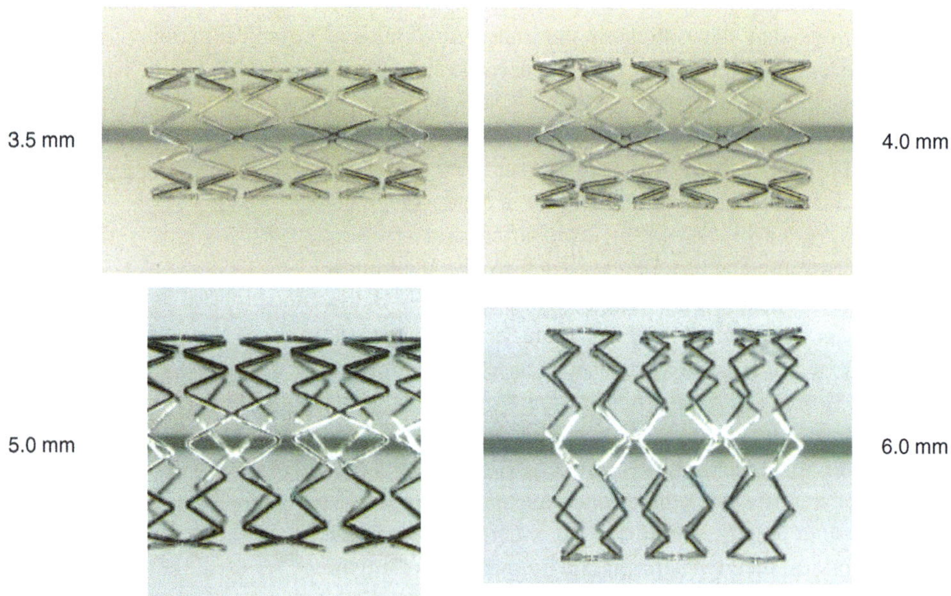

Expansion diameter	3.5 mm	4.0 mm	5.0 mm	6.0 mm
Radial force (N/cm)	10.3	11.9	12.9	15.2

Fig. 3.7 Bench testing of the Nobori 3.5-mm JV stent. The Nobori stent was designed with taller crowns and thus gains greater radial stiffness as it is expanded to a larger diameter

3.3.3 Characteristics of the Nobori 3.5-mm JV Stent

The Nobori 3.5-mm JV stent is prone to fracture but is unlikely to suffer deformation or in-stent restenosis. This stent does not have a particularly large radial stiffness (Fig. 3.7) or elastic limit. Based on the results of bench tests, the Nobori 3.5-mm JV stent is more likely to fracture at a link than at a strut. The stumps of a fractured link have few processes and rarely stimulate the vessel wall. Thus, this stent has links that are easily fractured and continues to function well after all of its links have been fractured. A no-link stent has the highest conformability and generates minimal shear stress at the point of fracture.

3.4 Positioning the Stent

Before the stenting procedure, you must never forget to obtain angiograms and IVUS images.

3.4.1 Position of the Distal Stent Edge

When implanting a stent in the RCA ostium, you should position the distal edge of the stent beyond the point where the descending limb of the RCA becomes relatively linear (Fig. 3.8). If the distal edge of a stent implanted in the RCA ostium is located at the first branch (sinoatrial node artery or conus branch), the body of the stent tends to shift horizontally. Such movement is likely to generate shear stress on the artery and thus cause stent edge restenosis.

If stent edge restenosis occurs and requires implantation of an additional stent overlapping the existing stent, existence of the branch vessel combined with stent overlap will considerably increase the risk of fracture at the edge of the overlapping strut layers.

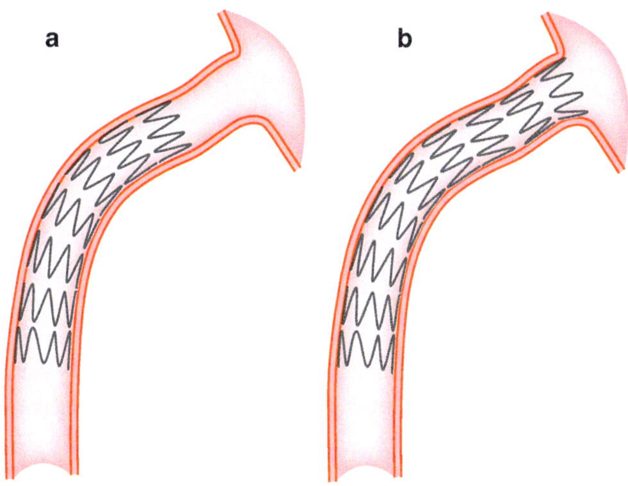

Fig. 3.8 Stenting RCA ostial lesions. The distal edge of the stent should be placed beyond the point where the descending limb of the RCA becomes linear. The proximal edge of the stent should not be distal to the RCA ostium (**a**), but should be located so that the stent covers the entire ostium (**b**)

3.4.2 Position of the Proximal Stent Edge

It may be difficult to determine the optimum position of the proximal edge of a stent after positioning its distal edge. The origin and shape of the RCA can vary considerably; it may arise directly from the sinus of Valsalva (Fig. 3.9b), or there may be a pouch between the sinus and the RCA ostium (Fig. 3.9a). The RCA may also begin to taper just after its origin (Fig. 3.9c). When determining the position of the proximal edge of the stent, you should consider the anatomy of the RCA ostium as well as the plaque burden and plaque distribution in this region.

Since the RCA shows considerable movement at a site several millimeters distal to its ostium, positioning the proximal edge of a stent in this region often results in stent edge restenosis and can even lead to dissection (if a Cypher stent is used) due to the mechanical stent edge effect. In addition, augmentation of the stent edge effect by the presence of plaque in this region is empirically known to occur. A stent with complete conformability would not have an edge effect, but such a stent has not been developed so far. Therefore, a stent with the maximum possible conformability should be implanted from the ostium to the distal landing zone (Fig. 3.8) to avoid the edge effect. Unless the RCA ostium has the morphology shown in Fig. 3.9a, the proximal edge of the stent should be positioned at the ostium, and the stent should be expanded to fit the ostial diameter. If the RCA ostium resembles that shown in Fig. 3.9a, the proximal edge of the stent should be positioned in the tapering, plaque-free region.

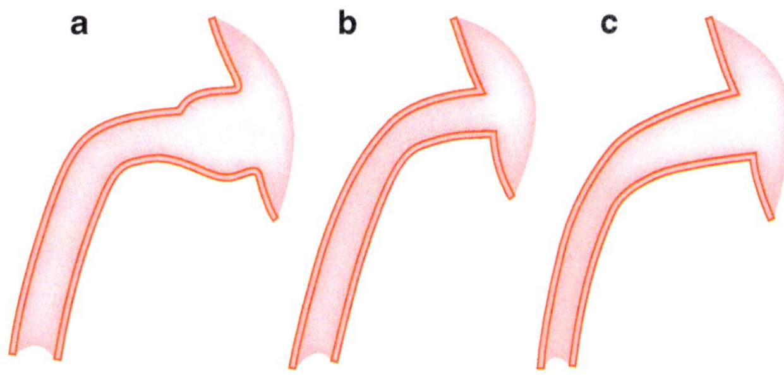

Fig. 3.9 Anatomy of the RCA ostium. (**a**) There may be a pouch between the sinus of Valsalva and the ostium of the RCA. (**b**) The RCA may arise directly from the sinus of Valsalva. (**c**) The RCA may begin to taper from its origin

3.4.3 Stenting of RCA Ostial Lesions (Fig. 3.10)

The potential for longitudinal deformation of 2-link stents has been a major limitation to their use for aorto-ostial lesions. Although a particularly high risk of such deformation has been suggested for specific stents, it should be recognized that there is some risk of longitudinal deformation with all 2-link stents, and you should take adequate precautions to prevent such deformation when using this type of stent.

To prevent longitudinal deformation, it is important to achieve complete apposition of the stent with the wall of the ostium by fully inflating a balloon that is compatible in size with the ostial diameter (EEM estimated by IVUS) as soon as possible after stent deployment without moving the guiding catheter. Even if there are plaques in the distal segment, this procedure can at least dilate the ostium to its normal external diameter. If a stent is placed at the ostium and only expanded to the internal (luminal) ostial diameter, it will often be displaced by subsequent contact with a post-dilatation balloon or the guiding catheter. Thus, an RCA ostial lesion should be managed by implanting a large-diameter stent from the ostium.

In Japan, the Promus PREMIER is the only DES with a 4.0-mm diameter that has been approved for marketing (as of 2015). Since the Promus PREMIER is unsuitable for aorto-ostial stenting, a DES pre-mounted on a 3.5-mm balloon is the only choice for this purpose. However, you may not achieve good apposition across a stenotic lesion with a 3.5-mm stent. In particular, lesion preparation by ostial dilatation may prevent optimal apposition of a 3.5-mm stent, potentially leading to deformation or migration during advancement of a post-dilatation balloon. Therefore, I try to expand the 3.5-mm stent to as large a diameter as possible. This improves apposition and also enlarges the stent lumen to minimize contact between the stent and the post-dilatation balloon, facilitating advancement of the balloon. For this purpose, I always draw back the stent delivery balloon after implanting the stent to a region where the RCA has a diameter greater than 4.0 mm, and then inflate the balloon at a high pressure (22 atm) to only expand the proximal part of the implanted stent (Fig. 3.10b).

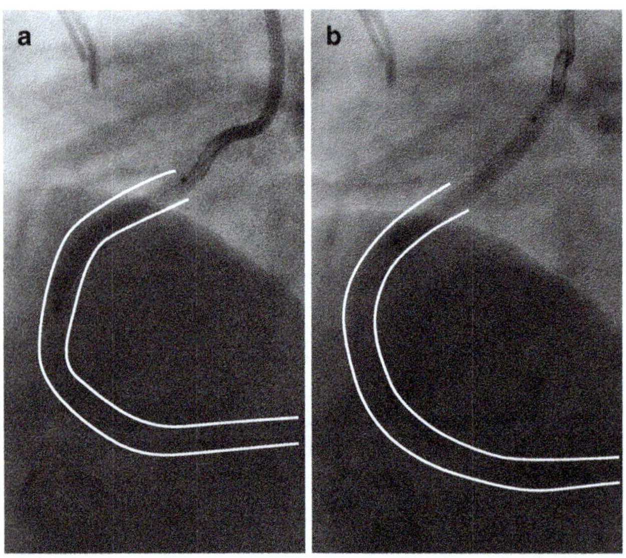

Fig. 3.10 Stenting of RCA ostial lesions. (**a**) A Nobori 3.5-mm stent has been deployed at 8 atm. (**b**) The proximal part of the stent was expanded by pulling the stent delivery balloon back and inflation at a high pressure (22 atm)

While withdrawing the balloon that is being/has been deflated, you should slightly advance the guiding catheter into the stent coaxial to the coronary artery so that it can enter the stent without causing deformation. You should adjust the position of the tip of the guiding catheter so as to keep the tip of the post-dilatation balloon coaxial with the vessel when advancing the balloon from the guiding catheter (Fig. 3.11).

In some situations, you should start inflation of the post-dilatation balloon while the proximal part is in the guiding catheter after advancing the guiding catheter several millimeters into the stent. If the guiding catheter is pulled back a little just as the distal part of the balloon has started to expand the implanted stent, the other part of the balloon will slide out of the catheter and the balloon will expand the entire stent. In most cases, inflating the balloon causes its proximal part to slide out of the guiding catheter, even if the catheter is not pulled back. However, the guiding catheter can sometimes push the balloon too away from the ostium to allow expansion of the entire stent. Therefore, a relatively long post-dilatation balloon should be selected for this technique, so that its previously inflated distal part maintains close contact with the stent struts before the proximal part slides out of the guiding catheter. This sliding movement is not due to advancing the balloon from the guiding catheter, but occurs because of disengagement of the guiding catheter as it is pushed back by the enlarging balloon. Thus, inflation of the balloon can reliably dilate the ostium. During inflation, the balloon spontaneously becomes coaxial with the vessel, and the tip of the guiding catheter is spontaneously lifted off the stent struts, so the guiding catheter will not deform the stent.

The RCA often begins to taper from its origin. If the patient has a tapering RCA ostium, rapid inflation of a post-dilatation balloon may cause the balloon to slip out of the

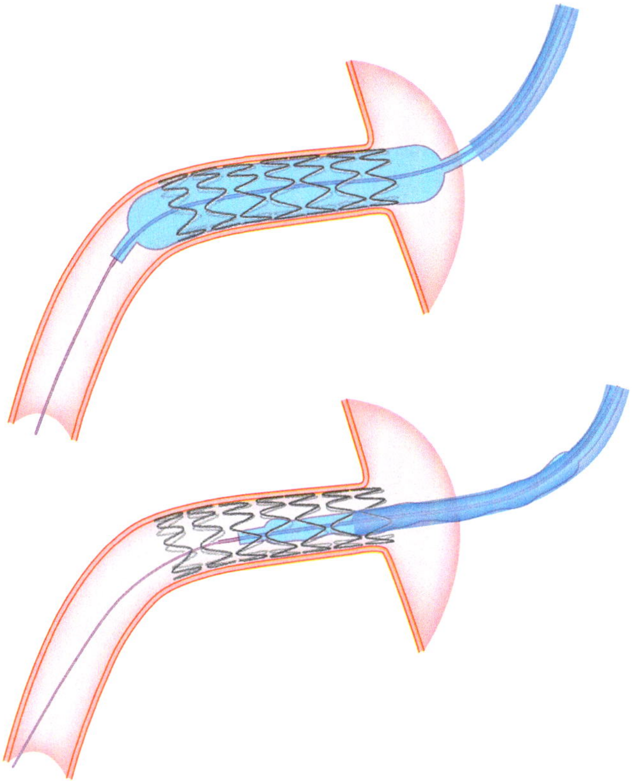

Fig. 3.11 Advancing the guiding catheter during balloon deflation. Withdrawing the balloon into the guiding catheter while keeping the balloon coaxial with the coronary artery introduces the guiding catheter into the stent implanted in the ostium while avoiding stent deformation

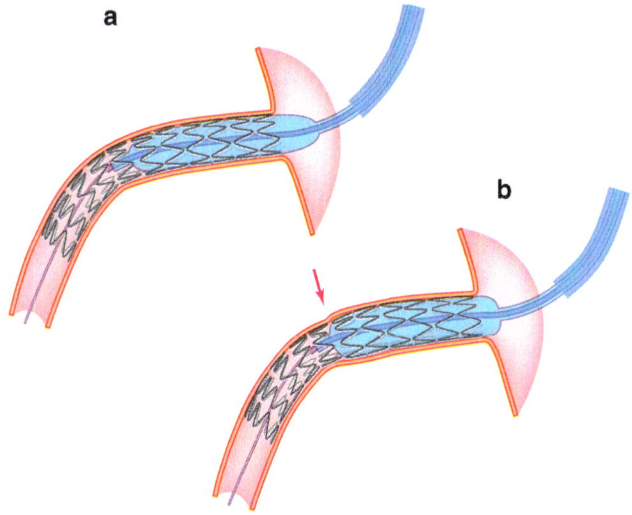

Fig. 3.12 Optimal balloon for RCA ostial stenting with a tapered ostium. The distal part of a tapered balloon (a balloon with long shoulders) achieves appropriate dilation of a tapered ostium and helps to preserve its anatomy (**a**). In contrast, inflation of a sandbag-shaped balloon to the ostial diameter may cause indentations in the tapered part of the vessel (**b**)

ostium. Therefore, if the ostium has this morphology, the balloon should be inflated slowly enough to allow gentle expansion of the stent from its distal part and to allow stable contact of the stent struts and balloon surface with the vessel wall.

In patients with a non-tapered RCA ostium (Fig. 3.9a, b), the balloon is inflated to the target diameter at a pressure near its RBP and then should be inflated at relatively high pressure for post-dilatation. If the RCA ostium is tapered (Fig. 3.9c), a balloon inflated to the ostial diameter may be oversized in the distal part of the landing zone. In this situation, a relatively large balloon that was inflated to the ostial diameter at a low pressure (about 10 atm) should also be inflated at relatively low pressure for post-dilatation.

Unlike LMT ostial stenting, the post-dilatation balloon for RCA ostial stenting may have long shoulders (the tapering parts of the balloon) (Fig. 3.12). For post-dilatation after LMT ostial stenting, a non-tapered, sandbag-shaped balloon should be inflated in the proximal part of the stent to prevent over-dilation of the LMT bifurcation. In contrast, a balloon with long shoulders (i.e., a tapered balloon) is a better choice for post-dilatation of an RCA ostial lesion when the ostium is tapered. This is because a tapered balloon will allow appropriate dilation of the tapered ostium and help to preserve its anatomy. I use a high-pressure balloon with long shoulders for post-dilatation after RCA ostial stenting.

One of the important reasons for dilating the ostium to its normal external diameter is to reduce the relative plaque burden. Assuming that the RCA ostium has a diameter of 5.5 mm and that the plaque has narrowed the lumen to 3.5 mm, inflating a 5.5-mm balloon in a stent placed at the ostium will dilate the lumen to nearly 5.5 mm (the diameter is slightly reduced by the plaque). If inflation of a 5.5-mm balloon dilates the vessel to an external diameter of 6.14 mm and an internal diameter of 5.5 mm, the relative plaque area is reduced from 60% to 37%.

Another important reason for dilating the ostium to its external diameter is to achieve complete stent apposition and thus prevent migration of the stent due to contact with the guiding catheter. In the presence of soft plaque with a smooth surface, a stent compatible with the luminal diameter of the vessel may easily be deformed by contact with a balloon or guiding catheter after deployment. Expansion of the stent by high-pressure balloon inflation will consolidate its apposition and minimize the risk of subsequent migration.

3.5 Necessity of Performing IVUS

As mentioned above, the strategy for RCA ostial stenting should be decided by considering the ostial diameter and the extent of ostial calcification, as well as the diameter, plaque burden, and extent of calcification of the vessel just distal to the ostium, all of which can be assessed by IVUS. The effect of scoring balloon angioplasty on calcification may also be taken into account when determining the sizes of the stent and balloon for post-dilatation.

Furthermore, IVUS guidance is sometimes very useful for positioning stents in the RCA ostium. Accordingly, I think IVUS is essential for PCI of LMT and RCA ostial lesions. I do not use OCT in these settings because it is not suitable for estimating the diameter of a large vessel in the presence of plaque.

3.6 Case Studies

Case 1 is a patient with a severely calcified RCA ostial lesion. Due to the abrupt edge of the calcified lesion, dilation with a large-diameter balloon might cause perforation. Inflation of a medium-diameter Lacrosse NSE balloon produced cracks in the calcified lesion. After stent implantation, post-dilatation was performed with a large-diameter balloon (Fig. 3.13).

Case 2 is a patient with a diffuse RCA lesion that could not be covered by a single stent. When multiple stents need to be implanted, a stent may be delivered to the ostium first (Fig. 3.14).

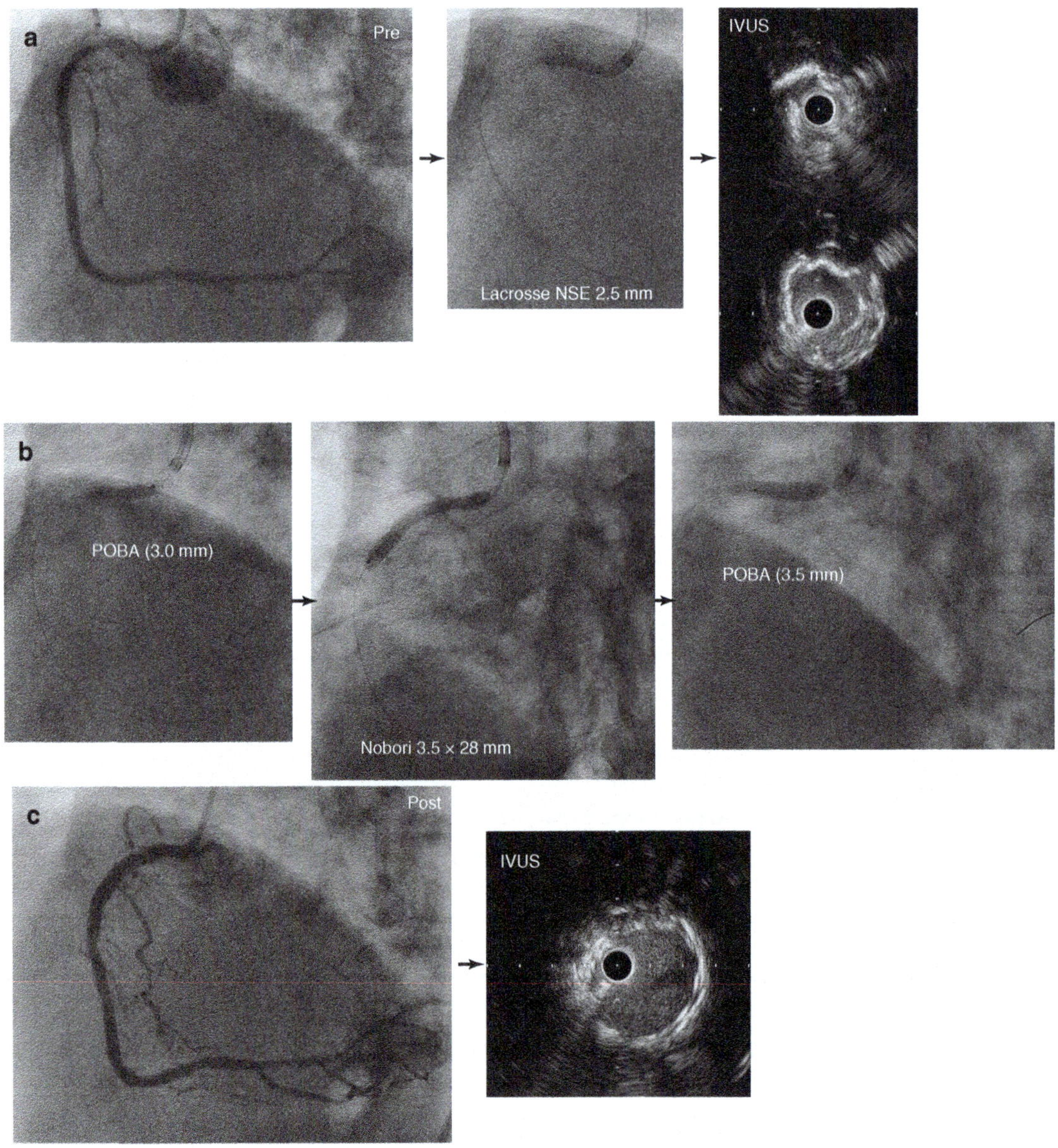

Fig. 3.13 Case 1. (**a**) A severely calcified RCA ostial lesion inaccessible to IVUS before balloon angioplasty was dilated with a 2.0-mm balloon and then with a 2.5-mm Lacrosse NSE balloon. IVUS showed that cracks had been made in the calcification by the balloon. (**b**) After high-pressure inflation of a 3.0-mm noncompliant balloon, a Nobori stent (3.5 × 28 mm) was implanted, and post-dilatation was performed with a 3.5-mm noncompliant balloon. (**c**) Optimal stent apposition was achieved

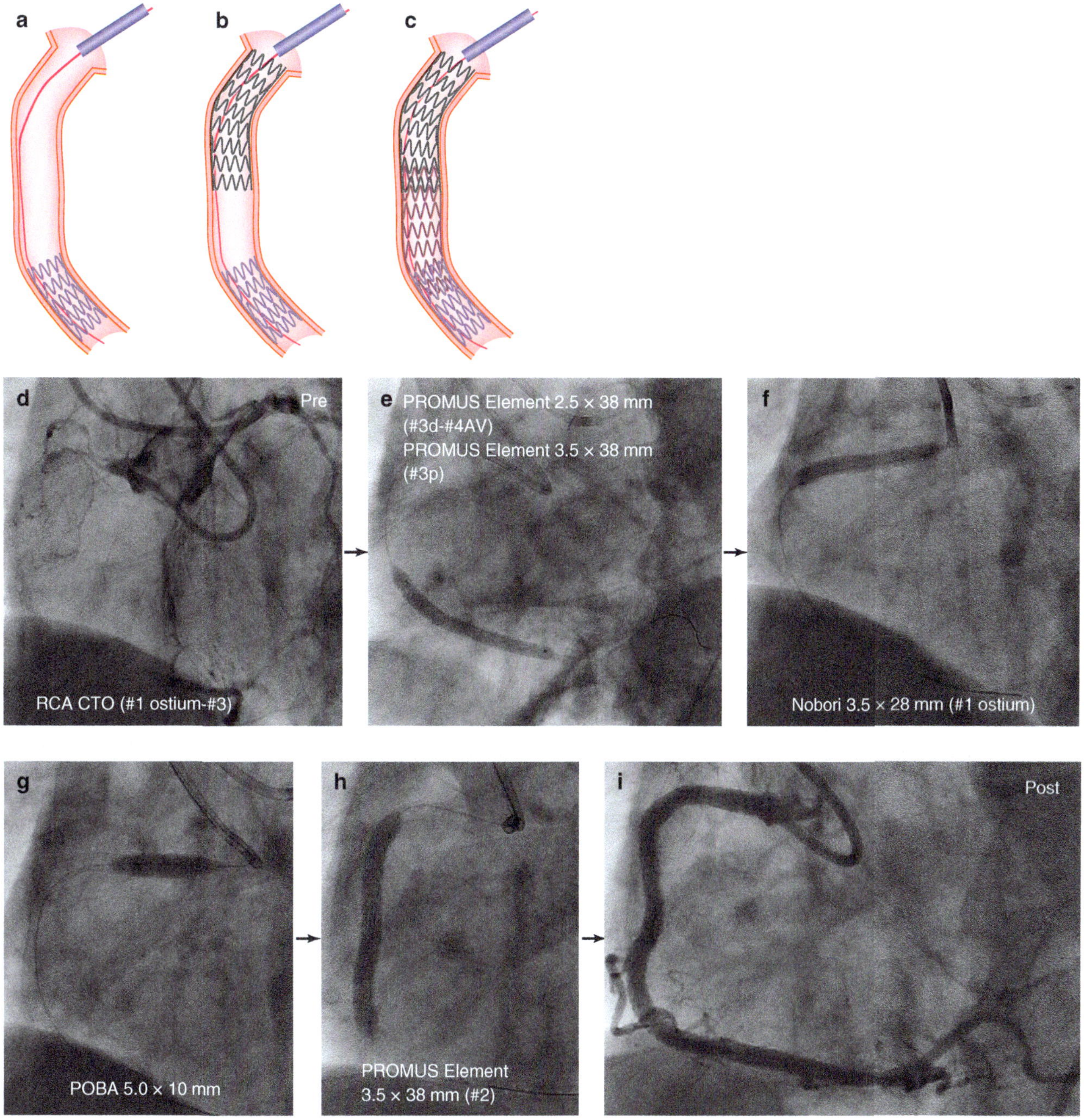

Fig. 3.14 Case 2. In a long RCA lesion that required multiple stents (**d**), two stents were first implanted in the distal RCA (Segments 3/4) (**a** and **e**). Subsequently, the third stent was implanted at the ostium (**b** and **f**), and a large-diameter balloon was inflated to the ostial diameter (**g**). Then the fourth (last) stent was implanted in the mid-RCA (**c** and **h**). Final CAG showed successful recanalization of the lesion (**i**). This stenting sequence allows a stent of the optimal size to be selected for the ostium and avoids unnecessary overlapping or gaps between stents

4 Stenting of Left Main Coronary Artery (LM) Lesions

As shown in Fig. 4.1, the survival of patients undergoing PCI for LM disease at my center was significantly worse than that of patients undergoing coronary artery bypass grafting (CABG) in the first-generation DES era (sirolimus-eluting stent: SES). However, survival has improved in the second-generation DES era to a level similar to that in patients undergoing CABG. Among several second-generation DES that are available, I use the Nobori 3.5-mm JV stent to treat almost all LM bifurcation lesions because it was developed with the aim of optimizing the stenting of such lesions. Before the Nobori stent became available, I used the Xience (an everolimus-eluting stent) for a while, but only in patients with a small- to medium-diameter LM. The outcomes shown in Fig. 4.1 were obtained with these stents and with other measures to solve various technical problems.

Since the second half of the SES era, it has generally been considered that CABG is indicated for patients with LM disease (particularly bifurcation lesions) requiring rotablation. However, in the last few years, PCI has been performed in some patients with LM disease that can be adequately prepared by rotablation and scoring balloon angioplasty (KBI with Lacrosse NSE balloons), as discussed later. If the LM lesion cannot be pre-dilated sufficiently, switching to CABG to prevent acute coronary occlusion should be considered, even if provisional stenting of the lesion is performed.

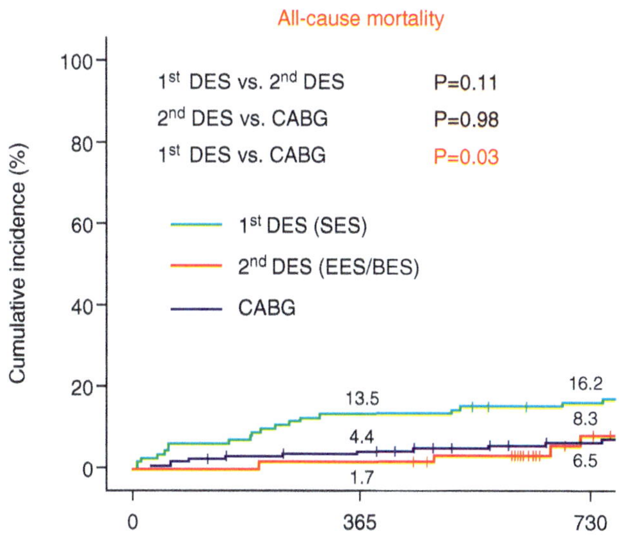

No. of patients at risk	Interval (days)		
1st DES (SES)	111	111	98
2nd DES (EES/BES)	58	58	42
CABG	159	154	136

Fig. 4.1 Survival of patients after PCI or CABG for unprotected LM lesions with a SYNTAX score ≤ 32 during the period from 2003 to 2012. Comparison of all-cause mortality after PCI with second-generation DES (everolimus-eluting stent [Xience] or biolimus-eluting stent [Nobori]) (n = 58) versus PCI with first-generation DES (SES [Cypher]) (n = 111) versus CABG (n = 159)

K. Mitsudo, *Non-Pushing PCI Techniques*, https://doi.org/10.1007/978-981-15-7043-8_4

4.1 Lesion Pathomorphology and Stenting Techniques

LM lesions vary with regard to anatomy and the indications for stenting. LM lesions can be classified as follows:

1. LM ostial lesions with little or no plaque in the trunk or bifurcation
2. Left main trunk lesions with no plaque in the ostium or bifurcation
3. LM bifurcation lesions involving the LAD and/or LCX ostium
4. LM lesions with severe calcification that requires rotablation
5. LM lesions that are expected to be difficult to dilate, but do not require rotablation

The outcome of PCI for these different LM lesions largely depends on the choice of stents and stenting techniques. If the lesion can be successfully recanalized by stenting of the ostium or trunk alone, the outcome will be favorable. What are the morphological characteristics of lesions in which such simple stenting is likely to be achieved?

A localized stenosis without significant plaque elsewhere (plaque area/cross-sectional vessel area $\leq$ 40%), as confirmed by IVUS (Fig. 4.2a or c), can be treated by implanting a short stent that covers the lesion. The LM can have an enormous plaque burden because of its large diameter, so post-stenting plaque shift may occur over a wider region. Hence, the stent should be 6 mm longer than the length of the stenosis to reliably cover the artery from 3 mm proximal to 3 mm distal to the lesion. For LM ostial lesions, the stent should be positioned so that its proximal part completely covers the entire ostium.

Left main trunk lesions with proximal plaque (Fig. 4.2e) should be treated by implanting a stent that can also cover the affected proximal segment, which is generally the entire ostium.

Bifurcation stenting is indicated for the left main trunk lesions approximating the bifurcation (Fig. 4.2d). Lesions such as those shown in this figure may be successfully treated by stenting with KBI, while culotte stenting may be indicated for some lesions depending on the expected extent of plaque shift and/or carina shift.

LM bifurcation lesions with diffuse plaque extending from the LM ostium to the proximal LAD and/or LCX (Fig. 4.2f or g) require both LM ostial stenting and bifurcation stenting.

When performing bifurcation stenting of the LM and LAD/LCX, the following points should be considered because of the unique anatomy of the LM:

1. As the LM (proximal main branch) has a large diameter, you should choose a stent that can be expanded to a suitably large diameter and should consider the possibility that some struts may lose radial strength after LM stenting with KBI (Fig. 4.3).
2. The LCX ostium is often difficult to dilate because this vessel can have a large take-off angle and because it may have undergone significant negative remodeling and may have severe fibrosis and/or calcification of its shoulders.
3. If the LM is severely calcified, the calcification will be thick and may be resistant to rotablation, as well as making the vessel difficult to dilate by POBA.
4. KBI is absolutely essential for adequate dilation of a stenotic LM bifurcation. In the presence of calcification, it may be necessary to perform KBI at a reduced pressure to prevent dissection of the LCX ostium or the LM, although stenting with reduced pressure KBI may only achieve suboptimal dilatation of a calcified bifurcation lesion.
5. Because the LCX ostium moves considerably during the cardiac cycle, you should take special care when choosing a stent for the LCX ostium and the technique for LCX ostial stenting.

To prevent acute adverse events and obtain favorable long-term outcomes, you should prepare the lesion as carefully as possible and optimize the stenting procedure. To achieve this objective, you should use an optimally designed stent and the optimal stenting technique when treating LM lesions, despite the potential for a longer procedural time and increased consumption of healthcare resources.

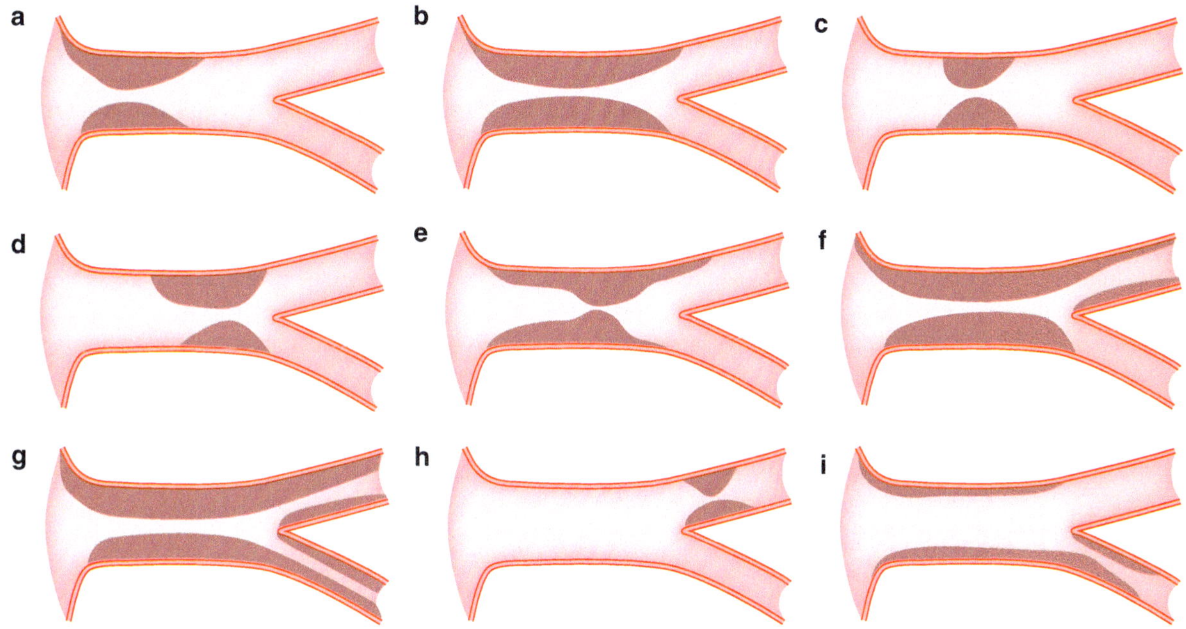

Fig. 4.2 Pathomorphology of LM lesions. (**a**) LM ostial lesion with plaque confined to the ostium (little or no or plaque elsewhere). (**b**) LM ostial lesion with diffuse plaque extending toward the bifurcation. (**c**) Left main trunk lesion with plaque confined to the trunk (the stent can also cover plaque-free segments proximal and distal to the lesion). (**d**) Left main trunk lesion that is too close to the bifurcation. (**e**) Left main trunk lesion with plaque extending to the ostium. (**f** & **g**) LM lesion involving the bifurcation. (**h**) LM bifurcation lesion with plaque confined to the LAD/LCX ostium. (**i**) Diffuse LM/LAD/LCX disease

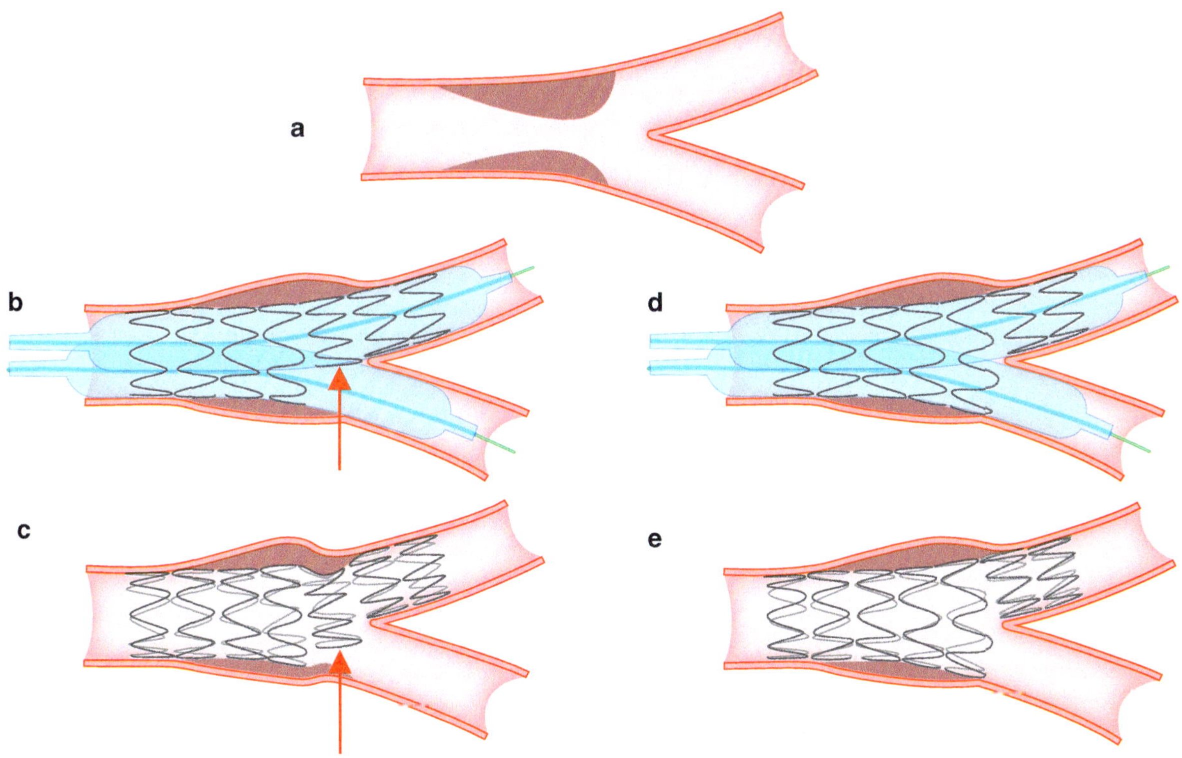

Fig. 4.3 Treatment of LM bifurcation lesions by stenting with KBI (**a**). If stenting with KBI causes partial jailing of the LCX (**b**), the culprit strut (red arrow) loses radial strength as it has no support at the site of the carina. This strut cannot resist vascular recoil due to plaque on the lateral side of the LCX (**c**; red arrow). Rewiring the LCX through the most distal cell at the carina to resolve jailing before KBI (**d**) results in all of the struts maintaining radial strength and resistance to vascular recoil (**e**)

4.2 Stent Design

The LM often has a large diameter of about 6 mm. For general balloon-expandable stents, the maximum diameter is calculated as the diameter of the SDB plus 1.0 mm. Until 2013, a 4.0-mm DES had not been approved in Japan, with the maximum diameter of the available stents being 4.5 mm after expansion (3.5 mm plus 1.0 mm). Apart from the specifications of the manufacturer, there are no data regarding the diameter to which a particular stent can be expanded. Currently, only one balloon-expandable coronary stent marketed in Japan can achieve a diameter of 6.0 mm without cracking or fracturing. This is the Nobori 3.5-mm JV stent, and it is the only stent in the world that is definitely expandable to 6 mm.

In addition to the maximum expansion diameter, the number of links is an important factor to be taken into account when designing a stent. For the reasons described in Chap. 2, it is desirable for a stent to have 0 to 2 links and for fracture to occur at a link rather than at a strut.

What is the optimal design of a stent for a bifurcation where the proximal MB has a large diameter and the SB shows extreme angulation (e.g., the LM bifurcation)? I would like to discuss this matter from several viewpoints.

4.2.1 Conformability

The term "stent conformability" encompasses both the concept of flexibility, which means the ability of a stent to flex when implanted in a tortuous vessel, and the concept of local conformability, which means the ability of a stent to achieve apposition to the walls of a tortuous and branching vessel.

4.2.1.1 Number of Links

Stenting of a bifurcation with a large branching angle should be done by using a stent that possesses particularly good flexibility. Flexibility is a synonym for the tendency to undergo longitudinal deformation. A stent with fewer links has greater flexibility, so stents can be ranked as follows in order of decreasing flexibility (increasing number of links): helical coil stents (no links) > one-link stents >two-link stents >three-link stents >six-link stents.

4.2.1.2 Stent Configuration and Strut Material

Every stent strut has a zigzag structure. Stents fit into two categories according to the basic design, which are slotted tube stents and ring/coil stents. Helical coil stents formerly marketed under the brand names of Wiktor, Cordis, or CrossFlex seem to have the greatest flexibility.

In this discussion, I will refer to one zigzag of the stent strut as a crown. A stent with a shorter crown has greater local conformability (Fig. 4.4). Among metal stents, those made of metals with greater elasticity generally have less conformability. If the design is similar, stents made of stainless steel (less elastic) are more conformable than those made of cobalt-chromium alloy (more elastic).

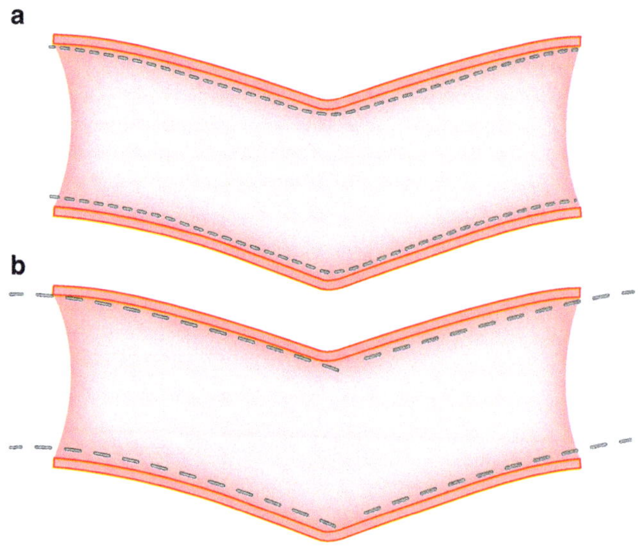

Fig. 4.4 Influence of the shape of the crowns. A stent with shorter crowns (**a**) shows better conformability to the vessel. Such a stent will rarely be affected by malapposition to the vessel wall as it maintains its initial alignment with the vessel despite vascular recoil. A stent with longer crowns (**b**) can only flex between the struts and expands discontinuously. Such a stent is more likely to develop malapposition when compressed by vascular recoil

4.2.1.3 Link Design

There are several link designs, including (1) inverse-phase links with peak-valley interconnections (Fig. 4.5a), (2) identical-phase links with peak-valley interconnections (Fig. 4.5b), and (3) identical-phase links with peak-peak interconnections (Fig. 4.5c). Among two-link stents, the highest flexibility is achieved by having struts linked by peak-valley interconnections and aligned in the identical phase with fewer longitudinal components in each link. The presence of a longer longitudinal link decreases the local conformability and flexibility of the stent.

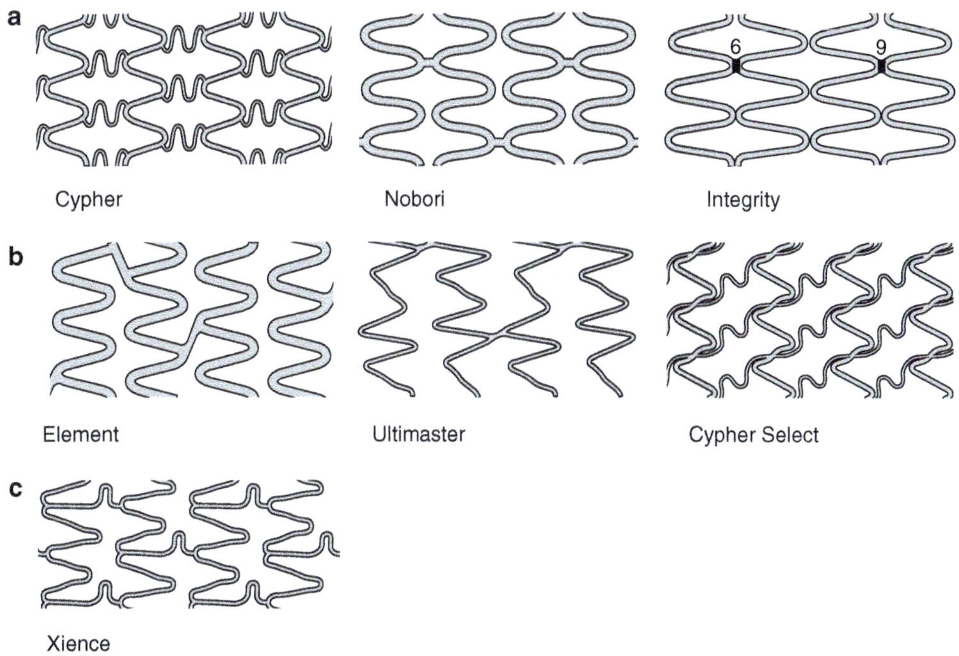

Fig. 4.5 Link designs. (**a**) Inverse-phase links with peak-valley interconnections. Adjacent struts are linked by peak-to-valley interconnections and are aligned inversely. (**b**) Identical-phase links with peak-valley interconnections. Adjacent struts are linked by peak-to-valley interconnections and are aligned in the same manner. (**c**) Identical-phase link with peak-peak interconnections. Adjacent struts are linked by peak-to-peak interconnections and are aligned in the same manner

4.2.2 Maximum Expansion Diameter

A stent for implantation in the ostium should be expandable to a diameter of about 6.0 mm in order to dilate the ostium to its normal external diameter and prevent malapposition at the lesion. To make a stent that can be expanded to such a large diameter, the number and height of the crowns are increased. For example, the Nobori 3.5-mm JV stent is designed with ten crowns that are 1.24 mm in height (i.e., higher than usual) to ensure that it can be expanded up to 6.0 mm in diameter. Currently, no other coronary stent (especially with two links) can be expanded to a diameter ≥ 5.5 mm.

4.2.3 Optimal Design of the Proximal Stent Edge for Ostial Stenting

A stent implanted in the ostium should have at least two links at its proximal edge. Focusing on this point, some stents have been developed with a larger number of links at the proximal edge. The proximal edge of the GFX stent (a two-link stent) often rolls up when it protrudes from the ostium (Fig. 4.6). The S-660 (another two-link stent) was designed with two links only at the edges to prevent such "roll-up" of the most proximal strut. Subsequently, the S-7 and Driver (2-link stents) were designed with three links only at the edges to further stabilize ostial dilatation.

However, two links at the edges is actually enough to prevent "roll-up" of the proximal edge. Even without apposition to the vessel wall, the proximal edge of a two-link stent will not roll up, although it may undergo slight deformation. If the ostium of the target vessel has been stented with a two-link stent and the most proximal strut is protruding from the ostium, you can insert a wire into the stent strut and advance a large-diameter balloon along the wire. Inflation of the balloon will never fail to dilate the ostium to its normal diameter (Fig. 4.7).

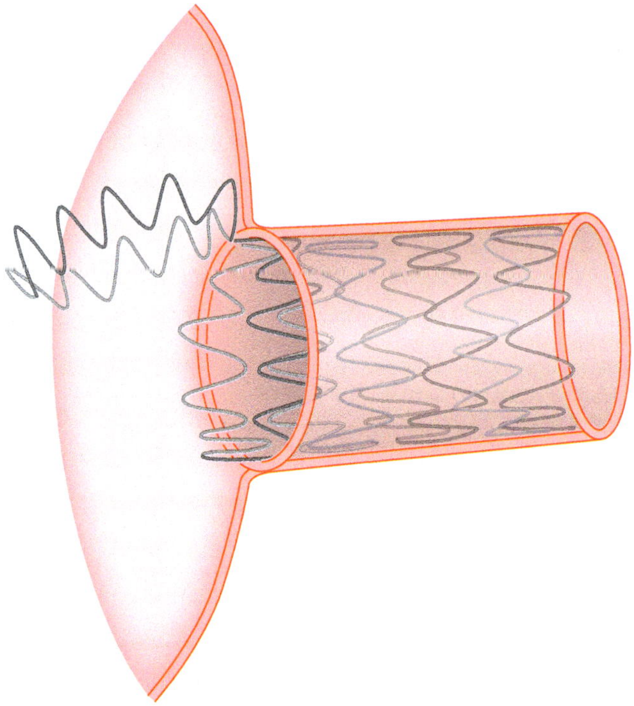

Fig. 4.6 Strut roll-up with a one-link stent. If the guiding catheter even comes into gentle contact with a two-link stent, its most proximal strut is likely to roll up

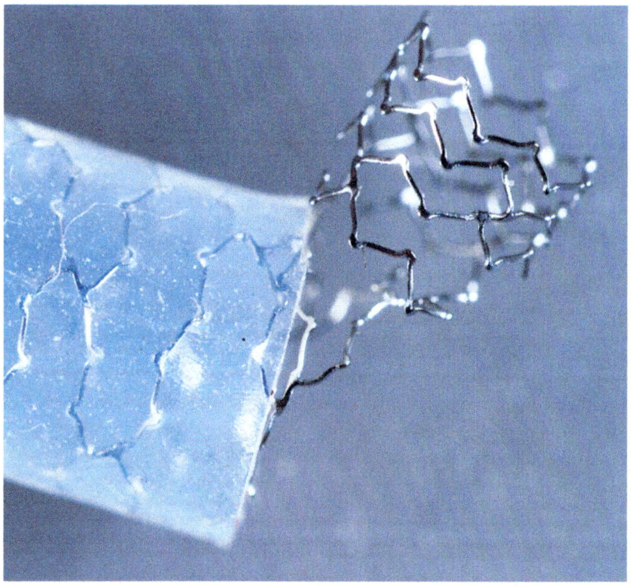

Fig. 4.7 A two-link stent (Nobori stent). A guidewire was inserted into the strut of a stent implanted in the LM ostium, and the ostium was dilated with a balloon to its external diameter (4.0 mm in this case). Because of its structural characteristics, a two-link stent does not induce SB jailing since the cells on the SB and MB sides can be enlarged to a similar extent. The most proximal strut of a two-link stent protruding into the sinus of Valsalva has gone outside the ostium so that the ostium is very accessible

Column 19 Promus PREMIER Stent

Here, I will make some comments about the Promus PREMIER stent, which is currently available. It would be correct to say that I want to give candid feedback to the interventionalists who assisted in the development of this product. As stated above, the Promus Element is a well-designed stent with high flexibility, which makes it prone to longitudinal deformation. If not manipulated carefully when performing ostial stenting, the Promus Element can be shortened when a guiding catheter, a balloon, or another stent comes into contact with its proximal edge.

Therefore, Boston Scientific Corp. developed the Promus PREMIER stent, in which the three most proximal struts are connected with four or five links to make the proximal part more resistant to deformation (Fig. 4.8). Despite advocating use of the Promus Element, I have never used the Promus PREMIER (as of September 2015), and I do not intend to use it in the future.

There are several reasons for this decision. First, the proximal part (4 mm long) of the Promus PREMIER is too rigid and its distal part is too flexible. The stent is likely to be fractured at the abrupt transition from the rigid part to the flexible part, applying excessive stress on the vessel. Second, there will be a greater difference in rigidity at the site two Promus PREMIER stents overlap with each other (four links plus two links). Third, during future intervention after ostial stenting has been done with a Promus PREMIER so that the proximal edge protrudes slightly into the sinus of Valsalva, POBA following wiring through a cell may not sufficiently dilate the cell. On the other hand, there are various effective interventional measures for preventing stent deformation.

For these reasons, I think that the 4-mm Promus Element stent should be approved for coronary ostial stenting. In Japan, the Nobori 3.5-mm JV stent is available and can meet the need for this indication. However, the 4.0-mm Promus Element may be sufficient for stenting a medium-sized coronary ostium (diameter ≤ 5.5 mm). Outside Japan, only 3.5- or 4.0-mm BioMatrix (9-crown and two-link) stents are available and not the Nobori 3.5-mm JV, so I have used the 4.0-mm Promus Element stent for a large coronary artery ostium. After stenting, CAG and IVUS generally show sufficient dilation and successful recanalization of the coronary ostium.

Although the Promus Element is not prone to fracture, it will undergo fracture at a strut more often than at a link (see Chap. 3 regarding the disadvantages of fracture at a strut). Better outcomes will be obtained with a modified stent that fractures at a link and minimizes vascular stimulation by the stumps of the broken link.

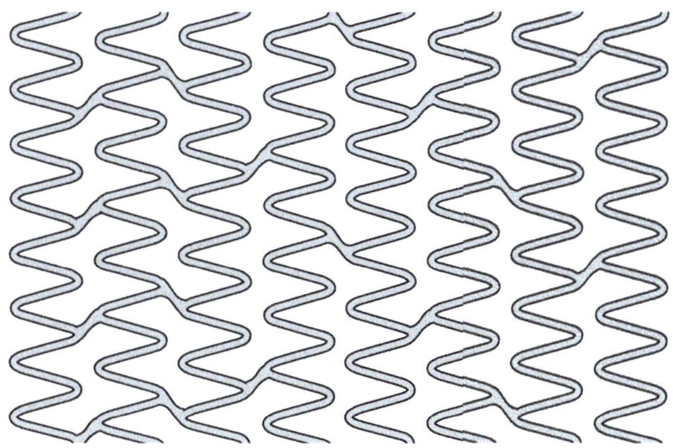

Fig. 4.8 Design of the Promus PREMIER stent

4.3 Lesion Preparation

It is essential to perform IVUS before PCI for LM lesions. As stated in Sect. I of this chapter (page 212), IVUS should be used to estimate the diameter of the target vessel and the overall plaque burden. In addition, IVUS is essential for assessing the extent and distribution of calcification and for quantifying plaque attenuation.

4.3.1 Preparation of the LM Ostium and Trunk

Most isolated LM ostial or trunk lesions are relatively soft and are not associated with severe calcification. Rotablation should be considered if there is circumferential calcification, while scoring balloon angioplasty (e.g., a Lacrosse NSE) or cutting balloon angioplasty should be considered when calcification is not circumferential. It is also important to perform scoring or cutting balloon angioplasty after rotablation in order to lessen vascular recoil.

The luminal diameter may be ≥2.25 mm at a calcified lesion in a large coronary artery (e.g., the LM or RCA). Since large-diameter (≥9 Fr) guiding catheters are no longer used, rotablation using a 2.38-mm or 2.5-mm burr is not feasible, which means that scoring or cutting balloon angioplasty should be considered.

4.3.2 Preparation of the Distal LM Bifurcation

It is well-known that an LAD ostium with plaques on the roof is difficult to dilate by POBA. Considering that the carina, the LCX ostium, and the distal LM are present on the contralateral side, inflation of a balloon that is sized to match the LAD diameter can easily displace the carina toward the LCX. Therefore, even if the balloon appears to have been inflated fully without indentations, it is unlikely to apply pressure to the roof of the LAD ostium (Fig. 4.9). Placing a stent from the LM to the LAD across the LCX ostium after POBA always causes carina shift and induces vascular recoil at the roof of the LAD ostium.

Debulking may be the optimal intervention to ensure sufficient dilation at the roof of the LAD ostium if a sufficient volume of plaque can be removed. At present, three debulking methods are available (Rotablator, excimer laser coronary angioplasty [ELCA], and directional coronary atherectomy [DCA]).

1. A Rotablator is used for debulking calcified tissue or other very hard tissue. Since it has become uncommon to use guiding catheters larger than 8 Fr, the maximum diameter of the Rotablator burr cannot exceed 2.25 mm. Consequently, the reduction of plaque volume after rotablation is relatively small compared to the LM diameter, and the residual thick layer of calcified plaque may resist POBA.

   Although some use can be made of the effect of guidewire bias, this method cannot completely ablate calcified plaque because the plaques are not always concentric with the vessel. Hence, complete debulking is difficult.

   However, even if debulking is not complete, subsequent KBI can apply pressure to plaques on the roof, thereby dilating the stenotic lesion to some extent (Fig. 4.9), and proper stent placement after KBI can optimally dilate the lesion. Thus, strategically adding rotablation to DES stenting with KBI will considerably improve the medium- to long-term outcome of PCI for LM disease.
2. ELCA may be effective for ablating thrombotic plaques in coronary arteries, but generally it cannot effectively ablate plaques in large vessels.
3. It has been suggested that DCA may achieve optimal debulking if performed by experienced interventionalists. However, we general interventionalists often find it difficult to sufficiently ablate plaques in the LM by DCA to avoid the need for stenting. This is because the LM arises in a leftward direction from the sinus of Valsalva and then runs almost straight until it branches into the LAD and LCX with extreme (left) anterior and posterior angulations, respectively. It should be noted that plaques which require debulking at the LM bifurcation exist in these extremely angulated vessels. It is almost impossible to accurately locate plaques at this angulated bifurcation by IVUS or to ablate plaques in such angulated vessels by using a linear debulking device.

Even when using DCA, I only expect to achieve a modest debulking effect with this device before implanting a DES.

Thus, the different debulking devices each have their own points. I regard them all as useful tools for lesion preparation to optimize stenting, and I think you should aim to achieve better long-term outcomes by combining optimal debulking and DES stenting with KBI.

Some interventionalists may recommend POT, i.e., dilation of the proximal vessel by a single large-diameter balloon, before stent implantation. However, it is very difficult to dilate the distal LM near the bifurcation to its normal diameter by inflating a single balloon (Fig. 4.10). Also, en face observation of the distal LM bifurcation by CAG is problematic due to the different angulations of the LAD and LCX. Taking these points into account, it is almost impossible to reliably dilate the distal LM bifurcation by using a single large balloon. In fact, a large balloon often fails to dilate an LM bifurcation lesion if it is inflated insufficiently

to prevent over-dilation of the distal MB (LAD) or if it slides back into the left main trunk or ostium.

This may occur not only during POBA but also during scoring or cutting balloon angioplasty. Even alternating inflation of balloons matching the diameters of the LAD and LCX, respectively, will fail to sufficiently dilate the LM bifurcation. KBI is eventually necessary, and high-pressure POBA often fails to dilate the bifurcation, even with KBI. In the first place, high-pressure KBI is not recommended at the distal LM bifurcation because it is associated with a risk of causing dissection in the LM bifurcation/trunk or in the LAD/LCX. When performing high-pressure KBI (≥14 atm) at the LM bifurcation, you must use balloons that are one quarter size smaller for both the MB and SB and slowly increase the pressure.

KBI cannot be done with cutting balloons, but can be performed with two scoring balloons (Fig. 4.11). To prepare a calcified lesion or some other hard lesion, I perform KBI with Lacrosse NSE balloons. Neither of the kissing Lacrosse NSE balloons will burst, even if inflated simultaneously at pressures up to the RBPs. Therefore, performing KBI with slightly undersized Lacrosse NSE balloons inflated sufficiently to remove indentations can crack calcification and achieve adequate dilation of the LM bifurcation, even by low-pressure inflation.

Performing additional KBI with two optimally sized balloons seems to ensure optimal stent deployment. This is probably because a stent cannot be deployed evenly if it is implanted after a single KBI procedure that has only cracked the calcification, since some of the struts may be blocked by calcified plaque(s) and may be deformed or deployed suboptimally. It is highly probable that post-dilatation, even at a high pressure, will fail to optimize stent implantation under such circumstances. In contrast, additional KBI with high-pressure balloons will temporarily dilate the vessel lumen to as cylindrical a shape as possible. Therefore, the pressure applied to the struts during implantation will be smaller, even if vascular recoil occurs subsequently. Accordingly, it is reasonable to think that performing additional KBI with high-pressure balloons will reduce the risk of uneven stent implantation compared with a single KBI procedure using Lacrosse NSE balloons.

The primary goals of lesion preparation are (1) to prevent plaque shift and carina shift after stent implantation in the MB (LM-LAD) and (2) to reduce the pressure of vascular recoil to ≤2.0 atm by dilating the (LM) bifurcation to its normal diameter.

I think that all interventionalists prepare LM lesions for PCI with these goals, although this cannot be verified objectively and the degree of commitment to the goals may vary. Those who have a particularly high commitment with a logical background may use a Rotablator or DCA for debulking, even in the absence of calcification. If these devices can be employed effectively to minimize the plaque burden, such preparation should lead to greater dilation of the lesion.

Nonetheless, the following points need to be considered before using either of these two devices. Regarding the Rotablator, can this device be optimally directed toward a non-calcified plaque by utilizing guidewire bias, and can a sufficient volume of plaque be ablated?

Regarding DCA, is it possible to definitely ablate plaques extending from the LM into the angulated proximal LAD or LCX with a DCA cutter, which can only be advanced linearly? In addition, it is doubtful whether CAG can accurately locate plaques that have been identified by IVUS, and it may be difficult for CAG to display the true take-off angle of the LCX. Accordingly, will the branching angle of the LCX observed in the RAO caudal view always correspond to the direction of the artery on IVUS? Is DCA a safe and effective debulking measure for LM bifurcation lesions, in principle? Convincing answers to these questions are required before commencing rotablation or DCA at the LM bifurcation.

Considering the risk/benefit ratio, it seems reasonable to think that it is not necessary to try such difficult debulking procedures as part of lesion preparation since the goal is to ensure optimal stent implantation.

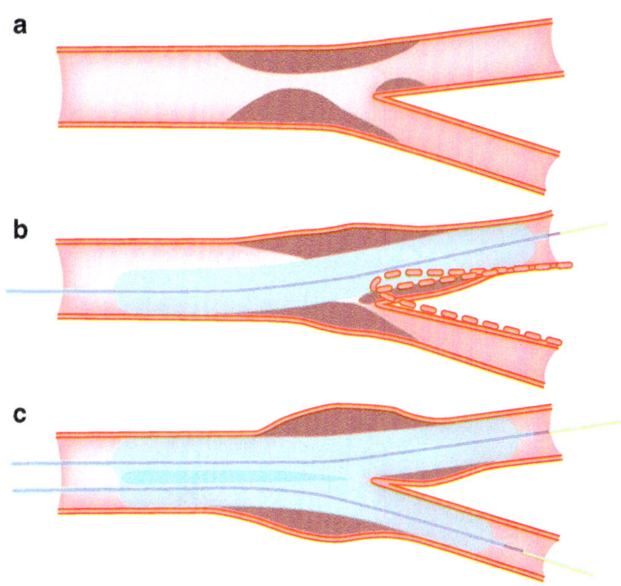

Fig. 4.9 KBI for bifurcation lesions. At a bifurcation stenosis (**a**), alternating balloon inflation appears to have sufficiently dilated the MB and the SB, as evidenced by the lack of indentations in either balloon (**b**). However, alternating balloon inflation has actually caused carina shift and deformation of the SB shoulder, which have transiently eliminated the indentations in the body of the SB balloon. During KBI, one or more indentations may reappear in the SB balloon, but can be eliminated by increasing the pressure to 8 atm. Accordingly, both the MB and SB will be dilated sufficiently and optimally prepared for stenting by KBI (**c**)

Column 20 Carina Shift

About 10 years ago, I participated in a live demonstration of PCI when I had not yet used IVUS, and I saw an operator protecting the SB during PCI of a non-LM bifurcation lesion after checking the IVUS findings. A commentator suggested that SB protection was unnecessary because plaque only existed on the contralateral side to the bifurcation. When consulted by the operator, I recommended that SB protection should be done because plaque on the contralateral side, if not effectively compressed by a stent implanted thereafter, might push the carina toward the SB, potentially causing SB stenosis or occlusion. SB occlusion did not occur after stent implantation, leading to the conclusion that this case did not require SB protection, although there was persistent mild stenosis of the SB. We understood the concept of "carina shift" in those days, although we had not coined the term, and we thought it was natural to take this phenomenon into account when performing bifurcation stenting. Several years ago, someone suddenly proposed the term "carina shift" as if it were a new concept, so we were initially somewhat confused, but we admired the term for its appropriateness. Our efforts to remind colleagues of the need for countermeasures against "carina shift" might have made a significant contribution to the coining of this term.

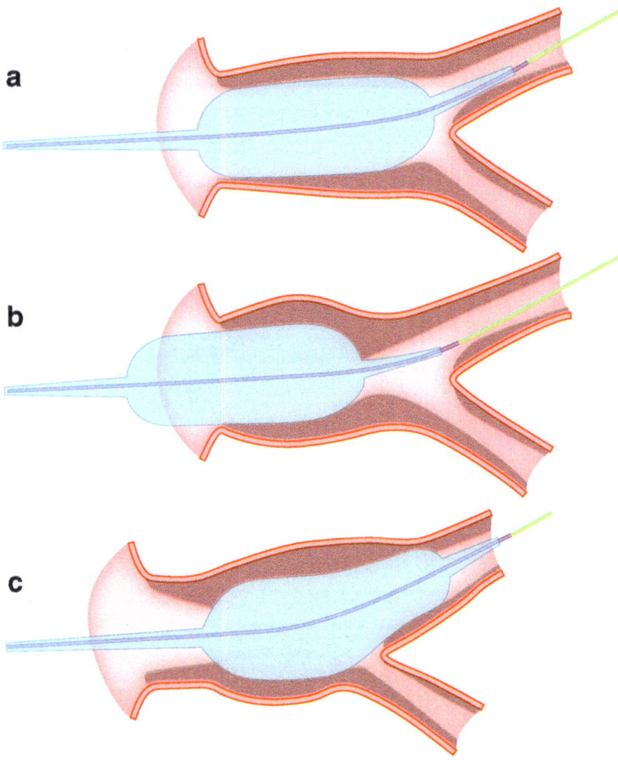

Fig. 4.10 Dilation of an LM lesion with a large-diameter balloon (POT). It is best to inflate a large-diameter balloon with the distal end just proximal to the carina (**a**). If the balloon slides back into the left main trunk, it cannot effectively dilate the lesion (**b**), while the balloon may injure the distal vessel if its distal end enters the distal MB (LAD) (**c**)

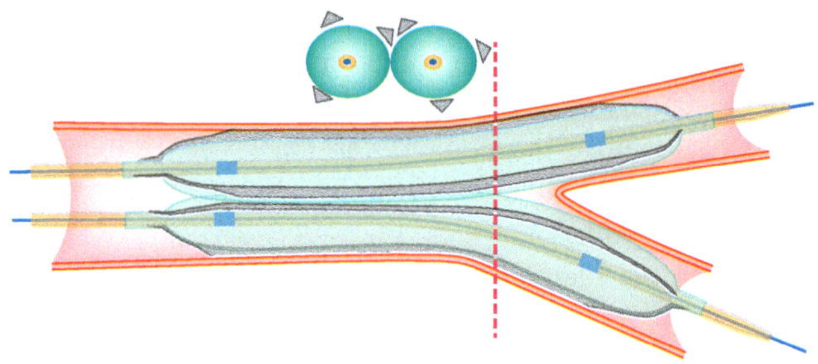

Fig. 4.11 KBI with Lacrosse NSE balloons. KBI can be performed with Lacrosse NSE balloons aligned so that they will not damage each other by their external scoring elements

Column 21 Selection of the Lacrosse NSE, AngioSculpt, and ScoreFlex® balloons (Fig. 4.12a–c)

I prefer the Lacrosse NSE balloon. It appears to me that IVUS shows better cracking of calcified plaques after inflation of the Lacrosse NSE balloon than the AngioSculpt balloon and there may be a good reason for this.

The scoring elements of these two balloons have different structures. The Lacrosse NSE balloon induces cracks in the longitudinal direction, while the AngioSculpt balloon induces cracks in both the longitudinal direction and obliquely (in the radial direction at points of inflection). Inflation of these balloons enlarges the cracks in calcified plaque, thereby increasing the luminal surface area in the radial direction and leading to dilation of the target vessel. Radial cracks can hardly contribute to dilation of the vessel in the radial direction, while cracks with both radial and longitudinal components will contribute to dilation with oblique distortion. Thus, it is clear that the Lacrosse NSE balloon will be more effective in achieving radial dilation of vessels because the scoring elements of this balloon are aligned parallel to its longitudinal axis.

In addition, both the AngioSculpt and ScoreFlex balloons have relatively fine metal cutting elements, while the Lacrosse NSE balloon had high plastic wedges as its cutting elements. These characteristic cutting elements of the Lacrosse NSE allow it to deform the vessel wall more extensively and crack plaques better during inflation. If the calcified plaque is eccentric, the plastic cutting elements are less likely to injure the relatively soft vessel wall on the opposite side.

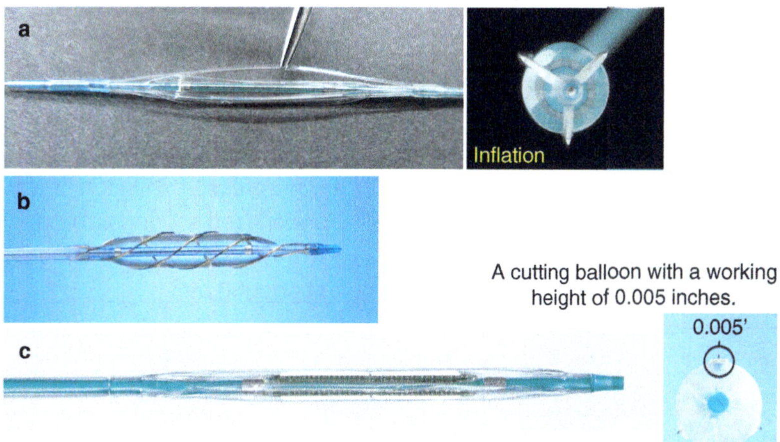

Fig. 4.12 Comparison of scoring/cutting balloons. (**a**) Lacrosse NSE ALPHA scoring balloon. (**b**) AngioSculpt scoring balloon. (**c**) FlexTome cutting balloon

4.3.3 Preparing the LAD/LCX Ostia and the Proximal LAD/LCX

Despite the smaller diameter of the LAD or LCX compared with the LM, a 3.5-mm stent is usually employed for crossover stenting from the LM to the LAD or LCX across the ostium of the other branch. If the LAD or LCX has a smaller diameter than 3.5 mm, the radial strength of the stent will be reduced. Accordingly, the region from the LAD/LCX ostium to the proximal LAD/LCX should be prepared with particular care to minimize vascular recoil. If there is any calcified plaque, scoring balloon angioplasty should be performed for pre-dilatation.

4.3.4 Practical Approach to Preparation

Figure 4.13 shows the algorithm used at my center when preparing LM bifurcation lesions for stenting.

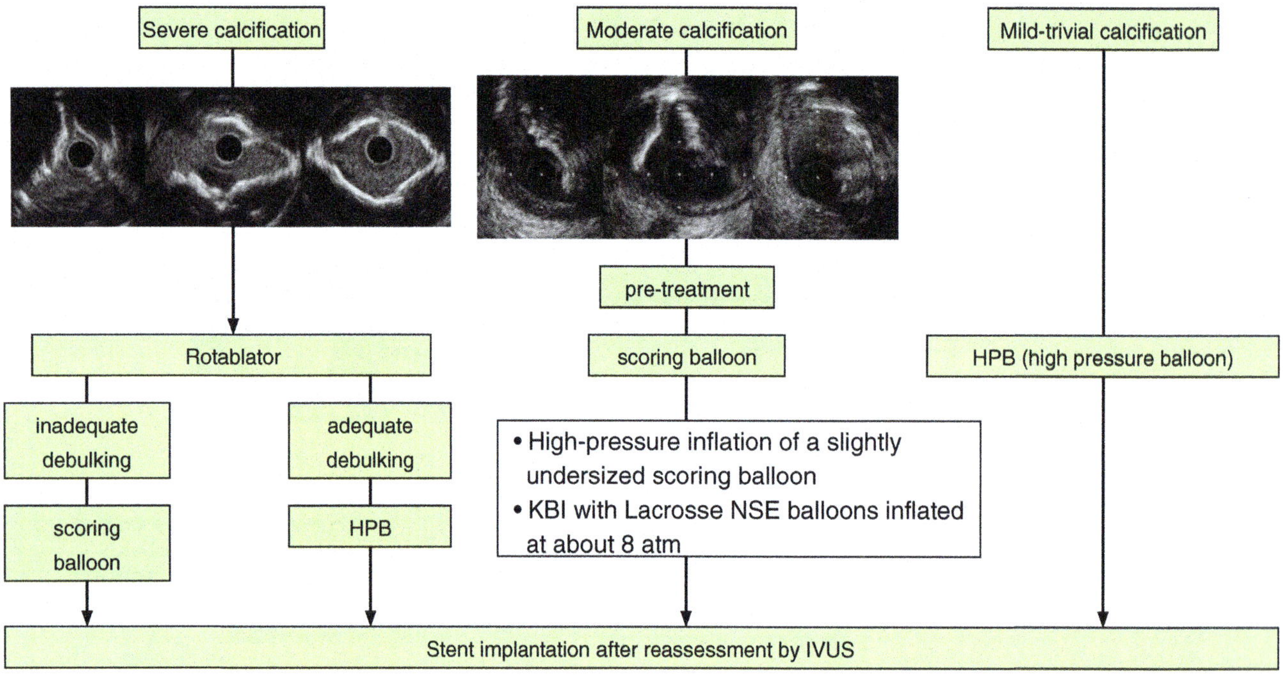

Fig. 4.13 Preparation of LM bifurcation lesions for stenting at my center

Before preparing an LM bifurcation lesion, I perform IVUS to estimate the vessel size, the extent of calcification, and the properties of the plaques. The approach to preparation of such lesions is stratified according to the extent of calcification.

4.3.4.1 Preparing a Bifurcation Lesion with Eccentric Calcification

Figure 4.14 shows an LM bifurcation lesion with markedly eccentric calcification on IVUS. Alternating high-pressure inflation was performed first, followed by simultaneous inflation (8 atm) of two 3.25-mm Lacrosse NSE balloons in the LM-LCX and LM-LAD, achieving dilation of the calcified region at the bifurcation (Fig. 4.15).

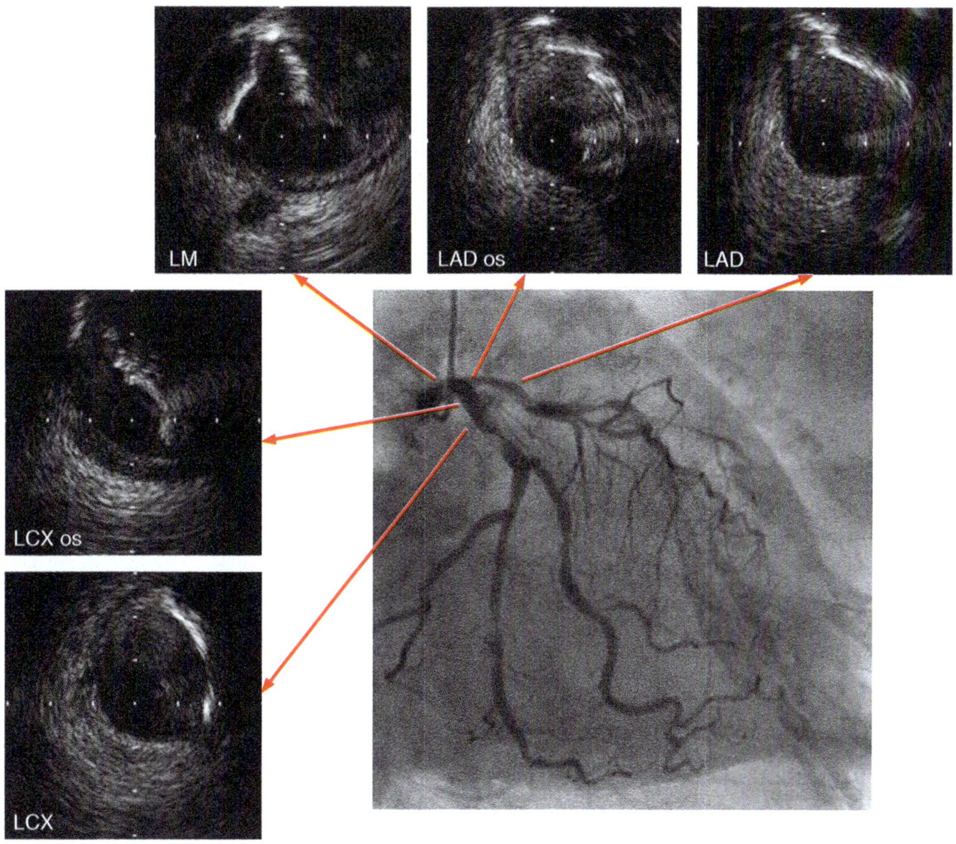

Fig. 4.14 LM bifurcation lesion with eccentric calcification. IVUS showed eccentric calcification in both the LAD and the LCX

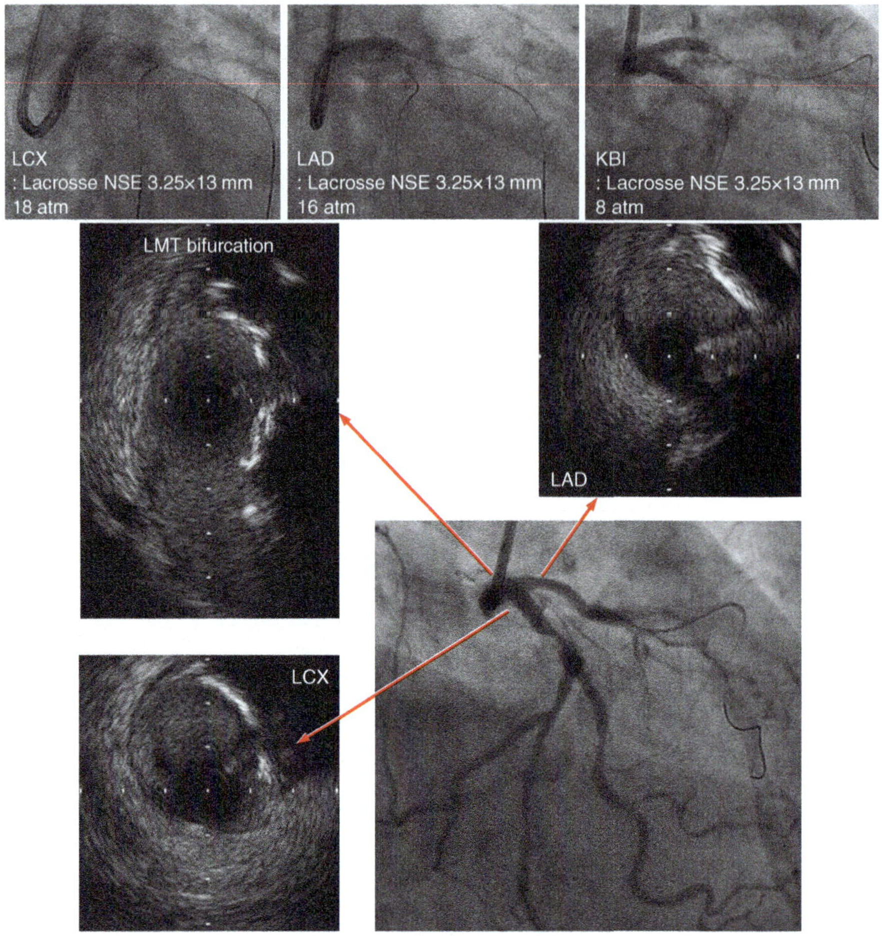

Fig. 4.15 Preparation of the lesion shown in Fig. 4.14. The LAD and LCX were pre-dilated by alternating high-pressure inflation, followed by KBI with slightly undersized Lacrosse NSE balloons

4.3.4.2 Preparing a Severely Calcified Bifurcation Lesion

Figures 4.16 and 4.17 show an LM bifurcation lesion in a dialysis patient with severe calcification in the LM-LAD and also in the LCX that prevented delivery of the IVUS catheter into the LAD.

Rotablation was performed with a 1.75-mm burr and then a 2.25-mm burr in the LAD, while a 2.25-mm burr was used in the LCX. Then both the LAD and LCX were dilated with a 4.0 mm cutting balloon. Subsequently, simultaneous inflation of 4.0 mm and 3.75 mm balloons in the LAD and LCX, respectively, achieved adequate preparation of the lesion for stenting.

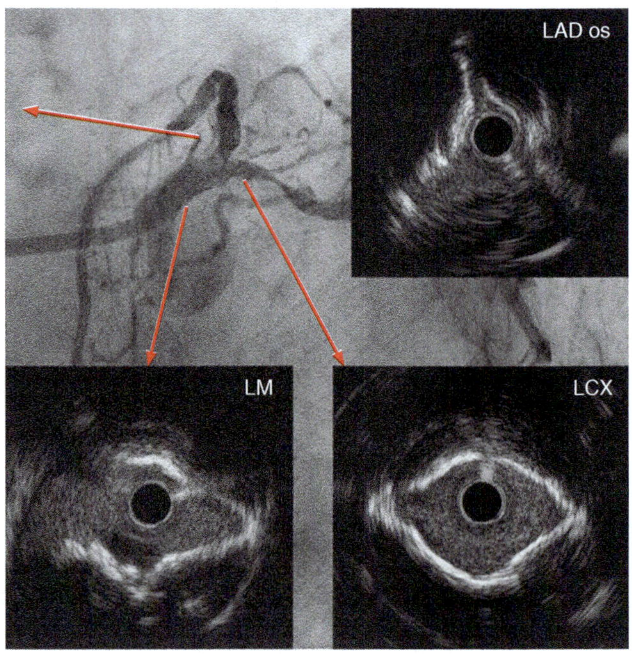

Fig. 4.16 LM bifurcation lesion in a dialysis patient. IVUS showed severe calcification in both the LAD and LCX

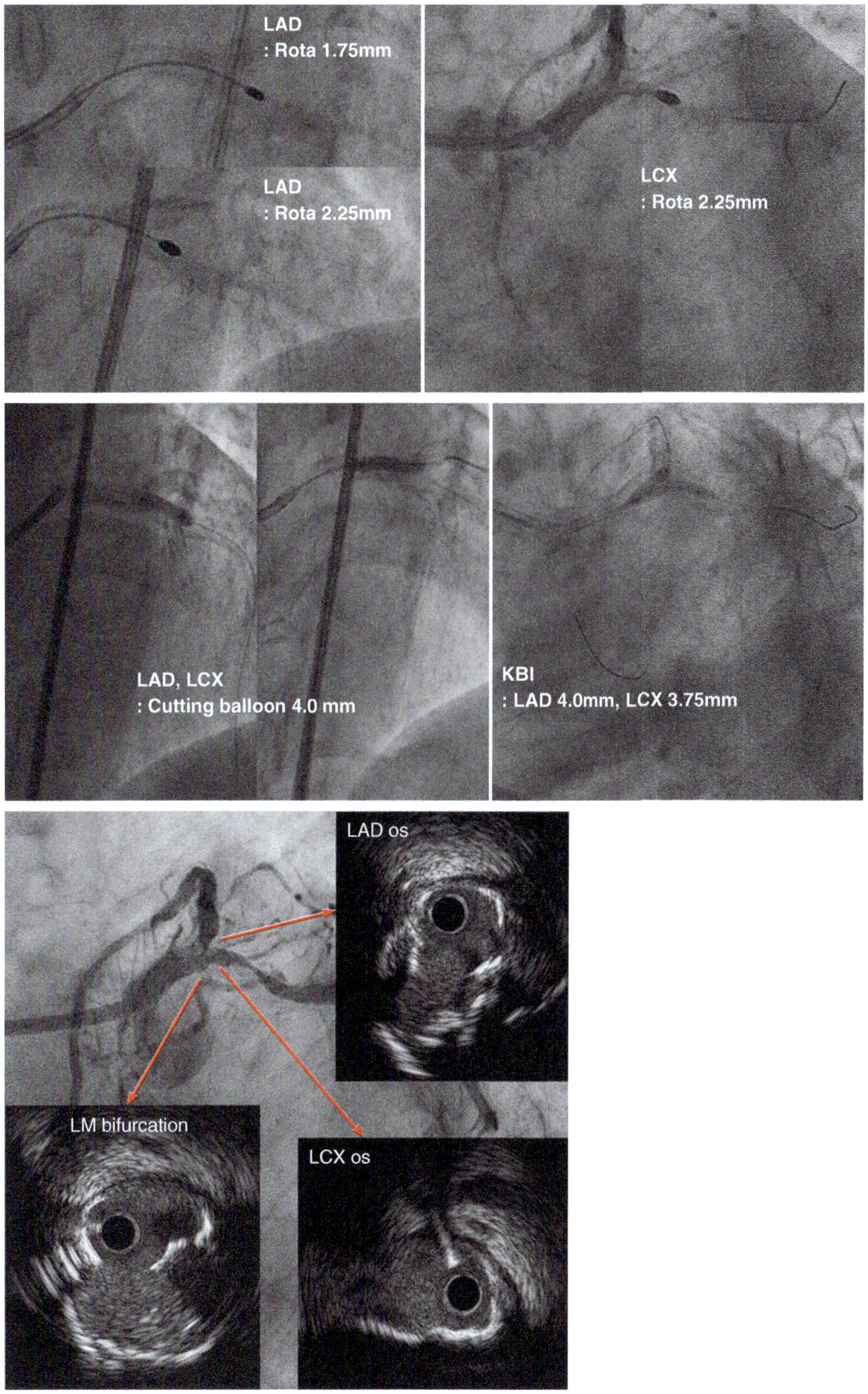

Fig. 4.17 Preparation of the lesion presented in Fig. 4.16. Rotablation with a 2.25-mm burr was followed by inflation of a 4.0-mm cutting balloon. Subsequently, simultaneous inflation of 4.0 mm (LAD) and 3.75 mm (LCX) balloons induced cracks in the calcified lesion, resulting in adequate preparation for optimal stent deployment

4.4 Stenting Strategy and Procedure

Stent implantation should only be done after adequate lesion preparation. Stenting should generally be provisional and should be performed on the basis of the following concepts and according to the following procedures.

4.4.1 Stenting a Relatively Long LM with Plaque Confined to the Ostium or Part of the Trunk (See Fig. 4.2a and c)

You should implant a two-link DES so that its distal edge is within the LMT. If the LM has a diameter > 3.5 mm and there are no calcified plaques so the vessel will only show modest recoil, pre-dilatation should be completed by inflating a balloon with a diameter of about 3.5 mm. If the lesion is pre-dilated to a diameter greater than 3.5 mm, a stent implanted by using a 3.5-mm SDB will show malapposition and will be likely to migrate immediately after implantation.

After a stent has been implanted, it may migrate or be deformed during withdrawal of the SDB or advancement of a post-dilatation balloon. To avoid this, the stent should be deployed to a diameter of 3.5 mm in order to create mild vascular recoil, since this will ensure that the stent becomes fixed and does not migrate from the landing zone.

If a 4 mm DES with 0 to 2 links is approved for use in the future, it should be used for the above procedures instead of a 3.5-mm DES.

4.4.2 Stenting the LM Bifurcation

In general, provisional stenting should be performed at the LM bifurcation, but a planned two-stent technique may be employed.

4.4.2.1 Stenting with KBI

Need for Post-stenting KBI

I think that stenting with KBI is the basic method of LM bifurcation stenting. This strategy is adopted for the following reasons: (1) to achieve optimal stent apposition, (2) to achieve sufficient dilation of the vessels around the carina to their normal diameters, and (3) to ensure good accessibility of the LCX if PCI needs to be performed in the future. Crossover stenting may sometimes be performed across the LCX ostium without post-stenting KBI, but is limited to cases where the LCX has a very small diameter and perfuses a very small territory of the left ventricle.

Stenting with KBI can only achieve favorable outcomes if the following requirements are met: (1) use of an optimally designed stent; (2) optimal guidewire routes; and (3) avoidance of stent deformation during balloon delivery.

If KBI is performed after implanting a two-link stent (e.g., a Cypher stent), it can actually lead to a worse outcome in many cases due to the stent design. Post-stenting KBI may also enhance jailing of the SB by a three-link stent. In contrast, post-stenting KBI is less likely to induce SB jailing and vascular stress if a two-link stent is used.

Stenting with KBI, especially at the LM bifurcation, should only be performed if the following requirements are met. First and most importantly, an optimally designed stent is needed. Second, the SB guidewire should cross the stent through the most distal cell at the carina and come into contact with the carina. After post-stenting KBI, you must check whether the SB guidewire has followed an appropriate route. Third, POT prior to SB wiring has recently become the standard intervention for preventing stent deformation. Fourth, if the SB balloon becomes blocked by a stent strut, it should not be advanced forcibly and must be delivered by a non-pushing technique (see Chap. 2). The anchor technique, in which an anchoring balloon is used to provide support for advancing the balloon, must not be employed.

I think that stenting with KBI is useful if it is performed appropriately when these requirements are met. It is doubtful whether previous studies that have found negative results for post-stenting KBI actually compared outcomes after KBI was performed with these requirements versus outcomes after stenting alone.

Practical Stenting with KBI

Crossover stenting is performed from the proximal MB to the distal MB or to the SB across the ostium of the other branch. In comparison with the proximal MB, the distal MB and the SB often have much smaller diameters. If the MB (LM) has a large diameter, a Nobori 3.5-mm JV stent needs to be implanted, even if the landing zone will be located in the distal MB (LAD) with a smaller diameter (about 3.0 mm). Because a Nobori 3.5-mm JV stent is usually deployed by inflating the SDB at 4.0 atm, the stent should be implanted by initial inflation at 4 to 5 atm. Subsequently, the SDB should be pulled back until its distal marker is at the carina and then inflated at a higher pressure of up to about 14 atm (Fig. 4.18).

The SDB should be withdrawn slowly so as to prevent the guiding catheter from becoming deeply engaged at the LM ostium and its tip from deforming a stent strut (Fig. 4.19). If the guiding catheter appears to spontaneously enter the LM ostium, you may need to pull it back slightly in order to prevent catheter advancement while withdrawing the SDB.

Note that pulling the guiding catheter back too far when attempting to prevent its advancement may result in loss of coaxiality with the LM (or the stent) after withdrawal of the SDB, which may prevent delivery of a post-dilatation (POT) balloon. If an attempt to regain coaxiality of the guiding catheter with the LM is made at this time, the tip of the guiding catheter often causes deformation of the proximal edge of the unapposed stent. Thus, it is important not to pull the catheter back excessively, and if the guiding catheter loses coaxiality with the LM, you should try to regain a coaxial position carefully without deforming the proximal edge of the stent.

In some cases, you can deliver a medium-sized balloon for pre-dilatation first and then move the guiding catheter to and fro or rotate it along the balloon catheter to regain coaxiality with the LM while avoiding stent deformation.

After withdrawing the SDB, you should immediately perform POT using a balloon that matches the diameter of the LM ostium. A new balloon should generally be used, but if the pre-dilatation balloon is reused, it should be reformed before introduction into the guiding catheter or rewrapped in the guiding catheter by inflation at about 10 atm before delivery into the stent. The POT balloon should be inflated at 14 atm inside the stent. In the presence of a jailed guidewire, the POT balloon should not be inflated at a pressure exceeding 14 atm to avoid trapping the guidewire. If symptoms and the hemodynamic profile permit, the POT balloon should be inflated at a rate of about 1 atm per second to prevent it from slipping out of the stent.

POT is often difficult to perform if the LM is less than 8 mm in length. In particular, when the LM ostium is tapered, the POT balloon and the stent are very likely to slip out of the ostium. As stent slippage toward the sinus of Valsalva may lead to excessive expansion of some of the stent struts, there is no use performing POT (Fig. 4.20).

If the LM is short (especially if it is tapered), it is better not to try POT and just perform KBI with great care. Since KBI can correct tapering of the LM to some extent, high-pressure POT can reliably dilate the LM after KBI (Fig. 4.21). In any case, bifurcation stenting should be accomplished by final KBI.

Subsequently, SB rewiring should be performed via the Crusade catheter according to the procedure described in Chap. 2 (see pages 155 to 157). Since the LM branches (LAD and LCX) do not lie in a single plane, it may be difficult to use CAG to determine whether the SB guidewire has crossed the stent through the most distal cell at the carina. In general, the LM bifurcation can be seen most clearly in a steep spider view, but this view does not always provide en face observation of the bifurcation. Since it is very hard to confirm the correctness of the guidewire route without an en face view of the bifurcation, you should perform provisional KBI.

Nonetheless, it is necessary to minimize SB jailing at the LM bifurcation. If severe SB jailing persists and culotte stenting has to be performed subsequently, you may have difficulty delivering a stent into the SB across the MB stent or may cause deformation of the MB stent. Since these events must particularly be avoided in LM bifurcation stenting, you should perform IVUS immediately after KBI to assess the extent of SB jailing. If necessary, you should attempt SB rewiring through the most distal cell of the MB stent at the carina and then repeat KBI (see Chap. 2 [pages 168 to 171]).

Before performing KBI, you need to withdraw the guidewire that has been jailed by the SB guidewire. For tips about withdrawing a jailed guidewire, please also refer to Chap. 2 (page 183). While withdrawing the jailed guidewire, you should take great care to prevent stent deformation.

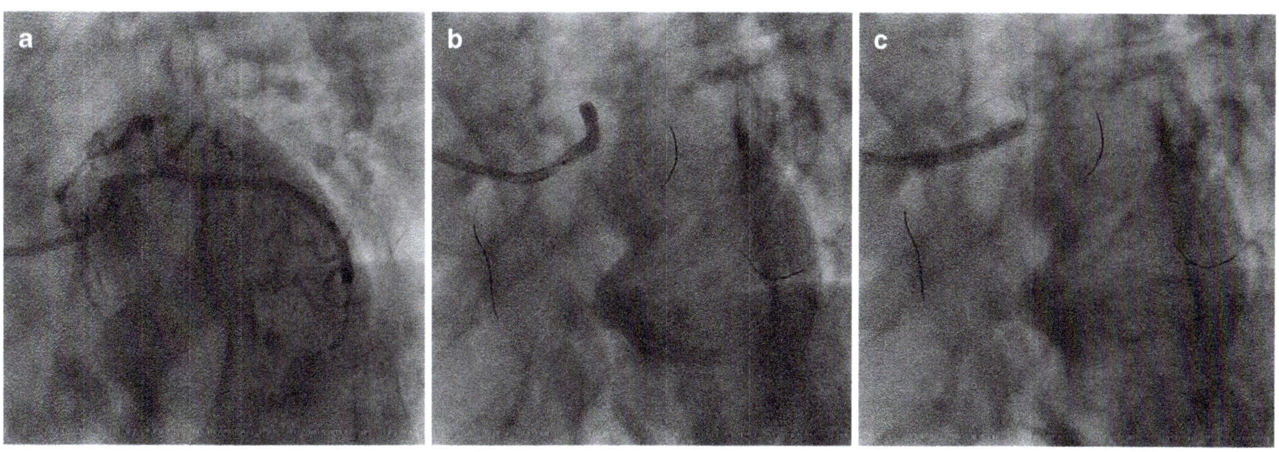

Fig. 4.18 Bifurcation stenting with a large-diameter proximal MB (LM) and small-diameter distal MB/SB. (**a**) Baseline CAG. (**b**) A Nobori 3.5-mm JV stent was implanted from the LM to the proximal LAD (Segment 6) with low-pressure (5 atm) expansion. (**c**) The SDB was pulled back to the LM trunk and inflated at a high pressure (16 atm)

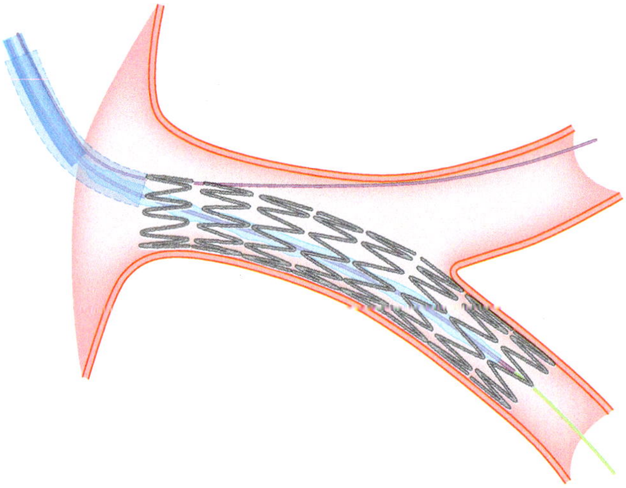

Fig. 4.19 Deformation of a stent implanted at the LM ostium. During withdrawal of the SDB, the guiding catheter may be advanced into the LM ostium, deforming the stent

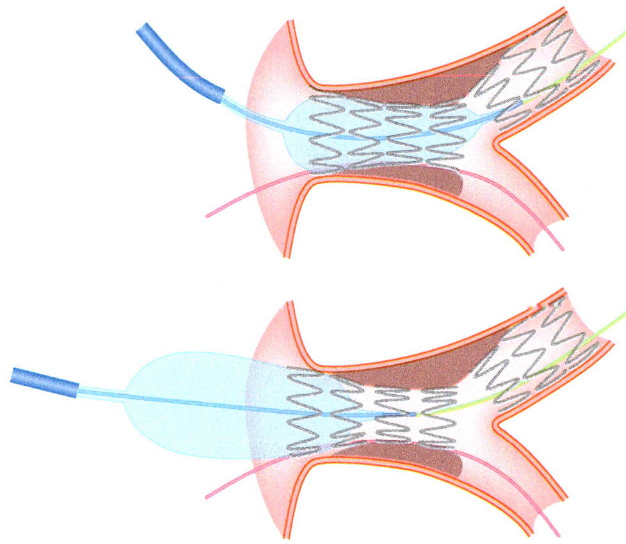

Fig. 4.20 Precautions when performing POT. As a result of the POT balloon slipping out of the ostium, the stent implanted in the LM has been deformed with overexpansion of its struts

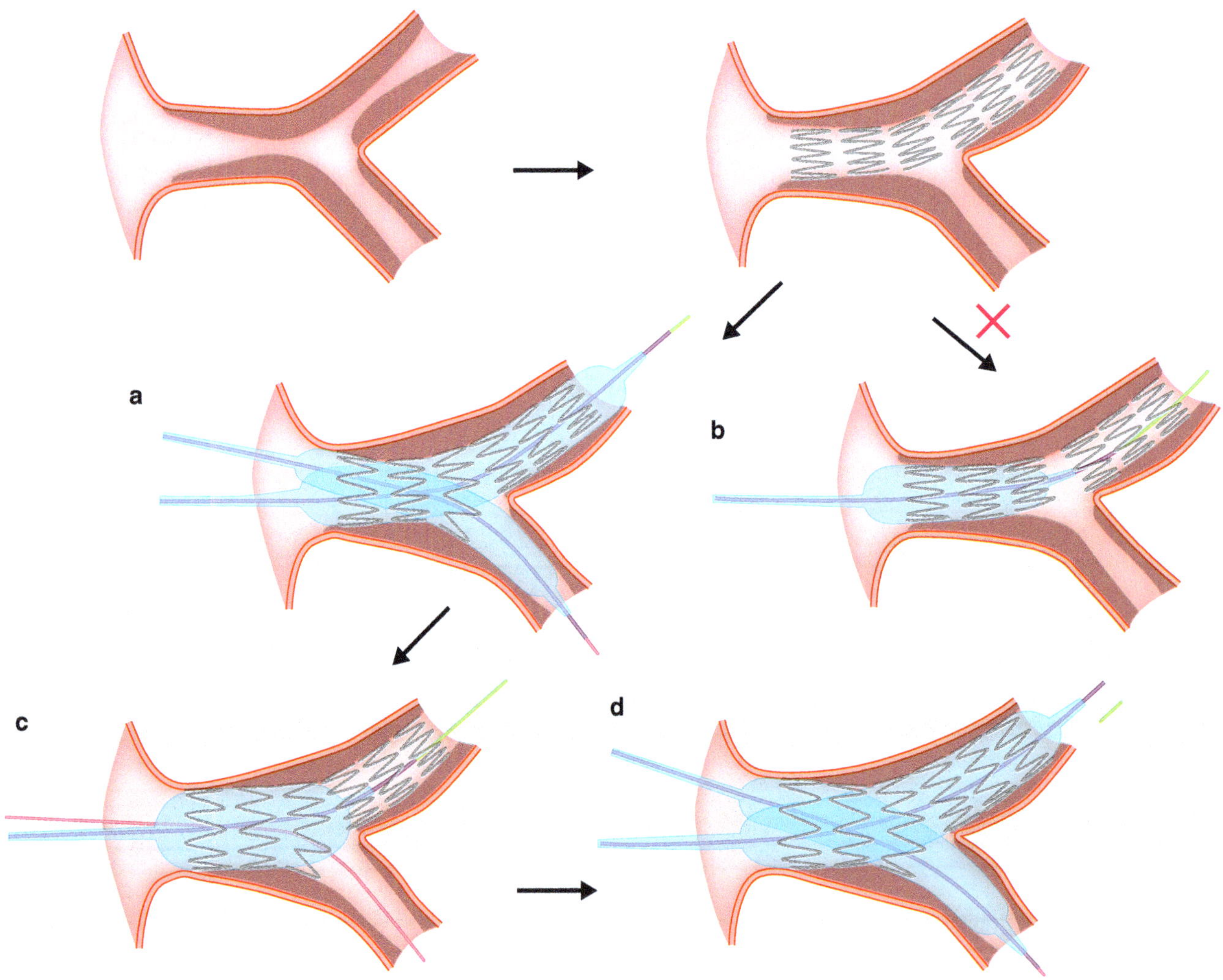

Fig. 4.21 Technique for performing POT and KBI in a short (tapered) LM. It is sometimes better to perform KBI first (**a** & **b**) and then POT (**c**). In any case, bifurcation stenting should be accomplished by final KBI (**d**)

4.4.3 Stenting up to the Ostium

If IVUS shows some plaque in the LMT, stenting should be performed up to the ostium to avoid positioning the stent edges in the trunk. If the LM is not too long for a stent ≤28 mm in length to easily cover the entire LM from its ostium to the LAD ostium, the LM should be stented up to the ostium even if the plaque burden is trivial.

To locate the proximal edge of a stent just at the ostium, it is generally recommended to position it at the end of the shoulders of the LM ostium in the AP cranial view (Fig. 4.22). However, it is sometimes impossible to distinguish the shoulders from the trunk on CAG, even after fine adjustment of the fluoroscopy angle. In such cases, you should introduce an IVUS catheter along the guidewire inserted into the LCX and use IVUS to locate the proximal edge of the stent and the LM ostium. Subsequently, you can adjust the position of the stent so that its proximal edge overlaps the LM ostium by advancing and withdrawing it repeatedly. When the proximal edge of the stent has been positioned to overlap the LM ostium, you should perform non-contrast CAG. While confirming that the stent remains in position, you should slowly withdraw the IVUS catheter, leaving only guidewires in the LM, and should then implant the stent. To prevent migration of the stent together with the IVUS probe, the LM should be pre-dilated to enlarge it enough to easily accommodate these devices.

This contrast-free method for accurately positioning a stent is very helpful for LM stenting in patients with chronic kidney disease.

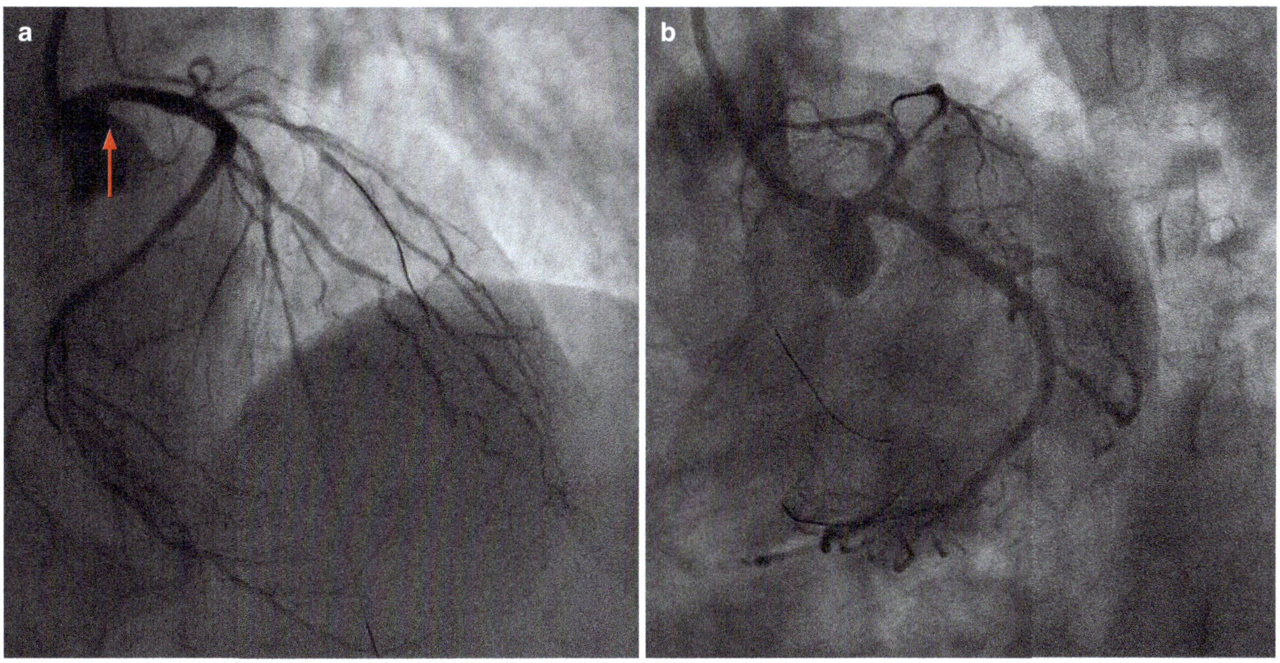

Fig. 4.22 Confirming the position of the stent edge. (**a**) AP and cranial 30° projection. (**b**) LAO 50° and caudal 29° projection. The AP cranial projection allows visualization of the LM ostium (red arrow). The stent should be implanted so that its proximal edge protrudes from the ostium. While the LAO caudal projection displays the LM bifurcation, it is not suitable for identifying the LM ostium

4.4.4 Stent Edge in the LMT

If the LM is too long to achieve complete coverage from its ostium to the LAD ostium with a 28-mm stent, you will need to choose between fully covering the LM or placing the stent edge in the LMT. If there is a significant plaque burden, chronic progression of stenosis at the proximal edge of a stent frequently occurs after stenting of other coronary arteries and similar outcomes are expected in the LM. Despite the lack of definite evidence, I think it is acceptable to implant the stent with its edge in the LMT if the LM is relatively long and has a relative plaque area of about ≤30%. If the LM is ≤10 mm long, it should be stented completely from its ostium to the LAD ostium.

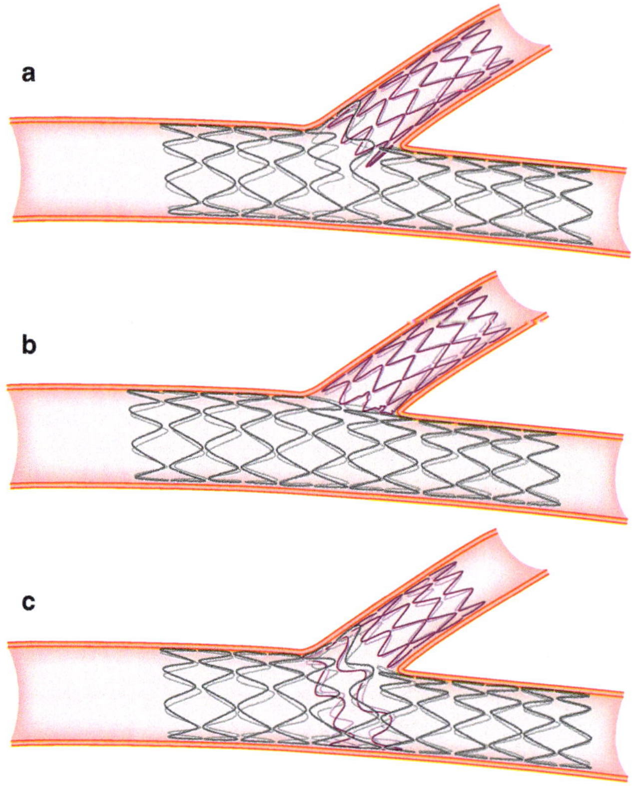

Fig. 4.23 T stenting versus culotte stenting. (**a**) Provisional T stenting. (**b**) Modified T stenting. (**c**) Culotte stenting. With provisional or modified T stenting, the stent struts may lose radial strength on the contralateral side

4.4.5 Culotte Stenting

4.4.5.1 Indications for Culotte Stenting

If provisional MB stenting with KBI leads to compromise of the SB, a second stent has to be implanted in the SB. There are two options for such two stenting, which are T stenting and culotte stenting. At the LM bifurcation, I often prefer culotte stenting for the following three reasons:

1. With T stenting, the proximal edge of the SB stent inevitably protrudes into the MB lumen and shows malapposition to the MB/SB wall.
2. With T stenting, the stent struts at the shoulders of the bifurcation receive no support from the contralateral wall and lose radial strength. In contrast, culotte stenting creates a double layer of struts at the bifurcation shoulders supported by the lateral wall of the proximal MB, thus leading to a twofold increase of radial strength (Fig. 4.23).
3. Culotte stenting is less complicated than T stenting. The only additional procedures required are SB rewiring and repeated POT plus KBI.

4.4.5.2 Practical Culotte Stenting

Additional stenting with KBI is all that is required to accomplish culotte stenting. When performing two stenting of the LM bifurcation, the aim is to completely eliminate SB jailing by the first stent. Note that to completely eliminate SB jailing, rewiring of the SB should be performed through the most distal cell at the carina and then KBI should be repeated.

If the LM has a large diameter and if a Nobori 3.5-mm JV stent has been implanted in the LAD, you should also implant a Nobori 3.5-mm JV stent in the LCX. If the LCX diameter is <3.5 mm, the stent should be deployed by inflating the SDB at a low pressure such as 4 to 5 atm. Subsequently, high-pressure post-dilatation should be performed with a balloon of the optimal size. When provisional culotte stenting is performed, it is ideal to limit protrusion of the SB stent to a distance of 6 to 8 mm into the MB (LM) lumen so as to minimize overlap between the two stents in the proximal MB (LM). You should position the POT balloon accurately to ensure safe and effective POT. If the POT balloon position is too proximal, it will have little effect when inflated, while the balloon may over-dilate and damage the ostium of the distal MB if its position is too distal.

As stated above, it is difficult to accurately position the POT balloon at the LM bifurcation with extreme angulation of the LAD or LCX. You do not need to worry about the distance for which the two stents appear to overlap. The most important objective of performing POT is to reliably achieve dilation of at least the proximal part of the LM in order to stabilize the stent prior to KBI.

Similar procedures apply to T stenting, except that the kissing balloons may be inflated at slightly higher pressures after two stenting. When KBI is done in the LMT, there is no problem with the proximal ends of the kissing balloons protruding into the sinus of Valsalva. To prevent distal dissection, the two kissing balloons should be inflated with their distal edges slightly proximal to the distal edges of the stents. High-pressure inflation of two optimally sized kissing balloons at the LM bifurcation is likely to cause dissection. Therefore, I generally limit the maximum pressure to about 14 atm when performing KBI. If a higher pressure is required, I try to inflate balloons one quarter size smaller at pressures escalating from 20 atm.

For two stenting, it is necessary to prepare the lesion sufficiently to eliminate the need for post-dilatation at very high pressures. Particularly if the LM is long, insufficient preparation will lead to luminal irregularity of the first stent, which may prevent advancement of a second stent through it. If the second stent is pushed forward forcibly when it becomes blocked, the stent often undergoes deformation and then is very difficult to advance further.

After implantation of the first stent, POT has to be performed in the presence of a jailed guidewire and therefore should be done by inflating the balloon at a relatively low pressure of about 14 atm. If high-pressure inflation is needed to sufficiently dilate the proximal MB, high-pressure POT may be performed before KBI after SB wiring. It is likely that high-pressure POT will smooth out irregularities in the first stent. If delivering the second stent into the SB is difficult, you should withdraw it and perform high-pressure POT along with relatively high-pressure KBI. This often facilitates delivery of the stent into the SB.

The second stent may also be blocked by the carina, but this can be prevented if KBI is performed using a guidewire that crosses the first stent into the LCX in contact with the carina. However, the second stent may sometimes be blocked by a "hard" carina. If this obstacle cannot be overcome by various efforts, you should remove the guidewire from the LAD and advance it into the LCX for use as a buddy wire. Then you should attempt to advance the second stent across the first stent. If this also fails, you should advance a balloon along the buddy wire across the point where the stent is blocked while slightly and gently pulling the SDB back. If the second stent is then advanced gently, it can often be delivered successfully.

If this technique also fails, you should inflate a balloon at 2 to 4 atm in the LCX to trap the guidewire along which the stent will be delivered. Then you should advance the stent while pulling the guidewire back slightly. After the stent has been advanced, you can remove the buddy wire or advance it into the LAD. If even this procedure cannot overcome stent blockage, it is a good idea to use a GuideLiner catheter. You should advance this catheter gently with the tip of the balloon protruding from the tip of the catheter. To facilitate passage of the catheter past the site of blockage, you should pull the preceding balloon back slightly. You should never apply strong force to the catheter. If this technique also fails, trapping the guidewire at a distal point by inflating a balloon at a low pressure will facilitate steady advancement of the stent.

When upfront culotte stenting is planned, the proximal edge of either stent is always positioned in the LMT. It is preferable to implant the first stent from the LMT to the LCX and the second stent from the LM ostium to the LAD, because this order of stenting will not induce indentations of the parts of the stents in the LM or LAD (Fig. 4.24).

Even if LAD stenting precedes LM-LCX stenting, placing the proximal edge of the stent in the LMT and covering the LM ostium with the second sent deployed in the LCX will avoid indentation of the stent in the LM. While inverse indentation may occur at the LAD ostium in this situation, the extent of indentation is usually acceptable.

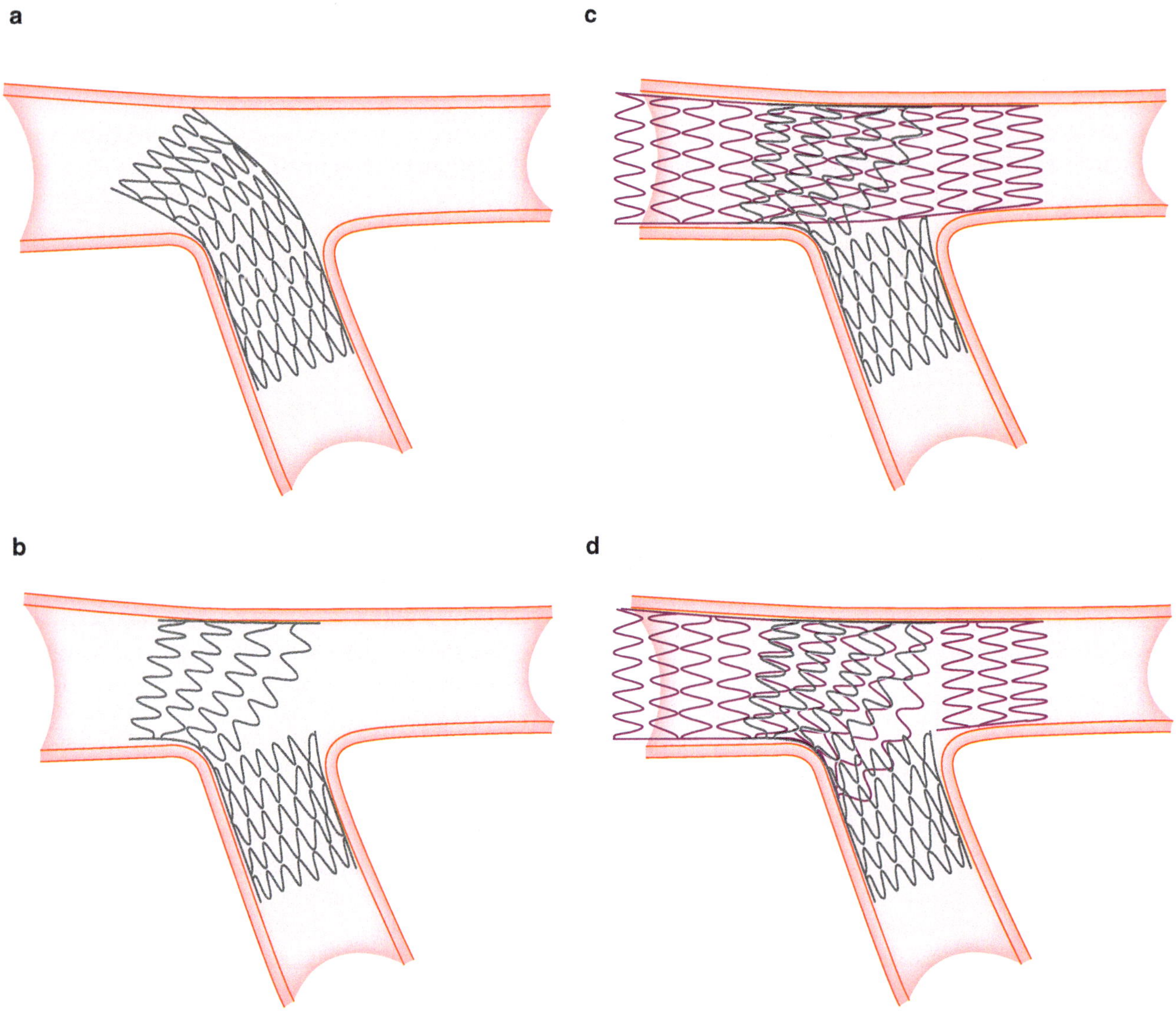

Fig. 4.24 Planned upfront culotte stenting. (**a**) When implanting the first stent in the LCX, protrusion of the proximal stent edge into the LM lumen should be limited to a distance of about 3 mm. (**b**) After initial POT and KBI. (**c**) After implanting the second stent from the LM to the LAD. (**d**) After repeat POT and KBI

4.4.6 T Stenting

T stenting of the LM bifurcation may be performed if the LCX has a take-off angle of nearly 90 degrees and particularly if there is a marked difference in diameter between the LAD and LCX (LAD > LCX). Under these circumstances, the struts of the stent implanted in the SB will not lose their radial strength (Fig. 4.25). You should implant the SB stent so that its proximal edge protrudes slightly into the MB lumen. IVUS guidance may assist with accurate positioning of the stent. The method of stent positioning is similar to that for accurately placing the proximal edge of a stent at the LM ostium. When stenting the SB, you should advance the IVUS probe along the guidewire inserted into the LAD and should confirm that the proximal edge of the stent is just at the LCX ostium. Since the SB stent will never cross over the LAD ostium, there is no need to remove the IVUS probe when inflating the SDB. If it is left in the LM/LAD, the IVUS probe will not interfere with advancement of the stent. Because of the large angle between the SB stent and the IVUS catheter, it is slightly difficult to visualize the proximal part of the stent by IVUS.

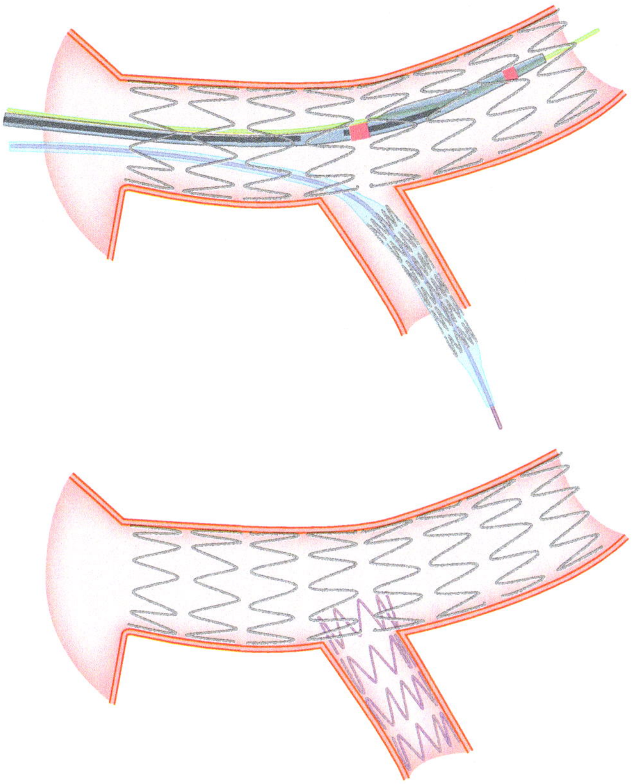

Fig. 4.25 T stenting. T stenting may be performed at the LM bifurcation if the SB (LCX) has a take-off angle of nearly 90 degrees and if the LCX has a small diameter

4.5 LM Trifurcation Stenting

Sometimes an additional artery arises at the bifurcation of the LM, forming a trifurcation. If this artery has a similar diameter to the LCX, it may be necessary to perform triple KBI and to implant stents in all three branches.

4.5.1 Stenting with (Triple) KBI

After stenting the LAD, you should perform KBI to achieve complete stent apposition and dilate the bifurcation to its normal diameter, as stated previously. As with bifurcation stenting, two-link stents should be implanted and the kissing balloons should be inflated at a relatively low pressure (8–10 atm) to avoid causing dissection/injury in non-stented segments of the SBs.

4.5.1.1 Lesion Preparation

You should follow the procedure recommended for bifurcation KBI. The individual branches should be adequately prepared to ensure that sufficient dilation can be achieved by low-pressure balloon inflation. The objectives of triple KBI are to reduce the risk of SB compromise by plaque shift or carina shift and to estimate the responsiveness of the distal LM bifurcation to low-pressure balloon angioplasty. When the LM bifurcation can be reliably expected to show low responsiveness, you should consider performing triple KBI with Lacrosse NSE balloons in order to optimize preparation of the trifurcation lesion.

4.5.1.2 Stent Placement

After implanting a stent in the LAD, you should perform POT and then triple KBI according to the following procedure (Fig. 4.26): (1) insert a new guidewire into the high lateral (HL) branch via the Crusade catheter; (2) perform KBI in the LAD and the HL branch; (3) insert a guidewire into the LCX via the Crusade catheter advanced along the HL guidewire; and (4) perform triple KBI. When wiring the SB, you should always pass the guidewire through the most distal cell at the carina.

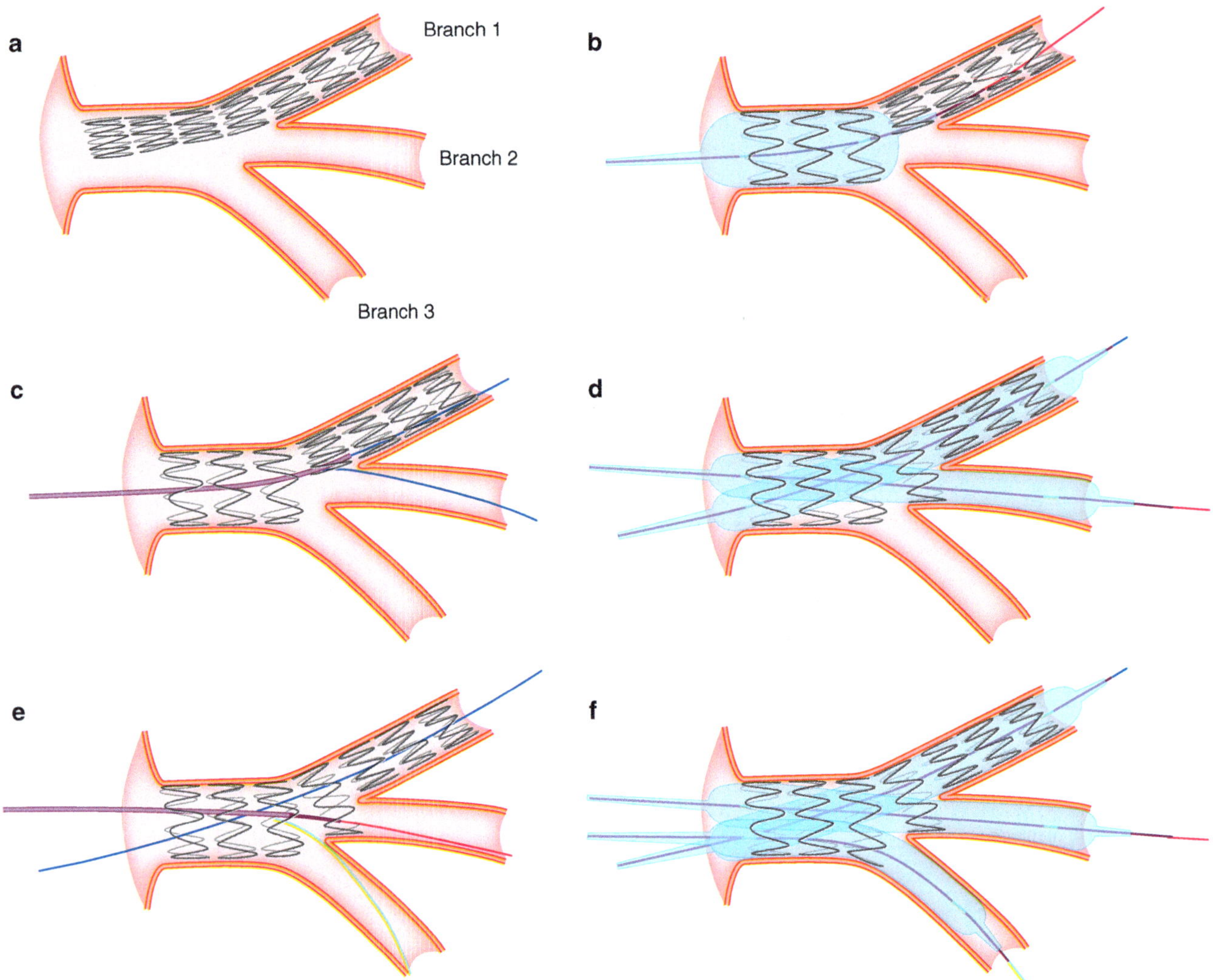

Fig. 4.26 Stent placement at the LM trifurcation. (**a**) Placing a stent in Branch 1. (**b**) POT. (**c**). Rewiring Branch 2 with the aid of the Crusade catheter. (**d**) Performing KBI in Branches 1 and 2. (**e**) Rewiring Branch 3 with the aid of the Crusade catheter advanced along the Branch 2 guidewire. (**f**) Performing triple KBI

4.5.2 Culotte Stenting at the LM Trifurcation

If lesions in the LAD and LCX are treated by culotte stenting, the HL branch will be compressed by both the LAD stent and the LCX stent, even if the culotte stenting is completed with triple KBI (Fig. 4.27). In other words, there will be dual carina shift toward the HL branch. If dual carina shift is considered to be approximately double that of a single carina, it is unlikely to be negligible, and persistent compression from dual carina shift may well increase the risk of restenosis at this branch.

Thus, a third stent needs to be implanted in the HL branch when treating LM trifurcation lesions because culotte stenting cannot prevent restenosis of the branch. An interventionalist who aims to recanalize all three branches at a trifurcation lesion should choose trifurcation stenting rather than culotte stenting. However, LM trifurcation stenting has been reported to achieve very poor mid-term outcomes with regard to patency of the HL branch.

The proximal HL largely overlaps the proximal LAD/LCX on CAG. If the HL branch is stented last, its ostium may not be covered sufficiently. Also, if triple KBI is only performed after stenting the HL branch following culotte stenting of the LAD/LCX, the guidewire inserted into the HL branch may bypass the culotte stents. On the other hand, if triple KBI is added to LAD stenting and to LCX stenting, trifurcation stenting will achieve full coverage of the three branches and ensure that all three stents obtain sufficient radial strength.

It is best to additionally perform triple KBI after HL stenting using the balloons maintained in the LAD and LCX. The stent in the HL branch should be positioned with its proximal edge protruding slightly into the LM lumen from the LAD-LCX carina (Fig. 4.28). IVUS can be used to confirm the position of the proximal edge of the stent.

Foreword

Dr. Kazuaki Mitsudo passed away due to sudden illness on October 18, 2015, to the immeasurable grief of his family. He was constantly striving to improve the outcomes of PCI, and we believe that he would have been incredibly disappointed at being deprived of the opportunity to completely fulfill this accomplishment.

Dr. Mitsudo had prepared a manuscript on PCI prior to his death, which was recently published as *Mitsudo's Non-Pushing PCI Techniques*. He was involved in the development of many devices of use in the PCI field and invented many novel techniques. He also made a significant contribution to the development of PCI through live demonstrations and technical training sessions. Among the many PCI fields, this book focuses on his techniques for chronic total occlusion and bifurcation lesions, including left main trunk lesions, which he described as the "final frontier of PCI." Based on his long experience, he also prepared a separate chapter on non-pushing PCI, which is considered to be the key to successful PCI.

Dr. Mitsudo previously published another book, *PTCA Technique* (Igaku Shoin), in 1995. The preface states that: "Technique is quite often based on experience. Indeed, there are techniques which are difficult to explain through words and photos. However, technique with a sound rationale can be explained." His PCI methods were not only based on excellent technique, but also on ample experience and clinical data, as well as a sound rationale. We have learned much directly from Dr. Mitsudo and have received invaluable instruction from him. This book explains the significance and background of each PCI technique, as well as its clinical application, in a logical manner. It conveys the essence of PCI as practiced by Dr. Mitsudo to all professionals in the field of interventional medicine.

To realize the publication of this book, staff members from the Department of Cardiovascular Medicine at Kurashiki Central Hospital have brushed up and summarized the manuscripts written by Dr. Mitsudo while remembering his lessons about PCI. We have tried to reflect his words as accurately as possible, but we ask for your understanding where we have failed to clearly portray his thinking.

Finally, this book has been made possible because of the strong desire of the family of Dr. Mitsudo to publish his manuscripts. We would like to express our sincere appreciation to the late Dr. Kazuaki Mitsudo and his family for the opportunity to be involved in the publication of this book.

May he rest in peace.

Kazushige Kadota
Kurashiki Central Hospital
Kurashiki, Japan
July 2016

Acknowledgments

I am delighted that this English edition of the work of my late husband has reached completion. I hope that this posthumous collection of his extensive experience and teachings reaches those professionals across the world undertaking their own endeavors in PCI, especially those who worked with and supported him.

Last of all, I would like to express my sincere gratitude to those involved in the translation.

Dr. Kazushige Kadota—Kurashiki Central Hospital
Dr. Takehiro Yamashita—Hokkaido Ohno Kinen Hospital
Dr. Jutaro Yamada—Saiseikai Shimonoseki General Hospital
Dr. Shingo Hosogi—Hosogi Hopital
Dr. Hiroyuki Tanaka—Kurashiki Central Hospital
Dr. Seiji Habara—Habara Heart Clinic
Ms. Makiko Kanaike—Kurashiki Central Hospital

Kazuyo Mitsudo
September 2020

Contents

Contributors

Seiji Habara Habara Heart Clinic, Kurashiki, Japan

Shingo Hosogi Hosogi Hospital, Kochi, Japan

Kazushige Kadota Department of Cardiology, Kurashiki Central Hospital, Kurashiki, Japan

Hiroyuki Tanaka Department of Cardiology, Kurashiki Central Hospital, Kurashiki, Japan

Jutaro Yamada Department of Cardiology, Saiseikai Shimonoseki General Hospital, Shimonoseki, Japan

Takehiro Yamashita Department of Cardiology, Hokkaido Ohno Kinen Hospital, Sapporo, Japan

Kazuyo Mitsudo, MD Health Care Plaza, Kurashiki Central Hospital, Kurashiki, Japan

List of Columns

These manuscripts of my late husband are being published as a result of the efforts of many people.

My husband was deeply committed to PCI. He was constantly focused on ways of spreading his technical knowledge and often spoke about writing new manuscripts for this purpose. He dedicated each moment of his spare time for writing this manuscript, even when it allowed for only a single additional line. On the eve of the completion of these manuscripts, he suddenly passed away due to illness, something for which I believe he would have shown terrible disappointment.

Those who were left behind following his death suddenly had the mission of transforming his manuscripts into a book that would fulfill his wishes of transmitting his wealth of ideas and techniques accumulated over many years of professional experience to as many people as possible. Over the years, he pushed his physiological limits in order to realize his potential from his commencement as a trainee physician and continued to work in this fashion right until his passing. In fact, the day before he was struck by sudden illness, he was working late into the night in order to prepare these manuscripts. It seemed to me that he would do whatever was possible in order to complete as many manuscripts as possible, despite this potentially shortening his life. He was unfortunately unable to finish all of his work, leaving some remaining areas in which his intentions may not be well understood. Despite this, we would be delighted if this book is widely read and significantly contributes to the development of PCI in the future.

I would like to deeply express my sincere appreciation to the many doctors who supported my husband in this publication, including members of the Department of Cardiovascular Medicine at Kurashiki Central Hospital. I am especially grateful to Dr. Hiroyuki Tanaka, Dr. Seiji Habara, and medical secretary Makiko Kanaike, who generously provided editorial support, case reports, and figures/tables despite their busy daily clinical practice.

July 2016
Kazuyo Mitsudo

Kazuaki Mitsudo
Department of Cardiology
Kurashiki Central Hospital
Kurashiki
Okayama
Japan

This English edition was published as a co-edition with its original Japanese language edition, Jutsusha MITSUDO no osanai PCI, copyright © 2016 by Igaku-Shoin Ltd., Tokyo Japan
ISBN 978-981-15-7042-1 ISBN 978-981-15-7043-8 (eBook)
https://doi.org/10.1007/978-981-15-7043-8

This Springer imprint is published by the registered company Springer Nature Singapore Pte Ltd.
The registered company address is: 152 Beach Road, #21-01/04 Gateway East, Singapore 189721, Singapore

Kazuaki Mitsudo

Non-Pushing PCI Techniques

Springer

Non-Pushing PCI Techniques